W9-CTH-456

Ritalin

Theory and Practice

Second Edition

Ritalin

Theory and Practice

Second Edition

Editors
Laurence L. Greenhill, M.D.
Betty B. Osman, Ph.D.

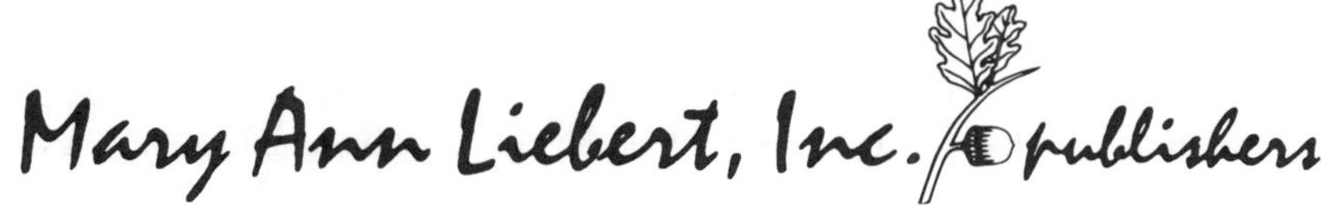

www.liebertpub.com

Library of Congress Cataloging-in-Publication Data

Ritalin: theory and practice/editors, Laurence L. Greenhill, Betty B. Osman. — 2nd ed.
p. cm.
Includes bibliographical references and index.
ISBN 0–913-113–82–4
1. Methylphenidate hydrocholoride—Therapeutic use. 2. Attention-deficit hyperactivity disorder—Chemotherapy. I. Greenhill, Laurence L. II. Osman, Betty B.
[DNLM: 1. Attention Deficit Disorder with Hyperactivity—drug therapy. 2. Methylphenidate—pharmacology. 3. Methylphenidate—therapeutic use. WS 350.8.A8 R598 1999]
RJ506.H9R57 1999
618.92′8589061—dc21
DNLM/DLC
for Library of Congress 99-36530
CIP

All papers, comments, opinions, findings, conclusions, or recommendations in *Ritalin: Theory and Practice*, Second Edition are those of the author(s), and do not constitute opinions, findings, conclusions, or recommendations of the Publisher, the Editors, and the editorial staff.

Printed in the United States of America

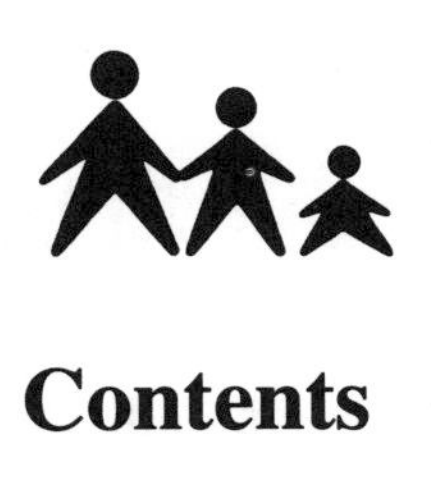

Contents

Contributors ix

Preface xiii

Pediatric Psychopharmacology in the United States: Issues and Challenges in the Diagnosis and Treatment of Attention Deficit Hyperactivity Disorder 1
Peter S. Jensen

Section 1
THE USE OF RITALIN

Pharmacoepidemiology of Methylphenidate and Other Stimulants for the Treatment of Attention Deficit Hyperactivity Disorder 7
Daniel J. Safer and Julie Magno Zito

Is Ritalin an Abused Drug? Does It Meet the Criteria of a Schedule II Substance? 27
Christine Sannerud and Gretchen Feussner

Section 2
DIAGNOSTIC ISSUES

Attention Deficit Hyperactivity Disorder and Methylphenidate: Assessment and Prediction of Clinical Response 45
Mark D. Rapport and Colin B. Denney

Ritalin: Comorbidity and Differential Clinical Response: The Role of Anxiety 71
Steven R. Pliszka

Section 3
CRITERIA FOR USE OF RITALIN

Combining Parent Training and Medication in the Treatment of Attention Deficit Hyperactivity Disorder 87
Russell Schachar and Richard Sugarman

Section 4
CLINICAL USE OF RITALIN

Rating Scales for Use in Assessment and Clinical Trials with Children 113
C. Keith Conners

Methylphenidate Versus Amphetamine: A Comparative Review 127
L. Eugene Arnold

Treatment of Adult Attention Deficit Hyperactivity Disorder 141
Thomas Spencer, Joseph Biederman, and Timothy Wilens

Psychostimulants in HIV-Infected Children and Adolescents: A Case Series 165
Jennifer F. Havens and E'Mett O. McCaskill

Coordinating Care in the Prescription and Use of Ritalin with Attention Deficit Hyperactivity Disorder Children/Adolescents 175
Betty B. Osman

Section 5
RITALIN EFFECTS IN CHILDREN WITH ATTENTION DEFICIT HYPERACTIVITY DISORDER

Prediction and Measurement of Individual Responses to Ritalin by Children and Adolescents with Attention Deficit Hyperactivity Disorder 193
William E. Pelham, Jr. and Bradley H. Smith

Dose-Response Effects of Ritalin on Cognitive Self-Regulation, Learning and Memory, and Academic Performance 219
Mary V. Solanto

Ritalin Effects on Aggression and Antisocial Behavior 237
Stephen P. Hinshaw and Steve S. Lee

Methylphenidate Treatment of *DSM-IV* Types of Attention Deficit Hyperactivity Disorder 253
Keith McBurnett

Methylphenidate: Effects on Language, Reading, and Auditory Processing 265
Rosemary Tannock

Attention Deficit Hyperactivity Disorder and Ritalin Side Effects: Is Sleep Delayed, Disrupted, or Disturbed? 287
Mark A. Stein and Maryland Pao

Methylphenidate Treatment for Children with Attention Deficit Hyperactivity Disorder and Tic Disorder: Inadvisable or Indispensible? 301
Jeffrey Sverd

Ritalin: An Energetic Factor? 321
Joseph Sergeant and Jaap J. van der Meere

Diagnostic Comorbidity, Attentional Measures, and Neurochemistry in Children with Attention Deficit Hyperactivity Disorder 341
Vanshdeep Sharma, Jeffrey H. Newcorn, and Jeffrey M. Halperin

Section 6
THE PHARMACOLOGY OF RITALIN AND FUTURE RESEARCH

Generic Methylphenidate Versus Brand Ritalin: Which Should Be Used? 363
Benedetto Vitiello and Laurie B. Burke

CONTENTS

Methylphenidate: The Role of the d-Isomer 369
Declan M.P. Quinn

Brain Imaging Studies of the Action of Methylphenidate and Cocaine in the Human Brain 375
Monique Ernst, Alyssa Earle, and Alan Zametkin

Randomized Clinical Trials of Long-Duration Stimulant Medications: Design Considerations 385
Laurence L. Greenhill, Jeffrey M. Halperin, and Howard Abikoff

Patterns of Use of Clonidine Alone and in Combination with Methylphenidate 401
Roland Regino, Martin Baren, Daniel F. Connor, and James M. Swanson

University of California, Irvine, Laboratory School Protocol for Pharmacokinetic and Pharmacodynamic Studies 405
James M. Swanson, Dave Agler, Erick Fineberg, Sharon Wigal, Dan Flynn, Katrina Fineberg, Yvonne Quintana, and Hani Talebi

Subject Index 433

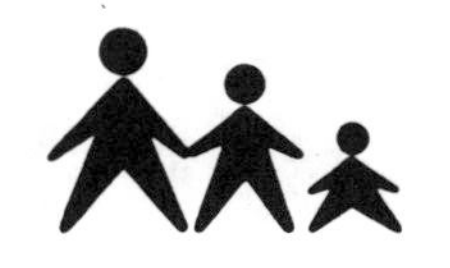

Contributors

Howard Abikoff, Ph.D.
New York University Child Study Center; and Division of Child and Adolescent Psychiatry, New York University Medical Center, New York, New York

Dave Agler, M.Ed.
Teacher, University of California, Irvine, Child Development Center, Centerpointe, Irvine, California

L. Eugene Arnold, M.Ed., M.D.
Professor Emeritus of Psychiatry, Ohio State University, Columbus, Ohio

Martin Baren, M.D.
Clinical Professor, Department of Pediatrics, University of California Medical Center, Irvine, California

Joseph Biederman, M.D.
Chief, Joint Program in the Pediatric Psychopharmacology Unit, Massachusetts General Hospital; and Professor of Psychiatry, Harvard Medical School, Boston, Massachusetts

Laurie B. Burke, R.Ph., M.P.H.
Senior Regulatory Research Officer, Center for Drug Evaluation and Research, Food and Drug Administration, Washington, D.C.

Daniel F. Connor, M.D.
Associate Professor, Department of Psychology, University of Massachusetts Medical Center, Worcester, Massachusetts

C. Keith Conners, Ph.D.
Professor of Medical Psychology, Department of Psychiatry, Duke University Medical Center, Durham, North Carolina

Colin B. Denney, Ph.D.
Post-Doctorate Fellow, Department of Psychology, University of Hawaii at Manoa, Honolulu, Hawaii

Alyssa Earle, B.A.
Office of Clinical Director, National Institutes of Health, Bethesda, Maryland

Monique Ernst, M.D., Ph.D.
Associate Director, NIDA Brain Imaging Center, National Institute on Drug Abuse, Baltimore, Maryland

Gretchen Feussner, B.S.
Pharmacologist, Drug and Chemical Evaluation Section, Office of Diversion Control, Drug Enforcement Administration, Washington, D.C.

CONTRIBUTORS

Erick Fineberg, M.Ed.
Teacher, University of California, Irvine, Child Development Center, Centerpointe, Irvine, California

Katrina Fineberg, B.A.
Research Coordinator, University of California, Irvine, Child Development Center, Centerpointe, Irvine, California

Dan Flynn, M.A.
Teacher, University of California, Irvine, Child Development Center, Centerpointe, Irvine, California

Laurence L. Greenhill, M.D.
Department of Psychiatry, Division of Child and Adolescent Psychiatry, New York State Psychiatric Institute; and Disruptive Behavior Disorders Clinic, Columbia-Presbyterian Medical Center, New York, New York

Jeffrey M. Halperin, Ph.D.
Professorial Lecturer, Department of Psychiatry, Division of Child and Adolescent Psychiatry, The Mount Sinai School of Medicine, New York, New York; and Professor of Psychology, Neuropsychology Graduate Program, Queens College, City University of New York, Flushing, New York

Jennifer F. Havens, M.D.
Director, Pediatric Psychiatry, Babies' and Childrens' Hospital, New York Presbyterian Hospital, New York, New York

Stephen P. Hinshaw, Ph.D.
Professor of Psychology; and Director of Clinical Psychology Training, Department of Psychology, University of California at Berkeley, Berkeley, California

Peter S. Jensen, M.D.
Senior Advisor to the Director, National Institute of Mental Health, Bethesda, Maryland

Steve S. Lee, B.A.
Graduate Student, Department of Psychology, University of California at Berkeley, Berkeley, California

Keith McBurnett, Ph.D.
Assistant Professor, Department of Psychiatry, University of Chicago, Chicago, Illinois

E'mett O. McCaskill, Ph.D.
Family Support Program Coordinator, The Special Needs Clinic, New York Presbyterian Hospital, New York, New York

Jeffrey H. Newcorn, M.D.
Associate Professor of Psychiatry and Pediatrics, Department of Psychiatry, Division of Child and Adolescent Psychiatry, The Mount Sinai School of Medicine, New York, New York

Betty B. Osman, Ph.D.
Psychologist, Department of Behavioral Health, White Plains Hospital Center, White Plains, New York

Maryland Pao, M.D.
Assistant Professor of Psychiatry and Pediatrics, Center for Neuroscience and Behavioral Medicine, Children's National Medical Center, Washington, D.C.

William E. Pelham, Jr., Ph.D.
Professor, Department of Psychology, State University of New York at Buffalo, Buffalo, New York

Steven R. Pliszka, M.D.
Associate Professor and Chief, Division of Child and Adolescent Psychiatry, The University of Texas Health Science Center at San Antonio, San Antonio, Texas

Declan M.P. Quinn, M.B., F.R.C.P. (C)
Associate Professor, Department of Psychiatry, College of Medicine, University of Saskatchewan, Saskatoon, Saskatchewan, Canada

Yvonne Quintana, B.A.
Research Assistant, University of California, Irvine, Child Development Center, Centerpointe, Irvine, California

Mark D. Rapport, Ph.D.
Chair, Graduate Studies and Professor of Clinical Child Psychology, Department of Psychology, University of Hawaii at Manoa, Honolulu, Hawaii

Roland Regino, B.A., B.S.
Researcher Associate, University of California, Irvine, Child Development Center, Centerpointe, Irvine, California

Daniel J. Safer, M.D.
Associate Professor, Departments of Psychiatry and Pediatrics, Johns Hopkins University School of Medicine, Baltimore, Maryland

Christine Sannerud, Ph.D.
Drug Science Officer, Drug and Chemical Evaluation Section, Office of Diversion Control, Drug Enforcement Administration, Washington, D.C.

Russell Schachar, M.D., F.R.C.P. (C)
Professor, Department of Psychiatry; and Senior Scientist, Research Institute, The Hospital for Sick Children, University of Toronto, Toronto, Ontario, Canada

Joseph Sergeant, B.A., M.A., Ph.D.
Professor, Department of Clinical Neuropsychology, Vrije Universiteit, Amsterdam, The Netherlands

Vanshdeep Sharma, M.D.
Assistant Professor, Department of Psychiatry, Division of Child and Adolescent Psychiatry, The Mount Sinai School of Medicine, New York, New York

Bradley H. Smith, Ph.D.
Assistant Professor, Department of Psychology, University of South Carolina, Columbia, South Carolina

Mary V. Solanto, Ph.D.
Associate Professor of Psychiatry, Division of Child and Adolescent Psychiatry, Mount Sinai Medical Center, New York, New York

Thomas Spencer, M.D.
Assistant Director, Pediatric Psychopharmacology Unit, Massachusetts General Hospital; and Associate Professor of Psychiatry, Harvard Medical School, Boston, Massachusetts

Mark A. Stein, Ph.D.
Professor of Psychiatry and Pediatrics, Center for Neuroscience and Behavioral Medicine, Children's National Medical Center, Washington, D.C.

Richard Sugarman, M.S.W., C.S.W.
Lecturer, Department of Psychiatry; and Social Worker, Neuropsychiatry Clinic, The Hospital for Sick Children, University of Toronto, Toronto, Ontario, Canada

Jeffrey Sverd, M.D.
Clinical Director, Sagamore Children's Psychiatric Center, State of New York Office of Mental Health, Dix Hills, New York

James M. Swanson, Ph.D.
Director, University of California, Irvine, Child Development Center, Centerpointe, Irvine, California

Hani Talebi, B.A.
Research Assistant, University of California, Irvine, Child Development Center, Centerpointe, Irvine, California

Rosemary Tannock, Ph.D.
Senior Scientist, Brain & Behavior Research Program, The Hospital for Sick Children; and Associate Professor of Psychiatry, University of Toronto, Toronto, Ontario, Canada

Jaap J. van der Meere, Ph.D.
Laboratory of Experimental Clinical Psychology, University of Amsterdam, Amsterdam, The Netherlands

Benedetto Vitiello, M.D.
Chief, Child and Adolescent Treatment and Preventive Intervention Research Branch, National Institute of Mental Health, Bethesda, Maryland

Sharon Wigal, Ph.D.
Director, Clinical Trials, University of California, Irvine, Child Development Center, Centerpointe, Irvine, California

Timothy Wilens, M.D.
Staff, Pediatric and Adult Psychopharmacology Clinic, Massachusetts General Hospital; and Associate Professor of Psychiatry, Harvard Medical School, Boston, Massachusetts

Alan Zametkin, M.D.
Office of Clinical Director, National Institutes of Health, Bethesda, Maryland

Julie Magno Zito, Ph.D.
Associate Professor of Pharmacy and Medicine, Department of Pharmacy Practice and Science, University of Maryland School of Pharmacy, Baltimore, Maryland

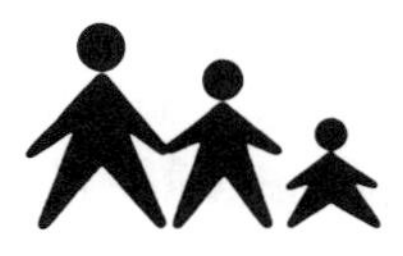

Preface

The first edition of this book was published in 1991 as a key reference and guide for professionals involved in research or in the clinical use and management of methylphenidate (Ritalin). At that time, there was no book available on the subject, so it was difficult for professionals to find detailed information on its efficacy, safety, and use. Our book was received with enthusiasm by the medical and research community, as well as by other professionals involved in treating children with attention deficit hyperactivity disorder (ADHD).

The current revision of this book was undertaken for four reasons:

1. Since the first edition was written, a larger body of research on ADHD has become available. This is represented in this volume by chapters on neuroimaging by Ernst et al. and by Quinn; on language processing in ADHD by Tannock; on the locus of methylphenidates in a cognitive model by Sergeant and van der Meere; on new findings in the psychopharmacology of methylphenidate by Rapport and Denney, Solanto, and Vitiello and Burke. Arnold contributes a scholarly review comparing Ritalin with amphetamine. Although the clinical use of Ritalin remains controversial and misconceptions prevail, its research knowledge base has grown significantly.
2. An ever-increasing number of youths are taking Ritalin to alleviate their symptoms, as Safer and Zito report in their chapter and Jensen in his introduction to this volume. This is shown by a 500% increase in Ritalin production, and a 2.5-fold increase in prescriptions since 1991. This is leading to concerns about diversion, use, and abuse, which are discussed in detail by Sannerud and Feussner in their chapter.
3. Commensurate with the developments in theory and pharmacokinetics of Ritalin, there have been a plethora of new clinical research reports. These include new data on adults' responses to Ritalin, as reported in Spencer et al.'s chapter and the response to Ritalin by children with congenital HIV, as reported by Havens and McCaskill. New information on side effects impacts clinical practice; Ritalin's effects on sleep are reported by Stein and Pao, and Ritalin's effects on tics by Sverd. Comorbid disorders may affect the response to Ritalin, as discussed by Pliszka, for children with ADHD and anxiety symptoms, and by Hinshaw and Lee for ADHD children with aggresive behaviors. Pelhams' previous chapter on the diversity of individual responses to Ritalin has been updated and supplemented by chapters on ADHD subtype response to Ritalin by MacBurnett. Schachar and Sugarman describe the effects of combining parent training with the administration of Ritalin in his chapter. Conners provides an update on the use of his well-known parent and teacher rating forms.
4. In the past four years, there has been a flood of information in the media about Ritalin, some that is incorrect. It is important to set the record straight about the current state of knowledge about this medication, while expanding the knowledge of people who live and work with ADHD children and adolescents.

Physicians—pediatricians in particular—increasingly are called on to prescribe Ritalin and to answer questions about the effects of the drug, its dosage, and its titration, as well as its case management. With the ever-expanding body of information on Ritalin, the practicing physician may have neither the time nor the resources to locate and review all the current data.

Other health care professionals as well, including nurses, psychologists, social workers, and educators, are confronted with requests for information about the appropriate use of Ritalin and its risks and side effects, as well as administration and dosage schedules of the drug. These professionals may also be in a position to help monitor and evaluate the treatment, particularly for school age children—the primary consumers of Ritalin in the United States today.

The updated revision of this book is designed to be a key reference and comprehensive resource for professionals involved in research or in the clinical use and management of Ritalin. Chief among them are child psychiatrists, pediatricians, family physicians, and pediatric neurologists who prescribe, administer, and monitor Ritalin therapy in their practices.

This volume is neither for or against the use of Ritalin. The need for logical and dispassionate information on the subject is evident. The articles in this volume are written from a variety of perspectives, covering a broad spectrum of topics. Chapters include issues of assessment and diagnosis, criteria for use and pediatric management of Ritalin, effects on children and adolescents with other disorders, ramifications for language and cognition, the pharmacology of Ritalin, and comparative studies.

Although some chapters in this edition have been updated, new sections have also been added to include current findings. *Ritalin: Theory and Practice, 2nd ed.,* is predicated on the idea that the use of Ritalin merits different approaches because of its multiplicity of roles: as a treatment modality for ADHD and other behavior disorders of childhood; for children with developmental disabilities; and for adults with ADHD and AIDS-related problems.

This book is a testament to the productivity, talent, and genuine concern for patient care found in the contributors to this volume, who so generously gave of their time, their expertise, and their clinical experience with children with ADHD. Special thanks, too, for the inspiration and encouragement of our publisher, Mary Ann Liebert, who recognized the need for this book and supported the endeavor. And to our families and those who assisted in the technical preparation of this book, we express our deepest gratitude.

Betty B. Osman, Ph.D.
Laurence L. Greenhill, M.D.

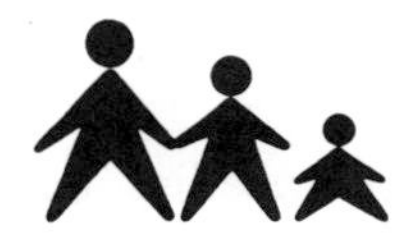

Pediatric Psychopharmacology in the United States: Issues and Challenges in the Diagnosis and Treatment of Attention Deficit Hyperactivity Disorder

PETER S. JENSEN

Given the heightened media interest in the use of Ritalin for the treatment of children with attention deficit disorder (ADD), it should come as no surprise that the prescribing of psychotropic agents for children and adolescents with psychiatric disorders has become relatively commonplace. For example, Pincus and colleagues (1998) have documented the increasing rate of prescribing of antidepressants for children and adults in the 10 years prior to 1994. Similarly, we have noted that in 1995, over 2 million visits to physicians resulted in prescriptions of psychostimulant medications, principally for attention deficit hyperactivity disorder (ADHD)—as many as 6 million prescriptions (Jensen et al., 1999a). In addition, we have found that the levels of visits to prescribing physicians for other psychotropic agents in 1995 were quite substantial: 300,000 visits resulting in the prescription of a serotonin reuptake inhibitor, another 300,000 resulting in prescription of a mood stabilizer; and over 250,000 visits resulting in prescriptions of tricyclic antidepressants.

In consequence of these increased rates of prescribing, great interest is evident among physicians, mental health professionals, and others interested in the public health and welfare of children about the appropriate and judicious use of psychotropic medications in this vulnerable age group. In the last decade, the number of peer-reviewed articles in the leading journal of the field, the *Journal of the American Academy of Child and Adolescent Psychiatry,* has doubled. Similarly, in the last decade, a new journal on child and adolescent psychopharmacology and a journal on attention disorders have been founded. All these factors translate into a heightened need for science-based information for health care providers and consumers, as well as an insatiable interest on the part of the media for information about the safety and efficacy of psychotropic medications in children.

What do increased medication rates of prescribing mean for children with ADD? While the exact rates of ADHD have not been firmly established, most experts place the national prevalence of ADHD at somewhere between 3% and 5% of children under age 18, roughly translating to about 4 million children. Nonetheless, given the estimates of 6 million prescriptions/mentions, if we assume that a given ADHD child receives one prescription per month over 9 months of the year, the data suggest that only as few as 650,000 children (6 million prescriptions divided by nine prescriptions per child = 650,000) are being actively treated for ADHD across the United States. Given such assumptions, we might conclude

Office of the Director, National Institute of Mental Health, Bethesda, Maryland.

The opinions and assertions contained in this chapter are the private views of the author and are not to be construed as official or as reflecting the views of the Department of Health and Human Services or the National Institute of Mental Health.

that, of the estimated 4 million children needing care and treatment for ADHD, only 1 in 6 children are actively being treated. On the other hand, some data suggest that many children with ADHD do not receive prescriptions throughout the year. Indeed, the modal number of prescriptions appears to be one to four prescriptions per child per year, according to data from the Suffolk county study by Sherman and Hertzig (1991). Assuming three prescriptions per child per year, such findings would translate to only 2 million children being treated for ADHD with psychostimulants (6 million prescriptions divided by three prescriptions per child) and that these same 2 million children are being inadequately (or at least inconsistently) treated, while the other 2 million are receiving even less care.

Thus, rather than children with ADHD being overtreated or even children being "overdiagnosed with ADHD," examination of the known facts suggests that the majority of children with ADHD are not recognized, evaluated, or adequately treated. In fact, in analyses that my colleagues and I have conducted on data collected in the Methodology of Epidemiology in Children and Adolescents (MECA) Study across four United States and Puerto Rican communities, we found that, among children determined to have ADHD within an epidemiologic sampling frame, only one in eight children with ADHD within a given year was actually being treated with ADHD medications (Jensen et al., 1999). I suggest that these data provide a more accurate picture, namely, that despite decreased stigma and greater public awareness, most children with ADHD are not receiving any medication treatment, perhaps in part because of the continuing effects of stigma and parental concerns about the use of psychostimulants.

These data indicate substantial reasons for concern about the actual assessment and diagnostic and prescribing practices in the community. As Sloan et al. have reported, primary care providers report that they have not had sufficient training in the diagnosis and treatment of ADHD. The amount of time allotted within a typical pediatric practice is frequently insufficient for an appropriate diagnostic evaluation, so it should not be surprising to find that many cases of psychiatric disorder (including ADHD) may not be identified in primary care practice. Even once a condition has been identified, many health care providers do not have the other necessary skills to provide parental guidance and behavioral training, much less the careful medication titration that may be required for the treatment of ADHD. Follow-up and monitoring of care is often scanty and insufficient (Jensen et al., 1989; Sloan et al., 1999). Diagnostic practices too commonly ignore the importance of assessments obtained from school personnel. Also, too many diagnostic decisions are still based on outdated thinking, (e.g., whether the child responds to a psychostimulant).

Fortunately, the last several years have witnessed the publication of treatment guidelines by professional associations, such as the American Academy of Child and Adolescent Psychiatry and the American Medical Association. Moreover, the Agency for Health Care Policy Research has worked with the American Academy of Pediatrics to better define the optimal treatment practices to guide physicians in their evaluation, diagnosis, and treatment of children with ADHD. While such guidelines are useful, clear consensus about what should constitute the best practices is not yet fully apparent. How should the diagnosis of the ADHD be established? What length of time is necessary for an adequate evaluation? What is the role of information obtained from parents and teachers or directly from the child in order to make a diagnosis? What are the necessary "rule ins" and "rule outs" as a part of the overall diagnostic and assessment procedure? What are the other required components of an evaluation, such as any laboratory work, hearing and vision testing, psychologic testing, and educational performance testing?

Actual treatment practices and what should constitute state-of-the-art treatment have also not been fully explicated. When medication is used, how should it be titrated? If the child does not respond to the first psychotropic agent, what treatment should be considered next? What other treatments, apart from medication, should be implemented as a part of the overall plan? Which child needs which treatments, and in which order and/or combination? How does this vary as a function of the child's age, gender, or parent and family preferences? Should psychostimulants be prescribed for children with comorbid ADHD and conduct disorder and/or substance use? How do factors such as comorbidity affect the choice of treatment or the likelihood of therapeutic response? When the physician decides to use a medication, what are the short-term and long-term effects of the medication, in terms of both its therapeutic benefits and its potential immediate and long-term side effects?

In light of this spate of questions, the need for information is all too apparent. Such information must be accurate, comprehensive, and, most importantly, accessible and understandable to providers. Such needs are particularly acute with ADHD, for which the majority of prescriptions are written by providers in primary care settings, including pediatricians and family practitioners. Consequently, this volume is timely and fills a critical need for up-to-date information by outstanding researchers and practitioners in the field of ADHD. Such a volume cannot replace the need for more adequate training within our pediatric, psychiatric, psychology, social work, and nursing training programs or the need for public information that is accurate and not sensationalist. Nonetheless, this volume goes a long way in bringing together, into one format and one place, a state-of-the-art statement about the diagnosis and treatment of ADHD. Dr. Greenhill and colleagues have done yeoman's service for the field, not just for the practitioners and treatment providers but also for the families who must rely upon sound knowledge and an informed medical care system. This volume is a remarkable contribution to that yet unrealized state of affairs. Nonetheless, given the prevalence of ADHD and the fact that it comprises the lion's share of mental disorder referrals in pediatric, psychiatric, and psychology mental health settings, this volume, if effectively implemented and used, will take us a long way toward realizing the objectives of a responsive health care system for children with mental and behavioral disorders.

REFERENCES

Jensen, P., Bhatara, V., Vitiello, B., Hoagwood, K., Feil, M. & Burke, L.B. (1999a), Psychoactive medication prescribing practices for US children: Gaps between research and clinical practice. *J. Am. Acad. Child. Adolesc. Psychiatry*, 38:557–565.

Jensen, P.S., Kettle, L., Roper, M.S., Sloan, M.T., Dulcan, M.K., Hoven, C., Bird, H.R., Bauermeister, J.J. & Payne, J.D. (1999b), Are stimulants overprescribed? Treatment of ADHD in four U.S. communities. *J. Am. Acad. Child Adolesc. Psychiatry*, 38:797–804.

Jensen, P.S., Xenakis, S.N., Shervette, R.S. & Bain, M.W. (1989), Diagnostic and treatment practices of ADD in the general hospital. *Hosp. Commun. Psychiatry,* 40:708–712.

Pincus, H.A., Tanielian, T.L., Marcus, S.C., Olfson, M., Zarin, D.A., Thompson, J. & Magno Zito, J. (1998), Prescribing trends in psychotropic medications: Primary care, psychiatry, and other medical specialties. *JAMA* 279:526–531.

Sloan, M., Jensen, P. & Kettle, L. (1999), Assessing services for children with ADHD: Gaps and opportunities. *J. Attention Disorders* 3:13–29, 1999.

Sherman, M. & Hertzig, M.E. (1991), Prescribing practices of Ritalin: The Suffolk County, New York study. In: *Ritalin: Theory and Patient Management,* eds. L.L. Greenhill & B.B. Osman. Larchmont, NY: Mary Ann Liebert, Inc., pp 187–193.

Section 1

The Use of Ritalin

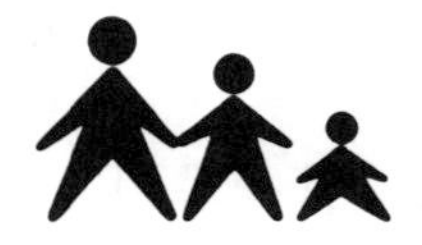

Pharmacoepidemiology of Methylphenidate and Other Stimulants for the Treatment of Attention Deficit Hyperactivity Disorder

DANIEL J. SAFER[1] and JULIE MAGNO ZITO[2]

INTRODUCTION

Before 1960, psychotropic medication was not commonly prescribed for children. Stimulant treatment was indeed described as beneficial for children with behavior problems as early as 1937, but only after medication treatment breakthroughs for adult schizophrenia, depression, and anxiety occurred in the 1950s did pharmacotherapy for youths become actively considered as a treatment option. Controlled trials of dextroamphetamine and methylphenidate in the mid- and late 1960s began the scientific legitimization of this new therapeutic direction.

Even in the 1970s, there was great caution because the idea of medicating children to alter their aberrant behavior struck most American adults as inappropriate. The media exaggerated the extent of the increasing psychiatric medication treatment for youths, inflammatory books were written on the subject, and even the U.S. Congress appointed a blue-ribbon panel to investigate the matter (Schrag and Divoky, 1975; Anonymous, 1971; Maynard, 1970).

Media criticisms and government cautionary moves concerning the stimulant treatment of youths have continued well into the 1990s. At the state level, legislative mandated panels submitted reports on stimulant treatment in Michigan (Goldstein, 1991), Virginia (ADHD Task Force, 1991), and Maryland (House Bill, 1997). Various legal efforts were undertaken to limit stimulant therapy, and the U.S. Drug Enforcement Administration has tried both to limit methylphenidate (Ritalin) production and to suggest that this drug has been frequently abused (U.S. Drug Enforcement Administration, 1995, 1996).

Nonetheless, over the years, prescribing physicians and researchers have found stimulants to be useful in the treatment of attention deficit hyperactivity disorder (ADHD), and committee reports from professional medical specialty organizations have concluded that such treatment is usually beneficial (Goldman et al., 1998; AACAP Work Group on Quality Issues, 1997; Committee on Children with Disabilities, 1996).

This chapter not only focuses on the increased use of stimulants since the 1970s but also describes the various factors that influence stimulant treatment. Among these are the research methods used to estimate drug prevalence, the specific drug therapy prescribed, the various settings in which treatment prevalence is measured (e.g., regular classroom versus special education classrooms), and the demographic, clinical, and broad social factors that influence the prevalence of this disorder and its drug treatment.

---

[1]Departments of Psychiatry and Pediatrics, John Hopkins University School of Medicine; and [2]Department of Pharmacy Practice and Science, University of Maryland School of Pharmacy, Baltimore, Maryland.

RESEARCH METHODS FOR POPULATION-BASED MEASURES

Epidemiology provides measures for describing disease according to person, place, and time patterns. In recent years, computers have made it possible to apply epidemiologic methods to the study of drug utilization and to create population-based estimates of drug use (Zito and Riddle, 1995; Zito and Craig, 1991; Strom, 1994). A more detailed review of the available data sources has recently been published (Zito and Safer, 1997). The advantages of using large community-based samples to estimate drug prevalence include: (1) providing more stable estimates that are reliable across patient subgroups, clinical settings, physician specialties, and geographic locale, in contrast to the convenience sampling typical of many clinical studies; (2) showing the variation that exists in practice; and (3) generating questions about whether certain treatment patterns are medically beneficial. Study designs that incorporate the usual practice setting into drug evaluation can: (1) show how patients in the usual practice setting are similar to or different from those in clinical trial populations; (2) aid in measuring treatment effectiveness, i.e., the outcome of therapy in the usual practice setting, as opposed to the more rigorously controlled but less generalizable measurement of treatment efficacy (Lehman, 1996); and (3) provide information on people who do *not* participate in clinical trials. This discussion stresses descriptive epidemiology, which uses drug prevalence as a quantitative measure of drug utilization. Drug prevalence as used herein is the frequency at which youths receive one or more prescriptions for the treatment of ADHD per 100 youths in the age group or school group under study.

Types of medication prescribed for ADHD

Methylphenidate accounts for most of the stimulant treatment for attentional problems in the United States. Marketing data from 1995 stimulant sales had the following distribution: methylphenidate (83%), dextroamphetamine (9.2%), and pemoline (7.8%) (Batoosingh, 1995). These data parallel data from the Baltimore County school survey, which assessed the growth of methylphenidate use over the last three decades. In 1971, methylphenidate accounted for only 40% of all medication prescribed for ADHD, but since then the rate has steadily increased. The percentage rose to 90% by 1983 and has subsequently remained near that level (Safer and Krager, 1988).

Dextroamphetamine (Dexedrine and Dextrostat) accounted for 29% to 36% of stimulant medication prescribed for ADHD in 1971–1973 in Baltimore County, but this agent's use gradually decreased to 3% to 5% of the total in the 1980s and 1990s. Pemoline (Cylert) accounted for 1% to 6% of stimulants prescribed for ADHD, although prescriptions for this drug have declined since the mid-1990s (Safer and Krager, 1994; Safer and Krager, 1992). The latter is probably accounted for by increased awareness of potentially serious liver toxicity that can occur during pemoline treatment (Pizzuti, 1996).

Combination medication therapy

Clinical recommendations for combination medication therapies have appeared in recent years (Wilens et al., 1995) despite the absence of rigorous data to support their efficacy or safety. There is, of late, an increased awareness of comorbid conditions that exist with ADHD (August et al., 1996), and it is likely that they result in increased psychotropic treatment. Unfortunately, as yet there are only meager epidemiologic data that measure the frequency of combined medication therapies and no rigorous data on their effectiveness.

Chapter overview

With these introductory concepts as background, this chapter details the prevalence of treatments for ADHD according to the following factors: educational settings, namely, parochial and private, special education, and public schools; patient demographic factors such as gender, ethnicity/race, age, and economic status; clinical characteristics that contribute to variations in the prevalence of medication usage, such as diagnostic issues, mental retardation, the medication administration regimen, duration of treatment, and patient adherence and satisfaction with treatment; and clinical system characteristics, including physician specialty, medical setting, payment source, and geographic variations that directly affect prevalence. Then, on a broader level, factors are discussed that indirectly affect the prevalence of ADHD treatment, including the role of pharmaceutical promotion and consumer advocacy groups, the impact of the media and threatened lawsuits, government regulation, and legislation and judicial decisions. Next, the size of the U.S. population of youths receiving drug treatment for ADHD is discussed, and international utilization patterns will be addressed.

PREVALENCE ESTIMATES OF MEDICATION USE FOR ADHD

Lifetime prevalence

Six studies reported that 52% to 71% of youths with a clinical diagnosis of ADHD were treated with stimulant medication for this disorder at some time before reaching adulthood (Cullinan et al., 1987; Copeland et al., 1987; Bosco and Robin, 1980; Barkley et al., 1991).

Point or period prevalence

The earliest prevalence surveys of medication treatment for ADHD were reported in the early 1970s (Krager and Safer, 1974; Stephen et al., 1973). Stephen et al. surveyed physicians (36% response rate) in the Chicago area in 1970–1971 and estimated that approximately 2% of public and private school students were receiving medication for hyperactivity. The Krager and Safer report of medication treatment for hyperactivity was based on 1971 and 1973 school nurse counts of Baltimore County elementary school students. In 1973, the nurses' count of elementary school students receiving medication treatment for hyperactivity resulted in a point prevalence of 1.7%.

In 1975 and 1977, surveys were performed at various geographic sites in the U.S. using different sources to gather the data. One study used reports from school psychologists, two used school guidance counselors, one queried parents, and one used school nurses. Their prevalence findings for students receiving medication for ADHD showed a threefold variation from 0.8% to 2.6% of the student population (Gadow, 1981).

Surveys in the 1980s were primarily from school children in Baltimore County (Safer and Krager, 1988; Safer and Krager, 1984), but in the 1990s the field of pharmacoepidemiology expanded dramatically, and now these data are being reported from a variety of sources (Table 1). Data sources are divided into two types: numerator sources (e.g., U.S. Drug Enforcement Administration [DEA], triplicate prescription databases, IMS America, and Scott Levin prescription surveys) and population-based sources, where both numerator and denominator data are available (e.g., Medicaid or epidemiologic surveys). The denominator consists of all enrollees, residents, or students of a defined region regardless of

TABLE 1. DATA SOURCES FOR MEASURING DRUG UTILIZATION PATTERNS AND CASE EXAMPLES

Data Sources	*Basis or Location*	*Time Frame*	*Description*
Prescription trends (numerator data only)			
DEA ARCOS database	Wholesale shipments of controlled substances to retail registrants	Annual	Kilograms of base weight (U.S. Drug Enforcement Administration, 1996)
DEA production quotas	Estimate of future need based on previous use	Annual	(U.S. Drug Enforcement Administration, 1996)
Triplicate (or duplicate) reporting to the state	Michigan, New York, (Rhode Island)	Various intervals	Michigan (Rappley et al., 1995) and New York (Sherman and Hertzig, 1991) studies developed population-based estimates from these numerator data and census data
IMS America	Proprietary audit of pharmacy prescription sales (NPA) or of clinical encounters (NDTA)	Various intervals	National sampling of prescription sales; 3.8 million prescriptions in 1993 for stimulants among 2–18-year-olds (Vitiello et al., 1994)
Scott Levin National Physician's Drug and Diagnosis Audit	Similar to IMS' NDTA approach; 2,400 U.S. physicians' reports	Various intervals	National sampling (Swanson et al., 1995a)
Population-based estimates (numerator and denominator)			
County data from ad hoc research or clinical surveys	Tennessee county; rural North Carolina county; Baltimore County school nurse surveys; Virginia school surveys	Various intervals	County epidemiologic study or school survey (LeFever et al., 1997; Safer and Krager, 1994; Angold and Costello, 1997; Wolraich et al., 1996)
Administrative claims data	Medicaid systems with noncapitated payment programs	Various intervals	Maryland stimulant use, 1988 through 1994 (Zito et al., 1995)
	HMO programs in which most prescriptions are dispensed at the HMO	Northwest region of Kaiser Permanente in Oregon & Washington	91% Caucasian membership (Zito et al., 1995)

DEA = Drug Enforcement Administration.

their health status. The fourth column of Table 1 lists published reports using these data sources. The collective data from these sources, particularly from the population-based estimates, allow for the assessment of numerous factors that, in themselves, contribute to variations in the prevalence of medication usage for ADHD.

Prevalence of ADHD treatment according to educational setting

Parochial and private schools

School surveys in Baltimore County, Maryland, recorded medication treatment prevalence for ADHD in parochial and private schools separately. These figures were available because, until 1992, county health department nurses were assigned to all schools and therefore participated in the county's biennial student medication surveys. Throughout the 1970s and 1980s, the rate of medication usage for ADHD in parochial and private schools in the county steadily rose, but its relative rate consistently averaged only one third that of its public school counterparts (Safer and Krager, 1992). The lower use may be attributed to fewer children in need of treatment (school selection bias), parental cultural differences, or differences in teachers' attitudes (Jerome et al., 1994).

Special education

Students in special education classes of public elementary schools have consistently had higher stimulant medication treatment rates for ADHD than students in regular classes. Since such findings were first reported in the early 1980s in Baltimore County, Maryland, additional estimates from that site have confirmed the higher ADHD medication prevalence (19% to 30% of self-contained class, special education students at the elementary school level) in these children (Safer and Krager, 1988; Safer and Krager, 1984). These figures are consistent with other special education samples, specifically, a 25% elementary school special education class ADHD medication rate (Bussing et al., 1996) and a 31% prevalence of psychotropic medication for ADHD (Hansen and Keogh, 1971). However, a 9% ADHD medication rate for special education students in northern Illinois was reported (Cullinan et al., 1987), but this relatively low rate may be accounted for by the fact that these students were older (average age = 12 years) and that 83% were mainstreamed, i.e., placed in regular classes. Special education students who were placed in off-site schools, comprising seriously handicapped and mentally retarded youths, had an ADHD medication rate in Baltimore County that has hovered around 15% over the last two decades (Safer et al., 1996).

In all, 27% to 30% of all students receiving medication for ADHD in the Baltimore County public schools have been in special education classes or schools. This is generally understandable when one considers that 33% to 42% of school-identified youths with ADHD in primary schools receive special education services, largely in association with learning disabilities (Lambert et al., 1981; Charles and Schain, 1981; Barkley et al., 1990a). The Baltimore County data may not generalize to other areas of the country and should not be interpreted as definitive, but two conclusions seem firm. First, parochial and private schools have had fewer medicated children, and second, special education classes have far more children medicated for ADHD than do regular public school classrooms.

Public schools

In three studies of public school populations, the percentage of youths diagnosed with ADHD who were receiving stimulant treatment was reported. In a 1978 survey of grades K–5 in two California counties, 17.4% of the students with ADHD had received medication for that disorder at some time during the study year (Lambert et al., 1981). According to a 1976–1977 survey of parents (67% response rate) and teachers (75% response rate) of children of elementary, middle, and junior high school age in Grand Rapids, Michigan, 23% with ADHD were being treated with stimulant medication (Bosco and Robin, 1980). Based upon teacher identification, 26% of the K–5 school children with ADHD features (n = 8258) in a middle Tennessee county in 1993–1994 were being treated with stimulant medication (Wolraich et al., 1996).

Stimulant treatment of public *elementary* students has plateaued since 1987 in Baltimore County, Maryland (see Table 1). It could be that the treatment population is nearly saturated. A likely contributing factor is the increased prescription of alternative nonstimulant medications, e.g., antidepressants and clonidine.

Public middle school students were not surveyed in Baltimore County until 1975 because very few of these students received medication for ADHD before then. But their numbers rose steadily and, by 1975, 0.59% of the county's middle/junior high school students were receiving medication for ADHD (Table 2). This treatment continued to expand so rapidly that the rate of medication for ADHD at this school level rose sevenfold between 1975 and 1997 (see Table 2).

The prevalence of medication usage for ADHD has increased even more rapidly in Baltimore County public high schools. Between 1983 and 1997, medication treatment for ADHD rose sevenfold in these schools (see Table 2). Because 97% of all students receiving stimulant medication were first prescribed that treatment before or during their elementary school years (Safer and Krager, 1994), the prominent secondary school increases in that treatment during the last two decades are largely due to the prolongation of that therapy.

Patient demographic factors

Gender-specific prevalence of drug therapy for ADHD

In Baltimore County public schools in the early 1980s, the gender ratio for youths with medication for ADHD was 1:6 female:male (F:M) in the elementary schools and 1:12 in the middle schools. Since then, the gender ratio has steadily narrowed. In the 1990s the F:M gender ratio dropped to 1:4 in the elementary schools and 1:5 in the high schools (Safer et al., 1996). In 1991, Maryland Medicaid 5- to 14 year-olds had an F:M ratio of 1:3.7 (Zito et al., 1997). The increased proportion of girls receiving medication for ADHD is now more in line with ADHD prevalence surveys based on school samples, which consistently report an F:M ratio for ADHD of 1:2 and 1:3 (Luk and Leung, 1989; McGee et al., 1987; Glow, 1980). In addition, the inclusion of the "predominantly inattentive" ADHD subcategory within *DSM-IV* has proportionally increased the number of treatment-eligible girls above that of earlier versions of the *DSM* (Gaub and Carlson, 1997).

TABLE 2. PREVALENCE OF MEDICATION FOR ADHD (%) AMONG BALTIMORE COUNTY SCHOOL CHILDREN DURING A 27-YEAR PERIOD

Public Schools	*1971*	*1975*	*1983*	*1987*	*1995*	*1997*
Elementary	1.07	2.08	3.61	5.96	5.23	5.76
Middle	—	0.59	1.50	3.68	4.25	5.64
High	—	—	0.22	0.40	1.21	1.64
Special education—off site	16.1	15.0	13.3	13.2	18.21	26.54
Total	—	—	2.29	3.93	4.10	4.80

Race/ethnicity-specific drug prevalence

Prescriptions for Maryland youths with Medicaid insurance have been tabulated by race and age (Zito et al., 1997). The data show that African-American youths had a rate of methylphenidate treatment 2.5-fold *lower* than that of their Caucasian Medicaid counterparts. Even when corrected for geographic variation, a 2.0-fold lower use among African-American Medicaid youths was observed (Zito et al., 1998a). A similar degree of relative undertreatment of African-American youths with ADHD was found in several Virginia school districts (LeFever et al., 1997), a phenomenon previously noted among special education students (Gadow, 1981; Cullinan et al., 1987).

Age-specific prevalence of stimulant therapy for ADHD

ADHD in youths. Among 5- to 14-year olds with Maryland Medicaid insurance, the peak medication usage occurred from 8 to 11 years of age (Zito et al., 1997). This is consistent with other epidemiologic studies (Safer and Krager, 1992; Rappley et al., 1995).

Adult ADHD. The number of U.S. adults identified as having ADHD has increased substantially, although this has not been documented by population-based epidemiologic studies. Regardless, the number of prescriptions for methylphenidate written for U.S. adults has increased nearly 2.5-fold between 1992 and 1997 (Morrow, 1997).

Of course, not all methylphenidate is being prescribed to adults for the treatment of ADHD. This agent has been promoted for unlabeled indications, including the augmentation of antidepressant medication effects, reversal of the sexual side effects of selective serotonin reuptake inhibitor antidepressants, treatment of fatigue in the elderly, and reversal of some of the concentration problems common with AIDS and chronic fatigue syndrome, in addition to treatment of narcolepsy, a labeled indication (Holmes, 1995). It is noteworthy that, in the Maryland Medicaid administrative claims dataset of 1988–1994, 46% (1070/2317) of the individuals over age 19 who were prescribed methylphenidate were 60 years or older, and more than 75% of them were women. Presumably, these older adults were not receiving methylphenidate for ADHD (Zito et al., 1998b).

Economic status

Baltimore County student surveys were analyzed since 1971 to compare the prevalence of medication treatment for ADHD in public elementary school districts above and below the county's family income. In the early 1970s, schools in those census tract areas that had a family income above the median income for the county had higher medication rates (Krager and Safer, 1974). A reversal of this relationship took place from the late 1970s until the late 1980s, presumably because of the development of county clinics to serve hyperkinetic children without medical insurance.

The medical literature is mixed on whether socioeconomic status alters the prevalence of stimulant treatment. Some reports indicate that youths in lower socioeconomic classes receive relatively less medication for ADHD (Ross, 1979; LeFever et al., 1997), whereas authors have noted no relationship between family income and the use of medication for ADHD (Safer and Krager, 1992; Bosco and Robin, 1980; Hansen and Keogh, 1971). In the more recent Virginia school study, there was a significantly greater probability of having ADHD medication at school for Caucasians residing in neighborhoods with a family income above the median ($p < 0.001$) and for African-American children without public assistance ($p < 0.01$). Clarification of the role of the family's socioeconomic status in decision making about the diagnosis and treatment for ADHD awaits better data.

Clinical factors influencing drug prevalence

Diagnostic changes from DSM III *to* DSM IV

The attention deficit without hyperactivity subgroup was not a major consideration in the 1970s because the diagnostic and treatment emphasis then was on hyperkinesis (American Psychiatric Association, 1968). In the *DSM-III* (American Psychiatric Association, 1980), attentional problems without hyperactivity became a separate subcategory, and then in the *DSM-III-R* (American Psychiatric Association, 1987) and the *DSM-IV* (American Psychiatric Association, 1994), inattentiveness increasingly intermeshed with hyperactivity/impulsiveness to become a very significant feature in the quasi-unified, tripartite diagnostic category ADHD.

During this period, several small studies reported that stimulant drugs improved attentional disorders *in children who did not have notable hyperactivity* (Lahey and Carlson, 1991). Probably as a consequence, stimulant treatment of inattentiveness began to rise. Baltimore County clinic surveys revealed that, whereas 7% of youths medicated for ADHD in the mid-1970s were primarily inattentive, this rate rose to 18% in the mid-1980s (Safer and Krager, 1989) and to 20% in 1990. The proportion of predominantly inattentive youths receiving stimulant medication relative to the total number of students medicated for ADHD, however, is still a good deal less than the inattentive/total ADHD proportion found in recent elementary school prevalence studies: 47% to 56% (Wolraich et al., 1996; Baumgaertel et al., 1995; Gaub and Carlson, 1997).

The predominantly inattentive *DSM-IV* (1994) subcategory, which now constitutes approximately half the ADHD student total, is also clearly larger than the proportion of students who were classified as ADD without hyperactivity—13% to 20%—under *DSM-III* (American Psychiatric Association, 1980; Ullmann et al., 1984; Szatmari et al., 1989; McGee et al., 1990; Costello et al., 1988; Anderson et al., 1987). In fact, now almost 5% of elementary school students are being classified in the predominantly inattentive subgroup of ADHD using *DSM-IV* criteria (Wolraich et al., 1996; Gaub and Carlson, 1997). Primarily as a result of the expansion that has occurred in the code 314 *DSM* diagnostic category, the total prevalence of ADHD has swelled, as is apparent in numerous comparative *DSM* classification studies of the same youths (Leung et al., 1996; Baumgaertel et al., 1995).

Thus, including inattentiveness in addition to hyperactivity as part of one multifaceted diagnostic pattern has broadened the code 314 *DSM* category and has heightened diagnostic variability (Barkley, 1996). In contrast, the latest version of the International Classification of Diseases (ICD) (World Health Organization, 1994) retained its ICD-9 *hyperkinetic* disorder category (314.0–314.9), even though it adopted several *DSM-IV* changes (Swanson et al., 1998).

Presumably, in response to more children being identified as having ADHD, more are being medicated. The threefold increase in the proportion of youths given stimulant medication for attention deficit without hyperactivity in Baltimore County schools since the mid-1970s gives support to this contention (Safer and Krager, 1989).

Persistence of the features of ADHD

In the 1970s, because ADHD was believed to be exclusively a childhood disorder, stimulant medication was generally stopped after the elementary school years, and the peak

TABLE 3. SUMMARY OF METHYLPHENIDATE (OR STIMULANT) PREVALENCE DATA FROM VARIOUS STUDIES

Study Authors	*Prevalence Estimate*	*Sampling, Design, Population*	*Implications*
Angold & Costello, 1997	7.7% 4-year stimulant prevalence	9- to 15-year-old rural North Carolina youths identified by telephone screening & parent/child interviews; yearly reassessment for 4 years.	Community-based screening, rediagnosis based on parent-only reports; self-report of medications any time during 4-year interval.
LeFever, et al., 1997	17% medication point prevalence among Caucasian boys; 90.3% methylphenidate	1995–1996 survey of grades 2–5 (7–10 years old) in 2 Virginia school districts (n = 27, 810)	Age range and mid-Atlantic region may explain higher prevalence.
Rappley, et al., 1995	2.0% 2-month methylphenidate prevalence	1992 2-month sampling of triplicate prescription database for the state of Michigan among 5- to 14-year-olds	Denominator is the census data for youths in the state.
Sherman & Hertzig, 1991	0.4% annual methylphenidate prevalence	1986 1-year sampling of triplicate prescription database for 1 semi-rural county in New York among 3–17-year-olds	Rate is driven down by the wide age range and probably by the community practices of the geographic area. Also 6 years earlier than the Rappley et al. (1995) study.
Safer, et al., 1996	4.6% methylphenidate point prevalence	1995 Baltimore County school children (5–14 years old)	Counts of school enrollees (numerator) per school census data (denominator).
Wolraich, et al., 1996	2.98% stimulant prevalence of teacher-identified sample of youths	K–5th grade, Tennessee county in 1993–1994	Rate is influenced by narrow age range and probably by the community practices of the area.
Zito, (cited in Safer et al., 1996)	4.7% annual methylphenidate prevalence	1994 Maryland Medicaid youths ages 5–14	Counts of individuals with any administrative claim for methylphenidate during the study year per 100 eligible individuals.
Zito et al., 1998b	1.1% annual methylphenidate prevalence	1991 HMO population from Northwest U.S. region, ages 5–14	Rate may be driven by regional training, practice setting, patient preference, and school policies.

time for ADHD medication treatment was the 3rd grade (Safer and Krager, 1984). In the 1990s, the trend has been to continue stimulant treatment for most positively responding youths, at least into their beginning secondary school years. Thus, instead of 3rd grade being the grade of peak use, the 4th through 6th grades have now become the most prominent period of stimulant use (Zito et al., 1997; Safer and Krager, 1992; Rappley et al., 1995).

Baltimore County students who were receiving stimulant medication in middle school when surveyed were found to have been receiving it for a median of 4–5 years. For high school students receiving methylphenidate for ADHD, the median duration of use was 7 years (Safer and Krager, 1988). From an overall perspective, this is probably skewed, because the average duration following the initiation of stimulant medication for all ADHD youths in treatment studies has been reported to vary from 1 year (Firestone, 1982) to 2 years (Solomons, 1973) to 2.5 years (Charles and Schain, 1981; Lambert et al., 1981; Riddle and Rapoport, 1976) to 3 years (Barkley et al., 1991).

Physician specialties

Most prescriptions for stimulants are written by pediatricians, followed by family practitioners and then by child psychiatrists (Wolraich et al., 1990; Rappley et al., 1995; Gadow, 1983). Moreover, Rappley and colleagues found in their 1992 study (1995) that 5% of pediatricians wrote 50% of the methylphenidate prescriptions written by that specialty. A decade earlier, a similar unevenness in the pattern of prescribing by pediatricians was described (Bennett and Sherman, 1983). Furthermore, prescribing patterns for ADHD differ by medical specialty, with psychiatrists prescribing more nonstimulant psychotropic medications than primary care physicians (Epstein et al., 1991).

Medical settings and payment sources

In the 1991 study of the prevalence of medication treatment for ADHD youths ages 5 through 14, the Northwest Kaiser Permanente HMO rate for methylphenidate treatment was approximately one half that of estimated rates from Baltimore County schools and Maryland Medicaid (Zito et al., 1998b). Although it is unlikely, it is possible that the lower prevalence of methylphenidate prescribing in that HMO is related to a lower prevalence of ADHD youths seen in HMOs, as was suggested by the data from another study (Costello et al., 1988). Somewhat more likely is the possibility that HMO patients are given fewer prescriptions than they receive in non-HMO settings because of the HMO emphasis on primary care (Rabin et al., 1978) and because Medicaid includes more impaired youths. The implications of differences in medication prevalence by medical setting relate to access to care and variations in treatment protocols and treatment outcomes. As the U.S. health care system embraces managed care systems, these questions will need to be addressed by research studies.

Geographic variations

In Michigan in 1992, prescription rates for methylphenidate varied tenfold from county to county (Rappley et al., 1995), and, in the DEA wholesale sales data of 1995, there were differences of up to fivefold in the amount of this drug that was shipped to states within the United States (Hancock, 1996). An eightfold variation across Australia was reported recently (Hazell et al., 1996). Some rural-urban differences have been reported in population-based studies (Zito et al., 1997; Szatmari et al., 1989; Conway, 1976), but from the meager data available, these differences appear to be relatively minor.

Special clinical groups: mentally retarded youths

The use of prescribed stimulants for ADHD in mentally retarded students in public school ranges from 3.4% among the moderately retarded (Gadow, 1985) to nearly 15% among the mildly retarded (Cullinan et al., 1987). Youths who are most severely retarded *seldom* respond favorably to stimulant treatment (Gadow, 1985), whereas mildly retarded youths with ADHD respond near the level of their nonretarded counterparts (Aman et al., 1991). Thus, the prevalence of treatment and the response rates appear to dovetail.

Medication regimen and dosage form

Although most youths receiving stimulant medication for ADHD take it only on school days and only twice daily (Kwasman et al., 1998; Ruel and Hickey, 1992), stimulant use on nonschool days and after school has increased (Stein et al., 1996). These broadened administration patterns increase drug mentions, prescriptions, and bulk sales, although they obviously do not increase the number of individuals taking the medication.

The relative use of sustained-release stimulant tablets and capsules has not been systematically reported in the medical literature, although notations by Baltimore County school nurses in recent surveys indicated that these tablets and capsules use for ADHD had been modest: less than 5% of the total. This is probably because their effects are similar to those of non–sustained-release stimulant tablets (Greenhill, 1995).

Patient adherence and satisfaction with treatment

Research indicates that patients' adherence to prescribed medications is less than complete. Generally, adherence rates for youths receiving methylphenidate range from 61% to 75% (Stine, 1994; Sleator et al., 1982; Johnston and Fine, 1993). Nonadherence increases over time as treatment proceeds (Brown et al., 1987; Firestone, 1982) and becomes most prominent during adolescence (Sleator et al., 1982; Safer and Krager, 1989; Brown et al., 1987; Barkley et al., 1990b). Given that the duration of treatment is being extended, adherence patterns should concern the clinical practitioner. Adherence is improved by regular review of teacher ratings and by monitoring dosing, side effects, and satisfaction with treatment (Weithorn and Ross, 1975). Parent survey data regarding youths medicated with stimulants in New South Wales, Australia, indicated that 31% of the respondents were neutral or dissatisfied with treatment management, and a similar proportion reported a lack of significant improvement. While a large majority of respondents reported considerable improvement, the fact that surveys overrepresent positive responders (responder bias) and that many adolescents are nonadherent suggests an important subgroup in need of close clinical monitoring (Hazell et al., 1996).

OTHER FACTORS THAT INFLUENCE THE PREVALENCE OF TREATMENT FOR ADHD

Pharmaceutical promotion, consumer advocacy groups, and academic thought leaders

The aggressive advertising campaign to market a mixed compound composed of four amphetamine salts (dextroamphetamine sulfate, saccharate, amphetamine sulfate, and aspartate), Adderall, for ADHD has sizably increased that drug's market share, even though no research has yet been done to determine whether this amphetamine combination has any merit over dextroamphetamine alone.

Several advocacy groups for youths and adults with attentional problems have emerged over the past decades. CHADD (Children and Adults with Attention Deficit Disorders) is the largest, with a membership of 38,000 across the United States. It provides useful local services in terms of resources for behavioral management, educational materials, and legal rights. The organization's indirect support of stimulants for the treatment of ADHD may be influencing its membership in this direction. Recently, CHADD has come under fire for accepting financial support from a major pharmaceutical manufacturer of ADHD medications, Ciba-Geigy (now Novartis), the maker of Ritalin (Glusker, 1997).

Academic thought leaders, through lectures and writing, have an effect on prescription practices that is rarely appreciated or noted. For example, publications alerting physicians about the potential lethality of high-dose desipramine treatment for children with ADHD (Riddle et al., 1991) probably reduced sales (Vitiello et al., 1994), although it took a few years to have this impact (Zito, unpublished 1990–1993 MD Medicaid data).

Impact of the media and threatened lawsuits

A campaign against Ritalin treatment for youths in the United States was spearheaded by a wing of the Church of Scientology in the late 1980s. As part of that campaign, media reports critical of Ritalin treatment appeared, and lawsuits were threatened or begun. In cities where lawsuits were begun, the anti-Ritalin media campaign had the effect of substantially reducing the number of youths prescribed stimulant treatment for ADHD. An analysis of wholesale pharmaceutical data on methylphenidate sales revealed that the simple initiation of lawsuits resulted in a far more profound effect on limiting that drug's usage than did media coverage without legal actions (Safer, 1994).

Government regulation

Methylphenidate (Ritalin), dextroamphetamine sulfate (Dextrostat, Dexedrine), and Adderall are Schedule II controlled drugs regulated by the DEA. The DEA sets aggregate production quotas and has made efforts to keep them low, which on one occasion resulted in an unsuccessful legal attempt (in 1986) to restrict production (U.S. Drug Enforcement Administration, 1995). In the mid-1990s, the DEA released an internal memo suggesting that abuse of methylphenidate was widespread and dangerous (U.S. Drug Enforcement Administration, 1995).

Access to medications for appropriate use should be balanced against the control of an abusable substance. Increased methylphenidate treatment of adolescents would be likely to increase the opportunity for abuse, as suggested by the anecdotes reported in the popular press (Stepp, 1996; Ruley, 1996). Nevertheless, school surveys of youths reporting on abusable substances show only a slight increase in the use of medically obtained stimulant drugs for the purpose of abuse among 8th and 10th graders (Johnston et al., 1995).

Legislation and judicial decisions

ADHD was not a bonafide handicapping condition under the Education for All Handicapped Children Act of 1975, and a later attempt by the U.S. Congress to include ADHD within the Individual Disability Education Act of 1990 failed. However, after a review by the U.S. Department of Education in 1991, an administrative decision was made to allow ADHD within the "other health impaired" category of the act (Swanson et al., 1995b; Davilla et al., 1991). The resulting qualification for special education services by youths with ADHD increased the recorded prevalence of the disorder within schools and is believed to be related to increased stimulant medication treatment (Swanson, 1997).

In 1990, two legal decisions in the United States increased the eligibility of youths with ADHD for Supplemental Security Income (SSI) from Social Security. One was the Zebly v. Sullivan decision by the U.S. Supreme Court, which loosened the criteria for children with disabilities to obtain SSI. The other was the amended Social Security Administration guidelines, which, for the first time included ADHD as a childhood mental health impairment (Hannsgen and Sandell, 1996). These moves, like those in special education (Davilla et al., 1991), increased the formal identification of ADHD and presumably influenced the rate of stimulant medication treatment. At a minimum, these events would account for an enhanced role for the educational system in gaining access to health care for those with attentional disorders.

ESTIMATING THE U.S. POPULATION OF YOUTHS WITH DRUG THERAPY FOR ADHD

Estimates of the total number of youths in the United States treated with stimulant medication for ADHD have increased over the years from 300,000 in 1974, 410,000 in 1981, 515,000 in 1979, 700,000 in 1976, and 750,000 in 1989 to 1.5 million in 1995 (Safer et al., 1996; Safer and Krager, 1984).

INTERNATIONAL PERSPECTIVES ON ADHD AND STIMULANT TREATMENT

The prevalence of the teacher-rated features of ADHD is generally similar in at least seven countries of the world (Taylor, 1987; Szatmari et al., 1989; Luk and Leung, 1989; Glow, 1980). However, the prescribed use of stimulant treatment is profoundly *lower* in countries other than the United States and Canada (Swanson, 1997). Also in the 1990s, while the rate of stimulant treatment for ADHD sizably increased in the United States, Canada, and Australia (Hazell et al., 1996; Swanson, 1997; Hollander et al., 1996), the rate has not increased to any substantial degree elsewhere (Swanson, 1997).

A factor that partially accounts for this trend is the reliance in the United States on the *DSM* classification. Several other countries use the ICD-10 classification, which compared to the *DSM* nomenclature uses a far more restrictive category: hyperkinetic disorder (Swanson et al., 1998). In evaluations of the same patients using the 314 DSM/ICD diagnostic code, prevalence rates using the *DSM-III*, *-IIIR*, or *-IV* have been consistently and substantially higher than those using the ICD 9 and 10 (Taylor et al., 1991; Prendergast et al., 1988).

Another reason for the low rate of stimulant treatment in most countries is tight legal restrictions (Simeon et al., 1995; Safer and Krager, 1984). But perhaps a more fundamental factor relates to cultural differences. Phytopharmaceuticals and homeopathic medicine in many countries present an alternative to stimulant use that is not as well accepted in the United States (Elliger et al., 1990). Unfortunately, there are little data to support the efficacy or safety of such alternative medicines, and signs of their popularity in the United States include the development of standards by the United States Pharmacopeia (USP) and a research office at the National Institutes of Health. The myth that natural products are not harmful should be dispelled when patients are counseled about these products.

FUTURE RESEARCH DIRECTIONS—BEYOND PREVALENCE

The next step in population-based information on drug use patterns is to develop effectiveness studies by measuring outcomes of treatment in the usual practice setting (Jensen et al., 1996; Greenhill et al., 1996; Jensen et al., 1994; Vitiello and Jensen, 1995). Models defining the scope of outcomes for child and adolescent emotional and behavioral health are being developed (Burns, 1996). High rates of premature termination of treatment, in the range of 30% to 50%, pose questions about the quality of services delivered, the success of integrative treatment plans (multimodal interventions), and the effectiveness and side effect profile of long-term drug treatment. Outcomes for female inattentive patients are particularly important because the clinical trial data supporting stimulant efficacy involved pre-1990 samples that consisted almost entirely of male hyperactive youths (Spencer et al., 1996). Another step involves regular monitoring of the use of drugs for unlabeled indications. For example, the controversy over the safety of high-dose desipramine for attentional disorders could have been resolved if there had been a case registry for psychiatric drug use in children. Finally, N-of-1 methods (Guyatt et al., 1986) can be applied to the nonresponder so that the increasingly complex therapies that are being recommended can be evaluated in a scientific manner.

SUMMARY AND CONCLUSIONS

There is no doubt that methylphenidate treatment of ADHD in the United States has risen dramatically in the last three decades and that it has been influenced by numerous factors. The major ones accounting for this trend have been increases in the duration of treatment; increases in the diagnostic pool, particularly the inclusion of more youths with predominantly inattentive ADHD; the greater number of girls receiving medication; and the greater public acceptance of psychopharmacologic treatment of youths.

Media reports of the increases in methylphenidate treatment for ADHD have frequently raised the question whether much of this is caused by the application of a "quick fix." Linked to this is an assumption that teacher referrals and physicians' diagnoses are occasionally hasty and careless and that the full spectrum of therapies is not being utilized. These issues merit study, and pharmacoepidemiologic approaches certainly can help, largely because the answers lie in outcomes research at the community level.

REFERENCES

AACAP Work Group on Quality Issues (1997), Practice parameters for the assessment and treatment of attention-deficit hyperactivity disorder. *J. Am. Acad. Child Adolesc. Psychiatry*, 36:10(Suppl.), 855–1215.

ADHD Task Force (1991), Final report of the Virginia Departments of Education, Health Professions, Mental Health, Mental Retardation and Substance Abuse Services on the effects of the use of methylphenidate to the Governor and the General Assembly of Virginia. House Document No. 28.

Aman, M.G., Marks, R.E., Turbott, S.H., Wilsher, C.P. & Merry, S.N. (1991), Clinical effects of methylphenidate and thioridazine in intellectually subaverage children. *J. Am. Acad. Child Adolesc. Psychiatry*, 30:246–256.

American Psychiatric Association (1968), *Diagnostic and Statistical Manual of Mental Disorders, 2nd ed.* Washington, DC: American Psychiatric Association.

American Psychiatric Association (1980), *Diagnostic and Statistical Manual of Mental Disorders, 3rd ed.* Washington, DC: American Psychiatric Association.

American Psychiatric Association (1987), *Diagnostic and Statistical Manual of Mental Disorders, 3rd revised ed.* Washington, DC: American Psychiatric Association.

American Psychiatric Association (1994), *Diagnostic and Statistical Manual of Mental Disorders, 4th ed.* Washington, DC: American Psychiatric Association.

Anderson, J.C., Williams, S., McGee, R. & Silva, P.A. (1987), *DSM-III* disorders in preadolescent children: Prevalence in a large sample from the general population. *Arch. Gen. Psychiatry*, 44:69–76.

Angold, A. & Costello, E.J. (1997), Stimulant medication: A general population perspective [abstr.]. *NCDEU Abstracts of the 37th Annual Meeting, May 27–30.*

Anonymous (1971), Report of the conference on the use of stimulant drugs in the treatment of behaviorally disturbed young school children. *Psychopharmacol. Bull.*, 7:23–29.

August, G.J., Realmuto, G.M., MacDonald, A.W., III, Nugent, S.M. & Crosby, R. (1996), Prevalence of ADHD and comorbid disorders among elementary school children screened for disruptive behavior. *J. Abnormal Child Psychol.,* 24:571–595.

Barkley, R.A. (1996), Research developments and their implications for clinical care of the ADHD child. *Psychiatric Times*, 38–41.

Barkley, R.A., Anastopoulos, A.D., Guevremont, D.C. & Fletcher, K.E. (1991), Adolescents with ADHD: Patterns of behavioral adjustment, academic functioning, and treatment utilization. *J. Am. Acad. Child Adolesc. Psychiatry*, 30:752–761.

Barkley, R.A., DuPaul, G.J. & McMurray, M.B. (1990a), Comprehensive evaluation of attention deficit disorder with and without hyperactivity as defined by research criteria. *J. Consult. Clin. Psychol.* 58:775–789.

Barkley, R.A., Fischer, M., Edelbrock, C.S. & Smallish, L. (1990b), The adolescent outcome of hyperactive children diagnosed by research criteria: I. An 8-year prospective follow-up study. *J. Am. Acad. Child Adolesc. Psychiatry*, 29:546–557.

Batoosingh, K.A. (1995), Ritalin prescriptions triple over last 4 years [abstr.]. *Clin. Psychiatry News*, 23:1–2.

Baumgaertel, A., Wolraich, M.L. & Dietrich, M. (1995), Comparison of diagnostic criteria for attention deficit disorders in a German elementary school sample. *J. Am. Acad. Child Adolesc. Psychiatry*, 34:629–638.

Bennett, F.C. & Sherman, R. (1983), Management of childhood "hyperactivity" by primary care physicians. *J. Dev. Behav. Pediatr.,* 4:88–93.

Bosco, J.J. & Robin, S.S. (1980), Hyperkinesis: Prevalence and treatment. In: *Hyperactive Children: The Social Ecology of Identification and Treatment*, eds. C.K. Whalen & B. Henker. New York: Academy Press, pp. 173–187.

Brown, R.T., Borden, K.A., Wynne, M.E., Spunt, A.L. & Clingerman, M.S. (1987), Compliance with pharmacological and cognitive treatments for attention deficit disorder. *J. Am. Acad. Child Adolesc. Psychiatry*, 26:521–526.

Burns, B.J. (1996), What drives outcomes for emotional and behavioral disorders in children and adolescents? In: *Using Client Outcomes Information to Improve Mental Health and Substance Abuse Treatment*, Nr. 71 Fall 1996 Ed., eds. D.M. Steinwachs, L.M. Flynn, G.S. Norquist & E.A. Skinner. San Francisco: Jossey-Bass, pp. 89–102.

Bussing, R., Perwien, B.A., & Belin, T. (1996), Predicting unmet service needs among children in special education: Who is at risk? [abstr.] *American Psychiatry Association Meeting*.

Charles, L. & Schain, R. (1981), A four-year follow-up study of the effects of methylphenidate on the behavior and academic achievement of hyperactive children. *J. Abnormal Child Psychol.,* 9:495–505.

Committee on Children with Disabilities (1996), Medication for children with attentional disorders. *Pediatrics*, 98:301–304.

Conway, A. (1976), An evaluation of drugs in the elementary schools: Some geographic considerations. *Psychol. Schools*, 13:442–444.

Copeland, L., Wolraich, M., Lindgren, S., Milich, R. & Woolson, R. (1987), Pediatricians' reported practices in the assessment and treatment of attention deficit disorders. *J. Dev. Behav. Pediatr.,* 8:191–197.

Costello, E.J., Costello, A.J., Edelbrock, C., Burns, B.J., Dulcan, M.K., Brent, D. & Janiszewski, S. (1988), Psychiatric disorders in pediatric primary care: Prevalence and risk factors. *Arch. Gen. Psychiatry*, 45:1107–1116.

Cullinan, D., Gadow, K.D. & Epstein, M.H. (1987), Psychotropic drug treatment among learning-disabled, educable mentally retarded, and seriously emotionally disturbed students. *J. Abnormal Child Psychol.*, 15:469–477.

Davilla, R.R., Williams, M.L. & MacDonald, J.T. (1991), Clarification of policy to address the needs of children with attention deficit hyperactivity disorders within general and/or special education. Memorandum from the U.S. Dept. of Education.

Elliger, T.J., Trott, G.E. & Nissen, G. (1990), Prevalence of psychotropic medication in childhood and adolescence in the Federal Republic of Germany. *Pharmacopsychiatry*, 23:38–44.

Epstein, M.A., Shaywitz, S.E., Shaywitz, B.A. & Woolston, J.L. (1991), The boundaries of attention deficit disorder. *J. Learn. Disabil.*, 24:78–86.

Firestone, P. (1982), Factors associated with children's adherence to stimulant medication. *Am. J. Orthopsychiatry*, 52:447–457.

Gadow, K.D. (1981), Prevalence of drug treatment for hyperactivity and other childhood behavior disorders. In: *Psychosocial Aspects of Drug Treatment for Hyperactivity*, eds. K.D. Gadow & J. Loney. Boulder, CO: Westview Press, pp. 13–76.

Gadow, K.D. (1983), Pharmacotherapy for behavior disorders. *Clin. Pediatr.*, 22:48–53.

Gadow, K.D. (1985), Prevalence and efficacy of stimulant drug use with mentally retarded children and youth. *Psychopharmacol. Bull.*, 21:291–303.

Gaub, M. & Carlson, C.L. (1997), Behavioral characteristics of *DSM-IV* ADHD subtypes in a school-based population. *J. Abnormal Child Psychol.*, 25:103–111.

Glow, R.A. (1980), A validation of Conners TQ and a cross-cultural comparison of prevalence of hyperactivity in children. In: *Advances in Human Psychopharmacology*, eds. G.D. Burrows & J.S. Werry. Greenwich, CT: JAI Press, pp. 302–320.

Glusker, A. (1997), Deficit selling. *Washington Post Magazine*, 13–27.

Goldman, L.S., Genel, M., Bezman, R.J. & Slanetz, P.J. (1998), Diagnosis and treatment of attention-deficit/hyperactivity disorder in children and adolescents (Report of AMA Council on Scientific Affairs). *JAMA*, 279:1100–1107.

Goldstein, E. (1991), Methylphenidate use in Michigan [letter]. *Am. J. Hosp. Pharm.* 48:2129.

Greenhill, L.L. (1995), Attention-deficit hyperactivity disorder. *Child Adolesc. Psychiatr. Clin. North Am.* 4:123–168.

Greenhill, L.L., Abikoff, H., Arnold, E., Cantwell, D.P., Conners, C.K., Elliott, G., Hechtman, L., Hinshaw, S.P., Hoza, B., Jensen, P.S., March, J.S., Newcorn, J., Pelham, W.E., Severe, J.B., Swanson, J.M., Vitiello, B. & Wells, K. (1996), Medication treatment strategies in the MTA study: Relevance to clinicians and researchers. *J. Am. Acad. Child Adolesc. Psychiatry,* 34:1304–1313.

Guyatt, G., Sackett, D., Taylor, D.W., Chong, J., Roberts, R. & Pugsley, S. (1986), Determining optimal therapy—randomized trials in individual patients. *N. Engl. J. Med.*, 314:889–892.

Hancock, L. (March 18, 1996), Mother's little helper. *Newsweek*, 127:51–56.

Hannsgen, G.P. & Sandell, S.H. (1996), Deeming rules and the increase in the number of children with disabilities receiving SSI. *Soc. Security Bull.*, 59:43–49.

Hansen, P. & Keogh, B.K. (1971), Medical characteristics of children with educational handicaps: Implications for the pediatrician. *Clin. Pediatr.*, 10:726–730.

Hazell, P.L., McDowell, M.J. & Walton, J.M. (1996), Management of children prescribed psychostimulant medication for attention deficit hyperactivity disorder in the Hunter region of NSW. *Med. J. Aust.*, 165:477–480.

Hollander, E., Quinn, D., Hunt, R.D. & Perry, P.J. (1996), The ADHD debate: Stimulants or alternative agents. *Primary Psychiatry*, 3:52–55.

Holmes, V.F. (1995), Medical uses of psychostimulants. *Int. J. Psychiatry Med.*, 25:1–19.

House Bill (1997), Task force to study the uses of methylphenidate and other drugs on school children. House Bill 971: Section 18–313.

Jensen, P.S., Hoagwood, K. & Petti, T. (1996), Outcomes of mental health care for children and adolescents: II. Literature review and application of a comprehensive model. *J. Am. Acad. Child Adolesc. Psychiatry*, 35:1064–1077.

Jensen, P.S., Vitiello, B., Leonard, H. & Laughren, T.P. (1994), Child and adolescent psychopharmacology: Expanding the research base. *Psychopharmacol. Bull.*, 30:3–8.

Jerome, L., Gordon, M. & Hustler, P. (1994), A comparison of American and Canadian teachers' knowledge and attitudes towards attention deficit hyperactivity disorder (ADHD). *Can. J. Psychiatry.*, 39:563–567.

Johnston, C. & Fine, S. (1993), Methods of evaluating methylphenidate in children with attention deficit hyperactivity disorder: Acceptability, satisfaction and compliance. *J. Pediatr. Psychol.*, 18:717–730.

Johnston, L.D., O'Malley, P.M. & Bachman, J.G. (1995), National survey results on drug use from the Monitoring the Future Study, 1975–1994. NIDA No. 95–4026.

Krager, J.M. & Safer, D.J. (1974), Type and prevalence of medication used in the treatment of hyperactive children. *N. Engl. J. Med.*, 291:1118–1120.

Kwasman, A., Tinsley, B.J. & Lepper, H.S. (1998), Pediatricians' knowledge and attitudes concerning diagnosis and treatment of attention deficit and hyperactivity disorders. *Arch. Pediatr. Adolesc. Med.*, 149:1211–1216.

Lahey, B.B. & Carlson, C.L. (1991), Validity of the diagnostic category of attention deficit disorder without hyperactivity: A review of the literature. *J. Learn. Disabil.*, 24:110–120.

Lambert, N.M., Sandoval, J. & Sassone, D.M. (1981), Prevalence of hyperactivity and related treatments among elementary school children. In: *Psychosocial Aspects of Drug Treatment for Hyperactivity*, eds. K.D. Gadow & J. Loney. Boulder, CO: Westview Press, pp. 446–463.

LeFever, G.B., Hannon, P.H., Dawson, K.V., Morrow, R.C. & Morrow, A.L. (1997), Prevalence of medication use for attention deficit hyperactivity disorder (ADHD): A population-based study of Virginia school children. *Pediatr. Res.*, 41:14 (Abstract).

Lehman, A.F. (1996), Evaluating outcomes of treatments for persons with psychotic disorders. *J. Clin. Psychiatry*, 57:Suppl 11:61–67.

Leung, P.W., Luk, S.L., Ho, T.P., Taylor, E., Mak, F.L. & Bacon-Shone, J. (1996), The diagnosis and prevalence of hyperactivity in Chinese schoolboys. *Br. J. Psychiatry*, 168:486–496.

Luk, S.L. & Leung, P.W. (1989), Conners' Teacher's Rating Scale—a validity study in Hong Kong. *J. Child Psychol. Psychiatry Allied Disciplines*, 30:785–793.

Maynard, R. (1970), Omaha pupils given "behavior" drugs. *Washington Post*, June 29, 1970.

McGee, R., Feehan, M., Williams, S., Partridge, F., Silva, P.A. & Kelly, J. (1990), *DSM-III* disorders in a large sample of adolescents. *J. Am. Acad. Child Adolesc. Psychiatry*, 29:611–619.

McGee, R., Williams, S. & Silva, P.A. (1987), A comparison of girls and boys with teacher-identified problems of attention. *J. Am. Acad. Child Adolesc. Psychiatry*, 26:711–717.

Morrow, D.J. (1997), Attention disorder is found in growing number of adults. *New York Times*, September 2, 1997, pp. A1–D4.

Pizzuti, D. (1996), Abbott Laboratories physicians warning letter: Important drug warning. Ref. 03-4735-R18.

Prendergast, M., Taylor, E., Rapoport, J.L., Bartko, J., Donnelly, M., Zametkin, A., Ahearn, M.B., Dunn, G. & Wieselberg, H.M. (1988), The diagnosis of childhood hyperactivity: A U.S.–U.K. cross-national study of *DSM-III* and ICD-9. *J. Child Psychol. Psychiatry Allied Disciplines*, 29:289–300.

Rabin, D.L., Bush, P.J. & Fuller, N.A. (1978), Drug prescription rates before and after enrollment of a Medicaid population in an HMO. *Public Health Rep.*, 93:16–23.

Rappley, M.D., Gardiner, J.R. & Jetton, R.C.H. (1995), The use of methylphenidate in Michigan. *Arch. Pediatr. Adolesc. Med.*, 149:675–679.

Riddle, K.D. & Rapoport, J.L. (1976), A 2-year follow-up of 72 hyperactive boys: Classroom behavior and peer acceptance. *J. Nerv. Ment. Dis.*, 162:126–134.

Riddle, M.A., Nelson, J.C., Kleinman, C.S., Rasmusson, A., Leckman, J.F., King, R.A. & Cohen, D.J. (1991), Sudden death in children receiving Norpramin: A review of three reported cases and commentary. *J. Am. Acad. Child Adolesc. Psychiatry*, 30:104–108.

Ross, R.P. (1979), Drug therapy for hyperactivity. In: *Drugs and the Special Child*, ed. M.J. Cohen. New York: Gardner Press, pp. 99–109.

Ruel, J.M. & Hickey, C.P. (1992), Are too many children being treated with methylphenidate? *Can. J. Psychiatry*, 37:570–572.

Ruley, M. (1996), Totally dope: High school students on the Ritalin buzz. *The Independent Weekly*, April 2, 1996, 8–10.

Safer, D.J. (1994), The impact of recent lawsuits on methylphenidate sales. *Clin. Pediatr.*, 33:166–168.

Safer, D.J. & Krager, J.M. (1984), Trends in medication therapy for hyperactivity: National and international perspectives. In: *Advances in Learning and Behavioral Disabilities*, ed. K.D. Gadow. Greenwich, CT: JAI Press, pp. 125–149.

Safer, D.J. & Krager, J.M. (1988), A survey of medication treatment for hyperactive/inattentive students. *JAMA*, 260:2256–2258.

Safer, D.J. & Krager, J.M. (1989), Hyperactivity and inattentiveness: School assessment of stimulant treatment. *Clin. Pediatr.*, 28:216–221.

Safer, D.J. & Krager, J.M. (1992), Effect of a media blitz and a threatened lawsuit on stimulant treatment. *JAMA*, 268:1004–1007.

Safer, D.J. & Krager, J.M. (1994), The increased rate of stimulant treatment for hyperactive/inattentive students in secondary schools. *Pediatrics*, 94:462–464.

Safer, D.J., Zito, J.M. & Fine, E.M. (1996), Increased methylphenidate usage for attention deficit disorder in the 1990s. *Pediatrics*, 98:1084–1088.

Schrag, P. & Divoky, D. (1975), *The Myth of the Hyperactive Child.* New York, NY: Pantheon.

Sherman, M. & Hertzig, M.E. (1991), Prescribing practices of Ritalin: The Suffolk County, New York study. In: *Ritalin Theory and Patient Management*, eds. L.L. Greenhill & B.B. Osman. Larchmont, NY: M.A. Liebert, Inc., pp. 187–194.

Simeon, J.G., Wiggins, D.M. & Williams, E. (1995), Worldwide use of psychotropic drugs in child and adolescent psychiatric disorders. *Prog. Neuropsychopharmacol. Biol. Psychiatry*, 19:455–465.

Sleator, E.K., Ullmann, R.K. & Von Neumann, A. (1982), How do hyperactive children feel about taking stimulants and will they tell the doctor? *Clin. Pediatr.*, 21:474–479.

Solomons, G. (1973), Drug therapy: Initiation and follow-up. *Ann. N.Y. Acad. Sci.*, 205:335–344.

Spencer, T., Biederman, J., Wilens, T., Harding, M., O'Donnell, D. & Griffin, S. (1996), Pharmacotherapy of attention-deficit hyperactivity disorder across the life cycle. *J. Am. Acad. Child Adolesc. Psychiatry*, 35:409–432.

Stein, M.A., Blondis, T.A., Schnitzler, E.R., O'Brien, T., Fishkin, J., Blackwell, B., Szumowski, E. & Roizen, N.J. (1996), Methylphenidate dosing: Twice daily versus three times daily. *Pediatrics*, 98:Pt 1:748–756.

Stephen, K., Sprague, R.L. & Werry, J. (1973), Drug treatment of hyperactive children in Chicago. NIMH Grant MH 18909.

Stepp, L.S. (1996), Ritalin, the newest available cheap high. *The Washington Post*, February 5, 1996, pp. A1–A6.

Stine, J.J. (1994), Psychosocial and psychodynamic issues affecting noncompliance with psychostimulant treatment. *J. Child Adolesc. Psychopharmacol.*, 4:75–86.

Strom, B.L. (1994), *Pharmacoepidemiology, 2nd ed.* New York: John Wiley and Sons, Inc., pp. 3–741.

Swanson, J.M. (1997), Hyperkinetic disorders and attention deficit hyperactivity disorders. *Curr. Opin. Psychiatry*, 10:300–305.

Swanson, J.M., Lerner, M. & Williams, L. (1995a), More frequent diagnosis of attention deficit-hyperactivity disorder [letter]. *N. Engl. J. Med.*, 333:944.

Swanson, J.M., McBurnett, K., Christian, D.L. & Wigal, T. (1995b), Stimulant medications and the treatment of children with ADHD. *Adv. Clin. Child Psychol.*, 17:265–322.

Swanson, J.M., Sergeant, J.A., Taylor, E.J., Sonuga-Barke, S., Jensen, P.S. & Cantwell, D.P. (1998), Attention-deficit hyperactivity disorder and hyperactive disorder. *Lancet*, 351:429–433.

Szatmari, P., Offord, D.R. & Boyle, M.H. (1989), Ontario Child Health Study: Prevalence of attention deficit disorder with hyperactivity. *J. Child Psychol. Psychiatry Allied Disciplines*, 30:219–230.

Taylor, E. (1987), Cultural differences in hyperactivity. *Adv. Dev. Behav. Pediatr.*, 8:125–150.

Taylor, E., Sandberg, S., Thorley, G. & Giles, S. (1991), *The Epidemiology of Childhood Hyperactivity.* Oxford: Oxford University Press.

U.S. Drug Enforcement Administration (1995), *Methylphenidate Review Document.* Washington, DC: U.S. Department of Justice.

U.S. Drug Enforcement Administration (1996), *Stimulant Use in the Treatment of ADHD.* Washington, DC: U.S. Department of Justice, pp 1–45.

Ullmann, R.K., Sleator, E.K. & Sprague, R.L. (1984), ADD children: Who is referred from the schools? *Psychopharmacol. Bull.*, 20:308–312.

Vitiello, B., Conrad, T., Burkhart, G. & Jensen, P.S. (1994), Survey of the use of psychotropic medication in children and adolescents [abstr.]. Presented at 19th CINP Congress, June 27–July 1, 1994, Washington, D.C.

Vitiello, B., & Jensen, P.S. (1995), Psychopharmacology in children and adolescents: Current problems, future prospects. Summary notes on the 1995 NIMH-FDA Conference. *J. Child Adolesc. Psychopharmacol.,* 5:5–7.

Weithorn, C.J. & Ross, R. (1975), Who monitors medication? *J. Learn. Disabil.,* 8:458–461.

Wilens, T.E., Spencer, T., Biederman, J., Wozniak, J. & Connor, D. (1995), Combined pharmacotherapy: An emerging trend in pediatric psychopharmacology. *J. Am. Acad. Child Adolesc. Psychiatry*, 34:110–112.

Wolraich, M.L., Hannah, J.N., Pinnock, T.Y., Baumgaertel, A. & Brown, J. (1996), Comparison of diagnostic criteria for attention-deficit hyperactivity disorder in a county-wide sample. *J. Am. Acad. Child Adolesc. Psychiatry*, 35:319–324.

Wolraich, M.L., Lindgren, S., Stromquist, A., Milich, R., Davis, C. & Watson, D. (1990), Stimulant medication use by primary care physicians in the treatment of attention deficit hyperactivity disorder. *Pediatrics,* 86:95–101.

World Health Organization (1994). *Pocket Guide to the ICD-10 Classification of Mental and Behavorial Disorders.* Washington, D.C.: Churchill Livingstone.

Zito, J.M. & Craig, T.J. (1991), Pharmacoepidemiology of psychiatric disorders. In: *Pharmacoepidemiology: An Introduction, 2nd ed.*, eds., A.G. Hartzema, M.S. Porta & H.H. Tilson. Cincinnati, OH: Harvey Whitney Books, pp. 270–288.

Zito, J.M., dosReis, S., Safer, D.J. & Riddle, M.A. (1998a), Racial disparity in psychotropic medications prescribed for youths with Medicaid insurance in Maryland. *J. Am. Acad. Child Adolesc. Psychiatry*, 37:179–184.

Zito, J.M. & Riddle, M.A. (1995), Psychiatric pharmacoepidemiology for children. *Child Adolesc. Psychiatry Clin. North Am.*, 4:77–95.

Zito, J.M., Riddle, M.A., Safer, D.J., Johnson, R., Fox, M., Speedie, S. & Scerbo, M. (1995), Pharmacoepidemiology of youth with treatments for mental disorders. *Psychopharmacol. Bull.*, 31:540 (Abstract).

Zito, J.M. and Safer, D.J. (1997), Sources of data for pharmacoepidemiology studies of child and adolescent psychiatric disorders. *J. Child Adolesc. Psychopharmacol.,* 7:237–253.

Zito, J.M., Safer, D.J., dosReis, S., Magder, L.S. & Riddle, M.A. (1997), Methylphenidate patterns among Medicaid youths. *Psychopharmacol. Bull.*, 33:143–147.

Zito, J.M., Safer, D.J., Riddle, M.A. Johnson, R.E. Speedie, S.M. & Fox, M. (1998b), Prevalence variations in psychotropic treatment of children. *J. Child Adolesc. Psychpharmacol.,* 8:99–105.

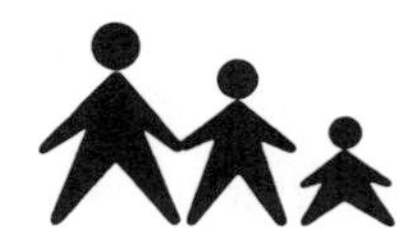

Is Ritalin an Abused Drug? Does It Meet the Criteria of a Schedule II Substance?

CHRISTINE SANNERUD and GRETCHEN FEUSSNER

Methylphenidate (MPH, Ritalin) is classified as a Schedule II stimulant under the Federal Controlled Substances Act (CSA). In order for any substance to be placed under control by the CSA, the law requires very specific findings. For a Schedule II classification, the drug or other substance must (1) have a high potential for abuse, (2) have a currently accepted medical use in treatment in the United States, and (3) show that abuse may lead to severe psychologic or physical dependence. Studies that address the abuse liability of a drug and data relating to the diversion of a drug from legitimate handlers, combined with clinical experience of actual abuse, provide critical information about the abuse potential and dependence profile for a drug. This chapter explores the scientific, medical, and law enforcement data that explain why MPH has been placed in the same classification as other highly abusable substances such as amphetamine, methamphetamine, and cocaine.

ABUSE LIABILITY

A good correlation exists between drugs that are abused by humans and those that maintain self-injection in laboratory animals (Schuster and Thompson, 1969; Griffiths et al., 1980). Several behavioral paradigms used in animals are sensitive models of human subjective and reinforcing effects. Specifically, preclinical evaluations of psychomotor stimulants in laboratory animals using drug discrimination and intravenous self-injection paradigms are considered useful for the prediction of human abuse liability of these compounds (Johanson and Balster, 1978; Preston et al., 1997).

Drug discrimination

Drug discrimination procedures provide an indirect measure of a drug's reinforcing effects and its abuse potential (Preston et al., 1997). The drug discrimination paradigm is based on the ability of psychoactive drugs to produce interoceptive stimuli and the ability of nonhuman and human subjects to identify the presence of these stimuli and to differentiate among the constellations of stimuli produced by different drug classes. In drug discrimination studies, the drug stimuli function as a cue to the subject to make an operant response in order to receive a reinforcer. Repeated pairings of a reinforcer with only the drug-ap-

Drug and Chemical Evaluation Section, Office of Diversion Control, Drug Enforcement Administration, Washington, D.C.

propriate response can produce reliable discrimination between drug and no-drug. This paradigm has been used extensively to characterize the behavioral profile of MPH.

Preclinical drug discrimination

Years of preclinical drug discrimination research show that MPH is (1) discriminable, (2) can be trained as a discriminative stimulus, and (3) generalizes to several psychomotor stimulants, including cocaine and d-amphetamine. Preclinical studies demonstrated that animals trained to discriminate d-amphetamine from saline showed generalization to MPH (Huang and Ho, 1974; Harris and Balster, 1971; Porsolt et al., 1982; Evans and Johanson, 1987; De la Garza and Johanson, 1987), animals trained to discriminate cocaine from saline showed generalization to amphetamine and MPH (McKenna and Ho, 1980; Silverman and Schultz, 1989), and animals trained to discriminate MPH from saline showed generalization to amphetamine and cocaine (Perkins et al., 1991; Silverman and Ho, 1980) (Table 1).

In rats, monkeys, and pigeons trained to discriminate d-amphetamine from saline, MPH produced d-amphetamine–like effects (Huang and Ho, 1974; Harris and Balster, 1971; Porsolt et al., 1982; Evans and Johanson, 1987; De la Garza and Johanson, 1987) (see Table 1). MPH and other psychomotor stimulants, including l-amphetamine, methamphetamine, cocaine, and ephedrine, all produced discriminative stimulus effects similar to those of d-amphetamine (Huang and Ho, 1974; Silverman and Ho, 1980; Porsolt et al., 1982; Rosen et al., 1986). However, MPH produced partial generalization to 2,5-dimethoxy-4-methylamphetamine (DOM) stimulus (Silverman and Ho, 1980). These data suggest that MPH produces amphetamine-like effects but not DOM-like hallucinogenic effects.

MPH also produced amphetamine-like effects in nonhuman primates and pigeons trained to discriminate d-amphetamine from saline (De la Garza and Johanson, 1987; Evans and Johanson, 1987). In these studies, MPH produced amphetamine-like discriminative stimulus effects without producing changes in general activity. Similarly, in animals trained to discriminate cocaine from saline under a variety of operant schedules of reinforcement, MPH shared discriminative stimulus effects with cocaine when tested for generalization. In rats, MPH, d-amphetamine, l-amphetamine, and methamphetamine all substituted for cocaine, suggesting that these drugs produce effects similar to those of cocaine (Colpaert et al., 1979; McKenna and Ho, 1980; Silverman and Schultz, 1989).

The discriminative stimulus effects of MPH appear to be robust; MPH generalizes to cocaine and d-amphetamine across several training dose conditions. Specifically, MPH generalized to cocaine when the training dose of d-amphetamine or cocaine was high or low (Wood and Emmett-Oglesby, 1988; Emmett-Oblesby et al., 1983; Rosen et al., 1986). Thus, regardless of training condition, MPH substituted for the cocaine discriminative stimulus.

In other studies, MPH produced stimulus effects similar to those of dl-cathinone (Goudie et al., 1986) in rats and of the selective dopamine uptake inhibitor (1-{2-[bis(4-fluorophenyl)-methoxyethyl}-4-(3-phenylpropyl)piperazine (GBR 12909) in monkeys (Melia and Spealman, 1991). MPH completely substituted for the GBR 12909 stimulus, as did high doses of cocaine, the cocaine analog (2β-carbomethoxy-3β-(4-fluorophenyl)tropane), and d-amphetamine. In addition to producing effects similar to those of cathinone, d-amphetamine, and cocaine in generalization tests, MPH will serve as a training stimulus in drug discrimination studies, demonstrating its ability to produce and maintain discriminable stimulant-like effects that can be used to guide behavioral choice under different operant schedules of reinforcement (Perkins et al., 1991; Overton 1982).

In summary, MPH produces discriminative stimulus effects similar to those of d-amphetamine, cocaine, and cathinone in laboratory animals (Table 1). Under cocaine and d-amphetamine training conditions, the stimulus effects produced by MPH completely sub-

Table 1. Discriminative Stimulus Effects of Methylphenidate (MPH) in Animals

Training/Species	*MPH Doses Tested (mg/kg/inj)*	*Like Training Drug?*	*Other Effects*	*Reference*
Amphetamine-Trained				
Rats	2.5 (ip)	Yes	MPH = methamphetamine = cocaine = ephedrine	Huang & Ho, 1974
Rats	0.5–2.0 (ip)	Yes	MPH = cocaine	Porsolt et al., 1982
Rats	0.1–10 (ip)	Yes		Rosen et al., 1986
Rhesus monkeys	1.0–30.0 (ig)	Yes	No changes in activity	De la Garza & Johanson, 1987
Pigeons	0.1–3.0 (im)	Yes		Evans & Johanson, 1987
Cocaine-Trained				
Rats	2.5 (ip)	Partial		McKenna & Ho, 1980
Rats	4.5 and 6.0 (ip)	Yes	MPH = amphetamine	Silverman & Schultz, 1989
Rats	0.31–1.25 (ip)	Yes	MPH = methamphetamine = cocaine	Colpaert et al., 1979
Rats	10 (ip)	Yes	MPH = d-amphetamine = cocaine	Emmett-Oglesby et al., 1983; Wood & Emmett-Oglesby, 1988
Cathinone-trained rats	0.5–4.0 (ip)	Yes	MPH = cathinone = cocaine = amphetamine	Goudie et al., 1986
GBR12909-trained rats	0.1–0.3 (ip)	Yes	MPH = GBR = cocaine = cocaine analogs = amphetamine	Melia & Spealman, 1991
DOM-trained rats	2.5 and 5.0 (ip)	Partial	MPH = amphetamine	Silverman & Ho, 1980
MPH-trained				
Rats	0.5–8.0 (ip)	Yes	Dose-related increases	Perkins et al., 1991
Rats	15 and 40 (ip)	Yes	Trained within 7–14 days	Overton, 1982

DOM = 2,5-dimethoxy-4-methylamphetamine.
inj = injection.
ip = intraperitoneal.
ig = intragastric.
im = intramuscular.

stituted for the cocaine or d-amphetamine training stimulus. The psychomotor stimulant effects of MPH are robust and can be demonstrated under many different training conditions, and when several different species of nonhuman animals are used.

Clinical drug discrimination studies

MPH produces stimulant-like discriminative stimulus effects in humans (Heischman and Henningfield, 1991) (Table 2). Male subjects who reported current stimulant abuse, were trained to discriminate 30 mg d-amphetamine taken orally from placebo. Physiologic measures, including blood pressure, heart rate, respiratory rate, oral temperature, and pupillary diameter, and subjective effects measures, including Addiction Research Center Inventory (ARCI), visual analog scales (VAS) and the Single Dose Questionnaire (SDQ) were completed 30 minutes and 1, 2, 4, 6, and 8 hours after drug administration. MPH and d-amphetamine produced dose-related increases in amphetamine responding. MPH and d-amphetamine produced similar profiles on the subjective effects measures. Both drugs produced significant dose-related increases in ratings on the Morphine-Benzedrine Group (MBG) and Amphetamine (A) scales of the ARCI, indicating stimulant effects. In addition, MPH increased reports of "high," and both drugs increased reports on the SDQ of drug liking, drive, and talkativeness. When asked to identify the drug (SDQ drug identification question), higher doses of MPH were identified as d-amphetamine or cocaine. Both MPH and d-amphetamine increased systolic and diastolic blood pressure, heart rate, and temperature. Thus, MPH substituted for d-amphetamine, and both drugs produced similar patterns of subjective effects, including increased ratings of euphoria, drug liking, and decreased sedation.

Drug self-administration

By use of several different types of intravenous self-administration procedures, the reinforcing effects of a drug and its relative abuse liability can be assessed. First, the substitution procedure is the most common and reliable method for evaluating whether a drug will maintain self-administration. It is used to evaluate the ability of a given dose of a test drug to maintain self-injection when substituted for a standard drug dose, which is known to maintain reliable rates and patterns of self-administration. Second, self-administration procedures can be used to assess the relative reinforcing efficacy of drugs that maintain self-administration. Observed differences in the reinforcing effects of drugs have been assumed to reflect the "strength," "efficacy," or "value" of the drug as a reinforcer. The methods used to evaluate relative reinforcing efficacy include progressive-ratio schedules, rates of drug-maintained responding, concurrent schedules, and discrete trials choice procedures. Third, another measure of reinforcing efficacy is the ability of drugs to induce self-administration behavior. By use of these procedures, the relative speed of acquisition of drug self-administration can provide information about their strength as reinforcers.

Preclinical self-administration

MPH maintained self-administration behavior in monkeys trained to self-administer intravenous cocaine under operant schedules of reinforcement (Bergman et al., 1989; Wilson et al., 1971; Wilson and Schuster, 1972; Aigner and Balster, 1979) and in rats trained to self-administer intravenous d-amphetamine under operant schedules of reinforcement (Nielsen et al., 1984). In these studies, MPH substituted for the cocaine or d-amphetamine training dose and continued to maintain self-administration behavior (Table 3).

TABLE 2. DISCRIMINATIVE, REINFORCING, AND SUBJECTIVE EFFECTS OF METHYLPHENIDATE (MPH) IN HUMANS

MPH Dose (mg)/ Population	*Results*	*Other Effects*	*Reference*
7.5–60 mg, oral	↑ "Positive" mood scores & drug liking ↑ Stimulant subjective effects	↑ Talkativeness, ↑ drive ↑ Blood pressure	Heischman & Henningfield, 1991
Stimulant abusers	Identified as amphetamine (44%) or cocaine (81%)	↑ Heart rate ↑ Temperature	
15–60 mg, subcutaneous	↑ "Positive" mood scores, ↑ drug liking	Low: ↑ relaxation, well-being, ↓ appetite High: Nervousness, anxiety, dysphoria	Martin et al., 1971
Narcotic abusers	MPH = d-amphetamine (7.5–30 mg) = methamphetamine (15–30 mg)		
20–40 mg oral (mean = 31 mg)	MPH chosen on 28% of sessions Placebo chosen on 9% of sessions MPH = amphetamine	↑ Activity level ↑ "Positive" mood scales ↑ Euphoria	Chait, 1994
Normal volunteers	No increase on drug liking	↑ Toxicity, dysphoria	
10 & 20 mg, oral	↑ Positive mood and subjective effects ↑ Talkative and friendly	↑ Activity, ↓ anxiety	Smith & Davis, 1977
Psychiatrists and psychologists	↑ Euphoria		
10 & 20 mg, oral	↑ Elation, ↑ euphoria	MPH = Amphetamine	Brown, 1977; Brown et al., 1978
Normal volunteers			
35 mg, intravenous	↑ "High," ↑ euphoria	MPH = Amphetamine	Huey et al., 1980
Psychiatric patients			
45–60 mg, subcutaneous	MPH: ↓ craving for cocaine	Self-administered MPH	Khantzian et al., 1984
Cocaine abusers			
60 mg	Disruptions in behavior Affective and thought disorders	Maintained on MPH dose	Keeley & Light, 1985
MPH dependent patients			

TABLE 3. REINFORCING EFFECTS OF METHYLPHENIDATE (MPH) IN ANIMALS

Training/Species	*MPH Doses Tested (mg/kg/inj) iv*	*Maintained Behavior*	*Other Effects*	*Reference*
Substitution: cocaine trained				
Squirrel monkeys	0.01–0.3	Yes	Psychomotor stimulant effects	Spealman et al., 1989
Rhesus monkeys	0.025–0.4	Yes	↑ MPH intake, ↓ food intake	Wilson et al., 1971
Rhesus monkeys	0.05	Yes	Blocked by chlorpromazine	Wilson & Schuster, 1972
Rhesus monkeys	0.01 and 0.1	Yes	↑ MPH intake, ↓ food intake	Aigner & Balster, 1979
Substitution: amphetamine trained				
Rats	4 and 8	Yes	MPH blocked amphetamine	Nielsen et al., 1984
Progressive ratio:			Increasing responses for MPH	Griffiths et al., 1975
Baboons	0.1–0.8	Yes	MPH ≈ Amphetamine	
Choice Paradigm:	0.1–0.8	Yes	MPH > Saline	
MPH vs. Cocaine	0.075 vs. 0.7	Yes	High MPH >> low MPH doses	Johanson & Schuster, 1975
Rhesus monkeys	0.075–0.7 MPH vs. 0.05 cocaine	Yes	High MPH >> cocaine 0.5 MPH = 0.5 cocaine	
Acquisition paradigm:				
Rhesus monkeys	0.1	Yes, MPH = cocaine = amphetamine	Cyclicity, ↑ stereotypies, ↓ weight, death	Downs et al., 1979
Dogs	0.025–0.4	Yes, MPH = amphetamine	Cyclicity, ↑ stereotypies and locomotor activity	Risner & Jones, 1975
Dogs	0.025–0.4	Yes, MPH > amphetamine	Cyclicity, ↑ stereotypies, locomotor activity and toxicity	Risner & Jones, 1976
Rats	1.0 and 0.32	Yes, MPH= cocaine = amphetamine		Collins et al., 1984
Rats	0.33	Yes, MPH > cocaine		Dworkin et al., 1993

iv = intravenous

In addition to a substitution procedure, the use of acquisition training for MPH shows its relative reinforcing efficacy in drug-naive animals with no previous drug training. The efficacy of drug reinforcers to maintain responding has involved comparing the relative rate of acquisition of self-administration, relative frequency, or rate of behavior each maintains, or by determining preference under a choice procedure. The reinforcing effects of MPH are potent, and it can be used to train naive animals to respond under operant schedules to receive an injection of MPH.

The reinforcing effects of MPH and several other psychomotor stimulants, including cocaine, methamphetamine, d-amphetamine, and phenmetrazine, was assessed in rats, dogs, and rhesus monkeys (Collins et al., 1984; Dworkin et al., 1993; Downs et al., 1979; Risner and Jones, 1975, 1976). In rats, the rate of acquisition of MPH was faster than those of d-amphetamine, nicotine, or caffeine. In dogs and monkeys, MPH, cocaine, d-amphetamine, and phenmetrazine produced a cyclic pattern of self-administration as well as weight loss, stereotypy, and death; this pattern of behavior and profile of effects is characteristic of psychomotor stimulant abuse. However, in the monkeys, unlimited access to MPH produced a higher rate of mortality than the other drugs; 75% of the monkeys that self-injected MPH died, compared with 66% and 25% of the monkeys that self-injected cocaine and d-amphetamine, respectively.

The reinforcing strength or reinforcing efficacy of MPH was evaluated in baboons trained to respond to cocaine using another self-administration procedure, called progressive-ratio procedure (Griffiths et al., 1975). This procedure involves systematically increasing the subject's response requirement until his or her responding falls below criterion (called the breaking point). In this study, MPH produced breaking points (1280 to 2400 responses per injection) that overlapped with those produced by cocaine (2400 to 4800 responses per injection).

Another method for comparing the relative efficacy of MPH and cocaine involved using preference procedures. Rhesus monkeys were given a choice between two doses of the same drug or doses of both drugs (Johanson and Schuster, 1975). When the monkeys were able to choose, both MPH and cocaine were chosen (more than 75%) over saline by all monkeys. In addition, higher doses of each drug were chosen over lower doses. However, when MPH was compared with cocaine, preference for cocaine decreased as the dose of MPH increased. At the highest dose of MPH versus cocaine, MPH was chosen by individual monkeys in 85% to 94% of the trials.

Reinforcing and subjective effects

In humans, MPH produces behavioral, physiologic, subjective, and reinforcing effects similar to those of d-amphetamine (Martin et al., 1971; Smith and Davis, 1977; Brown et al., 1978; Chait, 1994), including increases in rating of euphoria, drug liking, and activity, and decreases in sedation (see Table 3).

The physiologic, subjective, and behavioral effects of MPH were studied in narcotic abusers (Martin et al., 1971), psychiatric patients (Huey et al., 1980), and normal subjects (Chait, 1994; Brown, 1977; Brown et al., 1978; Smith and Davis, 1977). MPH increased "positive" mood scores and dose-dependently increased measures of "drug liking." In addition, subjects reported that low and intermediate doses of MPH produced feelings of relaxation, well-being, and contentment, whereas the highest dose intensified those feelings and produced dysphoria, nervousness, and anxiety. MPH also dose-dependently reduced appetite and decreased caloric intake. Similar subjective effects were seen with d-amphetamine and d-methamphetamine, suggesting that these drugs have similar mechanisms of action underlying their abuse potential.

In summary, MPH produces d-amphetamine-like and cocaine-like reinforcing effects in both humans and animals. Preclinical self-administration studies show that MPH is self-administered by animals under a variety of conditions, including when it is substituted for cocaine or d-amphetamine in drug-experienced animals or when it is begun in drug-naive animals. MPH has reinforcing efficacy similar to that of cocaine and d-amphetamine. In nonhuman primates, MPH can maintain high rates of self-injection in progressive ratio studies and is chosen over cocaine in preference studies. In clinical studies, MPH is self-administered by humans and produces patterns of reinforcing and subjective effects similar to those of d-amphetamine. MPH and d-amphetamine produce similar patterns of subjective effects, including increases in rating of euphoria, drug liking, and activity, and decreases in sedation.

Tolerance/sensitization

In preclinical studies, long-term administration of MPH produced tolerance to its disruptive and stimulus effects and showed cross-tolerance with d-amphetamine and cocaine (McNamara et al., 1993; Kolta et al., 1985; Emmett-Oglesby and Taylor, 1981; Emmett-Oglesby and Brewin, 1978; Wood et al., 1984, 1988; Leith and Barrett, 1981). Like d-amphetamine and cocaine, long-term administration of high doses of MPH produces psychomotor stimulant toxicity, including aggression, agitation, disruption in food intake, weight loss, stereotypic movements, and death (Downs et al., 1979; Wesson and Smith, 1978). This toxicity may be a result of sensitization (reverse tolerance) to the drug's effects during long-term use.

Dependence and withdrawal effects

In animals and humans, withdrawal from MPH has not been tested with behavioral paradigms. However, given the pharmacologic and behavioral similarities of MPH to cocaine and d-amphetamine, the preclinical data suggest that withdrawal from long-term MPH would result in an animal model of withdrawal "anxiety" similar to that demonstrated after withdrawal from long-term cocaine administration (Wood and Emmett-Oglesby, 1988, Wood et al., 1989).

In humans, abstinence from psychomotor stimulants such as d-amphetamine and cocaine after long-term use results in the appearance of withdrawal signs within 1 to 3 days, including depression, sleep disturbances, anxiety, fatigue, anger/hostility, dysphoria, psychomotor agitation, confusion, and drug craving (Gawin and Kleber, 1986; Gawin, 1989; Gawin and Ellinwood, 1988; Gawin et al., 1992; Weddington et al., 1990; Satel et al., 1991; Dackis and Gold, 1990; Watson et al., 1992).

In summary, methylphenidate is a psychomotor stimulant that is structurally and pharmacologically similar to the amphetamines. In preclinical and clinical studies, methylphenidate, like d-amphetamine and cocaine, was self-administered by laboratory animals, including rats, dogs, monkeys, and baboons (Wilson et al., 1971; Johanson and Schuster, 1975; Risner and Jones, 1975; Griffiths et al., 1975; Spealman et al., 1989). Methylphenidate produced discriminative stimulus effects similar to those of d-amphetamine and cocaine in laboratory animals (Huang and Ho, 1974; Evans and Johanson, 1987; Wood and Emmett-Oglesby, 1988). In preclinical and clinical studies, long-term administration of methylphenidate produced tolerance to its disruptive and stimulus effects and showed cross-tolerance with d-amphetamine and cocaine (Emmett-Oglesby and Taylor, 1981; Wood and Emmett-Oglesby, 1988; Leith and Barrett, 1981).

ACTUAL ABUSE

Some of the earliest published reports of MPH abuse came from Sweden (Borg, 1961; Jorgensen and Kodahl, 1961; Noriek, 1960), where widespread abuse and misuse of MPH led to its withdrawal from the Swedish market in 1968. Most of the U.S. literature cites case reports of individuals, where only a few studies describe abuse in certain groups or populations. The following discussion summarizes the patterns and severity of abuse associated with MPH and provides pertinent citations concerning the medical consequences associated with that abuse.

In the early 1960s, many members of the scientific community thought that stimulants produced a form of addiction that was relatively benign and infrequent (Kalant, 1972). Riox (1960) and McCormick and McNeal (1963) countered this view by providing detailed case reports of patients who abused MPH. These and subsequent case reports (Jaffe and Koschmann, 1970; Spensley and Rockwell, 1972; Brooks et al., 1974; Goyer et al., 1979; Keeley and Light, 1985; Jaffe, 1991) demonstrated that MPH is associated with patterns of abuse similar to those of other Schedule II stimulants. Like amphetamine and cocaine, abuse of MPH can lead to marked tolerance and severe psychologic dependence. The pattern of abuse is characterized by escalation in dose, binge use followed by severe depression, and an overpowering desire to continue the use of this drug despite negative medical and social consequences. The abuser may alter the mode of administration from oral use to intranasal or intravenous use to intensify the effects of the drug. Like other potent psychostimulants, high doses of MPH often produce euphoria as well as agitation, tremors, tachycardia, palpitations, and hypertension. Psychotic episodes with schizophrenic characteristics and paranoid delusions characteristic of amphetamine-like toxicity have been associated with MPH abuse (McCormick and McNeel, 1963; Spensley and Rockwell, 1972).

Throughout the 1970s and 1980s, several articles were published in the medical literature that documented the serious medical consequences associated with parenteral abuse of MPH. Large amounts of talc used as a filler in MPH tablets led to widespread obstruction of the pulmonary vascular bed when these tablets, intended for oral use, were crushed, diluted, and injected. Pulmonary hypertension brought on by repeated intravenous injections of MPH was strongly implicated in the deaths of several people in Oregon and Washington (Lewman, 1972); postmortem examination demonstrated a characteristic talc granulomatosis and morphologic evidence of severe hypertension. Other fatalities associated with intravenous MPH abuse have been reported (Levine et al., 1986; Lundquest et al., 1987). Brooks et al. (1974) provided case reports of MPH abusers who sought medical treatment for *Eikenella* abscesses at injection sites. Problems, such as vascular injury resulting in ischemia, created by intra-arterial injection of MPH were discussed by Lindell et al. (1972). Chillar et al. (1982) described two cases of hemiplegia brought on by intracarotid injection of MPH. Arnett et al. (1976) described a patient with staphylococcal tricuspid valve endocarditis with septic embolic pneumonia resulting from intravenous MPH abuse. Elenbaas et al. (1976) and Zemplenyi and Colman (1984) reported abscess formation as a complication of parenteral MPH abuse. Other serious complications of intravenous MPH abuse have included osteomyelitis (Abino and Pandarinath, 1977), precocious emphysema (Sherman et al., 1987), severe eosinophilia (Wolf et al., 1978), multiple organ failure (Stecyk et al., 1985), retinopathy (Gunby, 1979), and hepatic injury (Mehta et al., 1984). Carter and Watson (1994) conducted a study to characterize intravenous pentazocine/methylphenidate abuse in emergency department patients. This drug combination has been reported in other case studies (Bryan et al., 1973; Kishorekumar et al., 1985; Lundquest et al., 1987) and is referred to as "Ts & Blues" or "T & Rs" among street addicts in many areas of the United States and Canada.

The use of MPH by methadone clients has been studied by Lewman (1972), who estimated that about 20% of 360 addicts receiving methadone treatment at the Oregon Medical Center were injecting MPH regularly or on occasion. Raskind and Bradford (1975) found that methadone patients were more likely to abuse MPH than heroin street addicts. The methadone clients stated that MPH produced an intense "rush" that methadone did not, and that the "program" did not seem to know or care whether patients were using MPH. Haglund and Howerton (1982) assessed the use of MPH among 192 consecutive patients admitted to a central intake unit for drug abuse treatment. More than half of the clients seeking treatment reported using MPH, usually in combination with opioids. It is unknown whether MPH remains a popular drug among methadone patients, as routine testing does not screen for MPH use.

DIVERSION

Unlike cocaine, amphetamine, and methamphetamine where illicit manufacturing account for the vast majority of available drugs for abuse, pharmaceutical products diverted from legitimate channels are the only sources of MPH available for abuse. The Drug Enforcement Administration (DEA) is unaware of any clandestine production of MPH; this fact probably reflects its rather arduous chemical synthesis. Diversion of MPH has been identified by drug thefts, illegal sales, and prescription forgery. An analysis of drug thefts reported to the DEA indicates that MPH ranks in the top 10 most frequently reported controlled pharmaceuticals diverted from licensed handlers; most reports were generated by pharmacies, and most thefts occurred during break-ins at night. Data from state and local law enforcement agencies and DEA case files indicate that MPH is diverted in several ways by a wide range of individuals and organized groups, from health care professionals, including physicians, pharmacists, and nurses, to organized drug trafficking rings involving multistate distribution. This profile is consistent with other highly abusable pharmaceutical substances that are in Schedule II of the CSA.

MPH diversion has been a particular problem in some states. For example, in Nebraska, investigative services for the state reported that MPH ranked among the top three pharmaceutical drugs most frequently submitted to crime laboratories for analysis from 1991 through 1994, and from April 1992 through January 1995, MPH ranked sixth among drugs involved in incidents of forged or altered prescriptions. In Ohio, from March 1979 to January 1994, MPH ranked second among pharmaceutical drugs reported for false or forged prescriptions. The Ohio Board of Pharmacy reported 18 separate cases involving pharmacists who were diverting this drug for sale or personal use.

In recent years, data from prescription audits, production quotas, and sales figures from the manufacturers indicate that the use of MPH has increased significantly in the United States. In fact, the United Nations reported that in 1994, the United States produced and consumed 90% of the total world production of MPH (Figure 1). The primary use of this drug is for the treatment of attention deficit hyperactivity disorder (ADHD) in children, although there is a growing trend to use MPH for the treatment of ADHD symptoms in adults.

Because so many families with young children and adolescents are in daily contact with this drug, evidence of diversion and misuse/abuse in this setting is both noteworthy and alarming. Goyer et al. (1979), Fulton et al. (1988), and Jaffe (1991) are among the few who have addressed the abuse of MPH within the context of ADHD treatment. However, significant quantities of data from school surveys, emergency room reports, poison control centers, adolescent treatment centers, and law enforcement encounters all indicate a growing problem with the abuse of MPH among younger populations (DEA Reports, 1995, 1997). Since 1990, there has been a fivefold increase in the number of emergency room mentions for MPH in the Drug Abuse Warning Network (DAWN) and a tenfold increase

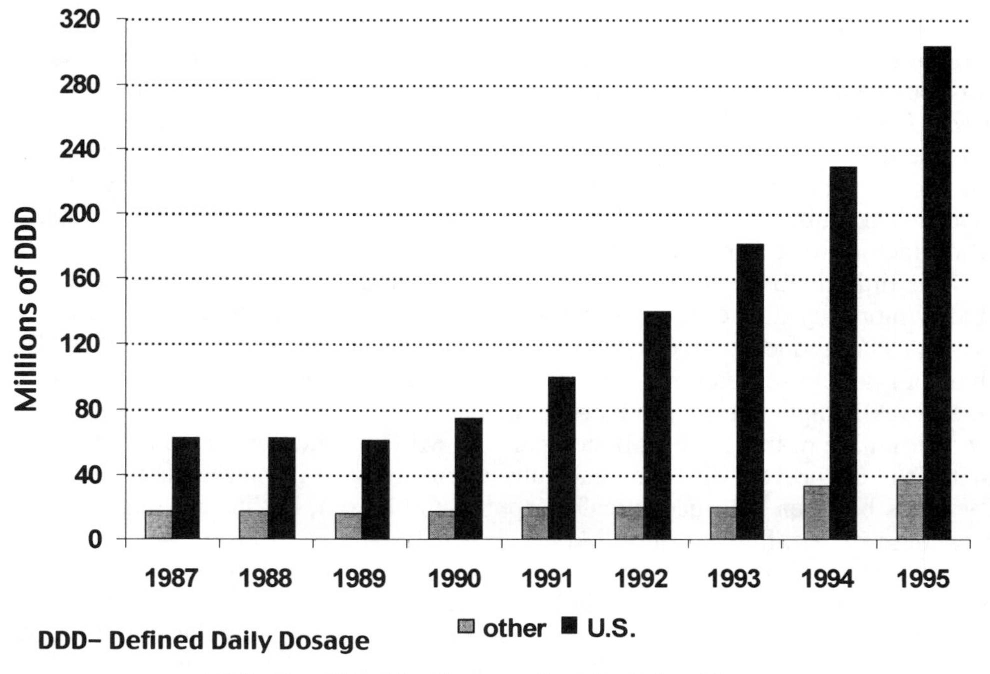

FIG. 1. Worldwide use of methylphenidate.

among children 10 to 14 years of age, who are just as likely to report abuse of MPH as of cocaine (Figure 2). The national survey Monitoring the Future, conducted by the Institute of Social Research at the University of Michigan (also referred to as the high school survey), indicated that about 1% of all 1994 and 1995 high school seniors had used Ritalin without a doctor's order during the previous year. In 1997, that percentage increased to 2.8. Adolescent treatment centers have uniformly reported an increase in abuse of MPH although few adolescents report this drug as their primary drug of abuse.

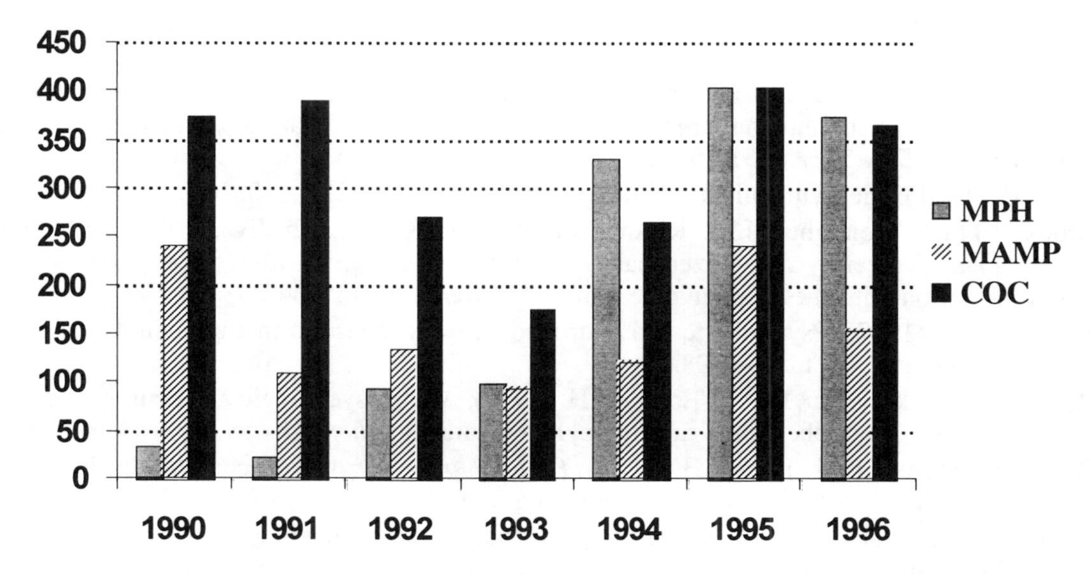

FIG. 2. Drug abuse of methylphenidate (MPH), methamphetamine (MAMP), or cocaine (COC) by children ages 10–14 as reported by U.S. emergency rooms to the Drug Abuse Warning Network (DAWN).

Four different types of cases centering on the use of MPH for ADHD treatment have been reported by law enforcement personnel throughout the United States: (1) parents who sell or abuse MPH medication prescribed to their children; (2) adolescents who sell their own MPH medication or siblings' medication to friends and classmates; (3) adolescents who abuse their own MPH medication or that of friends by crushing the tablets and snorting the powder; and (4) theft from home or school MPH supplies. The DEA held a conference in December, 1996, at which adolescent abuse was discussed and possible contributing factors were explored (DEA report, 1997).

There is little doubt that MPH is associated with significantly less abuse and associated morbidity/mortality than cocaine or methamphetamine (both classified as Schedule II stimulants). As a consequence, many people have used this information to argue that MPH does not have a high abuse potential. This disparity reflects the vastly different amounts of cocaine and methamphetamine produced by clandestine laboratories as well as uncontrolled street distribution of these drugs. In comparison, MPH production and distribution is highly regulated to help prevent diversion and subsequent abuse. It is interesting that the same disparity exists between pharmaceutical morphine and heroin, but no one suggests that morphine should be less highly controlled.

In conclusion, animal studies have shown that MPH has an abuse liability similar to that of other Schedule II stimulants, including amphetamine, methamphetamine, and cocaine. Actual data on abuse indicate that the pattern of MPH abuse is similar to that of other potent psychostimulants and that MPH is diverted and abused to a similar extent as other pharmaceutical Schedule II substances. Taken collectively, the data indicate that MPH fits the profile of a Schedule II substance.

REFERENCES

Abino, P.D. & Pandarinath, S. (1977), Methylphenidate (Ritalin) abuse. *J. Med. Soc. New Jersey*, 74:1061–1062.

Aigner, T.G. & Balster, R.L. (1979), Rapid substitution procedure for intravenous drug self-administration studies in rhesus monkeys. *Pharm. Biochem. Behav.*, 10:105–112.

Arnett, E.N., Battle, W.E., Russo, J.V. & Roberts, W.C. (1976), Intravenous injection of talc-containing drugs intended for oral use. *Am. J. Med.*, 60:711–718.

Bergman, J., Madras, B.K., Johnson, S.E. & Spealman, R.D. (1989), Effects of cocaine and related drugs in nonhuman primates: III. Self-administration by squirrel monkeys. *J. Pharmacol. Exp. Ther.*, 251:150–155.

Borg, E. (1961), Methylphenidate addiction. *Nord. Med.*, 65:211–213.

Brooks, G.F., O'Donoghue, J.M., Rissing, J.P., Soapes, K. & Smith, J.W. (1974), *Eikenella corrodens*, a recently recognized pathogen: Infections in medical-surgical patients and in association with methylphenidate abuse. *Medicine*, 53:325–342.

Brown, W.A. (1977), Psychologic and neuroendocrine response to methylphenidate. *Arch. Gen. Psychiatry*, 34:1103–1108.

Brown, W.A., Corriveau, D.P. & Ebert, M.H. (1978), Acute psychologic and neuroendocrine effects of dextroamphetamine and methylphenidate. *Psychopharmacology*, 58:189–195.

Bryan, V., Franks, L. & Torres, H. (1973), *Pseudomonas aeruginosa* cervical diskitis with chondro-osteomyelitis in an intravenous drug abuser. *Surg. Neurol.*, 1:142–144.

Carter, H.S. & Watson, W.A. (1994), IV pentazocine/methylphenidate abuse—the clinical toxicity of another Ts and Blues combination. *Clin. Toxicol.*, 32:541–547.

Chait, L.D. (1994), Reinforcing and subjective effects of methylphenidate in humans. *Behav. Pharmacol.*, 5:281–288.

Chillar, R.K., Jackson, A.L. & Alaan, L. (1982), Hemiplegia after intracarotid injection of methylphenidate. *Arch. Neurol.*, 39:598–599.

Collins, R.J., Weeks, J.R., Cooper, M.M., Good, P.I. & Russell, R.R. (1984), Prediction of abuse liability of drugs using IV self-administration by rats. *Psychopharmacology*, 82:6–13.

Colpaert, F.C., Niemegeers, C.J.E. & Janssen, P.A.J. (1979), Discriminative stimulus properties of cocaine: Neuropharmacological characteristics as derived from stimulus generalization experiments. *Pharm. Biochem. Behav.*, 10:535–546.

Dackis, C.A. & Gold, M.S. (1990), Addictiveness of central stimulants. In: *Addictive Potential of Abused Drugs and Drug Classes,* ed., C.K. Erikson, New York: Haworth Press, Inc., pp. 9–26.

De la Garza, R. & Johanson, C.E. (1987), Discriminative stimulus properties of intragastrically administered d-amphetamine and pentobarbital in rhesus monkeys. *J. Pharmacol. Exp. Ther.*, 243:955–962.

Downs, D.A., Harrigan, S.W., Wiley, J.N., Robinson, T.E. & Labay, R.J. (1979), Research communications in psychology. *Psychol. Behav.*, 4:39–49.

Drug Enforcement Administration (1995), *Methylphenidate Review: Eight-Factor Analysis.* Washington, DC: Office of Diversion Control.

Drug Enforcement Administration (1997), *Conference Report: Stimulants Used in the Treatment of ADHD.* Washington, DC: Office of Diversion Control.

Dworkin, S.I., Vrana, S.L., Broadbent, J. & Robinson, J.H. (1993), Comparing the reinforcing effects of nicotine, caffeine, methylphenidate and cocaine. *Med. Chem. Res.*, 2:593–602.

Elenbaas, R.M., Waeckerle, J.F. & McNabney, W.K. (1976), Abscess formation as a complication of parenteral methylphenidate abuse. *JACEP*, 5:977–980.

Emmett-Oglesby, M.W. & Brewin, A. (1978), Tolerance to the behavioral effects of methylphenidate after daily and intermittent administration. *J AOA*, 78:143–144.

Emmett-Oglesby, M.W., Mathis, D.A., Moon, R.T.Y. & Lal, H. (1990), Animal models of drug withdrawal symptoms. *Psychopharmacology*, 101:292–309.

Emmett-Oglesby, M.W. & Taylor, K.E. (1981), Role of dose interval in the acquisition of tolerance to methylphenidate. *Neuropharmacology*, 20:995–1002.

Emmett-Oglesby, M.W., Wurst, M. & Lal, H. (1983), Discriminative stimulus properties of a small dose of cocaine. *Neuropharmacology*, 22:97–101.

Evans, S.E. & Johanson, C.E. (1987), Amphetamine-like effects of anorectic and related compounds in pigeons. *J. Pharmacol. Exp. Ther.*, 241:817–825.

Fulton, A. & Yates, W.R. (1988), Family abuse of methylphenidate. *Am. Fam. Pract.*, 38:143–145.

Gawin, F.H. (1989), Cocaine abuse and addiction. *J Fam. Pract.*, 29:193–197.

Gawin, F.H. & Ellinwood, D.H. (1988), Cocaine and other stimulants. *N. Engl. J. Med.*, 318:1173–1182.

Gawin, F.H., Khalsa, H.K. & Anglin, M.D. (1992), Subjective symptoms of cocaine withdrawal. *NIDA Res. Mon.* Washington, DC: U.S. Government Printing Office, p. 442.

Gawin, F.H. & Kleber, H.D. (1986), Abstinence symptomatology and psychiatric diagnosis in cocaine abusers: Clinical observations. *Arch. Gen. Psychiatry*, 43:107–113.

Goudie, A.J., Atkinson, J. & West, C.R. (1986), Discrimination properties of the psychomotor stimulant dl-cathinone in a two-lever operant task. *Neuropharmacology,* 25:85–94.

Goyer, P.F., Davis, G.C. & Papoport, J.L. (1979), Abuse of prescribed stimulant medication by a 13-year-old hyperactive boy. *J. Am. Acad. Child Psychiatry*, 18:170–175.

Griffiths, R.R., Bigelow, G.E. & Henningfield, J.E. (1980), Similarities in animal and human drug-taking behavior. In: *Advances in Substance Abuse, vol 1*, ed., N.K. Mello. Greenwich, CT: JAI Press, pp. 1–90.

Griffiths, R.R., Brady, J.V. & Bradford, L.D. (1979), Predicting the abuse liability of drugs with animal drug self-administration procedures: Psychomotor stimulants and hallucinogens. In: *Advances in Behavioral Pharmacology, vol 2*, eds. T. Thompson & P.B. Dews. New York: Academic Press, pp. 163–208.

Griffiths, R.R., Findley, J.D., Brady, J.V., Dolan-Gutcher, K. & Robinson, W.W. (1975), Comparison of progressive-ratio performance maintained by cocaine, methylphenidate and secobarbital. *Psychopharmacology (Berl.)*, 43:81–87.

Griffiths, R.R., Winger, G., Brady, J.V. & Snell, J.D. (1976), Comparison of behavior maintained by infusions of eight phenethylamines in baboons. *Psychopharmacology*, 50:251–258.

Gunby, P. (1979). Methylphenidate abuse produces retinopathy. *JAMA*, 241–546.

Haglund, R.M. & Howerton, L.L. (1982), Ritalin: Consequences of abuse in a clinical population. *Int. J. Addict.*, 17:349–356.

Harris, R.T. & Balster, R.L. (1971), An analysis of the function of drugs in the stimulus control of operant behavior. In: *Stimulus Properties of Drugs*. eds., Thompson, T. & Pickens, R. New York: Appleton-Century Crofts, pp 111–132.

Heischman, S.J. & Henningfield, J.E. (1991), Discriminative stimulus effects of d-amphetamine, methylphenidate, and diazepam in humans. *Psychopharmacology*, 103:436–442.

Huang, J.T. & Ho, B.T. (1974), Discriminative stimulus properties of d-amphetamine and related compounds in rat. *Pharm. Biochem. Behav.*, 2:669–673.

Huey, L.Y., Janowsky, D.S., Judd, L.L., Roitman, N.A., Clopton, P.L., Segal, D., Hall,, L. & Parker, D. (1980), The effects of naloxone on methylphenidate-induced mood and behavioral changes: A negative study. *Psychopharmacology*, 67:125–130.

Jaffe, R.B. & Koschmann (1970), Intravenous drug abuse: Pulmonary, cardiac, and vascular complications. *A.J.R.*, 109:107–120.

Jaffe, S.L. (1991), Intranasal abuse of prescribed methylphenidate by alcohol and drug abusing adolescent with ADHD. *J. Am. Acad. Child Adolesc. Psychiatry*, 30:773–775.

Johanson, C.E. & Balster, R.L. (1978), A summary of the results of a drug self-administration study using substitution procedures in rhesus monkeys. *Bull. Narc.*, 30:43–54.

Johanson, C.E., Balster, R.L. & Bonese, K. (1976), Self-administration of psychomotor stimulant drugs: The effects of unlimited access. *Pharm. Biochem. Behav.*, 4:45–51.

Johanson, C.E. & Schuster, C.R. (1975), A choice procedure for drug reinforcers: Cocaine and methylphenidate in the rhesus monkey. *J. Pharmacol. Exp. Ther.*, 193:676–688.

Jorgenson, F. & Kodahl, T. (1961), On the abuse of Ritalin. *Ugeskr. Laeg.*, 123:1275–1279.

Kalant, O.J. (1972), *The Amphetamines: Toxicity and Addiction, 2nd ed.* Toronto: Addiction Research Foundation, University of Toronto Press.

Keeley, K.A. & Light, A.L. (1985), Gradual vs. abrupt withdrawal of methylphenidate in two older dependent males. *J. Subst. Abuse Treat.*, 2:123–128.

Khantzian, E.J., Gawin, F.H., Ricordan, C. & Kleber, H.D. (1984), Methylphenidate treatment of cocaine dependence: A preliminary report. *J. Subst. Abuse Treat.*, 1:107–112.

Kishorekumer, R., Yagnik, P. & Dhopesh, V. (1985), Acute myopathy in a drug abuser following an attempted neck vein injection. *J. Neurol. Neurosurg. Psychiatry*, 48:843–844.

Kolta, M., Shreve, P. & Uretsky, N.J. (1985), Effects of methylphenidate pretreatment on the behavioral and biochemical response to amphetamine. *Eur. J. Pharmacol.*, 117:279–282.

Levine, B., Caplan, Y.H. & Kauffman, G. (1986), Fatality resulting from methylphenidate overdose. *J. Anal. Toxicol.*, 10:209–210.

Leith, N.J. & Barrett, R.J. (1981), Self-stimulation and amphetamine: Tolerance to d and l isomers and cross tolerance to cocaine and methylphenidate. *Psychopharmacology*, 74:23–28.

Lewman, L.V. (1972), Fatal pulmonary hypertension from intravenous injection of methylphenidate (Ritalin) tablets. *Hum. Pathol.*, 3:67–70.

Lindell, T.D., Porter, J.M. & Langstron, C. (1972), Intra-arterial injections of oral medications: Complications of drug addiction. *N. Engl. J. Med.*, 287:1132–1133.

Lundquest, D.E., Young, W.K. & Edland, J.F. (1987), Maternal death associated with intravenous methylphenidate (Ritalin) and pentazocine (Talwin) abuse. *J. Foren. Sci.*, 32:798–801.

McCormick, T.C. & McNeel, T.W. (1963), Case report: Acute psychosis and Ritalin abuse. *Texas J. Med.*, 59:99–100.

McKenna, M.L. & Ho, B.T. (1980), The role of dopamine in the discriminative stimulus properties of cocaine. *Neuropharmacology*, 19:297–303.

Martin, W.R., Sloan, J.W., Sapira, J.D. & Jasinski, D.R. (1971), Physiological, subjective, and behavioral effect of amphetamine, methamphetamine, ephedrine, phenmetrazine, and methylphenidate in man. *Clin. Pharmacol. Ther.*, 12:245–258.

McNamara, C.G., Davidison, E.S. & Shenk, S. (1993), A comparison of the motor-activating effects of acute and chronic exposure to amphetamine and methylphenidate. *Pharmacol. Biochem. Behav.*, 45:729–732.

Mehta, H., Murray, B. & LoIudice, T.A. (1984), Hepatic dysfunction due to intravenous abuse of methylphenidate hydrochloride. *J. Clin. Gastroenterol.*, 6:149–151.

Melia, K.F. & Spealman, R.D. (1991), Pharmacological characterization of the discriminative stimulus effects of GBR 12909. *J. Pharmacol. Exp. Ther.*, 258:626–632.

Nielsen, J.A., Duda, N.J., Mokler, D.J. & Moore, K.E. (1984), Self-administration of central stimulants by rats: A comparison of the effects of d-amphetamine, methylphenidate and McNeil 4612. *Pharmacol. Biochem. Behav.*, 20:227–232.

Noreik, K. (1960), Methylphenidate addiction. *Tijdschr. Nor. Laeg.*, 80:442.

Overton, D.A. (1982), Comparison of the degree of discriminability of various drugs using a T-maze drug discrimination paradigm. *Psychopharmacology*, 76:385–395.

Parran, T.V. & Jasinski, D.R. (1991), Intravenous methylphenidate abuse: Prototype for prescription drug abuse. *Arch. Intern. Med.*, 151:781–783.

Perkins, A.N., Eckerman, D.A. & McPhail, R.C. (1991), Discriminative stimulus properties of triadimefon: Comparison with methylphenidate. *Pharmacol. Biochem. Behav.*, 40:757–761.

Porsolt, R.D., Pawelec, C. & Jalfre, M. (1982), Use of drug discrimination procedures to detect amphetamine-like effects of antidepressants. In: *Drug Discrimination: Applications in CNS Pharmacology*. eds., Colpaert, F.C. & Slangen, J.L. Amsterdam: Elsevier Biomedical Press, pp. 193–202.

Preston, K.L, Walsh, S.L. & Sannerud, C.A. (1997). Measures of interoceptive stimulus effects: Relationship to drug reinforcement. In: *Drug Addiction and Its Treatment: Nexus of Neuroscience and Behavior*, eds., B.P. Johnson, & J.D. Roache. Philadelphia: Lippincott-Raven, pp. 91–114.

Raskind, M.D. & Bradford, T. (1975), Methylphenidate (Ritalin) abuse and methadone maintenance. *Dis. Nerv. System* 36:285–289.

Rioux, B. (1960), Is Ritalin an addiction-producing drug? *Dis. Nerv. System*, 21:346–349.

Risner, M.E. & Jones, B.E. (1975), Self-administration of CNS stimulants by dogs. *Psychopharmacology*, 43:207–213.

Risner, M.E. & Jones, B.E. (1976), Characteristics of unlimited access to self-administered stimulant infusions in dogs. *Biol. Psychol.*, 11:625–634.

Rosen, J.R., Young, A.M., Beuthin, F.C. & Louis-Ferdinand, R.T. (1986), Discriminative stimulus properties of amphetamine and other stimulants in lead-exposed and normal rats. *Pharmacol. Biochem. Behav.*, 24:211–215.

Satel, S.L., Price, L.H., Palumbo, J.M., McDougle, C.J., Krystal, J.H., Gawin, F., Charney, D.S., Heniger, G.R. & Kleber, H.D. (1991), Clinical phenomenology and neurobiology of cocaine abstinence: A prospective inpatient study. *Am. J. Psychiatry,* 148:1712–1716.

Schuster, C.R. & Thompson, T. (1969), Administration of and behavioral dependence on drugs. *Ann. Rev. Pharmacol.*, 9:483–502.

Sherman, C.B., Hudson, L.D. & Pierson, D.J. (1987), Severe precocious emphysema in intravenous methylphenidate (Ritalin) abusers. *Chest*, 92:1085–1087.

Silverman, P.B. & Ho, B.T. (1980), The discriminative stimulus properties of 2,5-dimethoxy-4-methylamphetamine (DOM): Differentiation from amphetamine. *Psychopharmacology*, 68:209–215.

Silverman, P.B. & Schultz, K.A. (1989), Comparison of cocaine and procaine discriminative stimuli. *Drug Dev. Res.*, 16:427–433.

Smith, R.C. & Davis, J.M. (1977), Comparative effects of d-amphetamine, l-amphetamine, and methylphenidate on mood in man. *Psychopharmacology*, 53:1–12.

Spealman, R.D., Madras, B.K. & Bergman, J. (1989). Effects of cocaine and related drugs in non-human primates: II. Stimulant effects on schedule controlled behavior. *J. Pharmacol. Exp. Ther.* 251:142–149.

Spensley, J. & Rockwell, D.A. (1972), Psychosis during methylphenidate abuse. *N. Engl. J. Med.*, 286:880–881.

Stecyk, O., Loludice, T.A., Demeter, S. & Jacobs, J. (1985), Multiple organ failure resulting from intravenous abuse of methylphenidate hydrochloride. *Ann. Emerg. Med.*, 14:597–613.

Watson, R., Bakos, L., Compton, P. & Gawin, F. (1992), Cocaine use and withdrawal: The effects on sleep and mood. *Am. J. Drug Alcohol Abuse*, 18:21–28.

Weddington, W.H., Brown, B.S., Haertzen, C.A., Cone, E.J., Dax, E.M., Herning, R.I. & Michaelson, B.S. (1990), Changes in mood, craving, and sleep during short-term abstinence reported by male cocaine addicts: A controlled, residential study. *Arch. Gen. Psychiatry,* 47:861–868.

Wesson, D.R. & Smith, D.E. (1978), A clinical approach to diagnosis and treatment of amphetamine abuse. *J. Psychedelic Drugs*, 10:343–349.

Wilson, M.C., Hitomi, M. & Schuster, C.R. (1971), Psychomotor stimulant self-administration as a function of dosage per injection in the rhesus monkey. *Psychopharmacology*, 22:271–281.

Wilson, M.C. & Schuster, C.R. (1972), The effects of chlorpromazine on psychomotor stimulant self-administration in the rhesus monkey. *Psychopharmacology* (*Berl.*), 26:115–126.

Wolf, J., Fein, A. & Fehrenbacher, L. (1978), Eosinophilic syndrome with methylphenidate abuse. *Ann. Intern. Med.*, 89:224–225.

Wood, D.M. & Emmett-Oglesby, M.W. (1988), Substitution and cross-tolerance profiles of anorectic drugs in rats trained to detect the discriminative stimulus properties of cocaine. *Psychopharmacology*, 95:364–368.

Wood, D.M., Lal, H. & Emmett-Oglesby, M. (1984), Acquisition and recovery of tolerance to the discriminative stimulus properties of cocaine. *Neuropharmacology*, 23:1419–1423.

Wood, D.M., Laraby, P.R. & Lal, H. (1989), A pentylenetetrazol stimulus during cocaine withdrawal: Blockade by diazepam and haloperidol. *Drug Dev. Res.*, 16:269–276.

Zemplenyi, J. & Colman, M.F. (1984), Deep neck abscesses secondary to methylphenidate (Ritalin) abuse. *Head Neck Surg.*, 6:858–860.

Section 2

Diagnostic Issues

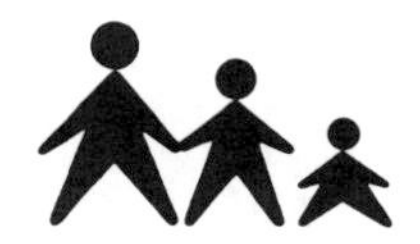

Attention Deficit Hyperactivity Disorder and Methylphenidate: Assessment and Prediction of Clinical Response

MARK D. RAPPORT and COLIN B. DENNEY

INTRODUCTION

Methylphenidate (MPH) is currently the most widely used drug for treating children with attention deficit hyperactivity disorder (ADHD). Its hard-earned reputation as the treatment of choice is well deserved. Over three decades of evidence attests to the therapeutic efficacy of MPH across broad-band domains of behavior and cognitive function.

Despite its demonstrated salutary effects, questions remain concerning the drug's long-term efficacy and the best way to define and measure clinical outcome. For example, some people have interpreted the rather dismal long-term outcome of children previously treated with MPH as indicative of the drug's impotence for altering the course of ADHD. Albeit reasonable, the argument is predicated on several assumptions, the most noteworthy being that the drug was carefully titrated and consistently administered, with clinical response authenticated, for a majority of children. Clearly, this reflects neither the reality of long-term investigations nor the practice parameters published to date.

Titration and measurement issues by nature are complex and multifaceted. Decisions must be made at a more detailed level concerning which behavior(s) to target for intervention, what constitutes an appropriate clinical response, whether dosage should be based on a child's body mass, and whether predictors of clinical response can be delineated. These issues constitute the basis of the present chapter.

We begin with a description of our clinical sample, procedures, and outcome measures. Subsequent sections of the chapter describe and discuss two clinical outcome studies. The first discusses body mass as a predictor of MPH response in children with ADHD. The second discusses the measurement of clinical outcome with specific emphasis on which behaviors should be targeted for intervention.

Clinical sample

One hundred thirty-four children with chronic problems of inattention, impulsivity, and overactivity were referred to the Children's Learning Clinic (CLC) by pediatricians, psychiatrists, and school system personnel over a 5-year period. All referred children and their parents participated in a detailed, semistructured clinical interview with the senior author (M.D.R.) at the CLC. The interview was adapted from the Schedule for Affective Disorders and Schizophrenia for School-Age Children (Orvaschel et al., 1982) and reviewed each of the disorders usually first evident in infancy, childhood, or adolescence as described in

Department of Psychology, University of Hawaii at Manoa, Honolulu, Hawaii.

the *Diagnostic and Statistical Manual of Mental Disorders (DSM)-III* (American Psychiatric Association, 1980). Seventy-six children met each of the following criteria and participated in the study: (1) an independent diagnosis by the child's referring physician and the CLC's directing clinical psychologist (M.D.R.) using *DSM-III* criteria for ADHD, (2) a maternal report of a developmental history consistent with ADHD and problems in at least 50% of the situations on Barkley's (1990) Home Situations Questionnaire, (3) a maternal rating of at least 2 standard deviations above the mean for the child's age on the Werry-Weiss-Peters Activity Scale (Routh et al., 1974), (4) a teacher's rating of at least 2 standard deviations above the mean on the Abbreviated Conners Teacher Rating Scale (ACTRS); Werry et al., 1975), and (5) the absence of any gross neurologic, sensory, or motor impairment as determined by pediatric examination.

By use of the described inclusion criteria, a total of 76 children with ADHD (66 boys, 10 girls) between the ages of 6 and 11 years (mean 8.51 years) participated in the study after informed consent had been obtained from their parents. All children were Caucasian, of at least average intelligence (mean IQ 102.17; SD 10.87) as assessed by the Peabody Picture Vocabulary Test—Revised, Form L (Dunn and Dunn, 1981), and from families of low to middle socioeconomic status. Eight children had experienced brief trials of psychostimulant within the past 4 years. All children were considered pervasively hyperactive according to the clinical interview and rating scale scores. A systematic review using recent diagnostic nomenclature indicates that each of the 76 children would currently be classified as meeting diagnostic criteria for attention deficit hyperactivity disorder—combined type as detailed in the *DSM-IV* (American Psychiatric Association, 1994).

Children who were comorbid for conduct disorder (CD) were purposely excluded from the study. Although the high degree of comorbidity between ADHD and CD has been well documented, there is sufficient evidence to suggest that the two disorders are at least partially independent (Abikoff and Klein, 1992; Blouin et al., 1989; Hinshaw, 1987) and are associated with different clinical presentations (Reeves et al., 1987; Werry et al., 1987) and patterns of parental psychopathology (Hinshaw, 1987; Lahey et al., 1988; Loeber et al., 1990). Whether children who are comorbid for ADHD and CD respond differently to psychostimulant therapy is presently unknown, although preliminary evidence suggests that children with CD may show similar behavioral improvement (Abikoff et al., 1987). Comorbidity for oppositional defiant disorder was not assessed, owing to the controversial nature of the disorder at the time when the study was initiated. Many children experienced symptoms of, but did not meet formal criteria for, anxiety and mood disorders.

Medication

A double-blind, placebo-controlled, within-subject (crossover) experimental design was used in which all ADHD children received each of five MPH (Ritalin) doses after baseline assessment. The order of drug administration was counterbalanced and determined by random assignment in such a way that an equal number of children received each dose during a given week of the study. MPH was prescribed by each child's physician in the following doses: placebo, 5 mg (range 0.10 to 0.26 mg/kg), 10 mg (range 0.20 to 0.52 mg/kg), 15 mg (range 0.30 to 0.79 mg/kg), and 20 mg (range 0.40 to 1.1 mg/kg). Fixed doses were used to reflect typical practice parameters in the United States and to permit direct comparison between absolute (kg) and mg/kg dosing methods. MPH and placebo doses were packaged in colored gelatin capsules by the clinic's pharmacist to avoid detection of dose and taste. Capsules were sealed in individual, daily envelopes to help control for accurate dose administration.

After baseline data collection (first week), parents were given 1 week's medication in predated envelopes at a single dose level (i.e., placebo, 5 mg, 10 mg, 15 mg, or 20 mg). This procedure continued until each child had received every dose for 6 consecutive days.

All weekly dose changes occurred on Sundays (i.e., no capsules were administered on Saturdays) to allow for "washout" and to control for possible rebound effects. Parents were instructed to give their child a capsule each morning, one-half hour before breakfast. Both used and unused envelopes were returned weekly to control for medication compliance. Medication was properly administered nearly 100% of the time. Makeup observation days were scheduled after rare occasions when compliance was not obtained.

Procedures

Children were observed in their regular classrooms for 20-minute intervals, 3 days per week across the 6-week (ADHD children) or 1-week (normal control group) evaluation period. No two children were in the same classroom. Observations were completed during the morning, owing to the behavioral time-response course of MPH and began 1.5 to 2 hours after children with ADHD had received their morning medication. Children in the normal control group were observed during the morning at a time that was held constant across all observation sessions. During each observation period, children completed their usual in-seat academic work assigned by the classroom teacher (e.g., mathematics or language arts worksheets).

Outcome measures

Teacher ratings

Classroom teachers completed the ACTRS each Friday throughout the study (i.e., 1 week for the normal control group and 6 consecutive weeks for the ADHD group). The outcome reflected the children's behavior during the morning hours (until 11:30 A.M.) only of that week. All teachers were blind as to when medication was administered and specific doses. The ACTRS was used because of its sensitivity in detecting MPH effects and ease of administration.

Attention

Children were observed by trained undergraduate and graduate-level research assistants for 60 consecutive intervals during each observation period throughout the study. Each interval was divided into 15 seconds of observation followed by 5 seconds for recording. A child's behavior was categorized as either on-task or off-task. Off-task behavior was defined as visual inattention to one's materials for more than 2 consecutive seconds within each 15-second observation interval, unless the child was engaged in an alternative task-appropriate behavior (e.g., sharpening a pencil). Observers were situated in the classroom in such a way as to avoid direct eye contact with the target child and were distanced from the child by approximately half the classroom size, while allowing for clear determination of task-related attention. Observers were blind to when medication was administered and specific doses for children in the ADHD group. For the normal control group, observers were blind to diagnosis and teacher ratings.

Academic efficiency

Children's performance on regularly assigned academic work during scheduled observation periods was used as a dependent measure to preserve ecological validity yet maintain adequate experimental control. Classroom teachers assigned academic seatwork consistent with the child's ability level, but with the stipulation that (1) the assignment be worked on during the optimal medication period (1.5 to 2 hours after medication), and (2) the assignment be gradable in terms of percentage completed and percentage accurate. Assignments were graded after class by either the teacher or the primary observer. Daily performance was recorded for both the percentage of problems completed and the percentage correct. The two scores were subsequently combined to calculate an academic efficiency score (AES). The score represents the percentage of academic assignments completed correctly.

Reliability

Interobserver reliability checks of each child's on-task behavior were obtained on 33% of the observation days and at least once per week for each participant in the study. Obtained and chance estimates were computed for occurrence, nonoccurrence, and overall agreement. Overall reliability was consistently above 85%, with a mean of 92.4% (range 86.3 to 99.8) across children. A mean kappa value of 0.84 was obtained across all observations. Overall reliability for AES data was consistently above 95%, with a mean of 97% and a kappa coefficient of 0.96.

Assessment of clinical MPH response

Control sample

Twenty-five normal children were evaluated to enable assessment of MPH response among clinical subjects using methods developed by Jacobson and Truax (1991) and Speer (1992). The normal control group consisted of 20 boys and 5 girls between the ages of 6 and 11 years (mean 8.56, SD 1.81) who were attending regular education classrooms in several public elementary schools in an urban district. These children were randomly selected from classroom rosters, did not evidence symptoms of ADHD or other problem behaviors according to parents' and teachers' reports, and had never been referred for evaluation of learning or behavior problems. The normal control children were of average or above average intelligence based on standardized test results provided by each child's school and from families of low to middle socioeconomic status. The teachers' ratings on the ACTRS for all members of this group were within 1.5 standard deviations of the mean for the child's age.

There were no significant differences between the ADHD and normal comparison groups with respect to age, IQ, and socioeconomic status. Learning disability was not directly assessed in either group. All children were currently attending regular elementary school classrooms, although several of the ADHD children concurrently received special education services (usually in reading and processing skills).

Determination of clinical responder status

Jacobson and Truax (1991) developed a method for evaluating the reliability and clinical significance of treatment gains among individual subjects. A modification of their procedure, designed to control for potential confounding influences of regression artifact, was used in the present series of investigations (Speer, 1992). The procedure assesses the extent to which individual subjects demonstrate change exceeding what would be anticipated on the basis of chance temporal variation (i.e., test-retest error). This is accomplished by first estimating the subjects' true initial scores based on their degree of pretreatment deviance from the normal population mean. An interval is subsequently constructed around each adjusted score, the width of which is equal to twice the standard of error of measurement associated with the instrument in question (the standard error of measurement is derived using the test-retest reliability coefficient). This interval represents the range in which scores are likely to fall 95% of the time under chance conditions.

Next, cutoff scores are derived for each measure that define entry into the normal range of functioning. The cutoff used in the present study was the midpoint between the clinical sample's pretreatment mean and the corresponding average for the control children as recommended by Jacobson and Truax (1991).

Clinical responder status is then evaluated for all individual subjects on each outcome measure by determining where treatment condition scores fall relative to the aforementioned interval and cutoff scores. Children whose scores fall outside and above the interval and above the normal-range cutoff are classified as "normalized." Those falling outside and above the interval but below the cutoff are categorized as "improved, not normalized." Those falling within the interval are described as "unchanged," and those falling outside and below it are characterized as "deteriorated."

BODY MASS AS A PREDICTOR OF MPH RESPONSE

Titrating MPH has become increasingly complex in recent years owing to advancements in clinical psychopharmacology. Sprague and Sleator's (1977) landmark study, for example, indicated that the dosage required for optimizing learning may be lower (0.3 mg/kg) than that required to produce optimal improvement in classroom behavior (1.0 mg/kg). Although the low-dose learning, high-dose behavior optimization hypothesis has not been supported by recent outcome studies (Douglas et al., 1986; DuPaul and Rapport, 1993; Pelham et al., 1985) or reviews (Rapport and Kelly, 1991), the implication that gross body weight or mass (kg) contributes to MPH response in children continues to influence clinical practice and controlled clinical trials.

The procedure of dosing on the basis of body mass has historical precedence. It is widely accepted in pharmacology and serves to address questions concerning whether standardized doses are functionally related to behavioral effects. Other people have disagreed with these premises, arguing that key pharmacokinetic factors (e.g., drug absorption, metabolism, and excretion rate) show such great interindividual variability for MPH that blood levels associated with the same dose per body mass are highly dissimilar (Shaywitz, 1984). In a similar vein, when behavioral and cognitive effects associated with MPH therapy are examined at the individual level (i.e., by plotting absolute dose in mg vs. dose in mg per kg on the abscissa), dose-response relationships are characterized by high interindividual and intraindividual variability that appears to be independent of gross body weight (Rapport et al., 1987; Rapport et al., 1989).

Three methodologic criteria must be satisfied for the rigorous evaluation of the postulated interaction between gross body mass and responsiveness to stimulant drugs. First, because age and weight are correlated, individual differences in age must be controlled in order to evaluate the independent influence of body mass on drug response.

Second, subjects must all receive multiple doses to enable explicit assessment of variations in the slope and shape of dose-response curves associated with individual differences in weight. Although dose-response profiles may vary incrementally as a function of weight, cogent arguments advanced by Kazdin and Kagan (1994) suggest that important etiologic and treatment-related differences are often evident among discrete subgroups within a sample. Consequently, evaluation of the dose × weight interaction should include comparisons of dose-response curves among discrete groups varying in mean body mass as well as corresponding analyses using weight as a continuous variable.

Finally, since the hypothesized dose × weight interaction implies that a child's body weight should guide the administration of MPH, it is important to assess the clinical importance of body mass as a moderator of drug response. Thus, analyses should examine the clinical predictive utility of body weight in distinguishing drug responders from nonresponders and/or identifying clinically beneficial doses.

Results

The hypotheses under consideration concern the impact of body weight on drug response rather than the influence of other variables correlated with age. Consequently, age effects were removed from individual differences in body mass. This was accomplished by regressing weight on age and transforming the resulting residuals to normalized *t* scores (mean 50, SD 10). These scores represent variations in body mass uncorrelated with age and were used in all subsequent data analyses.

The relationship between body mass and MPH response can assume several forms, as illustrated in Figure 1. First, continuous individual differences in weight may be associated with variations in dose-response curve parameters such as slope and shape (see Figure 1, A and B). Alternatively, such variations may be evident only in select ranges along the body weight continuum (see Figure 1, C and D). Finally, weight may distinguish between drug responders and nonresponders or enable categorization of children based on their optimal MPH dose.

Observed attention to task, academic efficiency, and teacher-rated behavior were subjected to a three-tier series of analyses to examine these possibilities. The first addresses the question whether incremental variations in body mass influence the slope or shape of the dose-response curves. The second series of analyses scrutinizes differences in dose-response curve parameters and rates of improvement across quartiles based on body mass. This approach evaluates whether variations in drug response are associated with select weight ranges. The third series of analyses assesses the clinical utility of body mass in predicting likelihood of response to at least one MPH dose as well as the dose required to yield optimal benefit.

Series I analysis

Dose-response profiles for the three dependent variables are depicted in Figure 2. The dose response curves were subjected to trend analysis (TA) with age-adjusted body mass entered as a continuous, between-subjects variable in order to characterize their slopes and shapes, and to determine whether trend properties were associated with incremental differences in weight. Attention was restricted to linear and quadratic trends, because no other components attained significance for the sample as a whole (Rapport et al., 1994).

The results are summarized in Table 1. Significant values of F_{lin} indicate the extent to which the treatment condition means fall along a straight line. F_{quad} assesses whether the slope of a dose-response curve changes systematically at any point along the dose range. R^2_{lin} and R^2_{quad} quantify the relative contributions of the corresponding trend components to the overall shape of a dose response curve. As shown in Figure 2 and Table 1, the three dose-response curves contain significant linear and quadratic components. The R^2 values

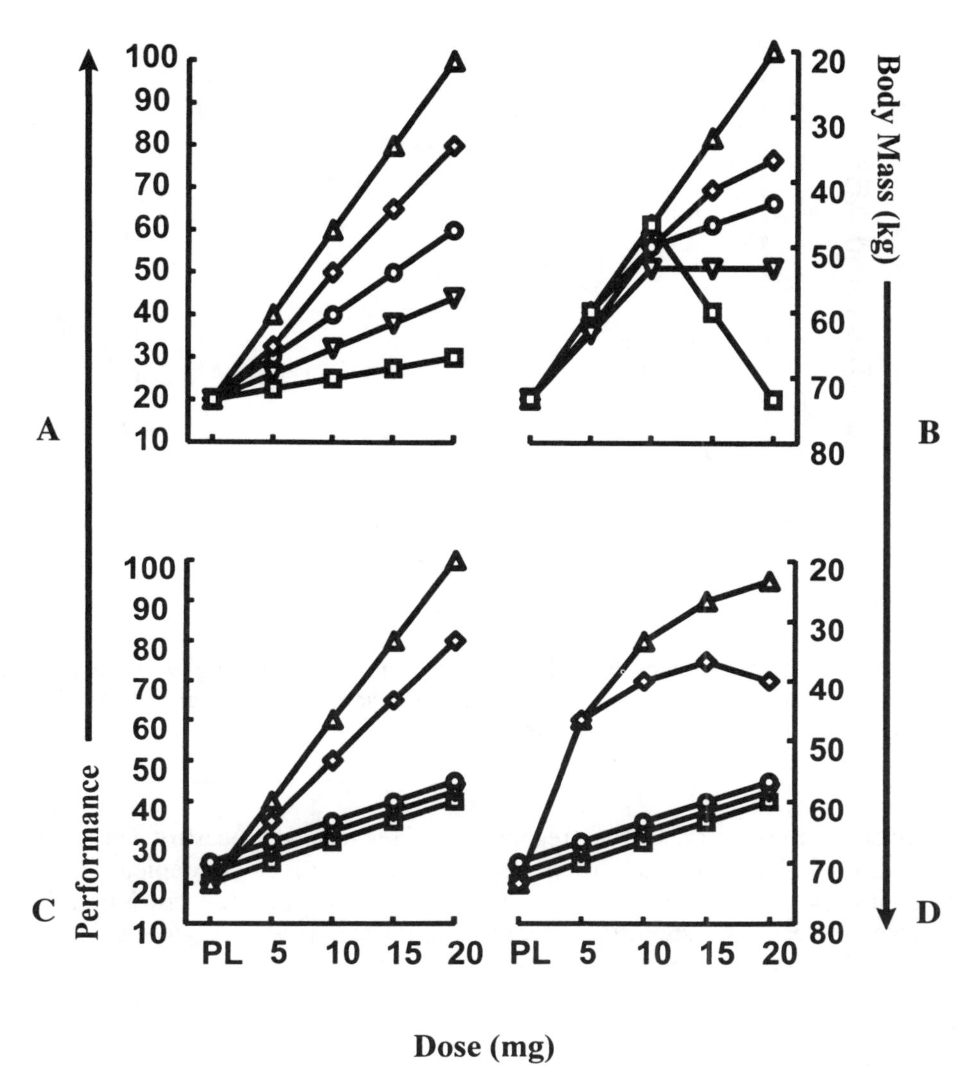

FIG. 1. Hypothetical variation in dose-response patterns as a function of body mass. **(A)** Incremental variations in slope as a continuous function of body mass. **(B)** Incremental variations in shape as a continuous function of body mass. **(C)** Variations in slope within discrete levels of body mass. **(D)** Variations in shape within discrete levels of body mass. Triangles = low weight; diamonds = moderately low weight; circles = medium weight; inverted triangles = moderately high weight; squares = high weight.

indicate that the dose-response curves are best characterized as largely linear, with rates of gain leveling off in the higher dose range. None of the linear and quadratic trend × weight interactions reached significance, indicating that the dose-response curve slope and curvature did not differ across children varying in body mass on any dependent measure.

Series II analyses

Subjects were grouped into quartiles on the basis of age-adjusted body mass to assess whether discrete subsets of children defined by mean differences in weight might exhibit

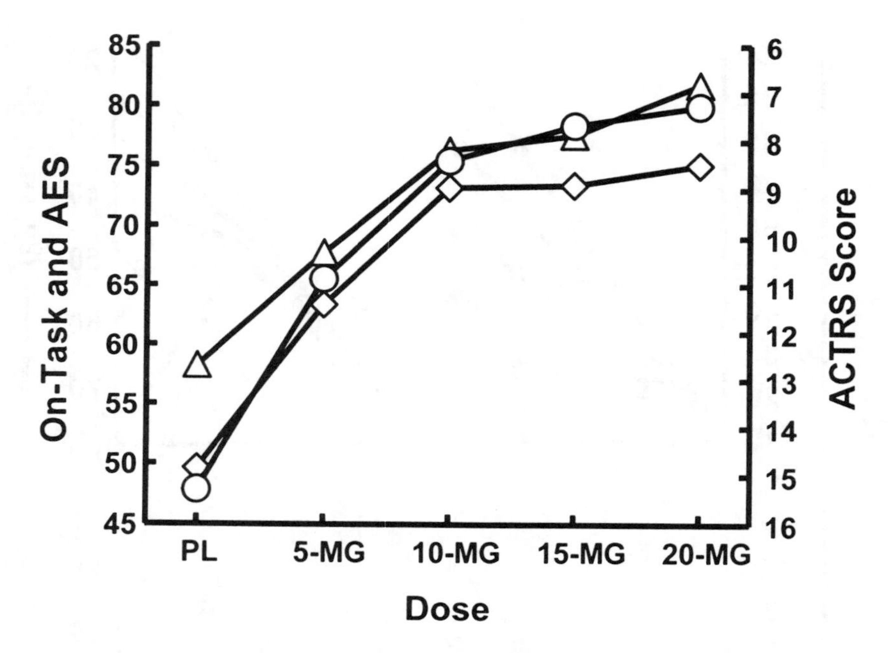

FIG. 2. Dose-response curves for all dependent measures. Triangles = percent on task; diamonds = academic efficiency; circles = ACTRS score. Improvement for all measures is indicated by upward movement on the ordinate.

different dose-response curves. Dose-response profiles for each measure were subsequently analyzed within and across these groups. Dose-response curves are depicted by quartile in Figure 3. Their parameters are described for each weight group (quartile) in Table 2.

The curves for each measure are generally similar across weight groups, although there are some subtle between-group differences in the degree of curvature for the on-task and academic performance domains (i.e., quartiles 1 and 2 showed evidence of curvature, whereas quartiles 3 and 4 did not).

TABLE 1. TREND ANALYSIS OF DOSE-RESPONSE CURVES

Measure	*Effect*	F_{lin}	R^2_{lin}	F_{Quad}	R^2_{quad}
% on-task	Dose	180.218***	0.92	23.02***	0.065
	kg	NS	—	NS	—
	Dose × kg	NS	—	NS	—
Academic efficiency	Dose	98.477***	0.81	23.712***	0.18
	kg	NS	—	NS	—
	Dose × kg	NS	—	NS	—
ACTRS	Dose	131.765***	0.84	23.828***	0.15
	kg	NS	—	NS	—
	Dose × kg	NS	—	NS	—

F_{lin} = significance test of linear trend component; R^2_{lin} = proportion of systematic dose variance accounted for by linear component; F_{quad} = significance test of quadratic trend component; R^2_{quad} = proportion of systematic dose variance accounted for by quadratic component; $***p < 0.001$; ACTRS = Abbreviated Connors Teacher Rating Scale; NS = not significant.

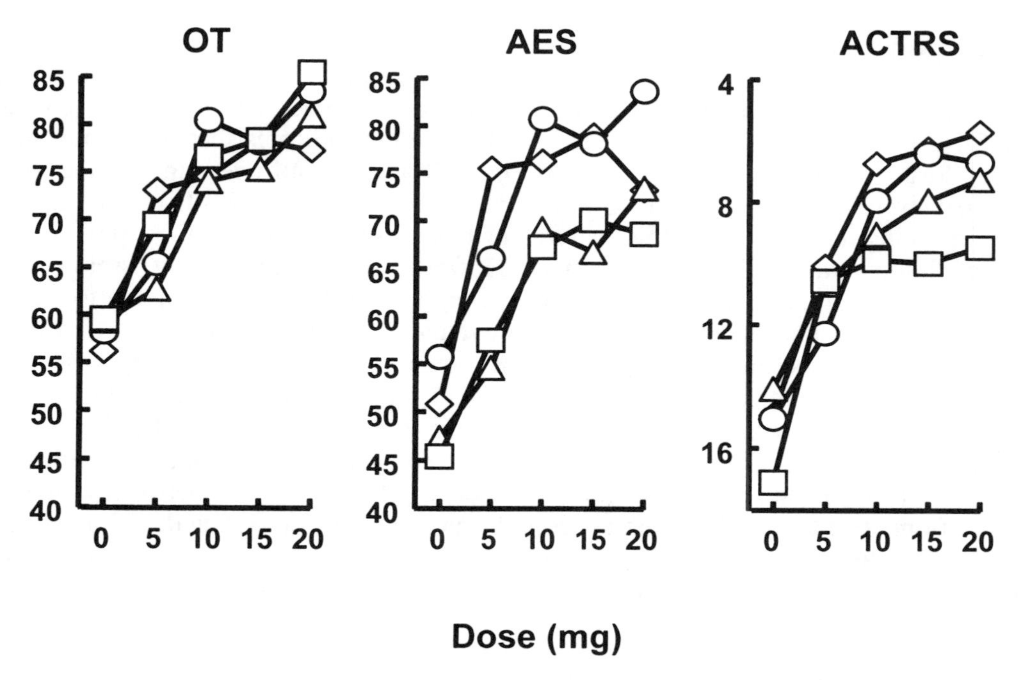

FIG. 3. Dose-response profiles among body mass quartiles. Diamonds = quartile 1; circles = quartile 2; triangles = quartile 3; squares = quartile 4; OT = % on task; AES = academic efficiency score; ACTRS = Abbreviated Conners Teaching Rating Scale score. On-task and AES scores are shown as percentages (left-hand ordinate). Raw score values are shown for the ACTRS. Improvement for the three measures is indicated by upward movement on the ordinate.

TABLE 2. DOSE-RESPONSE CURVE PROPERTIES ACROSS WEIGHT QUARTILES

Measure	*Quartile*	F_{lin}	R^2_{lin}	F_{quad}	R^2_{quad}
% on-task	1	32.93***	0.77	13.47***	0.18
	2	60.02***	0.85	5.99*	0.05
	3	35.50***	0.90	NS	—
	4	57.90***	0.94	NS	—
Academic efficiency	1	15.20***	0.66	7.780**	0.31
	2	35.94***	0.74	11.86***	0.23
	3	26.10***	0.85	NS	—
	4	23.73***	0.85	NS	—
ACTRS score	1	20.85***	0.80	5.976*	0.20
	2	47.01***	0.90	4.598*	0.08
	3	40.13***	0.89	5.430*	0.11
	4	28.35***	0.64	13.71***	0.27

OT = % on-task; F_{lin} = significance test of linear trend component; R^2_{lin} = proportion of systematic dose variance accounted for by linear component; F_{quad} = significance test of quadratic trend component; R^2_{quad} = proportion of systematic dose variance accounted for by quadratic component; $*p < 0.05$; $**p < 0.01$; $***p < 0.001$; ACTRS = Abbreviated Connors Teacher Rating Scale.

Linear and quadratic trend components were subsequently compared for all pairs of quartiles to evaluate whether these differences were of sufficient magnitude to discriminate the weight groups from one another. No significant differences emerged in terms of slope and shape for the pairs of dose-response curves. This finding indicates that the minor differences in dose-response patterns depicted in Figure 3 are of insufficient magnitude to justify their interpretation as evidence of weight-related differences in MPH response.

The preceding analyses show that patterns of dose-response were highly similar across groups of children varying in mean body mass. However, they do not directly assess whether group-level gains at each dose differed across weight quartiles. Gains relative to placebo at each dose were subsequently compared to evaluate this possibility. No differences in gain relative to placebo emerged across weight groups on any measure at any dose.

The preceding analyses evaluated whether incremental or discrete categorical differences in body mass were associated with differential patterns of response to MPH. Children differing widely in body mass consistently demonstrated comparable dose-response patterns with respect to both slope and shape. Moreover, no evidence of a relationship between weight and drug benefit relative to placebo emerged from the analysis. The preceding data, however, involve global statistics that do not directly assess the contribution of body mass to prediction of clinical responder status. This issue is addressed in the final series of analyses.

Series III analyses

The most global question raised by the purported interaction between body weight and drug response is whether body mass contributes to the identification of drug responders and non-responders. The relationship between body mass and responder status is illustrated in Figure 4.

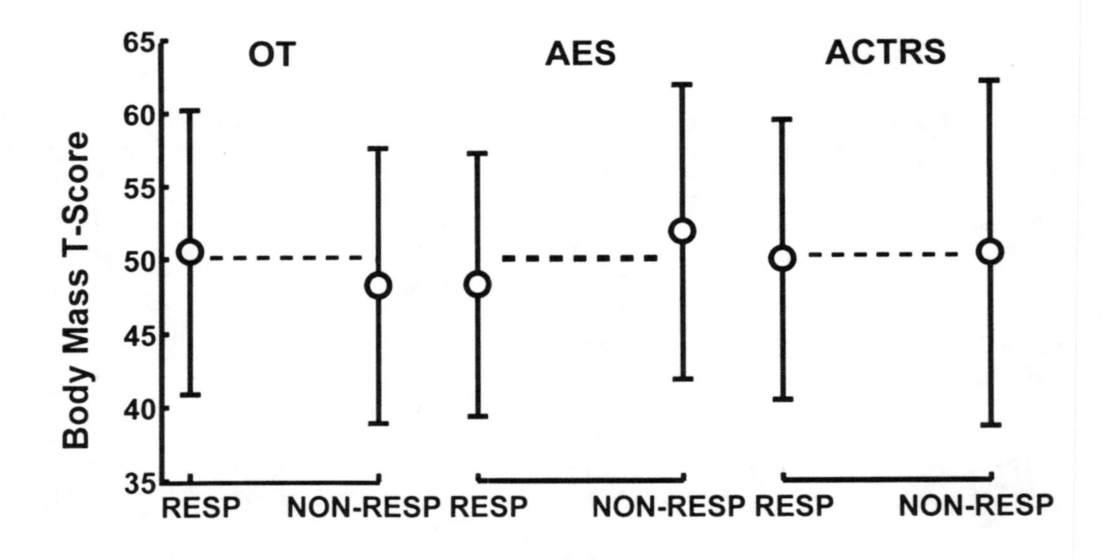

FIG. 4. Age-adjusted body mass (in standard T-scores) as a function of drug-response status. Resp = MPH responders; non-resp = MPH non-responders; OT = % on task; AES = academic efficiency score; ACTRS = Abbreviated Conners Teacher Rating Scale score.

Logistic regression analyses were performed to empirically examine whether body mass predicted membership in the responder and nonresponder categories for the three outcome variables. Logistic regression is a statistical technique explicitly designed for evaluating relationships involving categorical dependent measures. Body mass failed to predict responder status with respect to time on-task ($\chi^2(1) = 1.68$, NS), academic efficiency ($\chi^2(1) = 2.80$, NS), and ACTRS scores ($\chi^2(1) < 1$, NS).

The extent to which body mass could accurately identify children grouped on the basis of their optimal MPH dose was also of interest. Weight is plotted against optimal dose in Figure 5. A corresponding logistic regression analysis failed to show any systematic relationship between body weight and optimal dose for on-task ($\chi^2(3) = 4.17$, NS), academic efficiency ($\chi^2(3) = 3.28$, NS) and ACTRS score ($\chi^2(3) = 2.99$, NS).

The use of categorical rather than continuous outcome variables in the preceding analysis may have reduced statistical power sufficiently to enable otherwise significant relationships between clinical improvement on MPH and body mass to be overlooked. To evaluate this possibility, children's scores on their optimal MPH dose were expressed as a percentage of the change necessary to demonstrate clinical improvement. Standard regression analyses were subsequently used to determine whether these continuous improvement scores were related to body mass. The regression functions relating clinical improvement scores on each measure to body mass are depicted in Figure 6. None of the analyses yielded significant results (on-task: $R^2 = 0.0$, NS; academic efficiency: $R^2 = 0.029$, NS; ACTRS: $R^2 = 0.024$, NS).

In summary, the preceding analyses examined the extent to which body mass contributes to clinical prediction of MPH response in children. The data failed to reveal a significant relationship between weight and responder status, optimal MPH dose, or the degree of clinical improvement achieved at optimal dose.

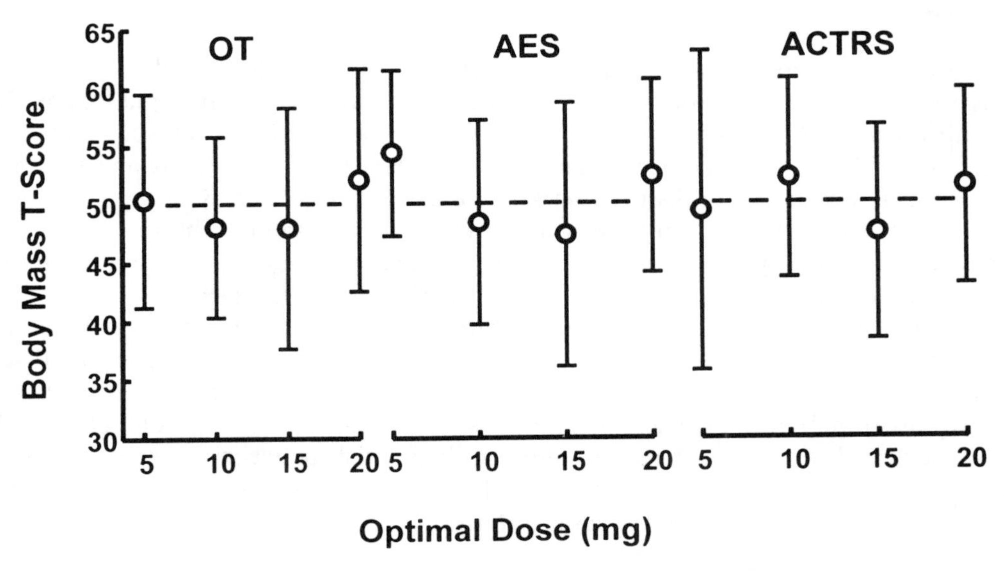

FIG. 5. Body mass as a function of optimal dose. Optimal dose = dose at which greatest clinical benefit observed; 5 = children showing largest MPH response at 5 mg; 10 = children showing largest MPH response at 10 mg; 15 = children showing largest MPH response at 15 mg; 20 = children showing largest MPH response at 20 mg; OT = % on task; AES = academic efficiency score; ACTRS = Abbreviated Conners Teacher Rating Scale score.

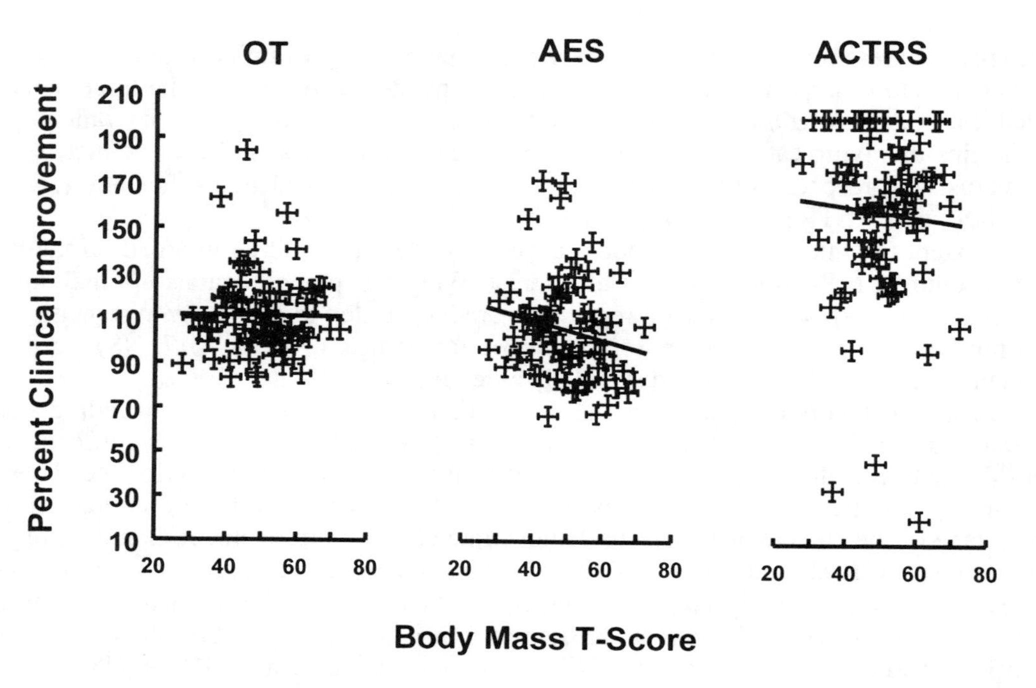

FIG. 6. Optimal improvement as a function of body mass. Percent clinical improvement = percentage of improvement necessary to show clinically significant change; OT = % on task; AES = academic efficiency score; ACTRS = Abbreviated Conners Teacher Rating Scale score; body mass T-score = age-adjusted body mass.

Comment

The mechanisms through which drugs exert their effects are multifaceted. The complexities involved have fueled attempts to identify moderator variables that might explain individual differences in response to similar drug doses. The practice of titrating medication on the basis of body weight emerged as one consequence of such efforts and was predicated on the assumption that distribution volume and other correlates of weight played a role in determining drug concentrations in targeted organ systems. The investigation described above was designed to comprehensively evaluate the degree to which weight contributes to methylphenidate response in children diagnosed with ADHD.

Dose-response profiles did not differ across children varying incrementally in body mass, nor were systematic variations in dose-response curve parameters observed across discrete groups of children differing in mean body mass. Neither did these groups differ with respect to gains from placebo at each dose. Finally, body mass failed to predict optimal dose or gains achieved at optimal dose, and did not distinguish between drug responders and nonresponders. Collectively, the findings fail to support the practice of titrating MPH on the basis of body weight in children with ADHD.

MEASURING CLINICAL OUTCOME IN CHILDREN RECEIVING MPH

The majority of treatment outcome research has emphasized three primary areas of inquiry: The effects of psychostimulants on (1) behaviors that are assumed to represent core components of the disorder itself such as attention, impulsivity, and overactivity; (2) interpersonal relationships or interaction styles; and (3) learning as it relates to classroom academic performance and achievement.

Findings representative of the latter area of inquiry have been equivocal and frequently debated over the past decade. The conundrum is embodied in the paradoxical findings that psychostimulants appear to enhance children's behavior on a short-term basis in both analog (Whalen et al., 1979) and natural classroom environments (Rapport et al., 1987), yet do not appear to translate into long-term gains related to academic achievement (Weiss and Hechtman, 1993). Conclusions drawn from long-term outcome studies have been criticized on methodological grounds, and numerous explanations have been offered to account for the paradoxical findings (Pelham and Murphy, 1986). Chief among the concerns is the traditional practice of evaluating treatment response on the basis of parents' and/or teachers' reports of children's social deportment. The practice has been questioned because of the inadequacy of such measures for establishing optimal dosage, especially with respect to cognitive and academic functioning (Rapport, 1990).

Questions concerning whether behavior and learning are affected at different dosage levels as proposed in the seminal study by Sprague and Sleator (1977) are also relevant to long-term outcome. Although most recent outcome studies have found similar dose-related effects on children's behavior and academic performance, their results have been limited by restricted dosage ranges and/or have been derived from analog settings using contrived rather than actual classroom academic assignments.

There is also relatively limited information available concerning the extent to which MPH-treated children approach normal levels of functioning. Previous outcome studies using standard statistical significance tests have reported enhanced attention (Loney et al., 1979; Whalen et al., 1979), reduced aggressiveness (Hinshaw et al., 1989), and improvements in some aspects of classroom behavior (Abikoff and Gittelman, 1985) sufficient to render MPH-treated children indistinguishable from normal control children. Standard analyses, notwithstanding, do not allow specifying the extent to which individual MPH-treated children attain levels of functioning comparable with those of their normal peers, improve while remaining impaired, or deteriorate during treatment.

The outcome study described below addresses questions concerning the measurement of MPH effects in the cohort of children with ADHD described earlier. More specifically, the effects of MPH on children's attention, academic efficiency (AES), and weekly teachers' ratings of classroom behavior (ACTRS) were subjected to a three-tier level of analysis. In the first series, broad effects of dose, between-dose differences, and trend analyses for the ADHD group are described. In the second series, responder status is evaluated within and across doses on each measure to assess the extent to which treated children approach normal levels of functioning. The third series examines relationships among responder status categories across three outcome measures to evaluate the utility of these different domains as broad indices of MPH response.

Results

Series I analysis: main effects, between-dose differences, and trend analyses

Broad dose effects. Children's attention (on-task), percentage of academic assignments completed correctly (AES), and weekly teachers' ratings (ACTRS) under baseline, placebo, and the four active MPH conditions (5 mg, 10 mg, 15 mg, 20 mg) were analyzed using a 6 (dose condition) × 3 (classroom measures) multivariate analysis of variance. A significant main effect emerged for dose condition (Wilks' lambda [5,71] = .185, $p < 0.001$), indicating that scores on the composite of the three classroom measures changed reliably as a function of dose.

Follow-up univariate analyses of variance (ANOVAs) with repeated measures across dose were performed to examine the overall effects of MPH on each dependent variable. Significant main effects of dose emerged for children's attention ($F[5,375] = 78.12$, $p < 0.00001$), academic efficiency ($F[5,375] = 43.46$, $p < 0.00001$), and teachers' ratings of classroom behavior ($F[5,375] = 65.26$, $p < 0.00001$). The two components of the academic efficiency measure were also analyzed to determine whether they were affected to a similar degree by MPH. Significant effects were observed for both the percent-complete ($F[5,375] = 34.59$, $p < 0.00001$) and percent-correct ($F[5,375] = 14.66$, $p < 0.00001$) components.

Magnitude of drug effects. Omega-squared values were calculated separately for the significant ANOVAs to determine the approximate percentage of variance of each dependent variable accounted for by MPH dose. These values indicated that dose accounted for a significant amount of variance for children's attention (46%), academic efficiency (32%), and teachers' ratings (41%). A stronger relationship was found between dose and the percent-complete (27%) than the percent-correct (13%) component of the academic efficiency measure.

Between-dose differences. Post hoc comparisons, using the Dunn (Bonferroni) correction to control for experiment-wise error rates, were conducted as a follow-up to all significant ANOVAs to elucidate specific between-dose differences for each measure. The results are summarized in Table 3. Children's attention, academic efficiency, and classroom behavior were significantly enhanced under all active medication conditions relative to baseline and placebo ($p < 0.00001$). Moreover, 10-mg, 15-mg, and 20-mg doses resulted in significant improvement for all three classroom measures compared with the 5-mg dose ($p < 0.0001$). Children's attention was also significantly enhanced under the 20-mg dose compared with the 10-mg ($p < 0.0001$) and 15-mg dose ($p < 0.01$). No additional between-dose differences were significant.

Different patterns of between-dose differences emerged for the percent-complete and percent-correct components of academic efficiency. Children completed a significantly greater percentage of academic assignments under the 10-mg, 15-mg, and 20-mg MPH conditions compared to baseline, placebo, and 5 mg ($p < 0.001$). In contrast, their accuracy on academic assignments was improved under all MPH conditions relative to baseline and placebo ($p < 0.001$), but no other differences between active drug conditions were evident (see Table 3).

Trend analyses. Analyses of trend were performed using placebo and active medication conditions to examine the shape of the relationships among dose and children's attention, academic efficiency, and ACTRS scores. The relative contributions of these trend components to the overall shape of each dose-response profile was evaluated by computing the proportion of the dose effect on each measure accounted for by each trend component (R^2_{trend}; Kepel, 1991).

As shown in Table 4, all three dose-response curves were characterized by both significant linear and quadratic trends. Higher-order trends (e.g., cubic) were not significant. The linear component accounted for the greatest percentage of explained variance for all three measures, indicating that classroom functioning improved as a linear function of increasing dose in the lower dose range, with rates of improvement decreasing slightly at doses exceeding 10 mg.

TABLE 3. SUMMARY OF BETWEEN-DOSE COMPARISONS

Measure	*Placebo*	*5 mg*	*10 mg*	*15 mg*	*20 mg*
Attention (on-task)					
Baseline	NS	****	****	****	****
Placebo	NS	****	****	****	****
5 mg	NS	NS	****	****	****
10 mg	NS	NS	NS	NS	***
15 mg	NS	NS	NS	NS	*
Academic efficiency					
Baseline	NS	****	****	****	****
Placebo	NS	****	****	****	****
5 mg	NS	NS	**	**	**
ACTRS scores					
Baseline	NS	****	****	****	****
Placebo	NS	****	****	****	****
5 mg	NS	NS	**	****	****

****$p < 0.00001$; ***$p < 0.0001$; **$p < 0.001$; *$p < 0.01$. All significant differences indicate that performance or behavior ratings under dose shown at the top of the table were superior to those shown along the left side of the table. ACTRS = Abbreviated Conners Teacher Rating Scale.

Series II analyses: evaluation of responder status

Responder status by dose. Children were categorized as normalized, improved, and unchanged on each measure as described previously. The percentages of the ADHD sample falling in these categories are shown in Figure 7 (see top three graphs of Figure 7). Inspection of the upper left-hand graph reveals that increasingly large proportions of treated children exhibited attention and classroom behavior falling within the normal range as an incremental function of dose. Children's AES scores, in contrast, showed an initially steep rise between placebo and 10-mg conditions, without substantial changes thereafter.

Rates of improvement without normalization are depicted in the upper center graph of Figure 7. Relatively few children fell in this category on measures of attention and academic efficiency across dose conditions. In contrast, modest percentages of the sample

TABLE 4. SUMMARY OF TREND ANALYSES

Measure	*Trend Component*	*F*	R^2_{Trend}	F_{res}
Attention (on-task)	Linear	182.02***	0.92	6.76*
	Quadratic	22.63**	0.07	NS
Academic efficiency score	Linear	99.77***	0.81	9.11*
	Quadratic	23.69***	0.18	NS
ACTRS Scores	Linear	132.92***	0.84	11.01*
	Quadratic	28.78***	0.15	NS

***$p < 0.00001$; **$p < 0.0001$; *$p < 0.001$; R^2_{Trend} = proportion of dose effect attributable to corresponding trend component; F_{res} = significance test determining whether variance remaining after extraction of trend justifies extraction of next higher order trend component. ACTRS = Abbreviated Connors Teacher Rating Scale.

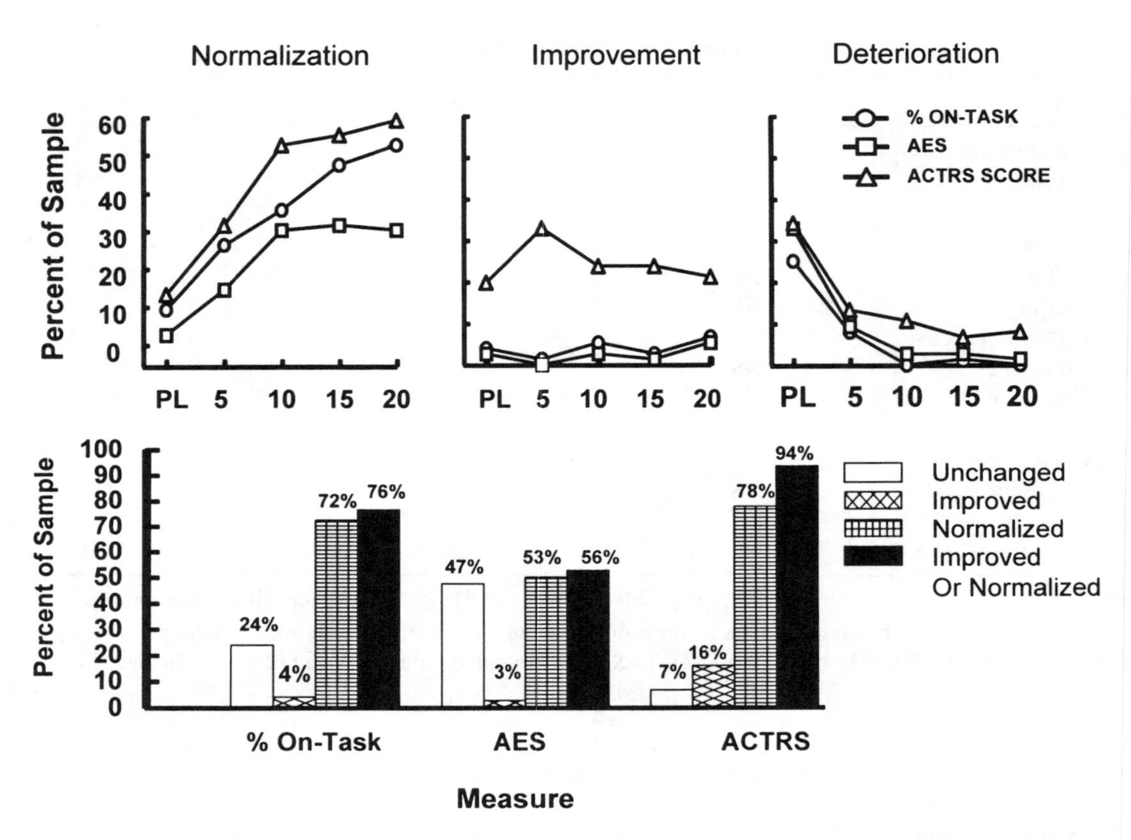

FIG. 7. Upper three graphs: clinical status of sample (n = 76) across MPH and placebo (PL) dose conditions; open circles = % on task; open squares = academic efficiency scores; open triangles = Abbreviated Conners Teacher Rating Scale scores (ACTRS). All categories referenced against baseline levels of functioning. Lower graph: Clinical status of sample collapsed across dose conditions: AES = academic efficiency scores; ACTRS = Abbreviated Conners Teacher Rating Scale Scores.

showed improvement without normalization in classroom behavior as a function of MPH treatment, with the largest percentage occurring with the 5-mg dose.

Between 25% and 35% of children in the sample significantly deteriorated in their classroom functioning under the placebo condition, as might be expected (see upper right-hand graphs in Figure 7). Deterioration rates declined subsequently with increasing dose. Approximately 10% of the ADHD children showed deterioration in their classroom behavior in several of the active medication conditions. One of these children showed deterioration relative to placebo at every dose on the teacher-rating measure, whereas all the others demonstrated improvement with or without normalization after receiving a higher MPH dose. This finding suggests that children showing deterioration at any given dose were not showing evidence of behavioral toxicity. Instead, it appears that the vast majority of them required higher doses of MPH.

Responder status across dose conditions. Responder-category membership rates collapsed across dose conditions are depicted in the bottom graph of Figure 7. Information contained in the figure addresses a more general, but practical clinical question: What is the likelihood that children will show normalization, significant improvement without normalization, or lack of change in different areas of their classroom functioning when prescribed a trial regimen of between 5 mg and 20 mg of MPH?

Inspection of Figure 7 reveals that nearly three fourths of the sample showed normalized attention in the classroom with at least one MPH dose, with 76% evidencing either normalized or significantly improved attention as a function of treatment. Teachers' ratings of classroom behavior showed even higher rates of clinical response, with 94% of the children exhibiting either significantly improved or normalized functioning. In contrast, only 53% of the children evidenced significantly improved or normalized academic functioning with treatment. A substantial number of those failing to show academic treatment benefit, however, were difficult to classify, as their scores fell above the cutoff defining the normal range of functioning despite their having not exhibited sufficient change from baseline to be categorized as improved.

Series III analyses: behavioral specificity and prediction of MPH response

A basic precept of behavioral assessment argues that evaluation and treatment should target variables that, when changed, promote gains in other areas. Applied to the clinical task of titrating MPH, the problem is reduced to the identification of central variables operative in children's daily lives that determine levels of functioning across a broad array of important domains.

This task is easier to describe than it is to achieve. Traditional parametric correlations between rates of change across measures are often low because of the poor reliability associated with change scores (Linn and Slinde, 1977). Even when reliability is adequate, however, there remains a potentially serious methodological problem. If improvement on a particular predictor is either necessary-but-not-sufficient or, conversely, sufficient-but-not-necessary to achievement of benefit in other areas, the linear relationship between predictor and outcome improvement score will be attenuated. For example, if attentional improvement is sufficient-but-not-necessary to yield changes in classroom behavior, then rates of change on this pair of measures will be in close agreement among children improving in attention but moderate or weak among those who do not. This will be reflected in a reduced correlation between gains on measures of attention and classroom behavior.

Analysis of positive and negative predictive power helps disentangle some of these complexities. These quantities are based on relationships between categorical outcomes such as "response" and "nonresponse." Positive predictive power (PPP) describes the conditional probability of a response on an outcome measure given a response on the predictor. Negative predictive power (NPP) refers to the converse probability: the likelihood of no-response on an outcome variable given a lack of response on a predictor. High values of both PPP and NPP indicate that change on a predictor is both necessary-and-sufficient to yield gains on the corresponding outcome variable. High values of PPP combined with low NPP suggest that gain on a predictor is sufficient-but-not-necessary to attain benefit of an outcome, whereas low PPP combined with high NPP values indicate that response on the predictor is necessary-but-not-sufficient to response on the outcome.

In order to assess the utility of the three classroom measures as indicators of broad-spectrum treatment benefit, children were categorized as either responders or nonresponders on the three classroom variables (percentage on-task, academic efficiency, and ACTRS scores) by use of methods described previously. In view of recent arguments concerning the potential etiologic significance of behavioral disinhibition in ADHD (Quay, 1988), children's responder status was also determined on the basis of total scores derived from the Teacher Self-Control Rating Scale (TSCRS; Humphrey, 1982). Responders were subjects showing either normalization or improvement with at least one active MPH dose. PPP and NPP were then computed for various pairs of the four measures.

Two analyses were conducted. The first assessed the relative predictive power of academic responder status relative to other classroom variables. The second analysis integrated the broad pattern of PPP and NPP rates for all combinations of the four variables in order to assess which variables were most appropriate as targets of MPH titration.

Analysis I. The positive and negative predictive power of attention, ACTRS scores, and ratings on the TSCRS (self-control) with respect to children's academic performance are depicted in the upper portion of Figure 8. PPP and NPP coefficients are shown as unbracketed and bracketed (parenthetical) values, respectively. Unidirectional arrows indicate that the two teacher rating scales (ACTRS, TSCRS) and direct observations of children's attention in class serve as the predictor variables for the academic performance outcome measure. The results shown in the figure reveal that changes in children's attention, general classroom behavior (ACTRS scores), and self-control all appear to be necessary-but-not-sufficient to yield commensurate benefit in the academic domain as indicated by the low to moderate PPP and relatively high NPP values. The attention measure, for example, reveals that there is a 60% probability (PPP = 0.60) of a child showing improved academic performance (i.e., is an academic responder) given improved attention with at least one of the active MPH doses. In a similar vein, there is a 72% probability (NPP = 0.72) that a child will fail to be an academic responder if his or her attention is not improved with at least one active dose. Notice that values associated with the two teacher rating scales (ACTRS, TSCRS) are remarkably similar to one another and can probably be used interchangeably.

The lower portion of Figure 8 shows PPP and NPP values when children's academic performance is used as the predictor variable. Interpretation of the values indicates that improved academic performance is sufficient-but-not-necessary for gains in other areas of classroom functioning. High PPP rates (0.88, 0.98, 0.93) indicate that there is an 88% to 98% probability of a child showing improved attention, classroom behavior and self-control, respectively, if the child shows significant improvement in academic performance (i.e., is an academic responder). NPP values indicate that a majority of children—1.0 minus 0.36, 0.11, and 0.22, or 64%, 89%, and 78%—will show improved attention, classroom behavior, and self-control, respectively, without evidencing improved academic performance. Thus, academic improvement is sufficient to yield improvement in other domains but is not necessary to them, since benefits in attention to task and general classroom behavior were frequently observed without corresponding academic gains.

Analysis II. The relationship among all possible pairs of measures, as both predictor and outcome variables, is shown in Figure 9. The results indicate that improvement in attention, classroom behavior, and self-control are likely to parallel one another regardless of which is used as a target for MPH titration. Positive changes in the three target measures, however, are unlikely to result in concomitant gains in the academic performance domain.

Examination of the ACTRS, one of the most widely used instruments for assessing MPH response in children, nicely illustrates this predicament. When used as a predictor measure, PPP and NPP values of 0.55 and 0.80 were observed, respectively (see values over unidirectional line drawn from ACTRS to Academic Performance in Figure 9). These values indicate that only 55% of children receiving improved ACTRS scores as a function of MPH therapy demonstrated corresponding improvement in academic performance. The NPP value of 0.80 indicates that 80% of children failing to evidence improved ACTRS scores also fail

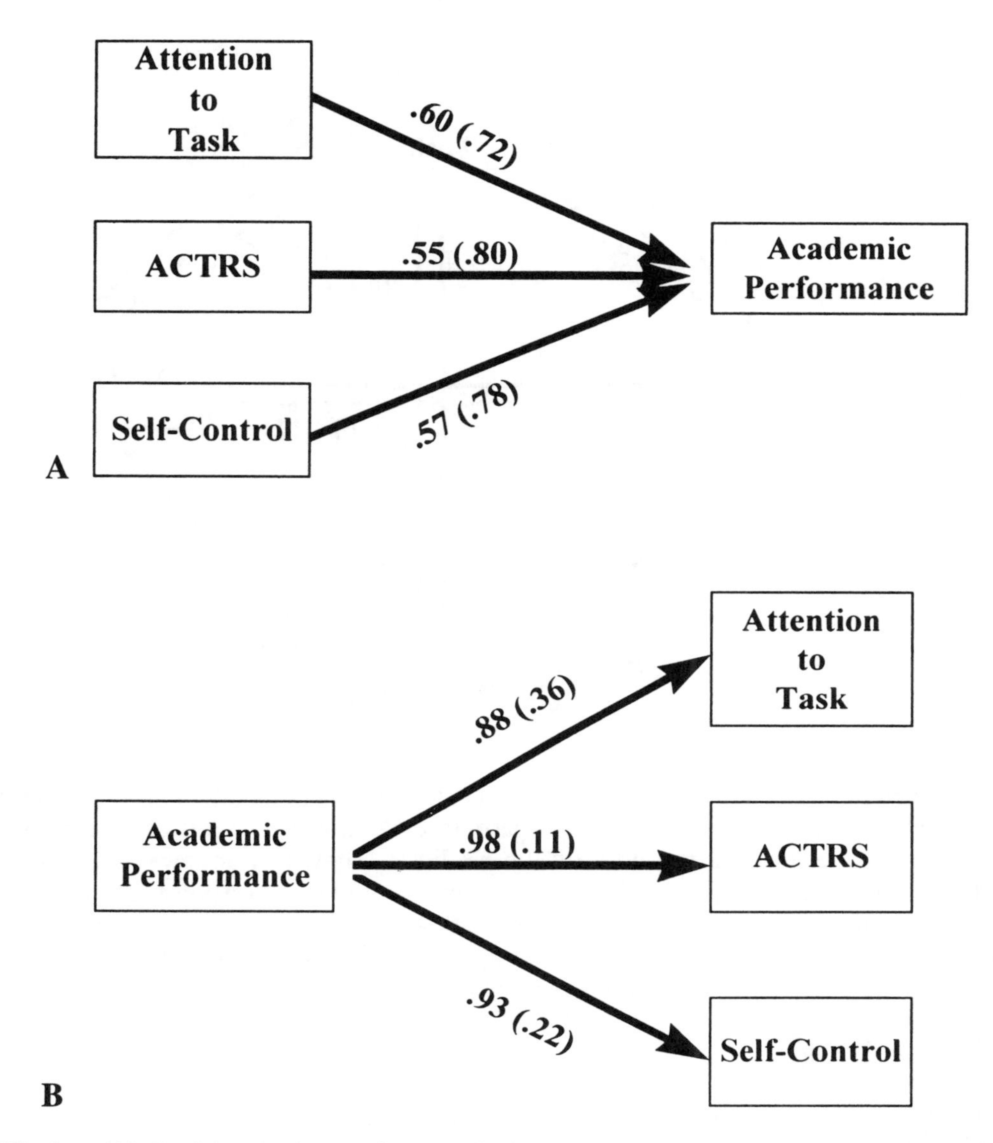

FIG. 8. **(A)** Positive and negative predictive powers of classroom attention, and teachers' ratings of behavior and self-control with respect to academic responder status. **(B)** Positive and negative predictive power of academic efficiency with respect to other classroom variables. Positive predictive power = conditional probability of a clinically significant response on an outcome variable, given a response on the predictor (shown as unbracketed values on arrows); negative predictive power = conditional probability of no response on an outcome variable, given no response on the predictor (shown as bracketed values); ACTRS = Abbreviated Conners Teacher Rating Scale.

to evidence improvement in their academic performance. Stated differently, only 20% of children who failed to show improved classroom conduct improved academically. Collectively, the values indicate that the ACTRS is not a particularly useful indicator of improvement in children's academic performance; however, it is nearly always a prerequisite for academic improvement (i.e., gains in this area are necessary-but-not-sufficient to yield academic improvement).

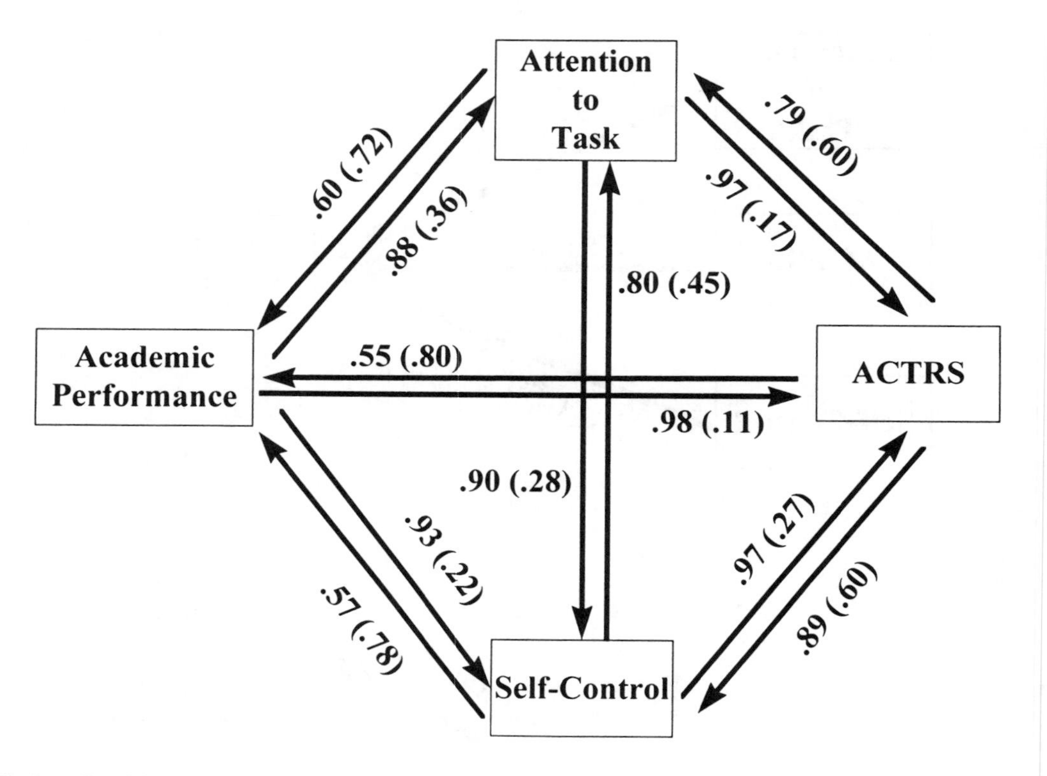

FIG. 9. Positive and negative predictive powers for combinations of classroom variables. Positive predictive power = conditional probability of a clinically significant response on an outcome variable, given a response on the predictor (shown as unbracketed values on arrows); negative predictive power = conditional probability of no response on an outcome variable given no response on the predictor (shown as bracketed values on arrows); ACTRS = Abbreviated Conners Teacher Rating Scale. Two-way arrows indicate bidirectional, sufficient-not-necessary relations between variables.

Examination of the converse relationship reveals a dramatically different picture. Using academic performance as the predictor variable results in PPP and NPP values of 0.98 and 0.11, respectively (see values below unidirectional line drawn from Academic Performance to ACTRS in Figure 9). The PPP coefficient indicates that 98% of the children demonstrating improved academic performance as a function of MPH therapy will show concomitant improvement in their classroom behavior. Conversely, the NPP coefficient indicates that 89% of children who fail to evidence improvement in their academic performance will nevertheless show improvement in classroom conduct.

Comment

Collectively, these results show that academic performance serves as an extremely useful target variable for purposes of titrating MPH among children with ADHD. Although not all children show a clinical response on this measure, it is highly probable that those who do will show commensurate gains in other areas. Moreover, those who do not show academic benefit are nevertheless very likely to improve in other domains when academic functioning is used as a target variable.

Evidence supporting the use of other variables as bellwethers of broad-spectrum change is not as compelling. Measures of classroom attention, self-control, and general deportment all reflect each other quite well, but none serves adequately as an index of academic performance. Although overt behavior problems often are the primary presenting problems at the time of clinical referral, children with ADHD are at high risk for academic failure and dropping out as they progress through their school years, and the latter outcomes impose barriers to adjustment that are at least as significant as overt behavior problems. These observations, combined with the expense in time and labor of controlled clinical drug trials, have a clear implication: Academic performance should serve as the primary target variable when MPH response is titrated in children with ADHD.

SUMMARY

Three complementary questions were addressed in the chapter. Is body mass a useful predictor of MPH response? Do children with ADHD derive significant clinical benefit from MPH therapy? And which behaviors should be targeted for intervention purposes? The first question was addressed by exploring the potential interaction between body mass and MPH response. The relationship was examined using body mass as (1) a continuous variable, (2) a discrete variable (predicated on the assumption that particular weight subgroups may show a unique response), and (3) an indicator for children evidencing a well-defined clinical response on various outcome measures. Collectively, the results revealed no evidence that body mass (weight in kgm) is associated with clinical response in children undergoing MPH therapy. Although one cannot prove the null hypothesis, there appears to be no compelling reason to titrate MPH on the basis of body mass.

The second question addressed in the chapter transcends the usual reporting of statistically significant change observed in children receiving MPH therapy by examining the extent to which this change is clinically meaningful. This was accomplished by comparing the ADHD sample with a matched control sample of normal children on three classroom outcome measures (attention, conduct, and academic efficiency), which in turn, enabled us to determine the degree to which ADHD children approached or achieved normal functioning. Our findings indicate that the attention span, or ability to pay attention in a regular classroom, is significantly improved or normalized in approximately 75% of children with ADHD taking at least one of four active MPH doses. Larger percentages of children benefit from MPH therapy in terms of their classroom conduct. Seventy-eight percent of the sample evidenced normal levels of classroom behavior as determined by teachers' ratings, whereas an impressive 94% of the sample showed either significantly improved or normal functioning in this domain. In contrast, only half of the sample significantly improved or reached normal levels of functioning in terms of their academic efficiency. Collectively, these findings shed some light on the apparent enigma between short-term MPH efficacy investigations and long-term follow-up studies. The latter are unanimous in demonstrating that children with ADHD are at continued risk for adult psychopathology, with an estimated 24% of children dropping out of school by the 11th grade because of their poor grades and collective academic failures (Mannuzza et al., 1993). Improved and even normalized levels of attention and behavior in the classroom, in and of themselves, may not be the most appropriate targets for titration purposes, as discussed below.

The third question addressed in the chapter has important implications for clinicians: Given the availability of different outcome measures commonly used for titrating MPH response in children with ADHD, can they be used interchangeably, or does one have particular benefits not shared by others? The answer to the question largely depends on the clinician's perspective concerning which domains of functioning are central to both the short-term and long-term well-being of the child being treated. Most children considered as candidates for MPH therapy are referred because of their disruptive conduct in and out of the classroom. As a result, conduct merits its rightful place as a primary target for MPH titration. The primary disadvantages encountered in targeting disruptive behavior, however, are that changes in this domain are unlikely to yield corresponding benefit with respect to a child's academic performance in the classroom and may mask learning difficulties when behavior control improves. This takes on additional importance in light of the robust relationship between academic performance and academic achievement in the short term, coupled with compelling evidence that academic achievement is one of the strongest predictors of adult adjustment and socioeconomic status. (Note: Academic achievement refers to information children can recall on a standardized test, whereas academic performance refers to how well children perform within a classroom setting on a day-to-day basis.) A reasonable compromise is to use an instrument such as the Academic Performance Rating Scale (APRS; DuPaul et al., 1991). The scale has sound psychometric properties, has proven sensitivity to overall and between-dose drug effects, requires minimal teacher time for completion, and includes factors covering both academic and behavioral domains.

There is a clear need to elucidate a comprehensive and integrated explanation of MPH effects that embraces multiple domains and levels of analysis. Although attempts have been made to derive predictive models of psychostimulant response on empirical (Buitelaar et al., 1995; Taylor et al., 1987) and theoretical grounds, they have yet to receive thorough and systematic evaluation. Until more comprehensive models enable refined prediction of response to MPH, optimal management of children receiving MPH should deemphasize weight-based titration. Systematic monitoring of emergent symptoms and response to a range of absolute doses across multiple domains using standardized instruments that target both behavioral control and academic performance is recommended. Even among MPH responders, large numbers of children with ADHD will require supplementary interventions if they are to succeed academically.

REFERENCES

Abikoff, H. & Gittelman, R. (1985), The normalizing effects of methylphenidate on the classroom behavior of ADDH children. *J. Abnorm. Child Psychol.*, 13:33–44.

Abikoff, H., Klein, R.G. (1992), Attention-deficit hyperactivity and conduct disorder: Comorbidity and implications for treatment. *J. Consult. Clin. Psychol.*, 60:881–892.

Abikoff, H., Klein, R.G., Klass, E., & Ganeles, D. (1987), Methylphenidate in the treatment of conduct disordered children. Presented at the American Academy of Child and Adolescent Psychiatry Annual Meeting, October, Washington, DC.

American Psychiatric Association (1980), *Diagnostic and Statistical Manual of Mental Disorders, 3rd ed.* (*DSM-III*). Washington, DC: American Psychiatric Association.

American Psychiatric Association (1994), *Diagnostic and Statistical Manual of Mental Disorders, 4th ed.* (*DSM-IV*). Washington, DC: American Psychiatric Association.

Barkley, R.A. (1990), *Hyperactive Children: A Handbook for Diagnosis and Treatment.* New York: Guilford Press.

Blouin, A.G., Conners, C.K., Seidel, W.T. & Blouin, J. (1989), The independence of hyperactivity from conduct disorder: Methodological considerations. *Can. J. Psychiatry*, 34:279–282.

Buitelaar, J.K., Rutger, J.V.G., Swaab-Barneveld, H. & Kuiper, M. (1995), Prediction of clinical response to methylphenidate in children with attention-deficit hyperactivity disorder. *J. Am. Acad. Child Adolesc. Psychiatry*, 34:1025–1032.

Douglas, V.I., Barr, R.G., O'Neill, M.E. & Britton, B.G. (1986), Dosage effects and individual responsivity to methylphenidate on the cognitive, learning and academic performance of children with attention deficit disorder in the laboratory and the classroom. *J. Child Psychol. Psychiatry*, 27:191–211.

Dunn, L.M. & Dunn, L.M. (1981), *Peabody Picture Vocabulary Test—Revised.* Circle Pines, MN: American Guidance Service.

DuPaul, J.G. & Rapport, M.D. (1993), Does methylphenidate normalize the classroom performance of children with attention deficit disorder? *J. Am. Acad. Child Adolesc. Psychiatry*, 32:190–198.

DuPaul, J.G., Rapport, M.D. & Perriello, L.M. (1991), Teacher ratings of academic skills: The development of the Academic Performance Rating Scale. *Sch. Psychol. Rev.*, 20: 284–300.

Hinshaw, S.P. (1987), On the distinction between attentional deficits/hyperactivity and conduct problems/aggression in child psychopathology. *Psychol. Bull.*, 101:443–463.

Hinshaw, S.P., Henker, B., Whalen, C.K., Erhardt, D.K. & Dunnington, R.E. (1989), Aggressive, prosocial, and nonsocial behavior in hyperactive boys: Dose effects of methylphenidate in naturalistic settings. *J. Consult. Clin. Psychol.*, 57:636–643.

Humphrey, L.L. (1982), Children's and teachers' perspectives on children's self-control: The development of two rating scales. *J. Consult. Clin. Psychol.*, 50:624–633.

Jacobson, N.S. & Truax, P. (1991), Clinical significance: A statistical approach to defining meaningful change in psychopathology research. *J. Consult. Clin. Psychol.*, 59:12–19.

Kazdin, A. & Kagan, J. (1994), Models of dysfunction in developmental psychopathology. *Clin. Psychol. Sci. Pract.*, 1:35–52.

Kepel, G. (1991), *Design and Analysis: A Researcher's Handbook, 3rd ed.* Englewood, NJ: Prentice-Hall, pp. 141–162.

Lahey, B.B., Piacentini, J.C., McBurnett, K., Stone, P., Hartdagen, M.A. & Hynd G. (1988), Psychopathology in the parents of children with conduct disorder and hyperactivity. *J. Am. Acad. Child Adolesc. Psychiatry*, 27:163–170.

Linn, R.L. & Slinde, J.A. (1977), The determination of the significance of change between pre- and post-testing periods. *Rev. Educ. Research*, 47:121–150.

Loeber, R., Brinthaupt, V.P. & Green, S.M. (1990), Attention deficits, impulsivity, and hyperactivity with or without conduct problems: Relationships and delinquency and unique contextual factors. In: *Behavior Disorders of Adolescence: Research Intervention and Policy in Clinical Practice and School Settings*, eds. R.J. McMahan & R.D. Peters. New York: Plenum Press.

Loney, J., Weissenburger, F.E., Woolson, R.F. & Lichty, E.C. (1979), Comparing psychological and pharmacological treatments for hyperkinetic boys and their classmates. *J. Abnorm. Child Psychol.*, 7:133–143.

Mannuzza, S., Klein, R.G., Bessler, A., Malloy, P. & LaPadula, M. (1993), Adult outcome of hyperactive boys: Educational achievement, occupational rank, and psychiatric status. *Arch. Gen. Psychiatry*, 50:565–576.

Orvaschel, H., Puig-Antich, J., Chambers, L.W., Tabrizi, M.A. & Johnson, R.A. (1982), Retrospective assessment of prepubertal major depression with the Kiddie-SADS-E. *J. Am. Acad. Child Adolesc. Psychiatry*, 21:392–397.

Pelham, W.E., Bender, M.E., Caddell, J.M., Booth, S. & Moorer, S. (1985), The dose-response effects of methylphenidate on classroom academic and social behavior in children with attention deficit disorder. *Arch. Gen. Psychiatry*, 42:948–952.

Pelham, W.E. & Murphy, H.A. (1986), Attention deficit and conduct disorders. In: *Pharmacological and Behavioral Treatment: An Integrative Approach*, ed., M. Hersen. New York: John Wiley & Sons, Inc., pp. 108–148.

Quay, H.C. (1988), Attention deficit disorder and the behavioral inhibition system: The relevance of the neuropsychological theory of Jeffrey A. Gray. In: *Attention Deficit Disorder, vol. 3*, eds., L.M. Bloomingdale & J. Sergeant. Oxford: Pergamon Press, pp. 117–125.

Rapport, M.D. (1990), Controlled studies of the effects of psychostimulants on children's functioning in clinic and classroom settings. In: *Attention Deficit Hyperactivity Disorder*, eds., K. Conners & M. Kinsbourne. Munich, Germany: MMV Medizin Verlag, pp. 77–111.

Rapport, M.D. (1995), Response to letter to the editor. *J. Am. Acad. Child Adolesc. Psychiatry*, 34:1559.

Rapport, M.D., Denney, C., DuPaul, G.J., & Gardner, M.J. (1994), Attention deficit disorder and methylphenidate: Normalization rates, clinical effectiveness, and response prediction in 76 children. *J. Am. Acad. Child Adolesc. Psychiatry*, 33:882–893.

Rapport, M.D., DuPaul, G.J. & Kelly, K.L. (1989), Attention deficit hyperactivity disorder and methylphenidate: The relationship between gross body weight and drug response in children. *Psychopharmacol. Bull.*, 25:285–290.

Rapport, M.D., Jones, J.T., DuPaul, G.J., Kelly, K.L., Gardner, M.J., Tucker, S.B. & Shea, M.S. (1987), Attention deficit disorder and methylphenidate: Group and single-subject analyses of dose effects on attention in clinic and classroom settings. *J. Clin. Child Psychol.*, 16:329–338.

Rapport, M.D., & Kelly, K.L. (1991), Psychostimulant effects on learning and cognitive function: Findings and implications for children with attention deficit hyperactivity disorder. *Clin. Psychol. Rev.*, 11:61–92.

Reeves, J.C., Werry, J.S., Elkind, G.S. & Zametkin, A. (1987), Attention deficit, conduct, oppositional, and anxiety disorders in children: II. Clinical characteristics. *J. Am. Acad. Child Adolesc. Psychiatry*, 26:144–155.

Routh, D.K., Schroeder, C.S. & O'Tuama, L. (1974), Development of activity level in children. *Dev. Psychol.,* 10:163–168.

Shaywitz, B.A. (1984), Pharmacokinetic, neuroendocrine, and behavioral substrates of ADD. In: *Attention Deficit Disorder: Diagnostic, Cognitive, and Therapeutic Understanding*, ed., L.M. Bloomingdale. New York: Spectrum Publications.

Speer, D.C. (1992), Clinically significant change: Jacobson and Truax (1991) revisited. *J. Consult. Clin. Psychol.*, 60:402–408.

Sprague, R.L. & Sleator, E.K. (1977), Methylphenidate in hyperkinetic children: Differences in dose effects on learning and social behavior. *Science*, 198:1274–1276.

Taylor, E., Schachar R., Thorley, G., Wieselberg, B.E. & Rutter, M. (1987), Which boys respond to stimulant medication? A controlled trial of methylphenidate in boys with disruptive behavior. *Psychol. Med.,* 17:121–143.

Weiss, G. & Hechtman, L. (1993), *Hyperactive Children Grown Up*. New York: Guilford Press.

Werry, J.S., Sprague, R.L. & Cohen, M.N. (1975), Conners Teacher Ratings Scale for use in drug studies with children: An empirical study. *J. Abnorm. Child Psychol.*, 3:217–229.

Werry, J.S., Reeves, J.C., & Elkind, G.S. (1987), Attention deficit, conduct, oppositional and anxiety disorders in children: I. A review of research on differentiating characteristics. *J. Am. Acad. Child Adolesc. Psychiatry*, 26:133–143.

Whalen, C.K., Henker, B., Collins, B.E., Finck, D. & Dotemoto, S. (1979), A social ecology of hyperactive boys: Medication effects in structured classroom environments. *J. Appl. Behav. Anal.*, 12:65–81.

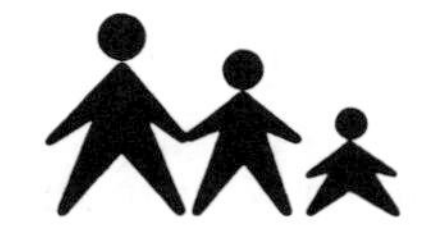

Ritalin: Comorbidity and Differential Clinical Response: The Role of Anxiety

STEVEN R. PLISZKA

INTRODUCTION

Before the publication of *Diagnostic and Statistical Manual of Mental Disorders (DSM), 3rd edition*, mental health clinicians rarely thought in terms of comorbidity of psychiatric disorders in childhood and adolescence. Some clinicians adopted a psychoanalytic perspective, viewing all behavior as arising from a particular unconscious emotional conflict, but even those who used a more medical model tended to classify children as hyperactive, unsocialized aggressive, or withdrawing, to use *DSM-II* labels. Only the first group was regarded as appropriate for psychotropic medication; the withdrawing group of children would today be viewed as either depressed or anxious. With *DSM-III*, the making of multiple diagnoses in children was encouraged if they indeed met the appropriate criteria. Furthermore, the 1980s saw the development of structured research interviews that queried parents and children about a wide range of psychiatric symptoms. For the first time, large-scale epidemiologic studies were performed with such interviews. These studies revealed a high degree of comorbidity for many DSM childhood disorders, particularly attention deficit hyperactivity disorder (ADHD) (Anderson et al., 1987; Bird et al., 1988). This raised the issue of how children with ADHD and a comorbid diagnosis differed from those with ADHD alone in terms of clinical course, etiology, or treatment response. This chapter focuses on children with ADHD who concurrently meet criteria for an anxiety disorder: How does their response to methylphenidate differ from that of children without anxiety? But first, several issues regarding the comorbidity of anxiety disorders and ADHD are briefly reviewed.

OVERVIEW OF ANXIETY DISORDERS

About 5%–15% of the childhood population meet the criteria for one of the anxiety disorders, with overanxious disorder (OAD) and separation anxiety being slightly more common than phobias in most studies (Klein, 1994; Cohen et al., 1993; Tannock, 1994). As with depressive disorders, parents may frequently be unaware of the child's anxiety symptoms (Pliszka, 1992). In a recent epidemiologic study (Cohen et al., 1993), 15% of the girls and 13% of the boys met the criteria for OAD at age 10. By age 18, only 5% of boys but 13% of the girls still met the criteria for the disorder. In contrast, about 12% of both sexes met criteria for separation anxiety at age 10, but by age 18 the prevalence of this disorder had fallen to less than 3%, regardless of gender. While the above anxiety disorders are common in childhood, panic disorder (in the absence of separation anxiety) is quite rare before

Division of Child and Adolescent Psychiatry, The University of Texas Health Science Center at San Antonio, San Antonio, Texas.

adolescence (Klein et al, 1992). Children with separation anxiety were younger at the time they were first evaluated and came from families lower on the socioeconomic scale than children with OAD (Last et al., 1987). Children with OAD had much higher rates of anxiety disorders among their first-degree relatives than did children with separation anxiety (Last et al., 1991). This study also uncovered the surprising finding that children with OAD, rather than those with separation anxiety, had a higher prevalence of panic disorder among their relatives. Previous indirect evidence had suggested that children with separation anxiety were more likely than children with other anxiety disorders to develop panic disorder (Klein, 1994), but at present the question remains unresolved. *DSM-IV* elected to merge OAD with generalized anxiety disorder (GAD), the criteria for which are shown in Table 1.

Notice that children need only meet one of the six symptoms of physical anxiety under Section C. The new GAD criteria may create new problems for clinicians dealing with anxious children with ADHD. Restlessness and poor concentration are symptoms of ADHD, and they should not count toward a GAD diagnosis unless the child is experiencing clear-cut anxiety and worry. As shown in Table 2, both epidemiologic and clinical studies find that about a quarter of ADHD children meet the criteria for a least one of the anxiety disorders (Anderson et al., 1987; Bird et al., 1988; Pliszka, 1989, 1992; Strauss et al., 1988; Last et al., 1987; Biederman et al., 1991, 1992; Faraone et al., 1991). When children with an anxiety disorder are identified, the overlap with ADHD is equally large. Children with any type of anxiety disorder (overanxious, separation anxiety, phobia) are equally likely to meet the criteria for ADHD (Last et al., 1987). Younger children with OAD are more likely to meet the criteria for ADHD than are adolescents with OAD (Strauss et al., 1988).

ISSUES IN CLINICAL DIAGNOSIS

Item A in the *DSM-IV* criteria for GAD is vague. Precisely what type of "worry or anxiety" about "events or activities" should be regarded as significant? The Diagnostic Interview Schedule for Children (DISC) uses several questions to make this item operational

TABLE 1. *DSM-IV* CRITERIA FOR GENERALIZED ANXIETY DISORDER (GAD)

A. Excessive anxiety and worry (apprehensive expectation), occurring more days than not for at least 6 months, about a number of events or activities (such as work or school performance).
B. The person finds it difficult to control the worry.
C. The anxiety and worry are associated with three (or more) of the following six symptoms (with at least some symptoms present for more days than not for the past 6 months). *Note*: Only one item is required in children.
   1. Restlessness
   2. Being easily fatigued
   3. Difficulty concentrating
   4. Irritability
   5. Muscle tension
   6. Sleep disturbance
D. Focus of anxiety and worry is not due to another Axis I disorder.
E. The anxiety, worry, or physical symptoms cause clinically significant distress or impairment in social, occupational, or other important areas of functioning.
F. The anxiety or worry is not directly due to substance/alcohol abuse.

(Shaffer et al., 1993; Jensen et al., 1995). For instance, does the child worry about:

1. upcoming tests or school projects?
2. his or her performance in upcoming sports events?
3. whether the family has enough money?
4. looking foolish when he or she does things?
5. dying or getting sick? Does the child exaggerate minor aches and pains?

These anxieties do not include simple fear of punishment for wrongdoing. Many children with ADHD have no foresight and lack the appropriate amount of anticipatory anxiety for events (such as studying for a test). When the test is over, and they are grounded for a poor grade, they may express dysphoria or nervousness. It is critical when taking a history from the parent to distinguish between true performance anxiety and unhappiness about the consequences of misbehavior. Next, the symptoms should have sufficient frequency to impair functioning. A child who is anxious for only a few minutes at a time should not be diagnosed as having GAD. For a correct diagnosis, anxiety should be present for at least an hour for three to five times per week.

Older children and adolescents may use the word *nervous* to describe their ADHD symptoms. How is this to be distinguished from true anxiety? There is no research on this matter, but clinical experience suggests that distinct qualitative factors separate the two feelings. When asked to give an example of their nervousness, ADHD adolescents describe a symptom more akin to motor restlessness or impatience. "When I'm in algebra class, it's so boring I want to jump up and scream," or "My mom says I bother the whole family the way I shake my leg when I'm sitting at the dinner table." One 16-year-old girl had a chief complaint of "being too nervous" as evidenced by her inability to stop talking in class or impulsively laughing at inappropriate times. Anxiety has a more painful quality; it is an internal experience as opposed to a reaction to immediate environmental stimuli.

Clinicians should avoid the error of assuming that because the child has experienced a life stressor, the ADHD symptoms are reflective of "unconscious conflicts." If children with psychodynamic conflicts caused by psychosocial stressors commonly developed "pseudo-ADHD," then one would expect that overall, children with ADHD and a history of such stressors would show a less robust response to stimulants. In fact, Taylor et al. (1987) did not find this to be the case. Hyperactive and inattentive boys with a wide variety of stressors such as single-parent families, placement in foster care, and parental separation responded just as well to stimulants as those without such histories. Children should

TABLE 2. OVERLAP OF ANXIETY DISORDERS AND ATTENTION DEFICIT HYPERACTIVITY DISORDER (ADHD)

Study	*ADHD Children Who Meet Criteria for Anxiety Disorder (%)*
Epidemiologic	
Anderson et al. (1987)	26
Bird et al. (1988)	23
Clinical	
Biederman et al. (1991)	30
Biederman et al. (1992)	29
Faraone et al. (1991)	29
Pliszka (1989)	28
Pliszka (1992)	39

not receive a diagnosis of anxiety disorder simply because they have experienced a psychosocial stressor.

This having been said, whose history of anxiety is most important: the parent's or the child's? Pliszka (1992) found that half of the ADHD children who met the criteria for OAD by their own report were not described as anxious by their parents, suggesting that parents may often be unaware of their child's internalizing symptoms. Bird et al. (1992) found that parents and children agree on the presence of anxiety symptoms only about half the time. They also found quite different prevalence rates for anxiety disorders, depending on whether the parent or the child was the informant. Based only on parents' report, the prevalence of separation anxiety in their sample was 6.3%, whereas if the diagnosis was based only on the child's report, 15% of the children had this disorder. If either a parent's or the child's report was accepted, then 19.2% of the sample met the criteria for separation anxiety disorder. A similar pattern was noted for OAD: According to the parents, only 3% of children were affected, but 6.9% met the criteria for OAD by child-only approach. If either the parent's or the child's report of symptoms was accepted, 11.4% of the sample met the criteria for OAD. Tannock (1994) compared two groups of ADHD/anxiety disorder children: One group met criteria by the children's report, while in the other group the children denied anxiety but the parents reported anxiety symptoms in the children. Only the children with ADHD/anxiety who themselves reported anxiety showed lower levels of self-confidence and impairment in daily activities. This suggests that the child's report, rather than the parent's report, is more important in making the diagnosis of anxiety, but further research is needed to resolve this issue.

CONTRASTING ADHD CHILDREN WITH AND WITHOUT ANXIETY DISORDERS

How are ADHD children with and without comorbid anxiety different? A body of research literature has emerged that examines this issue. Pliszka (1989; 1992) found that children with ADHD and OAD were older at the time of presentation than children with ADHD alone. An initial study (Pliszka, 1989) found that ADHD/OAD children were less likely to meet criteria for conduct disorder (CD) and had lower teacher ratings of inattention/hyperactivity than ADHD-only children. However, when a structured interview was used in a larger follow-up study, these findings were not confirmed (Pliszka, 1992). Biederman et al. (1991) also did not find differences in the rate of CD in ADHD and ADHD/anxiety children. In contrast, Tannock (1994) found higher rates of CD among ADHD/anxiety children. Neither Tannock (1994) nor Biederman et al. (1991) found differences between ADHD children with and without anxiety in terms of the prevalence of learning disabilities. While ADHD/anxiety and ADHD children were not found to be different in school performance (Biederman et al., 1991), ADHD/anxiety children reported more school problems than ADHD-only children; indeed, ADHD/anxiety children reported a wide variety of social difficulties beyond those reported by children with ADHD alone (Biederman et al., 1993b).

Mothers of children with ADHD/anxiety reported higher levels of problems during pregnancy, as well as developmental delays, than children with ADHD alone (Tannock, 1994). Children with ADHD/anxiety have generally experienced more stressful life events than ADHD-only children (Jensen et al., 1993; Tannock, 1994). Biederman et al. (1991) found much higher rates of divorce and separation among the families of ADHD/anxiety children (59%) than in ADHD-only children (27%). This suggests that ADHD/anxiety children may require, or be more likely to benefit from, psychosocial interventions, though no study has directly addressed this issue.

Pliszka (1989; 1992) used the observation technique of Barkley (1990) to assess the motor behavior of ADHD children with and without OAD. Children were placed in an observation room with a one-way mirror and required to perform arithmetic while being watched by a research assistant blind to the clinical information. Children were rated in terms of off-task behaviors: fidgeting, vocalizing, getting out of their seats, and playing with objects. In both studies, children with ADHD/OAD were less likely to display these impulsive-hyperactive behaviors than ADHD-only children. The second study (Pliszka, 1992) compared children in both ADHD groups with control subjects. When the total numbers of ADHD behavior were summed, the ADHD-only children were significantly more off-task and disruptive than the ADHD/OAD children, who in turn were significantly more disruptive than the control subjects.

The cognitive performances of ADHD children with and without anxiety have been compared by a variety of measures. Pliszka (1989) used the Memory Scanning Test. The child had to memorize four numbers, and then the computer screen presented one of three displays: a number by itself, a 4 × 4 grid of letters in which one number was embedded, or a 4 × 4 grid of numbers. The child had to scan the display and determine whether one of the four numbers he or she had memorized was present in the display. The child's reaction time was measured for each response. Normally, more time is required to respond to the number display than to the letter display, because in the latter the target is embedded in similar distracters. The single-number display produces the quickest responses. In the most difficult condition (number distracters), the ADHD group had shorter reaction times than the ADHD/OAD group and a higher number of errors. This suggested that as the task became more cognitively difficult the ADHD-only children became more impulsive, whereas the ADHD/OAD children slowed their reaction times.

In a follow-up study, Pliszka (1992) compared ADHD children with and without OAD to normal control subjects on the Inhibition version of the Continuous Performance Test (CPT). On this task, children were required to press a button every time a shape appeared on the screen, but if they saw a blue square, they had to withhold their response. Children with ADHD alone had a much higher number of errors of commission than children with ADHD/OAD, who in turn were not different from normal control subjects. Thus, the co-occurrence of OAD in ADHD appeared to attenuate impulsivity. This finding was confirmed in a follow-up study using an alternative measure of impulsivity, the Stop Signal Task (Pliszka et al., 1997). In both these studies, differences were obtained only when children were classified as anxious by their own report. No differences were found between anxious and nonanxious ADHD children if the anxiety diagnosis was based only on the parent's report.

Tannock et al. (1993) examined the differences between ADHD children with and without anxiety on a working memory task. In contrast to the CPT and the Stop Signal Task, which involve only simple inhibition and do not require active information processing, working memory tasks require the manipulation of information. ADHD children with and without anxiety performed the Children's Paced Auditory Serial Addition Task. Subjects were given a series of digits (i.e. 4, 5, 1, 7, etc.) by a tape recorder. They had to add the first two digits in the sequence (4 + 5 = 9). When they heard the third digit, they had to add it to the second (5 + 1 = 6), and when they heard the fourth digit, they had to add it to the third (1 + 7 = 8), and so on. The digits were presented in three different blocks of varying speeds. When the digits are presented at longer intervals, working memory is taxed because the information must be retained longer. The ADHD/anxiety children made more errors when the digits were presented at longer intervals, implying a greater impairment of working memory relative to the ADHD-only children. Reviewing the data on cognitive performance, Tannock (1994) suggested that the effect of anxiety in ADHD is to decrease impulsiveness but to increase difficulties with working memory and effortful processing. Clinically, therefore, ADHD/anxiety children are more likely to appear less overtly hyperactive and disruptive but more "slowed down" or inefficient.

Family studies

Biederman and colleagues (1991; 1992) have performed family studies to explore the pattern of inheritance of ADHD and anxiety. The relatives of ADHD-only and ADHD/anxiety probands were examined for ADHD and anxiety disorders. The relatives of children in a control group were similarly interviewed. ADHD and anxiety disorders are both familial; these studies address the genetic relationship between the two disorders. If they are independent of each other, then the rate of anxiety disorders should be elevated only in the families of the ADHD probands with anxiety disorders. Rates of ADHD should be elevated only in the relatives of the ADHD patients. In contrast, if children with comorbid ADHD/anxiety really have a genetically based anxiety disorder masquerading as ADHD, then one would expect the rate of anxiety disorders to be elevated only in the relatives of the ADHD/anxiety probands. The rate of ADHD among relatives of the comorbid group should not exceed that of the control group. The results of the studies by Biederman et al. (1992) are shown in Figure 1.

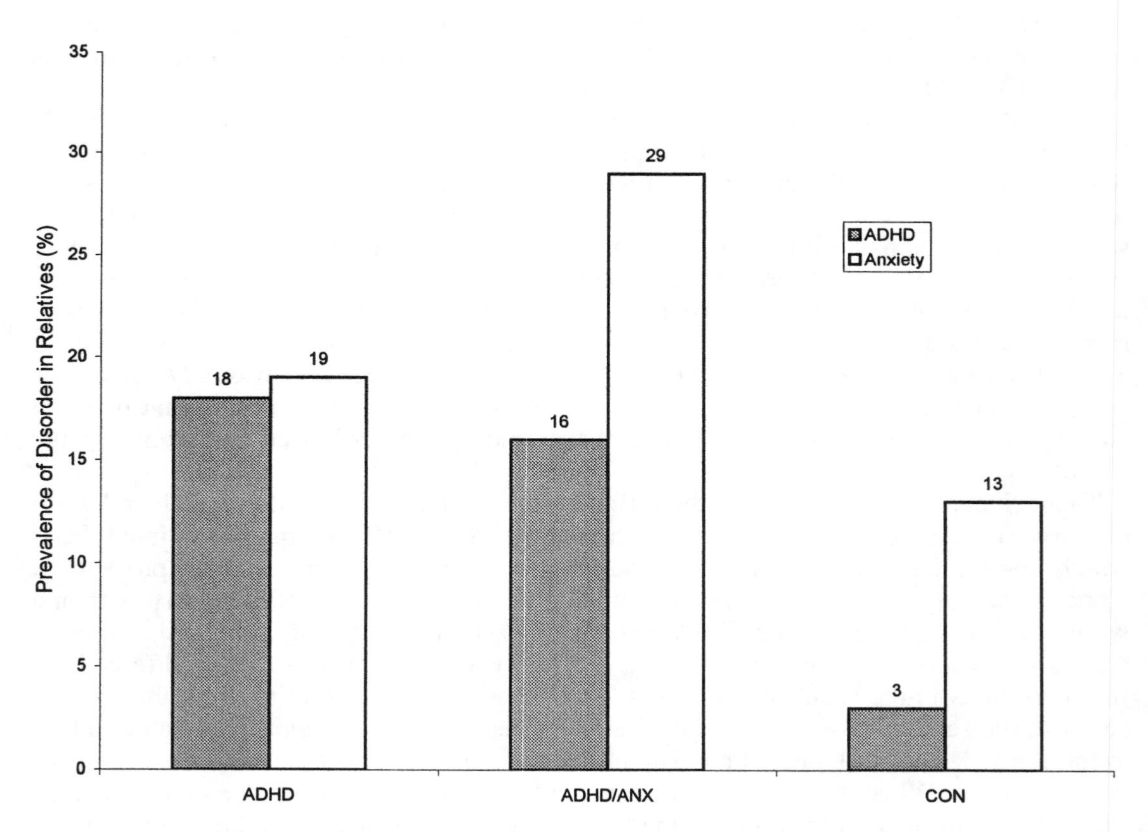

FIG. 1. Rate of disorders in relatives of children with attention deficit hyperactivity disorder (ADHD), with and without anxiety (Biederman et al., 1992). Anx = anxiety; con = control group.

In comparison with control subjects, the rate of anxiety disorders was elevated only in the relatives of ADHD/anxiety children, and not in the relatives of ADHD/only children. The rate of ADHD was equally elevated in both ADHD groups. Among the relatives of the ADHD/anxiety children, the two disorders did not cosegregate, meaning that an ADHD/anxiety child had relatives with ADHD alone as well as relatives with anxiety alone, but few relatives who had both disorders. This is most consistent with the hypothesis that ADHD and anxiety are separate disorders inherited independently of each other. A more recent family study from a different laboratory has confirmed this pattern (Perrin & Last, 1996).

Physiologic differences

ADHD children with and without anxiety do not show any baseline differences in heart rate, skin conductance, or blood pressure (Pliszka et al., 1993; Tannock et al., 1995; Urman et al., 1995). Pliszka et al. (1993) performed a classic conditioning experiment in which a video signal was paired with a presentation of aversive white noise. Control subjects, ADHD-only children, and ADHD/anxiety-disordered children all showed similar conditioning of heart rate and skin conductance to the conditioned stimulus. At the end of the paradigm, urine samples were collected and assayed for catecholamines (Pliszka et al., 1994). Children with ADHD, regardless of whether they had anxiety disorder, had elevated levels of normetanephrine (the principal metabolite of norepinephrine) relative to control subjects. ADHD children with anxiety disorder had elevated levels of epinephrine and metanephrine (the principal metabolite of epinephrine). More circulating epinephrine might suggest increased peripheral adrenal medulla activity in the ADHD/anxiety subgroup, which may explain some of the findings about response to psychostimulants in the ADHD/anxiety children reviewed next.

METHYLPHENIDATE IN COMORBID ADHD/ANXIETY

Pliszka (1987) suggested, based on a review of the literature, that children with comorbid ADHD and anxiety might show a less robust response to stimulant medications than ADHD children without internalizing disorders. In an attempt to determine predictors of response to stimulants, Taylor et al. (1987) treated a heterogeneous group of boys with behavior problems with a double-blind placebo-controlled trial of methylphenidate (MPH). Boys who at baseline had more symptoms of depression or anxiety were least likely to respond to the drug. This is consistent with other studies showing that baseline ratings of anxiety in hyperactive children predict poorer outcome of stimulant treatment (Swanson et al., 1978; Voelker et al., 1983; Zahn et al., 1975). Swanson et al. (1978) found that hyperactive children with a comorbid diagnosis of overanxious reaction were most likely to show deterioration during stimulant treatment as measured by the Paired Associates Learning Test, a laboratory measure of learning. Behavioral measures were not obtained in that study. Parents' ratings of hyperactive children's anxiety on the Personality Inventory for Children (PIC) predicted poor outcome to MPH treatment; indeed, this was the only factor on the PIC that had predictive value in terms of which subjects would respond to stimulant (Stein et al., 1996). Most recently, Buitelaar et al. (1995) treated 46 ADHD children with MPH and related baseline measures to stimulant response. High ratings on the anxiety factor of the Conners Parent Rating Scale was significantly associated with a poor outcome of MPH treatment.

Pliszka (1989) further examined this issue by treating 43 ADHD children (13 of whom had comorbid OAD) in a double-blind placebo-controlled trial of MPH. All children received a week of placebo and then were randomized to a 3-week double-blind crossover study of placebo and two doses of MPH. Teachers who were blind to the children's medication status rated the children each of the study weeks. Once a week, the children returned to the laboratory, where they performed arithmetic problems for 15 minutes while being observed through a one-way mirror. The observer was also blind to medication status. Over 80% of the nonanxious ADHD children were stimulant responders, while only 30% of the ADHD/OAD children were thought to clearly benefit from the drug. There were several placebo responders in the ADHD/OAD group, whereas there were no such responders in the nonanxious ADHD group. The effects of stimulants on the observation room ratings were particularly striking (Figure 2). Nonanxious ADHD children had a highly significant reduction in ratings of off-task and fidgeting behaviors in response to MPH, whereas ADHD/OAD children showed little improvement on this measure.

There was no evidence that the ADHD/OAD children suffered any unusual side effects, nor did they appear to become more anxious. Of course, 30% of the ADHD/OAD children did respond well to stimulants and continued treatment with MPH; thus, the study did not show that stimulants are absolutely contradicted in ADHD/anxiety.

In contrast, Tannock et al. (1991) did find that side effects of stimulants appear greater in the ADHD/anxiety group relative to the ADHD-alone group. Furthermore, these ADHD

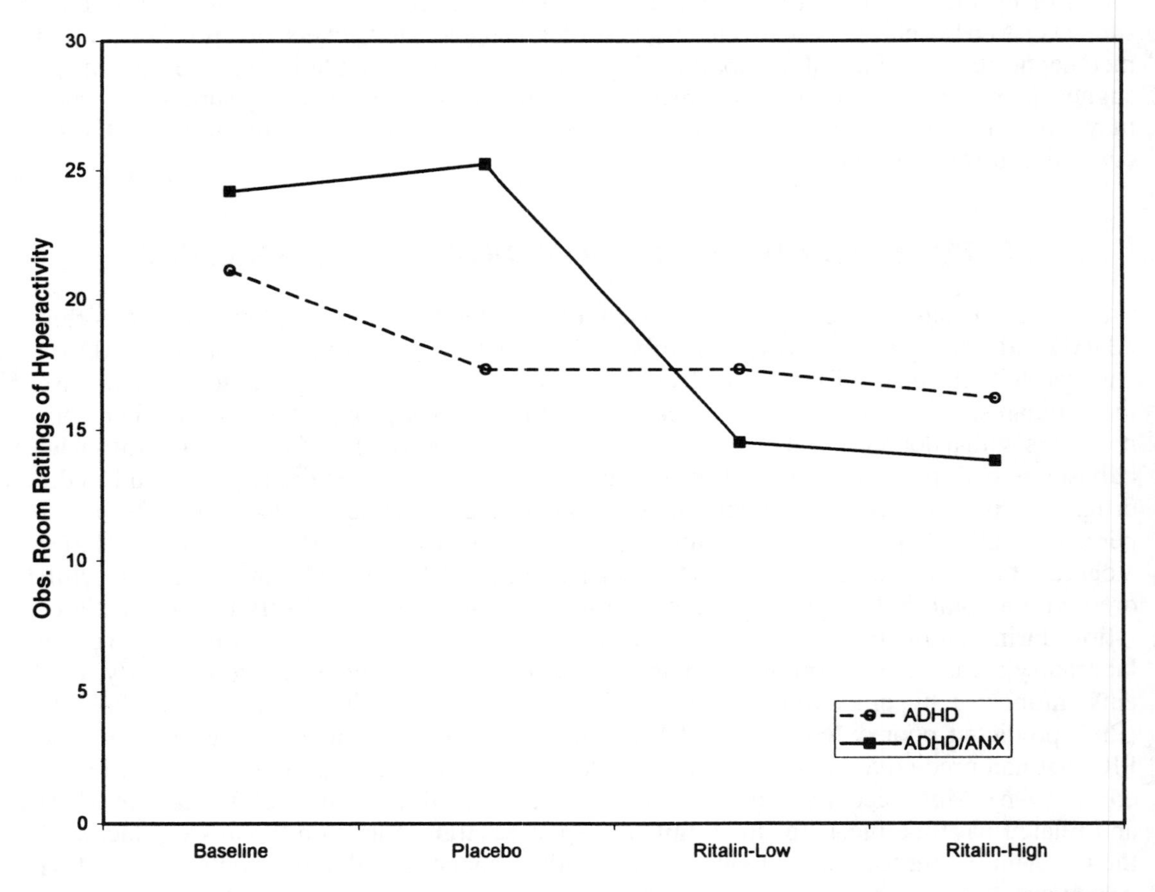

FIG. 2. Effects of methylphenidate on observation room ratings of behavior of children with attention deficit hyperactivity disorder (ADHD). Anx = anxiety.

children were monitored while receiving long-term MPH treatment (over 12 months). Not only did ADHD/OAD children have less behavioral improvement, but that what improvement there was tended to decline over time (Tannock, 1994). Tannock et al. (1995) compared ADHD/anxiety and ADHD children on the serial addition working memory task described earlier. Children performed the task while receiving placebo and three dosages of MPH (0.3, 0.6, and 0.9 mg/kg/dose). ADHD children without anxiety showed clear improvements in performance on the task while taking MPH; the improvements were linearly related to dose. In contrast, ADHD/anxiety children showed only modest improvements while taking the low dose, which were not enhanced by the higher dose. The ADHD/anxiety children did not show a deterioration in cognitive performance, however, and unlike those studied by Pliszka (1989), they did show significant reductions in motoric behavior during the cognitive task. While there were no baseline differences in heart rate, ADHD/anxiety children showed a much greater increase in pulse to the low MPH dose than did the nonanxious ADHD children. The ADHD/anxiety group also had an exaggerated increase in diastolic blood pressure to MPH (Urman et al., 1995). As noted above, Pliszka et al. (1994) found increased peripheral epinephrine in ADHD/anxiety children relative to ADHD-only children. Further MPH-related increases in circulating epinephrine in these children might lead to "overarousal" and less improvement in cognitive performance.

Finally, DuPaul et al. (1994) divided ADHD children into "internalizers" and "noninternalizers" according to the child's baseline Child Behavior Checklist score. Similarly to Pliszka (1989), they found that ADHD children with comorbid internalizing symptoms had a less robust response to stimulants than did nonanxious ADHD children. These findings suggest the need for caution in the use of stimulants in ADHD/anxiety-disordered children, but a significant minority of them will respond well to stimulant (Pliszka, 1989). Also, not all studies have found that ADHD/anxiety children have a less robust response to stimulants—in fact, Livingstone et al. (1992) found that ADHD children with comorbid internalizing disorders responded better to a higher dose of methylphenidate than did those without an internalizing disorder. Recently, Diamond et al. (1998) found anxious and nonanxious ADHD children to have an equally robust response to methylphenidate.

When stimulants are selected as the psychopharmacologic treatment, careful monitoring of behavior, and school performance in particular, is indicated. The child should be watched for signs of increased anxiety or overfocusing, and the medication should be discontinued if this occurs. On the other hand, if the stimulant response is robust, the clinician should inquire about the anxiety symptoms. If they have remitted along with the ADHD symptoms one would be justified in concluding that the anxiety was a result of the problems arising secondary to the ADHD. If stimulants are not effective, then one of the antidepressant medications may be considered.

ANTIDEPRESSANTS

Tricyclic antidepressants (TCAs) are superior to placebo but not as effective as stimulants in the treatment of ADHD, and thus they should always be viewed as drugs of second choice in the treatment of inattention and hyperactivity (Pliszka, 1987). One review suggested that TCAs might be more effective in ADHD children with comorbid anxiety; however, Biederman et al. (1993a) found that anxious and nonanxious ADHD children responded equally well to desipramine. Thus, while there is evidence that ADHD/anxious children have a less robust response to stimulants, there is no clear evidence that they respond better to TCAs. In addition, desipramine has recently been associated with sudden death in children (Biederman et al., 1995; Popper and Ziminitzky, 1995; Varley and McClellan, 1997). Thus, many clinicians have returned to imipramine as the principal TCA when a child does not respond to stimulants. Bupropion has been shown to be superior to placebo in the treatment of ADHD, though none of the subjects had comorbid anxiety disorders (Conners et al., 1996). If stimulants are not effective for a particular ADHD/anxiety patient, and side effects preclude the use of TCAs, bupropion might be a useful alternative.

Birmaher et al. (1994) treated 30 anxious children and adolescents (mean age 14) with an open trial of fluoxetine. The children, who were all nonresponders to psychotherapy, had a variety of anxiety diagnoses other than OCD; two-thirds had failed trials of tricyclics. The mean dose of fluoxetine was 25.7 mg/day. Only one patient received 10 mg/day; all the others were receiving 20–60 mg/day. The side effects were mild and transient, and none of the subjects had worsening of anxiety symptoms. Anxiety severity scores showed a highly significant reduction, with 56% of the patients rated as moderately or markedly improved. Gammon and Brown (1993) combined fluoxetine and stimulants in 32 patients with ADHD who had a variety of comorbid disorders. Many had symptoms of depression and anxiety. Doses of fluoxetine ranging from 2.5 to 20 mg a day were combined with the usual daily doses of MPH (10–60 mg/day). The side effects were minimal, with no cases of increased agitation, and most of the subjects showed a marked improvement over treatment with MPH alone. While controlled trials are needed, these studies suggest that stimulants may be combined with specific serotonin reuptake inhibitors in children with comorbid internalizing disorders.

SUMMARY

Children with ADHD/anxiety represent up to a quarter of the ADHD population. Overall, they are older at the time of presentation and may have fewer aggressive symptoms. Cognitively, they show somewhat less impulsiveness and hyperactivity but may have more impairment of working memory and other higher cognitive functions. ADHD and anxiety appear to be inherited independently of each other, so genetics does not explain the high degree of overlap between the disorders. Parent-reported and child-reported anxiety have different correlates; future studies should explore these differences more fully. In terms of psychopharmacologic management, the following strategy has been found useful:

1. Begin with stimulant treatment, but be aware that the rate of nonresponse may be higher in children with comorbid ADHD/anxiety disorder.
2. If a child has failed to respond to two different stimulants (MPH and dextroamphetamine), only then should the child be considered a stimulant nonresponder (Elia et al., 1991).
3. If a child has a marked adverse response to the first stimulant tried—increase in anxiety, adverse cognitive response, severe side effects—then the clinician is justified in moving to a nonstimulant medication without trying an alternative stimulant.
4. Either bupropion or imipramine is a reasonable alternative in the ADHD/anxiety child who is a stimulant nonresponder.
5. If a child has a positive response of the ADHD symptoms to stimulant medication, but remains highly anxious, an SSRI may be added to the stimulant, with careful monitoring of the side effects. Further controlled studies are needed to validate this strategy.

Further studies are needed to contrast ADHD children with and without anxiety in terms of long-term outcome, other associated comorbidities (learning problems, aggression), and biologic correlates. The clinician should be alert to comorbid anxiety symptoms in ADHD, as such symptoms may signal the need for a different approach to the treatment of the child, in terms of both psychotropic medications and psychosocial interventions.

REFERENCES

Anderson, J.C., Williams, S., McGee, R. & Silva, P.A. (1987), *DSM-III* disorders in preadolescent children: Prevalence in a large community sample. *Arch. Gen. Psychiatry*, 44:69–76.

Barkley, R.A. (1990), *Attention Deficit Hyperactivity Disorder: A Handbook for Diagnosis and Treatment.* New York: Guildford Press.

Biederman, J., Baldessarini, R.J., Wright, V., Keenan, K. & Faraone, S. (1993a), A double-blind placebo controlled study of desipramine in the treatment of ADD: III. Lack of impact of comorbidity and family history factors on clinical response. *J. Am. Acad. Child Adolesc. Psychiatry*, 32:199–204.

Biederman, J., Faraone, S.V. & Chen, W.J. (1993b), Social Adjustment Inventory for Children and Adolescents: Concurrent validity in ADHD children. *J. Am. Acad. Child Adolesc. Psychiatry*, 32:1059–1064.

Biederman, J., Faraone, S.V., Keenan, K., Benjamin, J., Krifcher, B., Moore, C., Sprich-Buckminster, S., Ugaglia, K., Jellinek, M.S. & Steingard, R. (1992), Further evidence for family-genetic risk factors in attention deficit hyperactivity disorder: Patterns of comorbidity in probands and relatives psychiatrically and pediatrically referred samples. *Arch. Gen. Psychiatry*, 49:728–738.

Biederman, J., Faraone, S.V., Keenan, K., Steingard, R. & Tsuang, M.T. (1991). Familial association between attention deficit disorder and anxiety disorders. *Am. J. Psychiatry*, 148:251–265.

Biederman, J., Thisted, R.A., Greenhill, L.L. & Ryan, N.D. (1995), Estimation of the association between desipramine and the risk for sudden death in 5 to 14 year old children. *J. Clin. Psychiatry*, 56:87–93.

Bird, H.R., Canino, G. & Rubio-Stipec, M. (1988), Estimates of prevalence of childhood maladjustment in a community survey in Puerto Rico. *Arch. Gen. Psychiatry*, 45:1120–1126.

Bird, H.R., Gould, M.S. & Staghezza, B. (1992), Aggregating data from multiple informants in child psychiatry epidemiological research. *J. Am. Acad. Child Adolesc. Psychiatry*, 31:78–85.

Birmaher, B., Waterman, G.S., Ryan, N., Cully, M., Balach, L., Ingram, J. & Brodsky, M. (1994), Fluoxetine for childhood anxiety disorders. *J. Am. Acad. Child Adolesc. Psychiatry*, 33:993–999.

Buitelaar, J.K., Van der Gaag, R.J., Swaab-Barneveld, H. & Kuiper, M. (1995), Prediction of clinical response to methylphenidate in children with attention-deficit hyperactivity disorder. *J. Am. Acad. Child Adolesc. Psychiatry*, 34:1025–1032.

Cohen, P., Cohen, J., Kasen, S., Velez, C.N., Hartmark, C., Johnson, J., Rojas, M., Brook, J. & Streuning, E.L. (1993), An epidemiological study of disorders in late childhood and adolescence: I. Age and gender specific pattern. *J. Child Psychol. Psychiatry*, 34:851–867.

Conners, C.K., Casat, C.D., Gualtieri, C.T., Weller, E., Reader, M., Reiss, A., Weller, R.A., Khayrallah, M. & Ascher, J. (1996), Bupropion hydrochloride in attention deficit disorder with hyperactivity. *J. Am. Acad. Child Adolesc. Psychiatry*, 35:1314–1321.

Diamond, I.R., Tannock, R., Rimer, S., Bockus, S. & Schachar, R. (1998), Extended methylphenidate treatment of ADHD with and without comorbid anxiety. Presented at the 45th Annual Meeting of the American Academy of Child and Adolescent Psychaitry, October 27–Nov 1, Anaheim, CA.

DuPaul, G.J., Barkley, R.A. & McMurray, M.B. (1994), Response of children with ADHD to methylphenidate: Interaction with internalizing symptoms. *J. Am. Acad. Child Adolesc. Psychiatry*, 33:894–903.

Elia, J., Borcherding, B.G., Rapoport, J.L. & Keysor, C.S. (1991), Methylphenidate and dextroamphetamine treatments of hyperactivity: Are there true nonresponders? *Psychiatry Res.*, 36:141–155.

Faraone, S.V., Biederman, J., Keenan, K. & Tsuang, M.T. (1991), A family-genetic study of girls with *DSM-III* attention deficit disorder. *Am. J. Psychiatry*, 148:112–117.

Gammon, G.D. & Brown, T.E. (1993), Fluoxetine and methylphenidate in combination for treatment of attention deficit and comorbid depressive disorder. *J. Child Adolesc. Psychopharmacol.*, 3:1–10.

Jensen, P., Roper, M., Fisher, P., Piacentini, J., Canino, G., Richters, J., Rubio-Stipec, M., Dulcan, M., Goodman, S. & Davies, M., et al. (1995), Test-retest reliability of the Diagnostic Interview Schedule for Children (DISC 2.1). *Arch. Gen. Psychiatry*, 52:61–71.

Jensen, P.S., Shervette, R.E., Xenakis, S.N. & Richters, J. (1993), Anxiety and depressive disorders in attention deficit disorder with hyperactivity: New findings. *Am. J. Psychiatry*, 150:1203–1209.

Klein, D.F., Mannuzza, S., Chapman, T. & Fyer, A.J. (1992), Child panic revisited. *J. Am. Acad. Child Adolesc. Psychiatry*, 31:112–116.

Klein, R.G. (1994), Anxiety disorders. In: *Child and Adolescent Psychiatry: Modern Approaches, 3rd ed.*, eds., M. Rutter, E. Taylor, L. Hersov. Oxford: Blackwell Scientific Publications, pp. 351–374.

Last, C.G., Hersen, M., Kazdin, A.E., Finkelstein, R. & Strauss, C.C. (1987), Comparison of *DSM-III* separation anxiety and overanxious disorders: Demographic characteristics and patterns of comorbidity. *J. Am. Acad. Child Adolesc. Psychiatry*, 26:527–531.

Last, C.G., Hersen, M., Kazdin, A., Orvaschel, H. & Perrin, S. (1991), Anxiety disorders in children and their families. *Arch. Gen. Psychiatry*, 48:928–934.

Livingstone, R.L., Dykman, R.A. & Ackerman, P.T. (1992), Psychiatric comorbidity and response to two doses of methylphenidate in children with attention deficit disorder. *J. Child Adolesc. Psychopharmacol.* 2:115–122.

Perrin, S. & Last, C.G. (1996), Relationship between ADHD and anxiety in boys: Results from a family study. *J. Am. Acad. Child Adolesc. Psychiatry*, 35:988–996.

Pliszka, S.R. (1987), Tricyclic antidepressants in the treatment of children with attention deficit disorder. *J. Am. Acad. Child. Adolesc. Psychiatry*, 26:127–132.

Pliszka, S.R. (1989), Effect of anxiety on cognition, behavior, and stimulant response in ADHD. *J. Am. Acad. Child Adolesc. Psychiatry*, 28:882–887.

Pliszka, S.R. (1992), Comorbidity of attention deficit hyperactivity disorder and overanxious disorder. *J. Am. Acad. Child Adolesc. Psychiatry*, 31:197–203.

Pliszka, S.R., Borcherding, S.H., Sprately, K.L., Leon, S.L. & Irick, S. (1997), Measuring impulsivity in children. *J. Dev. Behav. Pediatrics*, 18:254–259.

Pliszka, S.R., Hatch, J.P., Borcherding, S.H. & Rogeness, G.A. (1993), Classical conditioning in children with attention deficit hyperactivity disorder (ADHD) and anxiety disorders: A test of Quay's model. *J. Abnorm. Child Psychol.*, 21:411–423.

Pliszka, S.R., Maas, J.W., Javors, M.A., Rogeness, G.A. & Baker, J. (1994), Urinary catecholamines in attention deficit hyperactivity disorder with and without comorbid anxiety. *J. Am. Acad. Child Adolesc. Psychiatry*, 33:1165–1173.

Popper, C.W. & Ziminitzky, B. (1995), Sudden death putatively related to desipramine treatment in youth: A fifth case and a review of speculative mechanisms. *J. Child Adolesc. Psychopharmacol.*, 5:283–300.

Shaffer, D., Schwab-Stone, M., Fisher, P., Cohen, P., Piacentini, J., Davies, M., Conners, C.K. & Regier, D. (1993), The Diagnostic Interview Schedule for Children—Revised

Version (DISC-R): I. Preparation, field testing, interrater reliability, and acceptability. *J. Am. Acad. Child Adolesc. Psychiatry*, 32:643–650.

Stein, M.B., Walker, J.R., Anderson, G., Hazen, A.L., Ross, C.A., Eldridge, G. & Forde, D.R. (1996), Childhood physical and sexual abuse in patients with anxiety disorders and in a community sample. *Am. J. Psychiatry*, 153:275–277.

Strauss, C.C., Lease, C.A., Last, C.G. & Francis, G. (1988), Overanxious disorder: An examination of developmental differences. *J. Abnorm. Child Psychol.*, 16:433–643.

Swanson, J.M., Kinsbourne, M., Roberts, W. & Zucker, K. (1978), Time-response analysis of the effect of stimulant medication on the learning ability of children referred for hyperactivity. *Pediatrics*, 61:21–29.

Tannock, R. (1994), Attention deficit disorders with anxiety disorders. In: *Subtypes of Attention Deficit Disorders in Children, Adolescents and Adults*, ed., T.E. Brown. New York: American Psychiatric Press.

Tannock, R., Ickowicz, A. & Schachar, R. (1991), Effects of comorbid anxiety on stimulant response in children with ADHD. Presented at the 38th annual meeting of the American Academy of Child and Adolescent Psychiatry, San Francisco, October 16–20.

Tannock, R., Ickowicz, A. & Schachar, R. (1995), Differential effects of methylphenidate on working memory in ADHD children with and without comorbid anxiety. *J. Am. Acad. Child Adolesc. Psychiatry*, 34:886–896.

Tannock, R., Schachar, R. & Logan, G. (1993), Differential effects of methylphenidate on working memory in attention-deficit hyperactivity disorder with and without anxiety. Presented at the 40th annual meeting of the American Academy of Child and Adolescent Psychiatry, San Antonio, Texas, October 26–31.

Taylor, E., Schachar, R., Thorley, G., Wieselberg, H.M., Everitt, B. & Rutter, M. (1987), Which boys respond to stimulant medication? A controlled trial of methylphenidate in boys with disruptive behavior. *Psychol. Med.*, 17:121–143.

Urman, R., Ickowicz, A., Fulford, P. & Tannock, R. (1995), An exaggerated cardiovascular response to methylphenidate in ADHD children with anxiety. *J. Child Adolesc. Psychopharmacol.*, 5:29–37.

Varley, C.K. & McClellan, J. (1997), Case study: Two additional sudden deaths with tricyclic antidepressants. *J. Am. Acad. Child Adolesc. Psychiatry*, 36:390–394.

Voelker, S., Lachar, D. & Gdowski, C. (1983), The Personality Inventory for Children and response to methylphenidate: Preliminary evidence for predictive validity. *J. Pediatr. Psychol.*, 8:161–169.

Zahn, T.P., Abate, F., Little, B.C. & Wender, P.H. (1975), Minimal brain dysfunction, stimulant drugs, and autonomic nervous system activity. *Arch. Gen. Psychiatry*, 32:381–387.

Section 3

Criteria for Use of Ritalin

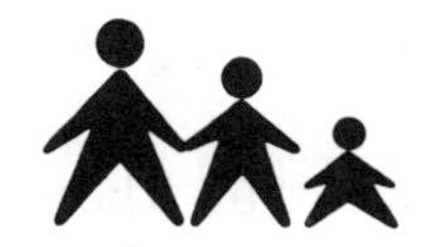

Combining Parent Training and Medication in the Treatment of Attention Deficit Hyperactivity Disorder

RUSSELL SCHACHAR[1] and RICHARD SUGARMAN[2]

INTRODUCTION

Attention deficit hyperactivity disorder (ADHD); American Psychiatric Association, 1994) is a common, impairing, and costly mental health condition occurring in approximately 5% of school-age children and adolescents and is a major reason for referral for children's mental health services (Szatmari et al., 1989b). Clinicians and researchers have been preoccupied with the effectiveness of pharmacologic and nonpharmacologic therapies administered individually and in diverse combinations (Richters et al., 1995). This chapter will illustrate the methodological and clinical implications of combined pharmacologic and nonpharmacologic treatments of ADHD by focusing on the combination of psychostimulants and behavioral parent training (PT). The primary reasons for focusing on PT are the widespread availability of this treatment modality, its established efficacy (Kazdin, 1997), and the complementary nature of PT and medications typically used for ADHD.

ADHD: A MAJOR PUBLIC HEALTH CONCERN

ADHD is a lifelong condition, first evident in the preschool years (Campbell, 1994) and persisting in approximately 50% of individuals throughout childhood, adolescence, and adulthood (Klein and Mannuzza, 1991; Hechtman et al., 1984). ADHD children are impaired in many aspects of their lives. Their relationships with peers, siblings, and parents and other adults are often characterized by aggressiveness and defiance. These children often perform poorly at school and may exhibit comorbid learning, mood, and anxiety disorders (Barkley, 1990; Biederman et al., 1991; Hinshaw, 1992). Their prognosis is characterized by an increased likelihood of delinquency, criminality, school suspensions, academic underachievement, demoralization, and substance abuse (Mannuzza et al., 1989; Mannuzza et al., 1991). Currently, ADHD is understood to be the behavioral manifestation of deficient self-regulation, in particular a deficit in inhibitory control, which may have a genetic or neurophysiologic basis (Barkley, 1997; Douglas, 1988; Quay, 1997). Although biologic factors clearly play a role, ADHD does not arise in a social vacuum. Families of ADHD children exhibit high rates of parental psychopathology, in particular ADHD and antisocial personality disorder, marital discord, and social isolation. The parenting practices of these families are frequently aversive, and their sense of parenting competence is low

Department of Psychiatry, [1]Research Institute, [2]Neuropsychiatry Clinic, The Hospital for Sick Children, University of Toronto, Toronto, Ontario, Canada.

(Mash and Johnston, 1983; Patterson, 1986). These social and psychologic factors shape the course of the disorder and are predictive of a poor outcome (Hechtman et al., 1984; Parker and Asher, 1987; Taylor et al., 1996; Weiss et al., 1985).

PHARMACOLOGICAL TREATMENT

Currently, as many 1.5 million children in North America receive medication for ADHD (Safer et al., 1996). The majority of prescriptions are for stimulants, in particular methylphenidate (MPH; Ritalin) and, to a lesser extent, dextroamphetamine (DEX) (Safer and Krager, 1988; Safer and Zito, 1996; Swanson et al., 1995). In most instances, medication is used as a sole intervention (Wolraich et al., 1990). In general, there is good reason for this therapeutic enthusiasm. Numerous studies attest to the effectiveness of both MPH and DEX in mitigating a range of the deficits associated with ADHD (Greenhill, 1992; Jacobvitz et al., 1990; Spencer et al., 1996).

Psychostimulant treatment rapidly reduces the severity of the core behavioral manifestations of the syndrome such as restlessness, inattentiveness, and impulsiveness (Schachar et al., 1997) and, in addition, improves many aspects of parent–child and peer interaction (Barkley and Cunningham, 1979; Schachar et al., 1987), including a reduction in aggression (Cunningham et al., 1991; Hinshaw et al., 1989a; 1992). Stimulants improve attention and inhibition, which are the supposed core executive function deficit in ADHD (Douglas et al., 1995; Tannock et al., 1989) and increase academic productivity (Famularo and Fenton, 1987; see also Solanto, this volume, pp. 219–235 for review). The literature supporting the use of medication in the treatment of ADHD is discussed in Pelham and Smith, this volume, pp. 193–217 as well as Greenhill et al., this volume, pp. 385–400.

Limitations of medication

Given the widespread enthusiasm for medication in the treatment of ADHD and the numerous benefits that drug treatment confers, one might think that drugs provide a rather complete therapy for ADHD. However, that does not appear to be the case. One limitation of medication is the substantial number of ADHD children who do not respond favorably to stimulants. Although there is no widely accepted definition of unfavorable response, the rate of nonresponse is estimated to be 25% of treated children (e.g., Spencer et al., 1996). Most children exhibit behavioral improvement if a range of doses and both MPH and DEX are tried (Arnold, 1996; Elia et al., 1991; Firestone, 1982). However, many children experience reasonable behavioral response only at a dose that engenders unacceptable side effects (Ahmann et al., 1993; Barkley et al., 1990b; Elia et al., 1991). These side effects result in discontinuation of medication in a substantial proportion of cases (10%; Schachar et al., 1997). Children with tics or high levels of concurrent anxiety also may experience a poor response and an increased risk of side effects (DuPaul et al., 1994; Lipkin et al., 1994; Pliszka, 1992; see Solanto, this volume).

Even for those who have a favorable behavioral response, medication does not normalize all aspects of the disorder. For example, stimulants do not necessarily normalize peer relationships (Hinshaw and McHale, 1991; Hinshaw et al., 1989b; Whalen et al., 1989), classroom behavior (Abikoff and Gittelman, 1984; Elia et al., 1991; Rapport et al., 1994), academic achievement (Barkley and Cunningham, 1979; Firestone et al., 1986; Rapport et al., 1994; Wolraich et al., 1978), or sense of personal competence (Pelham et al., 1992; Whalen and Henker, 1976). Moreover, various aspects of child behavior and adjustment may be affected differently by a particular dose of medication (Sprague and Sleator, 1977).

Doses that optimize a child's behavior may not also optimize his or her academic performance (Rapport et al., 1994). Consequently, medication is not a remedy that is simultaneously optimal for all aspects of a child's impairment.

Stimulants have very brief duration of action (2–4 hours for regular MPH and 6 hours for slow-release preparations) and are effective only when pharmacologically active with no carryover to the latter part of the day or weekends when homework must be done and when family and peer interactions are common (Gadow et al., 1990; Schachar et al., 1997). Typically, this means that if medication is taken twice daily, as is the case for most children, one can expect little direct impact of medication in the home setting (Schachar et al., 1997). Efforts have been made to expand the period of active medication by prescribing a third dose of MPH (Kent et al., 1995; Stein et al., 1996). To date, research has involved only very brief periods of three-times-daily administration of medication. Consequently, we do not know how many children will be able to tolerate a late-day dose for lengthy periods of time without an increase in the prevalence and severity of side effects and increased risk of termination of an otherwise helpful treatment.

Moreover, the effects of medication dissipate rapidly on discontinuation of treatment (Brown et al., 1986) suggesting that there is little lasting benefit for the child's self-regulatory capacity derived from a period during which symptoms are suppressed by medication. This is a serious deficiency of MPH, given that ADHD is a lifelong condition for many affected individuals (Klein and Mannuzza, 1991; Mannuzza et al., 1991), and medication may not be taken for very long periods of time. Adherence to drug treatment is surprisingly low (Brown et al., 1987; Firestone, 1982; Kauffman et al., 1981), many doses of medication are missed (Kaufman et al., 1981), and many individuals discontinue medication despite apparent continued benefit (Firestone et al., 1986). Even with optimal supervision in specialty clinics, treatment seems to be rather brief in relationship to the chronicity of ADHD (Barkley et al., 1990a). For example, Firestone (1982) found that after 10 months, as many as 50% of children had stopped taking their medication, and their decision to do so had been taken without consulting a physician. Similarly, Barkley et al. (1990a) reported that ADHD children originally assessed in a specialty clinic had received MPH for an average of 3 years out of the 8-year follow-up period. Dislike of taking medication (Sleator et al., 1982), habituation (Charles and Schain, 1981; Kupietz et al., 1988), side effects (Charles and Schain, 1981; Rie et al., 1976), and parental worry about side effects (Charles and Schain, 1981) account for many of these cases of early discontinuation. By contrast, those who discontinued therapy are not any less likely to have benefited from MPH (Firestone, 1982).

Even with continued administration and attendant suppression of core ADHD symptoms, there is little evidence that stimulant treatment improves *long-term* scholastic attainment or antisocial behavior (Hechtman et al., 1984; Schachar and Tannock, 1993 for review). However, it may also be the case that long-term outcome is simply not altered by drug treatment because the acute effects of MPH (e.g., reduction of core symptoms) are not those (e.g., impaired parent–child, adult, and peer relationships) that are crucial determinants of long-term outcome (Loney et al., 1978; Parker and Asher, 1987; Weiss et al., 1985).

Finally, for many families, medication is not an acceptable intervention for ethical, medical, or other reasons (e.g. Schachar et al., 1997). In a recent treatment study involving random assignment to MPH or placebo, we screened families applying for assessment to a child psychiatry department for their ADHD child. Of 210 cases meeting screening criteria, 27% refused participation because they felt that MPH was an unacceptable treatment, compared with 5% who refused to participate because they felt that it would be unacceptable to administer placebo to their children. Firestone (1982) encountered a similar rate of refusal (26% of families). Moreover, medication makes little sense as an intervention in the early stages of the development of ADHD because it is unlikely to be acceptable to the majority of parents of preschoolers and those whose children show early and mild symptoms of ADHD. For all these reasons, clinicians have continued to look toward alternatives to stimulant treatment, especially in the realm of nonpharmacologic interventions.

PSYCHOSOCIAL INTERVENTIONS

Various nonpharmacologic therapies have been used to treat ADHD. The prevalence of these interventions is far more difficult to determine than is the prevalence of drug use. The most common approaches are probably variations of PT, self-control training for children (Abikoff et al., 1988; Abikoff and Gittelman, 1984; Hinshaw et al., 1984b), and family therapy. Formal behavior modification programs in the classroom are probably less commonly administered because of difficulty in implementation (e.g., Pelham et al., 1993; Wolraich et al., 1978). There is considerable evidence to support the effectiveness of several of these nonpharmacologic interventions (Schachar et al., 1996).

This chapter focuses on PT because it is effective, is widely available in the community, and is a natural complement to stimulant medication. The rationale for PT rests on the link between family function and child outcomes. Among them are the links between marital conflict and child behavior problems (Grych and Ficham, 1990), the more specific association of family dysfunction and conduct disorder among ADHD children (Szatmari et al., 1989a), and an increase in prevalence of alcohol abuse (West and Prinz, 1987) and parental psychopathology, in particular ADHD, among the families of ADHD children (Biederman et al., 1992; Schachar and Wachsmuth, 1990).

THE NATURE OF PARENT TRAINING

The term PT is used in this chapter to refer to a range of behaviorally based psychotherapeutic techniques that focus on the parents' interactions with an ADHD child. PT programs share many features but may differ in ways that are important. Typically, PT programs for ADHD children are developments of programs used in the treatment of noncompliant, oppositional, and/or aggressive children (Forehand and McMahon, 1981; Patterson, 1986). Intervention is based on social learning principles and on the notion that parent–child interaction is bidirectional and that inappropriate and coercive parental responses to problematic child behavior serve to sustain maladaptive patterns of interaction (Patterson, 1976). The emphasis is typically on managing or coping with, rather than curing, problematic child behavior. PT programs provide a framework for understanding maladaptive parent–child interaction in terms of child and parental characteristics and the consequences of particular parental and child responses. The curriculum includes strategies for attending to and rewarding positive child behavior, the application of consequences for negative behavior, planning for transitions, and training in skills for increasing prosocial interactions between siblings, avoiding conflict, and responding effectively to noncompliant, aggressive behavior. PT programs have been adapted to focus on the acquisition of attentional skills (Pisterman et al., 1989).

PT directly targets aversive and negative parent–child interactions that are known to typify the families of ADHD children (Cunningham et al., 1988). PT enhances the parent's sense of competence, promotes acquisition of effective parenting strategies, decreases parenting stress, increases familiarity with community resources, and increases the family's sense of cohesion within the community (Dumas and LaFreniere, 1993). PT indirectly targets the core self-regulatory deficit in ADHD that is implicated in the development of aversive patterns of interaction between the ADHD child and others. In contrast to self-control training and other forms of behavior modification, with PT, parents rather than a therapist or teacher become the agents of change through educating their children in strategies that promote planning, self-evaluation, and self-regulation. The objective of PT is to establish parents as *long-term* agents of change who target failures of self-regulation in the very situations in which they arise rather than in analog situations that are constructed in the clinic or classroom.

Some PT groups are didactic in style (Anastopoulos et al., 1991; Horn et al., 1991), whereas others are more experiential (Cunningham et al., 1993b). Most include some role-playing (e.g., Horn et al., 1991) or modeling (Cunningham et al., 1993b). Some emphasize contingency-based reinforcement procedures (Abikoff and Gittelman, 1984). In some cases, PT has been combined with a parallel behavioral intervention applied at school (Abikoff and Gittelman, 1984). PT programs may also contain elements of education about the nature of ADHD (Anastopoulos et al, 1991; cf. Cunningham et al., 1993b).

Commonly, PT courses consist of about 12 sessions. They may be conducted with individual families or with groups of families and within a clinic (Anastouplos et al., 1991) or a community setting (Cunningham et al., 1995). Usually, participants have specific "homework" assignments to complete between sessions, and these assignments are reviewed within the sessions. Modeling of specific parenting strategies may occur within sessions, readings may be specified, and written handouts may be distributed (e.g., Abikoff and Gittelman, 1984). Some programs provide an opportunity for discussion of interpersonal family problems (e.g., Abikoff and Gittelman, 1984; Prinz and Miller, 1994). Booster sessions following completion of the PT program are commonly provided. PT programs can be delivered in a large group format within the community for low cost, compared to individually administered, clinic-based treatments (Cunningham et al., 1995).

PT has several potential advantages over pharmacologic treatment. PT may be a more acceptable intervention (Firestone, 1982; Kazdin, 1980). For example, 15% of families in the sample described by Firestone (1982) refused medication but accepted PT. PT has the added advantage of being well suited to programs of early intervention for children who might have only mild or moderate manifestations of ADHD or for young children who may be at risk for the development of more serious disturbance but who do not at the time of assessment have sufficient impairment to warrant more aggressive forms of intervention. In most treatment studies involving medication, a substantial proportion of clinic-referred cases are excluded because the child's presenting problems are not severe enough to warrant a diagnosis of ADHD or to justify treatment with medication. Even among clinic-referred cases, this is a substantial number of children (9%, Horn et al., 1991; 16%, Schachar et al., 1997). Many others may be excluded because the child has a comorbid condition (e.g., anxiety or tics) that is a relative contraindication to stimulant medications. Presumably, the families of these otherwise excluded children have sufficient concern about their children's adjustment to warrant contacting a treatment facility. Many of these families could be candidates for nonpharmacologic interventions.

Effectiveness of PT

Not only does PT make sense from a theoretical perspective as a treatment for ADHD, but it also appears to be effective. PT has been applied with reported success to preschool (Forehand and King, 1977; Pisterman et al., 1992b) and school-age children (Peed et al., 1977). PT improves parental behavior management skills (e.g., more consistent reinforcement of child compliance), increases child compliance, and enhances the parent's sense of competence (Cunningham et al., 1993a; Pisterman et al., 1992a, 1992c). These benefits persist for as long as 6 months following treatment (Cunningham et al., 1995; Pisterman et al, 1989). Some effects are not evident until later, for instance at a 6-month follow-up (Cunningham et al., 1995). PT is effective when administered in groups in the community as well as in clinic settings (Cunningham et al., 1995). The effect of PT increases with increasing attendance (Cunningham et al., 1995).

Generalization of the benefits of PT from the clinic to the home setting has been demonstrated (Peed et al., 1977; Forehand et al., 1981). But generalization to the school setting is inconsistent (McMahon and Davies, 1980), and generalization of effects to behaviors which were not specifically targeted by the PT is also inconsistent (Forehand and Atkeson, 1977; Wells et al., 1980; Pisterman et al., 1989). Parent training with preschoolers may improve child compliance but has little effect on the core deficits of ADHD (Pisterman et al., 1992c).

What is more important is the limited utilization and acceptability of PT reported in many studies. Some parents find PT or group treatment too involved or threatening and may prefer individual treatment (Pisterman et al., 1989; 1992b). And, some children find medication more acceptable than some behavioral interventions (Kazdin, 1984). Acceptability will have a direct effect on participation, enrollment, and adherence. Utilization rates for PT are approximately 50% in clinical settings (range of 28% to 50% Forehand et al., 1983) and slightly lower in groups conducted in the community (Cunningham et al., 1995; Firestone and Witt, 1982).

The typical family with an affected ADHD child has many of the characteristics that have been linked with low utilization, low responsiveness to parent training interventions, and high levels of dropout from treatment (Kazdin and Mazurick, 1994; Kazdin et al., 1997). For example, these families are characterized by parental depression (McMahon et al, 1981), low socioeconomic status (McMahon et al, 1981), low social support (Dumas and Wahler, 1983), low father involvement, and single-parent status (Patterson, 1976; Webster-Stratton, 1985). Even though utilization is greater among families with children who are highly disturbed than those with less disturbed children, fewer than half of families with highly disturbed children may enroll in PT programs (Cunningham et al., 1995).

Rationale for combined PT and medication

Even though PT is a theoretically appropriate and potentially effective treatment for ADHD in children, it has many limitations. However, the combination of medication with PT may compensate for many of these deficiencies. The question is, How might these two treatments work when combined? To answer this, we now turn to the possible effects of combining PT and MPH and the design requirements of any evaluation study before reviewing existing research evidence on the effectiveness of this combination. In general, combinations of interventions could have additive, nonadditive, positive, or negative synergistic, or positive or negative transactional effects.

Nonadditive effect

The first possibility is that the combination of two treatments may be no more effective than the most potent of the two individual treatments. Nonadditive effects could arise if one treatment on its own normalizes child behavior or if one intervention is essentially ineffective. Nonadditive effects might also arise as an artifact if a child reaches the ceiling on a particular outcome measure with one of the two treatments or if measures are not collected of the potential impact of each individual intervention. For example, it would be impossible for PT to enhance the effectiveness of MPH if MPH alone normalizes performance on a particular measure or if the study failed to include measures of treatment effects that are likely to emanate from PT (e.g., increase in compliance). Also, combined interventions might appear to have nonadditive effects if outcome measures are taken while one intervention is at the peak of its effects while the other is not.

Additive effect

Additive effects are evident when the impact of the combined intervention is greater than the effects of the individual interventions. Additive effects could arise when treatments operate primarily in different domains because of unique temporal effects. For example, MPH may affect daytime behavior and PT may affect behavior in the evening. Or each treatment may affect different symptoms. For example, MPH may reduce core ADHD symptoms and PT may improve the quality of parent–child interaction or reduce child aggression. Two treatments also could have quite distinct timing of onset: MPH effects may be observed almost immediately (Schachar et al., 1997), whereas PT effects may only be detected following completion of the intervention. Combined treatment could be more persistent and prevent relapse following termination of one or both components of treatment. This outcome would be particularly useful given the tendency for children to discontinue MPH, mentioned earlier. Persistence of treatment effects must be assessed in order to prove these hypotheses, given that ADHD is a chronic and persistent condition and that many of the impairments that are targeted in treatment do not arise until adolescence or adulthood.

Positive synergistic effect

PT and MPH could actually have mutually potentiating or synergistic effects, in which combined treatments could have effects that are greater than the sum of the effects of each individual treatment. A positive synergistic effect could arise if medication facilitates the acquisition of self-regulatory competence through improving attention, learning, memory or the capacity of the child for self-evaluation (e.g., Hinshaw et al., 1984a). Or, PT may train parents to identify and reinforce self-control skills acquired through use of medication. Although interactions between two types of intervention might yield greater effects than treatment on its own, two interventions might interact by achieving equivalent improvement at a lower dose of medication or with a less intensive family intervention. Lower doses of medication could mean fewer side effects and increased acceptability of medication. The use of less intense PT would reduce the cost and increase the availability of this intervention.

Negative synergistic effect

Not all interactions between interventions may be beneficial. For example, medication could undermine efforts to alter parenting practices by increasing the child's irritability, dysphoria, insomnia, or other side effects that might, in turn, have an adverse impact on child behavior. Adverse cognitive effects of MPH such as overfocusing might impair learning of new self-regulatory strategies.

Positive transactional effect

Transactional effects arise when one treatment effects the *process* of the other treatment. For example, rapid suppression of the core behavioral manifestations of ADHD resulting from administration of medication may make a family more likely to continue therapy because they will not be as discouraged with the slower pace of progress that can be associated with PT. Conversely, PT might enhance a family's sense of competence, which might otherwise be undermined by drug treatment. Or, PT could facilitate adherence to medication treatment through increasing awareness of the advantages of medication, knowledge of side effects and information about the nature of ADHD. These processes might allow parents to support the use of medication for longer periods of time.

Negative transactional effect

Just as one treatment might have a positive effect on the course of another treatment, so might one treatment have a negative effect on the other. For example, parents might feel that drug treatment would be premature as long as there are available psychosocial interventions they have not tried. Conversely, rapid improvement resulting from medication might undermine commitment to nonpharmacologic interventions by reinforcing the notion that ADHD requires a neurobiologic treatment, by relieving distress, by undermining readiness for change, or by providing a face-saving alternative to considering family factors in a child's difficulties. Or, medication might cause side effects that lead families to discontinue all forms of therapy, including parent training.

COMBINED TREATMENT STUDIES

Design and methodological considerations

A typical group design in combined treatment research is the single-factor design, in which two or more levels of one factor are varied, for example, pharmacotherapy, PT, and combined pharmacotherapy and PT. The relative effectiveness of each of these treatments is evaluated with a between-subject design, in which subjects are randomly assigned to receive one of the treatments, or a with-subject design, in which each subject receives all the treatments at different points in time. More powerful for evaluating synergistic effects are factorial designs, which involve simultaneous manipulation of two or more independent variables in a single study. The major advantage of the factorial design is that it permits examination of more than one treatment variable and their possible interactions in a more efficient and powerful manner than is possible with the single-factor designs (Ackles, 1986). An example would be random assignment to one of four treatment arms involving one of two levels of drug (e.g., MPH, placebo) or one of two levels of parent training (parent training, wait list control). Or, dose of medication (high versus low dose) might be varied to see if PT effects depended on the dose of medication. There are many variations on these basic group designs. All group designs require that there be random assignment to treatment conditions with concealment of condition.

In addition, single-case designs have been used to study the possible combined effects of medication and PT. Single-case designs, including withdrawal designs, multiple baseline designs, and alternating treatments designs (Ackles, 1986) present useful alternatives to the group designs and have many advantages (Barlow and Hersen, 1973).

Several requirements of a study that would be sensitive to combined treatment effect warrant particular mention. In order for evaluations of combined interventions to be sensitive to potential additive effects across situations or settings (e.g., in the school and in the home), subjects must exhibit pervasive symptoms. Many ADHD children exhibit their symptoms largely in the school setting (Szatmari et al., 1989b). In those cases, there may be relatively less behavioral disturbance in the home, resulting in a bias toward the effectiveness of MPH. It is necessary to use measures of treatment outcome that do not reach a ceiling with one of the two treatments in order to identify treatment interactions. Also, it is necessary to vary dose of medication in order to identify the possibility that combined treatments involving low doses of medication may be as effective as high doses of medication. Evaluations must be conducted over extensive periods of time to match the circumstances of typical practice.

The clinical significance of changes resulting from treatment cannot be established from mean or statistical difference between treatments alone but rather also require assessment of whether treated children behave similarly to normal children. As a result, it is ideal if normal comparison groups are included in combined treatment studies. Additionally, given the high prevalence of ADHD, the cost and utilization of treatments are important aspects of the evaluation of effectiveness.

Process and utilization measures are required in order to determine whether the provision of one treatment might have an impact on the provision of another. For example, does attendance at a PT group have an impact on medication compliance? Or, does medication treatment undermine commitment to nonpharmacologic interventions?

Identification of combined PT and medication treatment studies

Studies of combined PT and medication in the treatment of ADHD were identified through a search of Medline and PsychLit for English-language reports, followed by search for individual studies cited in those reports. The search method included ADHD treatment, combined treatments, parent training, and multimodal treatments. Comorbidity was not an exclusion. MPH and DEX were included. Few studies of combined PT and MPH were identified (Table 1). Uncontrolled cohort studies (e.g., Satterfield et al., 1982) were not included, although they suggest that multimodal interventions might enhance treatment outcome. Only studies that included some experimental control and a clear definition of ADHD were included. Three studies involved single-case designs (O'Leary and Pelham, 1978; Pelham et al., 1980; Pollard et al., 1983), and the remainder involved randomized control trials with either single-factor (Gittelman et al., 1980; Firestone et al., 1986) or factorial designs (Horn et al., 1991). In the study of O'Leary and Pelham (1978), MPH was withdrawn from seven ADHD subjects and nonpharmacologic treatment was given. There was no treatment condition in which MPH and PT were combined. Therefore, this study allows for comparison of MPH and PT but does not permit conclusions about the additive and synergistic effects of these two interventions. A total of 230 school-age subjects were involved in these studies. Meta-analysis was considered inappropiate because of the small number of subjects and the absence of a common outcome measure. Instead, a descriptive approach is taken in summarizing these studies.

In two studies (Firestone et al., 1981; Pollard et al., 1983), PT was the sole nonpharmacologic intervention, whereas in the other studies, PT was combined with self-control training (Horn et al., 1991) or classroom-based behavior modification conducted by a teacher (Gittelman et al., 1980; O'Leary and Pelham, 1978; Pelham et al., 1980). All these studies used MPH, usually administered twice per day for the most part. The dosing regimen was once per day in Pelham et al. (1980) and unspecified in Horn et al. (1991) and in O'Leary and Pelham (1978). The dose of MPH was manipulated systematically only in the studies of Pelham et al. (1980) and Horn et al. (1991). In the other studies, the dose of MPH was determined through clinical titration. In every study, the effects of the medication condition were assessed while the child was on active medication.

Two studies involved extensive follow-up periods of 12 months (Firestone et al., 1986) and 9 months (Horn et al., 1991; Ialongo et al., 1993). Only one study with a group design involved follow-up without medication in order to assess the effect of combined treatment on relapse prevention (Ialongo et al., 1993). Ialongo et al. (1993) monitored the subjects described in Horn et al. (1991) 9 months after the termination of the behavioral intervention *and* the withdrawal of stimulant medication.

Effects of combined treatment

Overall, the majority of studies have concluded that combinations of MPH and PT have nonadditive effects. When additive effects were detected, there is reason to believe that they were not primarily a result of PT. Firestone et al. (1986) observed that MPH resulted in greater improvement than did PT (PT + placebo condition) in classroom behavior, attention, and impulse control and that PT + MPH and MPH alone were approximately equivalent in effectiveness over the 2-year follow-up. Horn et al. (1991) identified some apparent evidence of additive effects. Combined treatment permitted the use of a lower dose of medication: Low-dose MPH (0.4 mg/kg) combined with PT was as effective in reducing teacher ratings of core ADHD symptoms as was high-dose MPH (0.8 mg/kg) when administered with or without PT. It is likely, however, that this apparent additive effect was a result of the self-control training that was combined with the PT, because no treatment effects of either MPH or PT were detected in the home. Gittelman et al. (1980) obtained a similar result. A positive interaction between MPH and PT was apparent for one observational measure. In-seat activity level showed greater improvement with combined PT + MPH treatment than with MPH alone, and the combined treatment produced the clearest *normalization* in comparison with a control group in classroom behavior. However, these apparent additive effects of combined treatment were likely a result of the behavior training strategies taught to classroom teachers, because no treatment effects of either MPH or PT were detected by parents.

Ialongo et al. (1993) were unable to demonstrate an additive effect of MPH and PT in terms of relapse prevention. They presented a 9-month follow-up of the children described in Horn et al. (1991) after MPH had been withdrawn following the acute phase of the intervention. Overall, they concluded that there was no evidence to support the hypothesis that PT enhanced maintenance of treatment gains. However, they did note (p. 188) that 25% of children treated initially in the combined treatment condition maintained their improvement on teacher ratings of core ADHD symptoms following discontinuation of MPH.

Pollard et al. (1983) reported that PT or MPH alone was sufficient to provide noticeable, clinically significant improvement in ratings of hyperactive behavior and in directly observed parent-child interactions. In general, combined intervention was not more effective than each individual treatment administered alone. However, additive effects were evident in that MPH and PT had somewhat *different* effects: MPH resulted in decreased maternal commands, whereas PT led to an increase in maternal positive responding. Pelham et al. (1980) reported that on-task behavior in the school setting was higher after intensive behavioral intervention than before, which argues for a positive interaction between school-based behavioral intervention and MPH.

Firestone et al. (1981; 1986) compared MPH + PT, placebo + PT, and MPH alone and found few differences in outcome. However, two aspects of their results could indicate a minimal *negative* interaction between MPH and PT. The MPH treatment group actually achieved greater gains in teacher-rated hyperactivity and academic performance than the placebo + PT or the MPH + PT groups.

In general, there is little evidence in this body of research to support any conclusions about the impact of one intervention on another. There is little evidence that adherence to

Table 1. Summary of Combined Treatment Studies of Attention Deficit Hyperactivity Disorder

Study	*Design*	*Age (years)*	*No.*	*Comparison*	*Duration (months)*	*Attrition (%)*	*Follow-up (months)*	*Attrition (%)*	*Dosing Schedule*	*Adjustment*	*Single Dose (mg/kg)*
Firestone et al. (1981)	SF	7	73	PT + PL, PT + MPH, MPH	3	50	12	62	BID	T	0.7
Gittelman et al. (1980)	SF	8	61	PT + PL, PT + MPH, MPH	2	5	0	NA	BID	T	0.7
Horn et al. (1991)	FD	9	78	PT + PL, PT + LO, PT + HI, PL, LO, HI	3	10	9	26	NS	F	0.4 & 0.8
O'Leary & Pelham (1978)	WD	8	7	PT, MPH, no med	4	12	1	12	NS	T	NS
Pelham et al. (1980)	MB	8	8	PT + MPH, MPH, PT, no treatment	3	0	5	0	OD	F	0.25, 0.75
Pollard et al. (1983)	NS	7	3	PT, MPH, PT + MPH	2	0	3	0	BID	T	0.35–0.6

SF = single factor; PT = parent training; PL = placebo; MPH = methylphenidate; T = titration; F = fixed dose; BID = twice daily; OD = once daily; NA = not applicable; NS = not specified; FD = factorial design; WD = withdrawal design; MB = multiple baseline; LO = low dose of MPH; HI = high dose of MPH.

combined and individual treatments differs from adherence to individual treatment conditions (e.g., Firestone et al., 1981; 1986). The only exception was the study by Horn et al. (1991), which found some evidence that families of children receiving medication may be *more* likely to discontinue a PT program; 8 of 32 assigned to MPH dropped out, versus 3 of 32 assigned to placebo.

DISCUSSION

The research reviewed in this chapter fails to support the hypothesis that the combination of MPH and PT has additive, synergistic, or transactional effects. Apparently, MPH treatment as a solo treatment achieves the same therapeutic result as it does when combined with PT. This observation is remarkable, given that PT, when administered by itself, is a demonstrably effective intervention for improving parenting practices and child behavior (see Kazdin, 1997, for review). How do we explain these results?

One set of explanations for these results may rest on the methodological limitations of the available research: PT and MPH may be effective in combination, but these combined effects may not be detectable within the limits of the available research. Perhaps better designed studies would reveal previously undetected effects of combined treatment. Methodological limitations in the body of the available research have been marked. Few children have been studied, and then only for relatively short periods of time. Potential interactions between PT and MPH have been studied inadequately because of the limited use of full factorial designs involving at least two levels of each treatment. Few studies have manipulated the dose of MPH to assess the possibility that combined treatment involving a low dose of MPH might achieve the same results as a high dose of MPH on its own. Relapse prevention has rarely been studied. While the positive effects of stimulants dissipate following termination of treatment, the beneficial effects of PT might emerge more gradually as parents acquire and practice more effective management skills. Consequently, longer periods of follow-up may be necessary to detect these effects.

Moreover, the effect of MPH is generally assessed under optimal conditions, that is, while medication is active. By contrast, PT is assessed some time after completion of the intervention. This comparison is fair in some ways, as it is predicated on the assumption that PT is sufficiently intense to achieve maximal and *persisting* effects. That is the stated goal of PT. However, these assumptions regarding PT are unproven. The effects of PT may take longer to develop. Although the doses of MPH is either manipulated in some studies or titrated to achieve optimal response in others, no similar procedure is used with PT. Neither duration, intensity, nor type of PT has been titrated in past combined treatment studies.

It is usual for research studies to adopt one type of parenting program for all parents (often for theoretical reasons rather than for reasons of specific efficacy or effectiveness). This strategy may miss the real differences that parents bring to the treatment. Although coping and mastery models of teaching parenting skills may work for many parents, other parents wish or require direct didactic instruction in order to understand their roles and choices. Although it is unlikely that one would suggest only one dosage of medication for all children (say 10 mg of MPH twice a day without regard to age, weight, comorbidity, or severity of impairments), research protocols typically offer one kind of parenting intervention with one kind of approach and intensity to the curriculum. While a great deal of time and energy has been devoted to optimizing the effects of medication, relatively less time has been spent in optimizing the effects of parenting programs in these studies.

The research studies reviewed here have generally made a strong case for the sophistication of the PT that was applied. Often PT was administered according to explicit manuals, by well-trained therapists, and in a reliable manner. However, it is far simpler to ensure the integrity of pharmacologic treatment than to ensure the integrity of PT, therapist commitment, and treatment potency. Perhaps this explains why PT in some treatment settings outperforms PT in others.

Methodological issues, such as pervasiveness of symptoms in study samples and ceiling effects on outcome measures, may have an impact on results. Low pretreatment levels of oppositional behavior may have precluded the detection of incremental effects of combined treatment in some studies (e.g. Horn et al., 1991). By contrast, most parental measures of child behavior have not been specifically tied to behavior in the home and may be influenced by "spillover" of perceived improvement at school. In other words, parents may be so relieved to receive reports of their child's improvement at school that they may actually report that the child is better at home. Sufficient care has not been taken to prevent this halo effect.

A second set of explanations for the apparent lack of incremental effect of PT and MPH may be attributed to the issue of treatment readiness. Studies of PT as a solo treatment have largely been conducted in specialized clinical settings, often those with a particular interest in PT. These studies would select families who were highly "ready" for PT. In sharp contrast, families attending settings in which combined treatment studies are typically conducted may be preoccupied with medication, may prefer neurobiologic explanations for ADHD, or may be less prepared for change. Exactly how these biases operate needs to be clarified. The mechanism may not be simple. There is evidence in some studies that parents acquire the social learning principles and practices that are taught in PT (see Ialongo et al., 1993, p. 186), and many studies record high attendance (Horn et al., 1991). However, high rates of attendance and assimilation of PT principles are not typical findings, suggesting that barriers to the success of PT certainly include suboptimal commitment to treatment.

In clinical practice rather than research protocols, client preferences are seen as integral and active parts of the treatment and its potential outcome. Client preferences for a particular style of treatment are included as factors in the selection and recommendation of specific treatments. In research studies, client preferences may be barriers to participation in a study, as clients must agree to random assignment. Randomization might impede commitment to the treatment and the development of a sense of ownership of the treatment. For some clients, being able to choose a treatment may be part and parcel of successful psychosocial treatment intervention (Prochaska et al., 1995).

Treatment implications

Does the conclusion reached in this review mean that clinicians should not recommend combined treatments and that researchers should not plan further combined treatment studies? Certainly not. To begin with, this review dealt only with the combination of MPH and PT. Combinations of medication and classroom management programs appear to yield additive and synergistic effects in measures of aggression (Abikoff and Gittelman, 1984; Carlson et al., 1992), academic achievement (Pelham et al., 1986; Richardson et al., 1988), and inattentive, overactive behavior (Christensen, 1975; Pelham et al., 1993). These combinations may permit the use of lower doses of medication, at least in the classroom (Abramowitz et al., 1992; Carlson et al., 1992) and may be more likely to achieve normalization in behavior (Hinshaw et al., 1984a). Moreover, classroom-based behavior intervention might target different behaviors than does medication (e.g. Wolraich et al., 1978).

The studies reviewed used only a limited range of PT programs. There are many strategies for enhancing the effectiveness of PT. For example, competency-based models of PT appear to be more potent than are didactic training methods (Rickert et al., 1988). For other families, PT may be enhanced through the provision of a systemic family intervention aimed at the identification and resolution of family issues before or after PT (Prinz and Miller, 1994). Besides providing an appropriate forum for the negotiation of family issues, this kind of systemic family intervention may serve to enhance the utilization of PT. Providing PT in a community setting rather than in specialized clinics may increase utilization, as community settings are typically seen as less stigmatizing (Cunningham et al., 1995; Szapocznik et al., 1980; Henggeler et al., 1995). When peer relationship skills are indicated as one of the child's major needs, combining PT with other psychosocial interventions, such as social skills groups, may be useful. This combination of social skills training and PT has shown some success (Frankel et al., 1997). Simultaneous treatment of children and parents through interrelated groups may have the effect of enhancing enrollment in both treatments.

PT may be rendered more effective if interventions are tailored to the characteristics and readiness of individual families. Families vary considerably in the extent to which they are ready to accept and commit to particular treatments. Treatment readiness varies with the severity of the child's disturbance, the extent to which the child's disturbance impairs family functioning, and the parental perception of the child's difficulties. These factors can change over time with the maturity of the child or, conversely, with the lack of it. The range of issues to be considered in creating the fit of parents to specific treatments includes not only the focus and relevance of the material to the child's situation but also the level of the language used and where the course takes place. Other factors that may have an impact on effectiveness and utilization are the style of the course (e.g., whether hands-on practice is required); the required commitment implied by the frequency, length, and total number of sessions; the costs of or the financial benefits of attending; and the distance that parents will have to travel as well as the time of day. Each of these logistic decisions has its own cascade of effects in enabling enrollment, attendance, and adherence or in creating additional barriers. Tailoring treatments to the needs of the family and layering them in time may have the effect of reducing dropouts from treatments and may yield more specific and meaningful results.

Readiness itself is not a static phenomenon. Consequently, various approaches may be used to move families along the continuum of treatment readiness. It may be possible to alter a family's decisional balance about a treatment (Prochaska et al., 1995) by increasing knowledge and opinions of ADHD as well as of PT and MPH. Education about various treatment options may be necessary before any particular treatment is begun.

The timing of the introduction of PT may be another crucial determinant of the utilization and effectiveness of PT. PT may be more effective once families have noticed the limitations of MPH. We often recommend all treatments simultaneously at the time of initial diagnosis or first intervention. This may short-circuit the process that the family must go through to find their own meaning from the diagnostic information. Complex ideas may need time to become personally meaningful. The hope for a "quick cure" may have to be explored first and exhausted before another treatment will be found to be worthy enough to be tried. If medication is very powerful in the short term, other treatments may look as if they are unnecessary. However, for some children, the "honeymoon period" of medication is followed by a period of less dramatic effectiveness. This kind of change may create a new platform of readiness that did not exist before the diagnosis and the initial medication trial. Families are ready for a particular treatment in the context of the information, distress, and motivation that they have at a particular time. The assumption cannot be made that one is ready for any or all treatments just because a problem exists. Given these potential changes in readiness, opportunities should be available for families to revisit treatments that they have previously attended and found to be of limited use. However, it must be noted that once a family has been offered a treatment and has not followed it, they tend to have the sense that they have "already been there and done that." Therefore, a treatment should be offered only when there is actually a reasonable probability of uptake.

Combined treatments may be rendered more effective if strategic therapeutic alliances between involved professionals are created and maintained. Typically, the professionals who provide PT are not the same people as those who assess children for this disorder and who prescribe and monitor medications. These alliances may require much preparation, as the goals, training, and paradigms that the two arms of these combined treatments use to assess their own outcomes and effectiveness may differ.

Given that the symptoms of ADHD persist over time, it is important for the clinician to maintain an ongoing relationship as a collaborator with the child and family in their struggle with ADHD. The goals in this relationship are not just related to the counting and influencing of discrete targets, such as in-seat behavior, but are also focused on the larger and longer-term issues of the quality of life of the child and family. The targets of our interventions and measured outcomes of our treatments must be relevant to the burden of suffering that ADHD can create for the child in the context of the family and community. This commitment to affecting quality-of-life issues requires a multimodal approach that can be adapted to the changing needs of the child and family as part of their long-term treatment and care.

CONCLUSION

ADHD is not cured by medication alone. Certainly medication is effective, particularly in the short term, for many aspects of an ADHD child's difficulties. Nevertheless, the medications so far available do not eliminate all impairments. In particular, problems remain in the relationship between the child and his or her parents. There is good reason to believe that these parent–child problems figure importantly in the poor outcome of many children. Furthermore, medication, as effective as it is, is typically used for brief periods of time in relationship to the chronicity of ADHD.

All these limitations provide compelling logic for the combination of pharmacologic and nonpharmacologic interventions. Although this review finds little support for the effectiveness of combined MPH and PT treatments, the combination has been studied little, and many methodological problems hamper the possibility of detecting combined effects. There is an urgent need to investigate various means of enhancing PT and methods for combining interventions. Typically, all interventions are offered at the same time. This may not be the optimal method. In some cases, it may be preferable to offer PT after a period of treatment with medication. By that time, families may be more aware of the limitations of medication and be ready for alternatives. Therapists need to consider treatment planning in relationship to the family's readiness for treatment. Practical means of assessing and enhancing readiness need to be developed.

Finally, new methods of evaluating efficacy that allow for choice of treatment need to be explored. This might be done by segmenting the population at the outset into those wishing to choose a specific treatment and those who are willing to be randomized to the various treatments. This method approximates the way in which people typically approach treatment. Some have a specific idea in mind and are searching for specific treatment resources, whereas others are willing to put their trust in the process and will follow "what the doctor orders." Neither stance is necessarily right or wrong, but the former is not very often represented in well-designed controlled treatment studies. The challenge is to find research methodologies that allow for treatment selection in a naturalistic manner that fosters commitment to treatments and supports clients becoming ready for these treatments while still being part of treatment effectiveness studies.

ACKNOWLEDGMENT

The authors acknowledge the assistance of Suzanne Bojthy in the preparation of the manuscript for this chapter.

REFERENCES

Abikoff, H., Ganeles, D., Reiter, G., Blum, C., Foley, C. & Klein, R.G. (1988), Cognitive training in academically deficient ADDH boys receiving stimulant medication. *J. Abnormal Child Psychol.,* 16:411–432.

Abikoff, H. & Gittelman, R. (1984), Does behavior therapy normalize the classroom behavior of hyperactive children? *Arch. Gen. Psychiatry*, 41:449–454.

Abramowitz, A.J., Eckstrand, D., O'Leary, S.G. & Dulcan, M.K. (1992), ADHD children's responses to stimulant medication and two intensities of a behavioral intervention. *Behav. Modification*, 16:193–203.

Ackles, P.K. (1986), Evaluating pharmacological–behavioral treatment interactions. In: *Pharmacological and Behavioral Treatment: An Integrative Approach*, ed., M. Hersen. New York: John Wiley & Sons, Inc., 54–86.

Ahmann, P.A., Waltonen, S.J., Olson, K.A., Theye, F.W., Van Erem, A.J. & LaPlant, R.J. (1993), Placebo-controlled evaluation of Ritalin side effects. *Pediatrics*, 91: 1101–1106.

American Psychiatric Association (1994), *Diagnostic and Statistical Manual of Mental Disorders, 4th ed.* (*DSM-IV*). Washington, DC: American Psychiatric Association.

Anastopoulos, A.D., DuPaul, G.J. & Barkley, R.A. (1991), Stimulant medication and parent training therapies for attention deficit-hyperactivity disorder. *J. Learning Disabil.*, 24:210–218.

Arnold, L.E. (1996), Responders and nonresponders. *J. Am. Acad. Child Adolesc. Psychiatry*, 35:1569–1570.

Barkley, R.A. (1990), *Attention-Deficit Hyperactivity Disorder: A Handbook for Diagnosis and Treatment.* New York: Guilford Press.

Barkley, R.A. (1997), Behavioral inhibition, sustained attention, and executive functions: Constructing a unifying theory of ADHD. *Psychol. Bull.,* 121:65–94.

Barkley, R.A. & Cunningham, C.E. (1979), The effects of methylphenidate on the mother–child interactions of hyperactive children. *Arch. Gen. Psychiatry*, 36:201–208.

Barkley, R.A., Fischer, M., Edelbrock, C.S. & Smallish, L. (1990a), The adolescent outcome of hyperactive children diagnosed by research criteria: I. An 8-year prospective follow-up study. *J. Am. Acad. Child Adolesc. Psychiatry*, 29:546–557.

Barkley, R.A., McMurray, M.B., Edelbrock, C.S. & Robbins, K. (1990b), Side effects of methylphenidate in children with attention deficit hyperactivity disorder: A systemic, placebo-controlled evaluation. *Pediatrics*, 86:184–192.

Barlow, D.H. & Hersen, M. (1973), Single-case experimental designs: Uses in applied clinical research. *Arch. Gen. Psychiatry*, 29:319–325.

Biederman, J., Faraone, S.V., Keenan, K., Benjamin, J., Krifcher, B., Moore, C., Sprich-Buckminster, S., Ugaglia, K., Jellinek, M.S., Steingard, R. et al. (1992), Further evidence for family-genetic risk factors in attention deficit hyperactivity disorder: Patterns of comorbidity in probands and relatives psychiatrically and pediatrically referred samples. *Arch. Gen. Psychiatry*, 49:728–38.

Biederman, J., Newcorn, J. & Sprich, S. (1991), Comorbidity of attention deficit hyperactivity disorder with conduct, depressive, anxiety, and other disorders. *Am. J. Psychiatry*, 148:564–577.

Brown, R.T., Borden, K.A., Wynne, M.E., Schleser, R. & Clingerman, S.R. (1986), Methylphenidate and cognitive therapy with ADD children: A methodological reconsideration. *J. Abnorm. Child Psychol.*, 14:481–497.

Brown, R.T., Borden, K.A., Wynne, M.E., Spunt, A.L. & Clingerman, S.R. (1987), Compliance with pharmacological and cognitive treatments for attention deficit disorder. *J. Am. Acad. Child Adolesc. Psychiatry*, 26:521–526.

Campbell, S.B. (1994), Hard-to-manage preschool boys: Externalizing behavior, social competence, and family context at two-year followup. *J. Abnorm. Child Psychol.*, 22:147–166.

Carlson, C.L., Pelham, W.E. Jr., Milich, R. & Dixon, J. (1992), Single and combined effects of methylphenidate and behavior therapy on the classroom performance of children with attention-deficit hyperactivity disorder. *J. Abnorm. Child Psychol.* 20:213–232.

Charles, L. & Schain, R. (1981), A four-year follow-up study of the effects of methylphenidate on the behavior and academic achievement of hyperactive children. *J. Abnorm. Child Psychol.*, 9:495–505.

Charles, L., Schain, R.J., Zelniker, T. & Guthrie, D. (1979), Effects of methylphenidate on hyperactive children's ability to sustain attention. *Pediatrics*, 64:412–418.

Christensen, D.E. (1975), Effects of combining methylphenidate and a classroom token system in modifying hyperactive behavior. *Am. J. Ment. Defic.*, 80:266–276.

Cunningham, C.E., Benness, B.B. & Siegel, L.S. (1988), Family functioning, time allocation, and parental depression in the families of normal and ADDH children. *J. Clin. Child Psychol.*, 17:169–177.

Cunningham, C.E., Bremner, R. & Boyle, M. (1995), Large group community-based parenting programs for families of preschoolers at risk for disruptive behaviour disorders: Utilization, cost effectiveness and outcome. *J. Child Psychol. Psychiatry Allied Disc.*, 36:1141–1159.

Cunningham, C.E., Bremner, R. & Secord-Gilbert, M. (1993a), Increasing the availability, accessibility, and cost efficacy of services for families of ADHD children: A school-based systems-oriented parenting course. *Can. J. School Psychol.*, 9:1–15.

Cunningham, C.E., Davis, J.R., Bremner, R., Dunn, K.W. & Rzasa, T. (1993b), Coping modeling problem solving versus mastery modeling: Effects on adherence, in-session process, and skill acquisition in a residential parent-training program. *J. Consult. Clin. Psychol.*, 61:871–877.

Cunningham, C.E., Siegel, L.S. & Offord, D.R. (1991), A dose-response analysis of the effects of methylphenidate on the peer interactions and simulated classroom performance of ADD children with and without conduct problems. *J. Child Psychol. Psychiatry Allied Disc.*, 32:439–452.

Douglas, V.I. (1988), Cognitive deficits in children with attention deficit disorder with hyperactivity. In: *Attention Deficit Disorder*, eds., L.M. Bloomingdale & J. Sergeant. Great Britain: Pergamon Press, pp. 65–82.

Douglas, V.I., Barr, R.G., Desilets, J. & Sherman, E. (1995), Do high doses of stimulants impair flexible thinking in attention-deficit hyperactivity disorder? *J. Am. Acad. Child Adolesc. Psychiatry*, 34:877–885.

Dumas, J.E. & LaFreniere, P.J. (1993), Mother-child relationships as sources of support or stress: A comparison of competent, average, aggressive, and anxious dyads. *Child Dev.*, 64:1732–1754.

Dumas, J.E. & Wahler, R.G. (1983), Predictors of treatment outcome in parent training: Mother insularity and socioeconomic disadvantage. *Behav. Assess.*, 5:301–313.

DuPaul, G.J., Barkley, R.A. & McMurray, M.B. (1994), Response of children with ADHD to methylphenidate: Interaction with internalizing symptoms. *J. Am. Acad. Child Adolesc. Psychiatry*, 33:894–903.

Elia, J. Borcherding, B.G., Rapoport, J.L. & Keysor, C.S. (1991), Methylphenidate and dextroamphetamine treatments of hyperactivity: Are there true nonresponders? *Psychiatry Res.*, 36:141–55.

Famularo, R. & Fenton, T. (1987), The effect of methylphenidate on school grades in children with attention deficit disorder without hyperactivity: A preliminary report. *J. Clin. Psychiatry*, 48:112–114.

Firestone, P. (1982), Factors associated with children's adherence to stimulant medication. *Am. J. Orthopsychiatry*, 52:447–457.

Firestone, P., Crowe, D., Goodman, J.T. & McGrath, P. (1986), Vicissitudes of follow-up studies: Differential effects of parent training and stimulant medication with hyperactives. *Am. J. Orthopsychiatry*, 56(3):413–423.

Firestone, P., Kelly, M.J., Goodman, J.T. & Davey, J. (1981), Differential effects of parent training and stimulant medication with hyperactives: A progress report. *J. Am. Acad. Child Adolesc. Psychiatry*, 20:135–147.

Firestone, P. & Witt, J.E. (1982), Characteristics of families completing and prematurely discontinuing a behavioral parent-training program. *J. Pediatr. Psychol.*, 7:209–222.

Forehand, R. & Atkeson, B.M. (1977), Generality of treatment effects with parents as therapists: A review of assessment and implementation procedures. *Behav. Ther.*, 8:575–593.

Forehand, R., Breiner, J., McMahon, R.J. & Davies, G. (1981), Predictors of cross-setting behavior change in the treatment of child problems. *J. Behav. Ther. Exp. Psychiatry*, 12:311–313.

Forehand, R. & King, H.E. (1977), Noncompliant children: Effects of parent training on behavior and attitude change. *Behav. Modification*, 1:93–108.

Forehand, R., Middlebrook, J., Rogers, T. & Steffe, M. (1983), Dropping out of parent training. *Behav. Res. Ther.*, 21:663–668.

Forehand, R., Rogers, T., McMahon, R.J., Wells, K.C. & Griest, D.L. (1981), Teaching parents to modify child behavior problems: An examination of some follow-up data. *J. of Pediatr. Psychol.*, 6:313–322.

Forehand, R.L. & McMahon, R.J. (1981), *Helping the Noncompliant Child: A Clinician's Guide to Parent Training.* New York: Guilford Press.

Frankel, F., Maytt, R., Cantwell, D. & Feinberg, D. (1997), Parent-assisted transfer of children's social skills training: Effects on children with and without attention-deficit hyperactivity disorder. *J. Am. Acad. Child Adolesc. Psychiatry*, 36:1056–1064.

Gadow, K.D., Nolan, E.E., Sverd, J., Sprafkin, J. & Paolicelli, L. (1990), Methylphenidate in aggressive-hyperactive boys: I. Effects on peer aggression in public school settings. *J. Am. Acad. Child Adolesc. Psychiatry*, 29:710–718.

Gittelman, R., Abikoff, H., Pollack, E., Klein, D.F., Katz, S. & Mattes, J. (1980), A controlled trial of behavior modification and methylphenidate in hyperactive children. In: *Hyperactive Children: The Social Ecology of Identification and Treatment*, eds., C. Whalen & B. Henker. New York: Academic Press, Inc.

Greenhill, L.L., (1992), Pharmacologic treatment of attention deficit hyperactivity disorder. *Psychiatr. Clin. North Am.*, 15:1–27.

Grych, J.H. & Fincham, F.D. (1990), Marital conflict and children's adjustment: A cognitive-contextual framework. *Psychol. Bull.*, 108:276–290.

Hechtman, L., Weiss, G. & Perlman, T. (1984), Hyperactives as young adults: Past and current substance abuse and antisocial behavior. *Am. J. Orthopsychiatry*, 54:415–425.

Henggeler, S.W., Schoenwald, S.K. & Pickrel, S.G. (1995), Multisystemic therapy: Bridging the gap between university- and community-based treatment. *J. Consult. Clin. Psych.*, 63:709–717.

Hinshaw, S.P. (1992), Externalizing behavior problems and academic underachievement in childhood and adolescence: Causal relationships and underlying mechanisms. *Psychol. Bull.*, 111:127–155.

Hinshaw, S.P. Buhrmester, D. & Heller, T. (1989a), Anger control in response to verbal provocation: Effects of stimulant medication for boys with ADHD. *J. Abnormal Child Psychol.*, 17:393–407.

Hinshaw, S.P., Heller, T. & McHale, J.P. (1992), Covert antisocial behavior in boys with attention-deficit hyperactivity disorder: External validation and effects of methylphenidate. *J. Consult. Clin. Psychol.*, 60:274–281.

Hinshaw, S.P., Henker, B., Whalen, C.K., Erhardt, D. & Dunnington, R.E. (1989b), Aggressive, prosocial, and nonsocial behavior in hyperactive boys: Dose effects of methylphenidate in naturalistic settings. *J. Consult. Clin. Psychol.*, 57:636–643.

Hinshaw, S.P., Henker, B. & Whalen, C.K. (1984a), Cognitive-behavioral and pharmacologic interventions for hyperactive boys: Comparative and combined effects. *J. Consult. Clin. Psychol.*, 52:739–749.

Hinshaw, S.P., Henker, B. & Whalen, C.K. (1984b), Self-control in hyperactive boys in anger-inducing situations: Effects of cognitive-behavioral training and of methylphenidate. *J. Abnormal Child Psychol.*, 12:55–77.

Hinshaw, S.P. & McHale, J.P. (1991), Stimulant medication and the social interactions of hyperactive children. In: *Personality, Social Skills, and Psychopathology: An Individual Differences Approach*, eds., D.G. Gilbert & J.J. Connolly. New York: Plenum Press.

Horn, W.F., Ialongo, N.S., Pascoe, J.M., Greenberg, G., Packard, T., Lopez, M., Wagner, A. & Puttler, L. (1991), Additive effects of psychostimulants, parent training, and self-control therapy with ADHD children. *J. Am. Acad. Child Adolesc. Psychiatry*, 30:233–240.

Ialongo, N.S., Horn, W.F., Pascoe, J.M., Greenberg, G., Packard, T., Lopez, M., Wagner, A. & Puttler, L. (1993), The effects of a multimodal intervention with attention-deficit hyperactivity disorder children: A 9-month follow-up. *J. Am. Acad. Child Adolesc. Psychiatry*, 32:182–189.

Jacobvitz, D., Sroufe, L.A., Stewart, M. & Leffert, N. (1990), Treatment of attentional and hyperactivity problems in children with sympathomimetic drugs: A comprehensive review. *J. Am. Acad. Child Adolesc. Psychiatry*, 29:677–688.

Kauffman, R.E., Smith-Wright, D., Reese, C.A., Simpson, R. & Jones, F. (1981), Medication compliance in hyperactive children. *Pediatr. Pharmacol.*, 1:231–237.

Kazdin, A.E. (1980), Acceptability of alternative treatments for deviant child behavior. *J. Appl. Behav. Anal.*, 13(2):259–273.

Kazdin, A.E. (1984), The acceptability of aversive procedures and medication as treatment alternatives for deviant child behavior. *J. Abnormal Child Psychol.*, 12:289–301.

Kazdin, A.E. (1997), Parent management training: Evidence, outcomes, and issues. *J. Am. Acad. Child Adolesc. Psychiatry*, 36:1349–1356.

Kazdin, A.E., Holland, L. & Crowley, M. (1997), Family experience of barriers to treatment and premature termination from child therapy. *J. Consult. Clin. Psychol.*, 65:453–463.

Kazdin, A.E. & Mazurick, J.L. (1994), Dropping out of child psychotherapy: Distinguishing early and late dropouts over the course of treatment. *J. Consult. Clin. Psychol.*, 62:1069–1074.

Kent, J.D., Blader, J.C., Koplewicz, H.S., Abikoff, H. & Foley, C.A. (1995), Effects of late-afternoon methylphenidate administration on behavior and sleep in attention-deficit hyperactivity disorder. *Pediatrics*, 96:320–325.

Klein, R.G. & Mannuzza, S. (1991), Long-term outcome of hyperactive children: A review. *J. Am. Acad. Child Adolesc. Psychiatry*, 30:383–387.

Kupietz, S.S., Winsberg, B.G., Richardson, E., Maitinsky, S. & Mendell, N. (1988), Effects of methylphenidate dosage in hyperactive reading-disabled children: I. Behavior and cognitive performance effects. *J. Am. Acad. Child Adolesc. Psychiatry*, 27:70–77.

Lipkin, P.H., Goldstein, I.J. & Adesman, A.R. (1994), Tics and dyskinesias associated with stimulant treatment in attention-deficit hyperactivity disorder. *Arch. Pediatr. Adolesc. Med.*, 148:859–861.

Loney, J., Prinz, R.J., Mishalow, J. & Joad, J. (1978), Hyperkinetic/aggressive boys in treatment: Predictors of clinical response to methylphenidate. *Am. J. Psychiatry*, 135:148–191.

Mannuzza, S., Klein, R.G., Bonagura, N., Malloy, P., Giampino, T.L. & Addalli, K.A. (1991), Hyperactive boys almost grown up: V. Replication of psychiatric status. *Arch. Gen. Psychiatry*, 48:77–83.

Mannuzza, S., Klein, R.G., Konig, P.H. & Giampino, T.L. (1989), Hyperactive boys almost grown up: IV. Criminality and its relationship to psychiatric status [see comments]. *Arch. Gen. Psychiatry*, 46:1073–1079.

Mash, E.J. & Johnston, C. (1983), Parental perceptions of child behavior problems, parenting self-esteem, and mothers' reported stress in younger and older hyperactive and normal children. *J. Consult. Clin. Psychol.*, 51:86–99.

McMahon, R.J. & Davies, G.R. (1980), A behavioral parent training program and its side effects on classroom behavior. *J. Special Educ.*, 4:165–174.

McMahon, R.J., Forehand, R., Greist, D.L. & Wells, K.C. (1981), Who drops out of treatment during parent behavioral training? *Behav. Counseling Q.*, 1:79–85.

O'Leary, S.G. & Pelham, W.E. (1978), Behavior therapy and withdrawal of stimulant medication in hyperactive children. *Pediatrics*, 61:211–217.

Parker, J.G. & Asher, S.R. (1987), Peer relations and later personal adjustment: Are low-accepted children at risk? *Psychol. Bull.*, 102:357–389.

Patterson, G.R. (1976), *Living With Children*. Champaign, Illinois: Research Press.

Patterson, G.R. (1986), Performance models for antisocial boys. *Am. Psychologist*, 41:432–444.

Peed, S., Roberts, M. & Forehand, R. (1977), Evaluation of the effectiveness of a standardized parent training program in altering the interaction of mothers and their noncompliant children. *Behav. Modification*, 1:323–350.

Pelham, W.E. Jr., Carlson, C., Sams, S.E., Vallano, G., Dixon, M.J. & Hoza, B. (1993), Separate and combined effects of methylphenidate and behavior modification on boys with attention deficit-hyperactivity disorder in the classroom. *J. Consult. Clin. Psychol.*, 61:506–515.

Pelham, W.E., Milich, R. & Walker, J.L. (1986), Effects of continuous and partial reinforcement and methylphenidate on learning in children with attention deficit disorder. *J. Abnorm. Psychol.*, 95:319–325.

Pelham, W.E., Murphy, D.A., Vannatta, K., Milich, R., Licht, B.G., Gnagy, E.M., Greenslade, K.E., Greiner, A.R. & Vodde-Hamilton, M. (1992), Methylphenidate and attributions in boys with attention-deficit hyperactivity disorder. *J. Consult. Clin. Psychol.*, 60:282–292.

Pelham, W.E., Jr., Schnedler, R.W., Bologna, N.C. & Contreras, J.A. (1980), Behavioral and stimulant treatment of hyperactive children: A therapy study with methylphenidate probes in a within-subject design. *J. Appl. Behav. Anal.*, 113:221–236.

Pisterman, S., Firestone, P., McGrath, P., Goodman, J.T. et al. (1992a), The effects of parent training on parenting stress and sense of competence. *Can. J. Behav. Sci.*, 24:41–58.

Pisterman, S., Firestone, P., McGrath, P., Goodman, J.T. et al. (1992b), The role of parent training in treatment of preschoolers with ADDH. *Am. J. Orthopsychiatry*, 62:397–408.

Pisterman, S., McGrath, P.J., Firestone, P. & Goodman, J.T. (1989), Outcome of parent mediated treatment of preschoolers with attention deficit disorder with hyperactivity. *J. Consult. Clin. Psychol.*, 57:628–635.

Pisterman, S., McGrath, P., Firestone, P., Goodman, J.T., Webster, I., Mallory, & Goffin, B. (1992c), The effects of parent training on parenting stress and sense of competence. *J. Behav. Sci.*, 12:41–58.

Pliszka, S.R. (1992), Comorbidity of attention-deficit hyperactivity disorder and overanxious disorder. *J. Am. Acad. Child Adolesc. Psychiatry*, 31:197–203.

Pollard, S., Ward, E.M. & Barkley, R.A. (1983), The effects of parent training and Ritalin on the parent–child interactions of hyperactive boys. *Child Fam. Behav. Ther.*, 5:51–69.

Prinz, R.J. & Miller, G.E. (1994), Family-based treatment for childhood antisocial behavior: Experimental influences on dropout and engagement. *J. Consult. Clin. Psychol.*, 62:645–650.

Prochaska, J., Norcross, J. & Di Clemente, C. (1995), *Changing for Good: The Revolutionary Program That Explains the Six Stages of Change and Teaches You How to Free Yourself from Bad Habits*. New York: William Morrow.

Quay, H.C. (1997), Inhibition and attention deficit hyperactivity disorder. *J. Abnorm. Child Psychol.*, 25:7–13.

Rapport, M.D., Denney, C., DuPaul, G.J. & Gardner, M.J. (1994), Attention deficit disorder and methylphenidate: Normalization rates, clinical effectiveness, and response prediction in 76 children. *J. Am. Acad. Child Adolesc. Psychiatry*, 33:882–893.

Richardson, E., Kupietz, S.S., Winsberg, B.G., Maitinsky, S. & Mendell, N. (1988), Effects of methylphenidate dosage in hyperactive reading-disabled children: II. Reading achievement. *J. Am. Acad. Child Adolesc. Psychiatry*, 27:78–87.

Richters, J.E., Arnold, L.E., Jensen, P.S., Abikoff, H., Conners, C.K., Greenhill, L.L., Hechtman, L., Hinshaw, S.P., Pelham, W.E. & Swanson, J.M. (1995), NIMH collaborative multisite multimodal treatment study of children with ADHD: I. Background and rationale. *J. Am. Acad. Child Adolesc. Psychiatry*, 34:987–1000.

Rickert, V., Sottolana, D., Parrish, J., Riley, A., Hunt, F. & Pelco, L. (1988), Training parents to become better behavior managers: The need for a competency-based approach. *Behav. Modification*, 12:475–496.

Rie, H.E., Rie, E.D., Stewart, S. & Ambuel, J.P. (1976), Effects of Ritalin on underachieving children: A replication. *Am. J. Orthopsychiatry*, 46:313–322.

Safer, D.J. & Krager, J.M. (1988), A survey of medication treatment for hyperactive/inattentive students. *JAMA*, 260:2256–2258.

Safer, D.J. & Zito, J.M. (1996), Increased methylphenidate usage for attention deficit disorder in the 1990s. 43rd *Annual Meeting of the American Academy of Child & Adolescent Psychiatry*, Washington, DC: American Academy of Child & Adolescent Psychiatry.

Safer, D.J., Zito, J.M. & Fine, E.M. (1996), Increased methylphenidate usage for attention deficit disorder in the 1990s. *Pediatrics*, 98:1084–1088.

Satterfield, J.H., Hoppe, C.M. & Schell, A.M. (1982), A prospective study of delinquency in 110 adolescent boys with attention deficit disorder and 88 normal adolescent boys. *Am. J. Psychiatry*, 139:795–798.

Schachar, R. & Tannock R. (1993), Childhood hyperactivity and psychostimulants: A review of extended treatment studies. *J. Child Adolesc. Psychopharmacol.*, 3:81–97.

Schachar, R., Tannock, R. & Cunningham, C. (1996), Treatment. In: *Hyperactivity Disorders of Childhood*, ed., S. Sandberg. Cambridge, Cambridge University Press.

Schachar, R., Tannock, R., Cunningham, C. & Corkum, P. (1997), Behavioral, situational, and temporal effects of treatment of ADHD with methylphenidate. *J. Am. Acad. Child Adolesc. Psychiatry*, 36:1–10.

Schachar, R., Taylor, E., Wieselberg, M., Thorley, G. & Rutter, M. (1987), Changes in family function and relationships in children who respond to methylphenidate. *J. Am. Acad. Child Adolesc. Psychiatry*, 26:728–732.

Schachar, R. & Wachsmuth, R. (1990), Hyperactivity and parental psychopathology. *J. Child Psychol. Psychiatry Allied Disciplines*, 31:381–392.

Sleator, E.K., Ullmann, R.K. & von Neumann, A. (1982), How do hyperactive children feel about taking stimulants and will they tell the doctor? *Clin. Pediatr.*, 21:474–479.

Spencer, T., Biederman, J., Wilens, T., Harding, M., O'Donnell, D. & Griffin, S. (1996), Pharmacotherapy of attention-deficit hyperactivity disorder across the life cycle. *J. Am. Acad. Child Adolesc. Psychiatry*, 35:409–432.

Sprague, R.L. & Sleator, E.K. (1977), Methylphenidate in hyperkinetic children: Differences in dose effects on learning and social behavior. *Science*, 198:1274–1276.

Stein, M.A., Blondis, T.A., Schnitzler, E.R., O'Brien, T., Fishkin, J., Blackwell, B., Szumowski, E. & Roizen, N.J. (1996), Methylphenidate dosing: Twice daily versus three times daily. *Pediatrics*, 98:748–756.

Swanson, J.M., Lerner, M. & Williams, L. (1995), More frequent diagnosis of attention deficit-hyperactivity disorder. *N. Engl. J. Med.*, 333:944.

Szapocznik, J., Perez-Vidal, A., Hervis, O., Brickman, A. & Kurtines, W. (1980), Innovations in family therapy: Strategies for overcoming resistance to treatment. In: *Hyperactive Children: The Social Ecology of Identification and Treatment*, eds., C. Whalen & B. Henker. New York: Academic Press.

Szatmari, P., Boyle, M. & Offord, D.R. (1989a), ADHD and conduct disorder: Degree of diagnostic overlap and differences among correlates. *J. Am. Acad. Child Adolesc. Psychiatry*, 28:865–872.

Szatmari, P., Offord, D.R. & Boyle, M.H. (1989b), Correlates, associated impairments and patterns of service utilization of children with attention deficit disorder: Findings from the Ontario Child Health Study. *J. Child Psychol. Psychiatry Allied Disciplines*, 30:205–217.

Tannock, R., Schachar, R.J., Carr, R.P., Chajczyk, D. & Logan, G.D. (1989), Effects of methylphenidate on inhibitory control in hyperactive children. *J. Abnorm. Child Psychol.*, 17:473–491.

Taylor, E., Chadwick, O., Heptinstall, E. & Danckaerts, M. (1996), Hyperactivity and conduct problems as risk factors for adolescent development. *J. Am. Acad. Child Adolesc. Psychiatry*, 35:1213–1226.

Webster-Stratton, C. (1985), The effects of father involvement in parent training for conduct problem children. *J. Child Psychol. Psychiatry*, 26:801–810.

Weiss, G., Hechtman, L., Milroy, T. & Perlman, T. (1985), Psychiatric status of hyperactives as adults: A controlled prospective 15-year follow-up of 63 hyperactive children. *J. Am. Acad. Child Psychiatry*, 24:211–220.

Wells, K.C., Forehand, R. & Greist, D.L. (1980), Generality of treatment effects from treated to untreated behaviors resulting from a parent training program. *J. Clin. Child Psychol.*, 9:217–219.

West, M.O. & Prinz, R.J. (1987), Parental alcoholism and childhood psychopathology. *Psychol. Bull.*, 102:204–218.

Whalen, C.K. & Henker, B. (1976), Psychostimulants and children: A review and analysis. *Psychol. Bull.*, 83:1113–1130.

Walen, C.K., Henker, B., Buhrmester, D., Hinshaw, S.P., Huber, A. & Laski, K., (1989), Does stimulant medication improve the peer status of hyperactive children? *J. Consult. Clin. Psychol.*, 57:545–549.

Wolraich, M.L., Lindgren, S., Stromquist, A., Milich, R., Davis, C. & Watson, D. (1990), Stimulant medication use by primary care physicians in the treatment of attention deficit hyperactivity disorder. *Pediatrics*, 86:95–101.

Wolraich, M., Drummond, T., Salomon, M.K., O'Brien, M.L. & Sivage, C. (1978), Effects of methylphenidate alone and in combination with behavior modification procedures on the behavior and academic performance of hyperactive children. *J. Abnorm. Child Psychol.*, 6:149–161.

Section 4

Clinical Use of Ritalin

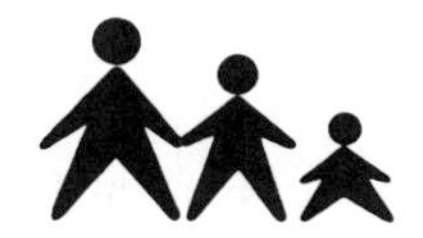

Rating Scales for Use in Assessment and Clinical Trials with Children

C. KEITH CONNERS

INTRODUCTION

Rating scales play an important role in clinical practice and in clinical trials with medications and other forms of treatment. In clinical practice, rating scales help guide the clinician toward correct diagnosis as well as providing coverage of relevant comorbid conditions. Rating scales also provide a convenient method of communicating findings to patients, parents, and teachers. They can be useful in documenting assessment and treatment outcome for managed care. Rating scales should be treatment-sensitive and provide clinicians with a means of tracking drug or psychosocial interventions over time.

In clinical trials, rating scales are useful in characterizing the samples being studied, documenting initial severity levels for different behavioral domains, recording progress during the trial, and providing endpoints for efficacy and behavioral side effects. Rating scales have the virtue of providing a common vocabulary across multiple sites in clinical trials, thereby reducing variance in sample description, entry criteria, and outcome measures. These scales can provide data from different sources (patient, parents, teachers, significant others) to aid the clinical trial investigator in reaching overall global decisions regarding efficacy and safety.

Desirable features of rating scales include reliability, validity, representative norms, sensitivity, specificity, and overall good predictive power. Ease of use, broad coverage of symptoms, and narrow-band measures of specific syndromes are additional features by which scales should be judged.

In this chapter I comment on both strengths and weaknesses of rating scales and describe a new set of scales covering child, adolescent, and adult psychopathology for the most common behavior disorders. Specific scales for monitoring drug treatment in clinical practice and clinical trials are highlighted. Comprehensive reviews of rating scales are available elsewhere (Conners, 1973; Conners, 1979; Conners and Barkley, 1985; Barkley, 1990; Achenbach et al., 1991).

WHY USE RATING SCALES IN CLINICAL PRACTICE OR CLINICAL TRIALS?

As noted in an early review (Conners & Barkley, 1985, p. 809), ratings can draw on a rater's often substantial previous experience with a child over long time intervals and diverse situations and circumstances; permit data to be gathered on rare and infrequent behaviors likely to be missed by *in vivo* assessments; are inexpensive to collect and extremely efficient in the time needed to gather information; have normative data available for comparative purposes to show whether a drug or other treatment has brought the child's be-

Department of Psychiatry, Duke University Medical Center, Durham, North Carolina.

havior closer to normal; have information regarding their psychometric and practical properties; incorporate the opinions of significant others in a patient's life whose ratings, regardless of accuracy or reliability, have substantial ecologic importance as they reflect perceptions of parents, teachers, or significant others; and permit the quantification of qualitative aspects of child behavior not readily gathered by other means. Rating scales have also proven to be drug-sensitive, both with respect to dose- and time-action phenomena.

CAUTIONARY REMARKS ON THE USE OF RATING SCALES

Because of their simplicity, ease of use, and utility, it is tempting to elevate rating scales to the status of gold standards of diagnosis or treatment response. However, although rating scales have many psychometric and practical advantages, they also are subject to errors, misuse, and misinterpretation. Several common errors affect most rating scales (for a thorough discussion, the reader is referred to Aiken, 1996). *Leniency error* refers to the tendency to judge the behavior too leniently with respect to its severity or frequency, and *severity error* is the opposite. Positive or negative *halo errors* occur when the rater gives an unfair positive or negative slant to items based on the judgment of one or more particular behaviors. It is known, for example, that teachers will rate children as deviant across a wide range of behaviors because of particularly disruptive classroom behaviors. These rating biases inflate the degree of attentional or nonaggressive hyperactivity (Abikoff et al., 1993; Schachar et al., 1986; Siegel et al., 1976). When raters make a *logical error*, they will give a rating on one occasion because they made a particular rating on another that they feel must logically follow. Thus, parents might say that the child is "restless and on the go" because they previously said the child was fidgety, despite the fact that these are qualitatively different behaviors. *Contrast errors* refer to errors caused by comparisons or contrasts with a particular person (often the self). Fathers or mothers often deny that current behavior problems of their child are significant, saying, "I was like that as a child, so it's probably just normal." When the parent contrasts the subject with a sibling rather than with normal children of the same age, or when the parent uses a particular referent of what is "normal," a contrast error may occur. The prevalence rate of ADHD varies dramatically as a function of contrast phenomena (Holborow et al., 1984). The *recency error* refers to the tendency to rate the child according to the most recent episodes of behavior. Thus, parents or teachers may rate the child as much more deviant following a particularly bad episode in school or at home.

These errors can be minimized by follow-up interviews that probe for possible leniency, recency, or severity errors. For example, when parents or teachers rate many behaviors as deviant, they may in fact be doing so because the child recently had a particularly egregious episode that stands out in their minds. When a parent comes to a clinical setting but has checked off very few behaviors on a rating scale, one must determine whether the problems are situation-specific (e.g., occur only in school) or in fact are being minimized or denied for psychologic reasons. It often happens, for example, that parents have been urged to receive help by the school when they themselves have no problem with the child at home, or perceive that there is no problem.

Adolescents often pose a particular assessment problem because they are frequently in the midst of normal separation from the nuclear family and rejection of many parental values, and they may be very resistant to revealing or admitting to problems in themselves. It is essential, therefore, that rating scales filled out by adolescents be preceded by reassurance, the development of trust, and a discussion of confidentiality. It is well to remember that rating scales normed on adolescents are usually collected under conditions of anonymity, so that they are more likely to reveal unflattering behaviors in themselves than the patient dragged to the office for psychiatric or psychologic evaluations.

These considerations emphasize the point that rating scales are not meant to stand alone, either in the diagnostic or in the treatment evaluation process. It is a perversion of their use to collect such information without adequate knowledge of the informants, and to use them in a mechanical way without consideration of their limitations or possible biases. Nevertheless, used conservatively and with appreciation for their limitations, rating scales are an invaluable complement to other clinical tools and treatment-monitoring methods.

RELATIONSHIP BETWEEN CONTINUOUSLY DISTRIBUTED RATING DOMAINS AND CATEGORICAL DIAGNOSTIC CRITERIA

There are two major problems with Diagnostic and Statistical Manual of Mental Disorders (*DSM*), *4th edition*—based categorical symptomatic criteria:

1. *DSM-IV* is based, among other things, on diagnostic symptom criteria that must reach a certain level of severity or frequency to count toward a particular diagnosis. For example, "often fidgets with hands or feet or squirms in seat" is one of the *DSM-IV* symptoms of ADHD. Typically, the answer to this question must be sought from parent, teacher, or other informants during the clinical interview. But variations in meeting this symptom criterion will occur because what counts as "often" must be subjectively determined. Since there are no normative criteria for symptoms or behaviors, it is difficult to know what should count as a "normal" amount of fidgeting or squirming. Moreover, there are gender and age differences in what is normative for most child behaviors. Most clinicians are not likely to accurately adjust their judgements of what counts as "often" for symptomatic behaviors according to age- and gender-specific norms.

However, with adequate representative samples in the population, it is possible to set the symptom cutoff according to a statistical decision. Without a normative reference, it may be difficult to discern whether the observer or reporter of behavior is making a judgment that is too lenient or severe compared with the average child of that age, gender, and situation. Rating scales can ask this question of thousands of parents or teachers, and determine statistically how the answers vary with age, gender, or other factors. Fidgeting or leaving one's seat, like most childhood behaviors, fall along a continuum of frequency or severity, with no clear demarcation between an abnormal and a normal state. In certain cases of what used to be called the "driven hyperkinetic child," the behavior is apparent in all situations. But for most children, one must rely on the observer's intrinsic averaging process, whereby the individual in question is compared with one's experience of all children at the appropriate developmental stage.

Since the *DSM*-based criteria were often rephrasing of items commonly found on rating scales, it is not surprising that rating scales have in turn used *DSM* phraseology in a normative context. Thus, *DSM* was strongly influenced by the empirical experience with rating scales, and the latter in turn have been shaped by the specific behaviors chosen to represent symptomatic criteria in diagnostic algorithms. However, one of the difficulties with the frequent revisions of *DSM* has been that carefully developed norms on *DSM* items have been outdated by newer criteria. For example, Pelham et al. (1992a) collected teacher information on the *DSM-III-R* symptoms among a special education sample as well as among a large normative sample (Pelham et al., 1992b). DuPaul (1991) also carried out a large study (729 children) of a *DSM-III-R* symptom list. As expected, the list produced Restlessness/Impulsivity and Inattention factors (though inexplicably, restlessness was common to both factors). A major limitation of this study was the 18% return rate and the limited social-class and ethnic composition of the sample. A large body of reliability and validity data from 30 years of research has been summarized for the pre-*DSM-IV* versions of the

Conners Scales (Conners, 1994; Wainright, 1996). I shall therefore describe the most recent restandardization, as well as newer scales that include the *DSM* items.

2. The cutoff thresholds for the items and the groupings to which they are assigned are based on relatively small and unrepresentative samples, and therefore the subtypes identified by particular symptom lists are somewhat arbitrary. The *DSM* subtypes for ADHD do not necessarily reflect empirical reality with respect to factor coherence. More recent, large-scale studies of representative samples in North America provide an age-based, gender-based, and statistically based complement to the threshold or categorical approach to diagnosis. By providing data on the frequency and severity of a wide pool of behaviors, these studies allow clinicians to check the more impressionistic symptom criteria obtained in face-to-face interviews with data that have demonstrated construct validity, reliability, and diagnostic sensitivity.

HISTORICAL DEVELOPMENTS LEADING TO A NEW GENERATION OF RATING SCALES

The Achenbach, Conners, and Quay (ACQ) Project

Many investigators carried out factor analytic investigations of child behavior problems and developed a variety of rating instruments. This literature suggested that approximately 11 syndromes were reliably identified across the various studies, but none of the studies had the requisite sample size, representative sampling, or statistical sophistication to definitively identify the major dimensions. This situation led Thomas Achenbach to obtain funding from the American Psychological Foundation to carry out a nationwide study of parent-based symptom ratings. That study incorporated representative items from prior investigations as well as most of the items from the three most widely used scales by Achenbach, Conners, and Quay: items suggested by an international panel of experts. A large representative sample of parent raters from nonreferred and clinical sources was obtained through a census tract survey conducted by a professional survey research team. The parent rating instrument (dubbed the ACQ) was administered to over 8500 normal and 8500 clinic parents. The results are described in publications (Achenbach et al., 1989; Achenbach et al., 1991).

On the basis of previous factor analytic studies, 12 syndromes were hypothesized: aggression, anxious/depressed, ADD with and ADD without hyperactivity, delinquent, mean (in girls only), obsessive-compulsive, schizoid, sex problems, social ineptness, somatic complaints, and unresponsive/uncommunicative/withdrawn. Clear evidence for eight of the factors emerged from factor analyses: withdrawn, somatic, anxious/depressed, thought problems, social problems, attention problems, delinquent, and aggressive. Of note was the finding that the expected factors of attention deficit disorder (ADD) with and without hyperactivity (based on then-current *DSM-III* concepts) did not appear as separate factors. Instead, an "attention" factor included a mixture of immature behavior, poor concentration, impulsivity, restlessness, and poor school work.

The ACQ Behavior Checklist included 23 competence items, three competence scales, 216 problem items, the eight syndrome scales, internalizing, externalizing, and total competence and problem scores. These were compared in large demographically matched samples of normal subjects and clinic patients. Most items and scales discriminated significantly ($p < 0.01$) between referred and nonreferred subjects. There were important sex and age differences in problem patterns, but regional and ethnic differences were minimal. Somewhat more problems and fewer competencies were reported for lower- than for upper-socioeconomic-status children. Referral rates were similar in most urban and rural areas, but they were significantly higher in areas of intermediate urbanization. Correlations of problem scores with those obtained 10 years earlier in a regional survey and with surveys in other countries showed considerable consistency in the rank order of prevalence rates among specific problems.

Interview data from the survey sample yielded significantly higher ACQ problem scores for children who had fewer related adults in their homes, more unrelated adults in their homes, or biologic parents who were unmarried, separated, or divorced; children in families on public assistance; and children whose household or family members had received mental health services: Children who scored higher on externalizing than internalizing problems tended to have unmarried, separated, or divorced parents and to come from families receiving public assistance. However, among children whose household or family members had received mental health services, there were greater proportions of both externalizing and internalizing patterns than among other children.

The ACQ made an important empirical contribution to understanding of replicable child dimensional syndromes. The large representative normal sample and the large clinic sample ensured that potentially important demographic phenomena could be examined for the first time in a scientifically acceptable manner. The finding that regional and ethnic effects were minimal is particularly useful in view of the claims to the contrary based on the small, regionally biased samples previously available. However, there were important limitations of the research version of the scale: It employed items from the then recently developed *DSM-III* criteria, and its extreme length made it unwieldy as a clinical instrument. Nevertheless, this study supplied an important background for more recent developments.

Restandardization of the Conners scales

Although the original Conners scales are still widely used in a variety of clinical and research settings, the various scales were created before the *DSM-IV* criteria and were constructed and standardized on somewhat restrictive samples. The original teacher and parent scales were standardized on relatively small clinic and local Baltimore school samples. The first revision (Goyette et al., 1978) was standardized on a representative sample of census tract–identified families but was restricted to urban Pittsburgh. The most popular scale, the brief 10-item subset known as the Hyperactivity Index, and the Teacher Rating Scale, were standardized on over 10,000 normal schoolchildren (Trites et al., 1979; Trites, 1988; Trites et al., 1982). Although large, this sample was the entire school population of but one Canadian city (Ottawa).

Moreover, this early work was characterized by item and factor analysis methodology of an earlier era. A particularly important limitation was the high intercorrelation of subscales caused by allowing items with high loadings on more than one factor. Some investigators became convinced that hyperactivity and conduct disorder dimensions were measuring the same thing (Sandberg et al., 1978). However, using a normative sample of 683 psychiatric and normal children (ages 4–15 years), we were able to demonstrate that high intercorrelations of these scales is of purely methodological origin. Basically, when items that load highly on more than one factor are allowed, the factors will be correlated. When this built-in factor correlation is corrected by removing dually loaded items, the results support the idea that hyperactivity and conduct disorder are independent behavioral dimensions (Blouin et al., 1989).*

*When factor analyses are carried out with orthogonal rotation of factors, the factors are by definition as uncorrelated as the data will permit. If the exact weights that emerge from the analysis for each item are used to weight the items in creating factor scores, then this uncorrelated property will be retained. However, for convenience, one often simply sums the raw item scores to get total factor scores, which are then usually standardized (e.g. with T-scores). To the extent that the same items are used in different factors, the factors will be correlated. If one's purpose is to provide an instrument with relatively independent factors, it behooves one to include items on a factor that have negligible loadings on all other factors.

Several methodological refinements were included in the new restandardization of the Conners rating scales. Data for the child and adolescent versions of the scales were collected from over 200 sites in the United States and Canada (a total of about 11,000 ratings on approximately 5000 children), selected to cover both urban and rural areas of all states and Canadian provinces, with a good representation of social class, ethnicity, age, and gender (Conners, 1997). The item pools were created using previous versions, but many new items were added as well. For example, the item pool for the teacher and parent scales started with 192 symptoms.

An important issue is the replicability of the factor structure. Usual approaches to factor analysis of symptom ratings extract factors according to a single criterion (such as the Eigenvalues or Scree Test). In our restandardization, the sample was split into a derivation sample and a cross-validation sample. The correlation matrix from the derivation sample was subjected to principal axis factoring, and a series of factor analyses was conducted to determine what items to retain. Items had to load significantly ($r > 0.30$) on a given factor and lower than r 0.30 on the other factors. Following the rational approach to scale construction, an item was eliminated if it lacked conceptual coherence with its factor, and standard Scree test criteria (Scree > 1.0) applied to select the number of factors for rotation. In addition, we employed the split-half factor comparabilities method (Everett, 1983) to determine the most reliable factor solution. Finally, the factor analysis was repeated on the cross-validation sample using confirmatory factor analysis, and multiple criteria were used to assess the goodness-of-fit of the predicted model.

A further aim of the restandardization was to retain the useful properties of long and short scales. Long scales are particularly useful for initial characterization of a child, adolescent, or adult when the broadest descriptive characterization is required, such as during an initial assessment. Shorter scales are useful for repeated measures, or when time availability for the raters is limited. The aim was to have equally powerful psychometric properties for the long and short scales so that no sacrifice in reliability or validity would occur between the different versions. In contrast to previous research with our scales, the shorter versions contained items that were an exact subset of the longer form but had equally good reliability.

It is of interest to ascertain how *DSM* items relate to the empirically derived factors, so the 18 criterion items for ADHD and the eight items for oppositional defiant disorder (ODD) were included in the item pool and subsequent analyses. Because these items are part of the new scales, ADHD subtypes can be measured both quantitatively and categorically. Those items can be administered separately as an 18-item set, or as part of the long form. Because the 18 ADHD items are normed, they can be used as a separate "ADHD rating scale" similar to the now outdated versions of the SNAP (Pelham et al., 1992). When they are administered as part of the long form, one can determine not only whether the child has met criteria for ADHD but also whether any of the most important comorbidities are present. Factor analyses showed that although several of the *DSM-IV* items loaded on expected factors of hyperactivity, impulsivity, and inattention, not all such items loaded on the expected subtype factors, and other, non-*DSM* items did (Conners et al., 1998a; Conners et al., 1998b).

Past research indicated that the so-called Hyperactivity Index was among the most consistent treatment-sensitive scales (see Wainright, 1996 for an annotated bibliography). This brief, 10-item scale was shown to do better than scales such as the Achenbach CBCL and Kendall and Wilcox's Self-Control Rating Scale in differentiating ADD from psychiatric and normal controls (Zelko, 1991). This scale was created from ten items showing the highest loading on each of the main factors from the long parent and teacher scales. Thus, it was more of a general psychopathology scale than a hyperactivity scale per se. Users sometimes mistakenly complained that this scale was not unidimensional but complex, and therefore argued that it was not useful (Ullman et al., 1985). A reanalysis of this scale using the large restandardization sample shows two clear factors, essentially internalizing and externalizing, or hyperactive-impulsive and emotional lability (Parker et al., 1996). Many drug studies relied on this index as a key outcome measure, both because of its brevity (which allows frequent readministration without a high user burden), and because of its drug sensitivity and ability to discriminate well-diagnosed ADHD from other samples (Conners, 1994). It may well be that it is precisely the combination of externalizing and internalizing behavior that has made this instrument so useful in diagnostic and treatment studies, since it covers the symptoms of disruptive behavior as well as the emotional lability so characteristic of ADHD children. This index has been restandardized on the new normative sample, but a new index has also been added using an entirely different methodology.

A true ADHD index was created by using discriminant function analysis of carefully diagnosed ADHD children and adolescents compared with age- and gender-matched subsamples of the standardization sample. This new 12-item index has high reliability and cross-validated sensitivity (98.2% and 97.1% in samples with n = 114 and 206 for the teacher scale, 92.3% and 100% in samples with n = 104 and 80 for the parent scale, and 90.7% and 90.7% in adolescent self-report scale with n = 86 and 86). Specificity figures are of the same general magnitude (77%–98%). Overall classification rates for both the initial and cross-validation samples range from 84%–96%.

One caution is that these high diagnostic sensitivity/specificity figures do not imply the stand-alone diagnostic utility of the scales. Since the discriminant analyses were based on clinical samples identified by diagnostic interviews that necessarily included many of the same symptom behaviors (how could they *not*?), the results merely show that the scales performed as expected when common sources of information were used in both the diagnostic process and in the ratings themselves. Although there was no "criterion contamination" in the sense that these were independent data sources, one simply could not avoid obtaining similar information from each source. Diagnostic accuracy with the scales, although well validated by cross-sample replication, will be less when the clinical diagnosis fails to use the appropriate symptomatic data from an interview that covers all the relevant symptoms, or when informants are less forthcoming than usual.

A new self-report adolescent scale

Relatively little work has been done on adolescents with ADHD. As children enter middle school, reports of teachers become less satisfactory, and there are more areas of function that are likely to escape the perusal of parents. Although self-report is subject to the adolescent's proclivity to "fake good," it is generally accepted that self-report is useful as a complement to parent and teacher scales, particularly with regard to internalizing states (Klorman, 1985). Moreover, there are important developmental differences that require a different set of items for adolescents than for younger children. At a National Institute of Mental Health conference on ADHD in adolescents, we presented an adolescent self-report scale based on our clinical experience of the unique presentation of problems in adolescents being evaluated for behavior and learning problems (Conners and Wells, 1985). We believed that in addition to the obvious areas of concentration, restlessness, and self-control, there were important symptom domains involving anger, social interactions, self-esteem, learning, mood states, and family problems. This new scale was standardized on 3486 adolescents between the ages of 12 and 18. Using a similar methodology as in the parent and teacher scales described above, the original item set was reduced from 100 to 87 items for the long form and 27 items for an abbreviated version. Six replicable factors emerged with good reliability and excellent sensitivity and specificity (Robin, 1994; Conners et al., 1997c).

Table 1 shows the composition of the child and adolescent scales, factor names, and number of items for the revised Conners Scales from the restandardization studies. The oppositional factor contains items that closely follow the content of *DSM-IV*. The cognitive/inattention factor includes traditional items associated with inattention and distractibility but also includes items relating to homework, reading, spelling, handwriting, and math performance. This indicates that the *DSM* practice of separating learning problems into a separate category is empirically invalid. Although we wrote a dozen or so items to capture both depression and anxiety as possibly separate scales, the analyses uniformly indicated that these rational scales coalesced into a single anxiety-shyness dimension, which, along with the psychosomatic factor, forms an internalizing dimension. Perfectionism could be considered a form of obsessive-compulsive personality, but because the full set of criterion items for that diagnosis did not load on the scale, we prefer a more neutral designation. This is a useful scale because it tends to be very low in ADHD children (consistent with their disorganization and messiness) but also because some of the anxious and compulsive behaviors are sometimes confused with ADHD behaviors. Notice that the teacher analyses produced parallel factors with the parent analyses, with the exception of psychosomatic complaints, which are not readily identified by teachers.

The family problems scale was created from items derived from current theory and data regarding the sources of conduct, delinquent, and other externalizing behaviors in adolescents. It includes items relating to parental monitoring and discipline, family cohesion and shared activities, and parental demands and expectations. Again, as in younger children, the adolescent "emotionality" scale includes items that reflect both anxious and depressed moods. Of interest is the emergence of a strong and clear-cut anger-control dimension, which may be the adolescent extension of earlier symptoms of verbal and behavioral impulsivity, tinged with affect. Also of interest is that the adolescent factor for hyperactivity includes items of "inner restlessness" as well as more traditional motoric restlessness.

TABLE 1. CONNERS RATING SCALES: REVISED CHILD AND ADOLESCENT SCALES (LONG VERSIONS)

Parent Scales		*Teacher Scales*		*Adolescent Self-Report Scale*	
Factor	*Items*	*Factor*	*Items*	*Factor*	*Items*
Oppositional	10	Oppositional	6	Family problems	12
Cognitive problems	12	Cognitive problems	7	Emotionality	12
Hyperactivity	9	Hyperactivity		Cognitive problems	12
Anxious/shy	8	Anxious/shy	7	Conduct problems	12
Perfectionism	7	Perfectionism	6	Anger control problems	8
Social problems	5	Social problems	6	Hyperactivity	8
Psychosomatic	6	N/A	5		
		Specialty Scales			
ADHD Index	12	ADHD Index	12	ADHD index	12
Global Index: restless-impulsive	6	Global Index: restless-impulsive	6	*DSM-IV* inattentive,	9
Global Index: emotional lability	6	Global Index: emotional lability	6	*DSM-IV* hyperactive-impulsive	9
Global Index: total score	12	Global Index: total score	12	*DSM-IV* total	18
DSM-IV inattentive	9	*DSM-IV* inattentive	9		
DSM-IV hyperactive-impulsive	9	*DSM-IV* hyperactive-impulsive	9		
DSM-IV total score	18	*DSM-IV* total score	18		

TABLE 2. DIAGNOSTIC UTILITY OF EMPIRICALLY DERIVED ADHD INDEX FOR TEACHER, PARENT, AND ADOLESCENT SELF-REPORT RATINGS

	Teacher Rating Scale		*Parent Rating Scale*		*Adolescent Self-Report Ratings*	
	Original	*Replication*	*Original*	*Replication*	*Original*	*Replication*
Sensitivity	98.2	97.1	92.3	100	90.7	90.7
Specificity	82.5	81.6	98.1	92.5	88.4	76.7
Positive predictive power	84.8	84.0	98.0	93.0	88.6	79.6
Negative predictive power	97.9	96.6	92.7	100	90.5	89.2
False positive rate	17.5	18.4	1.9	7.5	11.6	23.3
False negative rate	1.8	2.90	7.7	0.0	9.3	9.3
Kappa	.807	.786	.904	.925	.791	.674
Overall classification rate	90.4	89.3	95.2	96.3	89.5	83.7
No.	114	206	104	80	86	86

Table 2 shows the original and replication samples for the discriminant function analyses with each of the instruments.

Symptom dimensions in adult ratings

Several authors have shown the usefulness of symptom ratings with adults suspected of the adult form of ADHD (Spencer et al., 1995; Barkley, 1990; Ward et al., 1993). However, the earlier *DSM-III* concepts and the somewhat small and unrepresentative samples render those scales of doubtful validity.

Recent concepts of adult ADHD suggest an important role for executive functions, working memory, interpersonal relationships, and self-esteem in the symptom picture. In creating a new adult scale, we considered 19 such symptom categories and devised about 10 items per category for the initial pilot studies. The derivation sample consisted of 840 normal adults between the ages of 18 and 81. Results from this normative sample were cross-validated on a clinical sample consisting of 167 adults referred to an outpatient clinic for ADHD. These patients all had early histories of onset of ADHD symptoms, and met no other *DSM-IV* diagnoses. Approximately half of the original referral set was eliminated on the basis of other diagnoses (primarily panic anxiety or major affective disorders). A large set of items was created based on recent literature and recommendations by a number of clinicians, and ultimately reduced in preliminary analyses to a set of 42 items. (Again, since we were interested in *independent* dimensions, we did not allow items to load more than 0.40 on more than one factor, and retained only factors that met criteria for factor comparability in split-half samples.) The four replicable factors that emerged included inattention/memory problems, hyperactivity/restlessness, impulsivity/emotionality, and self-esteem. The dual names for three of the factors is indicative of their somewhat complex nature and indicates that purely rational concepts of factor composition often become tempered by empirical reality. The scales show good reliability, sensitivity, and specificity. As with the children's scales, a highly efficient ADHD index showed excellent sensitivity, specificity, and overall classification power (Conners 1999, submitted).

RATING SCALES IN DRUG TRIALS WITH CHILDREN

Rating scales have been used as subject selection and outcome measures since the 1960s. A large body of data has been collected on hundreds of drug trials. Several meta-analyses are in agreement in showing very large effect sizes of drug versus placebo comparisons using parent and teacher rating scales (Kavale, 1982; Ottenbacher and Cooper, 1983; Thurber and Walker, 1983). Scales such as the Hyperactivity Index show very good sensitivity to dose effects. However, careful analysis of individual cases reveals that at least three different patterns of dose-response effect are evident. The most typical is a linear effect of increasing benefit with increasing dose. Less common is a threshold effect, in which nothing happens with increasing dose until a given level, when suddenly improvement occurs. Finally, there is the classic quadratic effect, in which there is first an improvement with each dose, and then a worsening, sometimes to a level worse than in the placebo phase (Rapport et al., 1989; Rapport, 1990; Sprague and Sleator, 1977). These studies suggest the importance of individualizing each child's drug dose rather than relying on preestablished criteria based on group outcome studies.

The recently developed ADHD Index for parents, teachers, and adolescents should provide a sensitive measure of drug changes on the symptoms that most clearly discriminate ADHD children from normal subjects. Because of their brevity (12 items) and excellent psychometric properties, they are well suited for repeated measures in clinical drug trials. Similarly, the *DSM-IV* scales now provide, for the first time, a standardized measure for the criterion symptoms of the *DSM-IV* definition of ADHD. When a Food and Drug Administration drug trial explicitly targets ADHD, it seems important to include both the categorical and dimensional measures of the concept.

In clinical practice, it is often helpful to plot behavioral response as a function of time and drug dose. Figure 1 shows a tracking form with data from a drug trial for a 10-year- old boy. The form in this case plots the *DSM* symptom scores as well as the ADHD Index based on the Teacher Rating Scale. The data indicate that little change occurred with the 5-mg dose of Ritalin, and that increase of the dose beyond 10 mg had little effect. The clinical effect from the 10-mg dose is approximately 1.5 standard deviations (going from T-scores of 70–78 to 56–58). Because T-scores have a standard deviation of 10 points, it is relatively easy to judge the impact of the medication in relation to standing with respect to the normative population. In this case, the youngster approximated the normal range on the 10-mg dose.

Typically, drug trials with newer agents will need to ascertain the impact of the drug on other targets besides those most associated with ADHD. For example, anxiety, depression, perfectionism, and somatic complaints as well as ADHD symptoms may also increase or decrease with certain dosages or drugs. In those cases, it seems judicious to use the longer scales as baseline and end-of-treatment measures so that all dimensions of behavior are covered.

There is little experience with symptom changes caused by drugs in adolescent trials involving self-report. However, one study found similar drug effects from self-report as from parent and teacher report; but different patterns of side effects were obtained from the self- and other-reports (DuPaul et al., 1996). Because adolescents may be better reporters of internal states than either parents or teachers, it seems useful to include a self-report measure in trials with adolescents.

SUMMARY

As we have stated in earlier reviews (Conners and Barkley, 1985), no single rating instrument meets the needs of all investigators or clinicians. With the current generation of new instruments, there are both greater psychometric sophistication and more representative normative and clinical samples than were available in the past. Of particular interest is the fact that relatively brief forms are now available that retain the psychometric power of much longer and more cumbersome forms. This minimizes subject burden and user time.

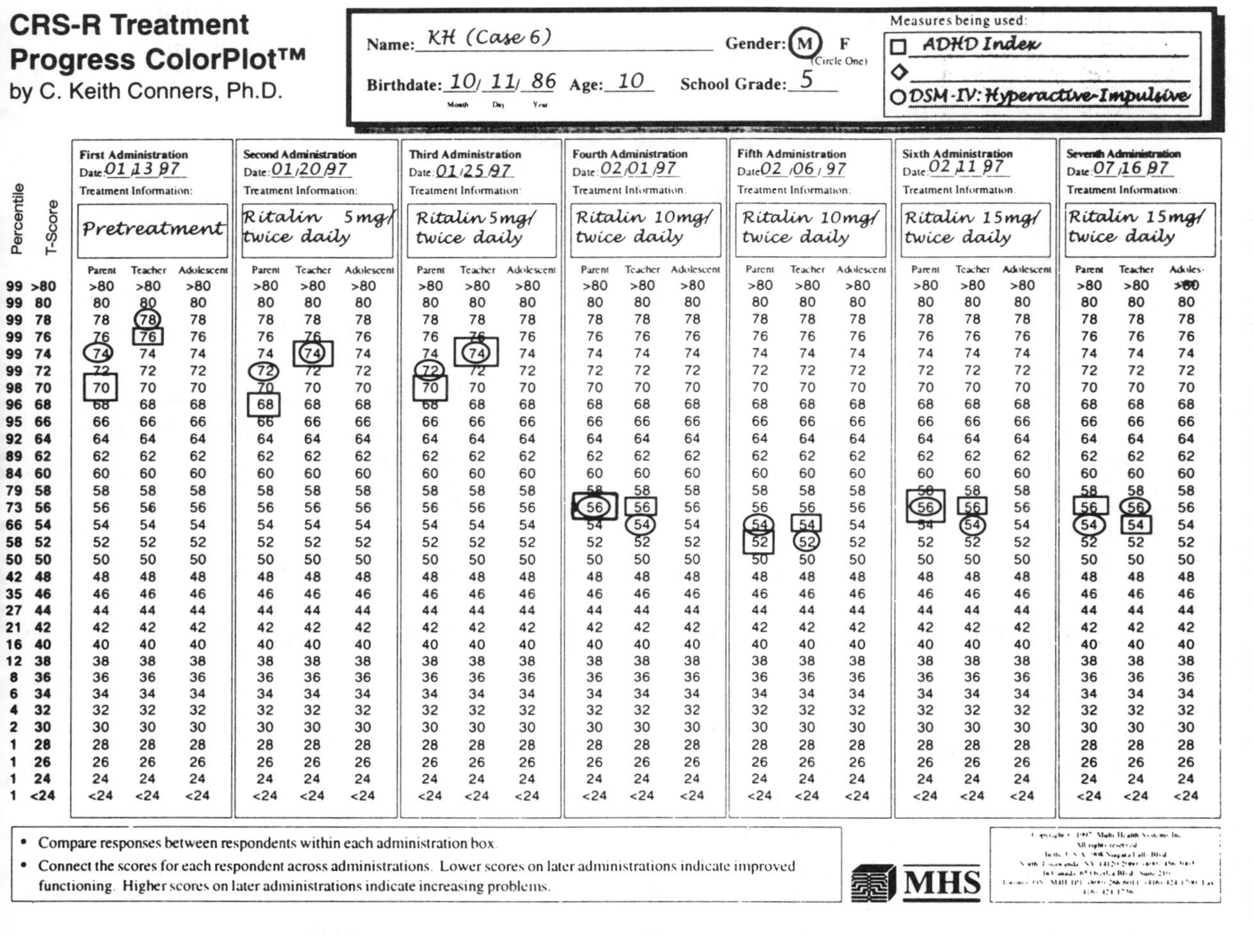

FIG. 1. Progress chart for recording a medication trial. The chart provides columns for parent, teacher, and adolescent self-report scores. T-scores for each instrument are plotted beginning with the pretreatment baseline and continuing for six different dosage adjustment phases. The left-hand column provides conversion factors for T-scores into percentiles. Different symbols indicate the type of scale (in this case the ADHD Index and *DSM-IV* Hyperactivity-Impulsivity scales. Alternatively, one might include the older Global Index subscales and/or the Inattention subscale of *DSM-IV*.

On the other hand, given the current state of child psychiatric nosology, there are occasions when broader coverage is important because of the ever-present comorbidities that affect both subject selection and response to treatment. The new scales, like the previous versions, cover conduct problems, hyperactivity/impulsivity, and inattention, but with refinements based on more recent concepts and a broader item pool. In addition, internalizing states such as perfectionism, anxiety, and shyness, and what is considered a somatizing anxiety dimension, continue to be represented. But adolescent data introduce new dimensions, and adult ratings reveal distinctive clusters of items that have no exact counterparts in younger samples.

Rating scales offer important information on dimensionalities of behavior that have been well established by decades of empirical work. But these data should always be seen in the context of several clinical operations such as interview, history, and other kinds of documentation. They are not meant to stand on their own or to relieve clinicians of the burden of careful synthesis of all information, and the informed use of intuition and clinical judgment.

REFERENCES

Abikoff, H., Courtney, M., Pelham, W.E.J. & Koplewicz, H.S. (1993), Teachers' ratings of disruptive behaviors: The influence of halo effects. *J. Abnorm. Child Psychol.*, 21:519–533.

Achenbach, T.M., Conners, C.K., Quay, H.C., Verhulst, F.C. & Howell, C.T. (1989), Replication of empirically derived syndromes as a basis for taxonomy of child/adolescent psychopathology. *J. Abnorm. Child Psychol.*, 17(3):299–323.

Achenbach, T.M., Howell, C.T., Quay, H.C. & Conners, C.K. (1991), National survey of problems and competencies among four- to sixteen-year-olds: Parents' reports for normative and clinical samples. *Monogr. Soc. Res. Child Dev.*, 56:1–131.

Aiken, L.R. (1996), *Rating Scales and Checklists: Evaluating Behavior, Personality, and Attitude.* New York: John Wiley & Sons, Inc.

Barkley, R.A. (1990), *Attention Deficit Hyperactivity Disorder: A Handbook for Diagnosis and Treatment.* New York: Guilford Press.

Blouin, A.G., Conners, C.K., Seidel, W.T. & Blouin, J. (1989), The independence of hyperactivity from conduct disorder: Methodological considerations. *Can. J. Psychiatry*, 34:279–282.

Conners, C.K. (1973), Rating scales for use in drug studies with children. *Psychopharmacol. Bull.* (Special issue on children): 24–42.

Conners, C.K. (1979), Rating scales. In: *Handbook of Child Psychiatry*, vol. 1, ed., J. Noshpitz. New York: Basic Books, pp. 675–691.

Conners, C.K. (1994), The Conners Rating Scales: Use in clinical assessment, treatment planning and research. In: *Use of Psychological Testing for Treatment Planning and Outcome Assessment*, ed., M. Maruish. Hillsdale, NJ: L. Erlbaum Associates, pp. 550–578.

Conners, C.K. (1997), *The Conners Rating Scales (Revised): Technical Manual.* Toronto: Multi-Health Systems.

Conners, C.K. (1999), *Conners' Adult ADHD Rating Scales (CAARS): Technical Manual.* Toronto, Ontario: Multi-Health Systems.

Conners, C.K. & Barkley, R.A. (1985), Rating scales and checklists for child psychopharmacology. *Psychopharmacol. Bull.*, 21:809–838.

Conners, C.K., Erhardt, D., Parker, J.D.A., Sitarenios, G., Epstein, J. & Sparrow, E. (1999), (submitted), Dimensions of psychopathology in adults: A new rating scale for adult ADHD.

Conners, C.K., Sitarenios, G., Parker, J.D.A. & Epstein, J.N. (1998a), The Revised Conners' Parent Rating Scale (CPRS-R): Factor structure, reliability, and criterion validity. *J. Abnorm. Child Psychol.*, 26(4), 257–268.

Conners, C.K., Sitarenios, G., Parker, J.D.A., & Epstein, J.N. (1998b), Revision and restandardization of the Conners Teacher Rating Scale (CTRS-R): Factor structure, reliability, and criterion validity. *J. Abnorm. Child Psychol.*, 26(4), 279–291.

Conners, C.K. & Wells, K.C. (1985) ADD-H adolescent self-report scale. *Psychopharmacol. Bull.* 21:921–922.

Conners, C.K., Wells, K.C., Parker, J.D.A., Sitarenios, G., Diamond, J.M. & Powell, J.W. (1997c), A new self-report scale for assessment of adolescent psychopathology: Factor structure, reliability, validity and diagnostic sensitivity. *J. Abnorm. Child Psychol.*, 25:487–497.

DuPaul, G.J., Anastopoulos, A.D., Kwasnik, D., Barkley, R.A. & McMurray, M.B. (1996), Methylphenidate effects on children with attention deficit hyperactivity disorder: Self-report of symptoms, side effects, and self-esteem. *J. Attention Dis.*, 1:3–15.

DuPaul, G.J. (1991), Parental teacher rating of ADHD symptoms in a community-based sample. *J. Clin. Child Psychol.,* 20:245–253.

Everett, J. (1983), Factor comparability as a means of determining the number of factors and their rotation. *Multivariate Behav. Res.*, 18:197–218.

Goyette, C.H., Conners, C.K. & Ulrich, R.F. (1978), Normative data on revised Conners Parent and Teacher Rating Scales. *J. Abnorm. Child Psychol.*, 6:221–236.

Holborow, P.L., Berry, P. & Elkins, J. (1984), Prevalence of hyperkinesis: A comparison of three rating scales. *J. Learning Disabil.*, 17:411–417.

Kavale, K. (1982), The efficacy of stimulant drug treatment for hyperactivity: A meta-analysis. *J. Learning Disabil.*, 15:280–289.

Klorman, R. (1985), Some thoughts on the diagnosis of ADD/H in adolescence. *Psychopharmacol. Bull.*, 21:913–914.

NIMH (1985), *Psychopharmacol. Bull.* (Special issue on rating scales and assessment instruments for use in pediatric psychopharmacology research), 21.

Ottenbacher, J.J., & Cooper, H.M. (1983), Drug treatment of hyperactivity in children. *Dev. Med. Child Neurol.*, 25:358–356.

Parker, J.D.A., Sitarenios, G. & Conners, C.K. (1996), Abbreviated Conners' Rating Scales revisited: A confirmatory factor analytic study. *J. Attention Disorders*, 1:55–62.

Pelham, W., Evans, S., Gnagy, E. & Greenslade, K. (1992a), Teacher ratings of *DSM-III-R* symptoms for the disruptive behavior disorders: Prevalence, factor analyses, and conditional probabilities in a special education sample. *School Psychol. Rev.*, 21:285–299.

Pelham, W.E., Gnagy, E.M., Greenslade, K.E., & Milich, R. (1992b), Teacher ratings of *DSM-III-R* symptoms for the disruptive behavior disorders. *J. Acad. Child Adolesc Psychiatry,* 31:210–218.

Rapport, M., Stoner, G., DuPaul, G., Kelly, K. & Schoeler, T. (1989), Attention deficit disorder and methylphenidate: A multilevel analysis of dose-response effects on children's impulsivity across settings. *J. Am. Acad. Child Adolesc. Psychiatry*, 27:60–69.

Rapport, M.D. (1990), Controlled studies of the effects of psychostimulants on children's functioning in clinic and classroom. In: *ADHD: Attention Deficit Disorder,* eds., C.K. Conners & M. Kinsbourne. Munich: MMV Medizin Verlag.

Robin, A.L. (1994), Adolescent self-report of ADHD symptoms. *ADHD Rep.*, 2:4–6.

Schachar, R.J., Sandberg, S. & Rutter, M. (1986), Agreement between teachers' ratings and observations of hyperactivity, inattentiveness, and defiance. *J. Abnorm. Child Psychol.*, 14:331–345.

Siegel, L.J., Dragovich, S.L. & Marholin, D.I. (1976), The effects of biasing information on behavioral observations and rating scales. *J. Abnorm. Child Psychol.*, 4:221–233.

Sandberg, S.T., Rutter, M. & Taylor, E. (1978), Hyperkinetic disorder in psychiatric clinic attenders. *Dev. Med. Child Neurol.*, 20:279–299.

Spencer, T., Wilens, T., Biederman, J., Faraone, S.V., Ablon, J.S. & Lapey, K. (1995), A double-blind crossover comparison of methylphenidate and placebo in adults with childhood-onset attention-deficit hyperactivity disorder. *Arch. Gen. Psychiatry*, 52:434–443.

Sprague, R.L. & Sleator, E.K. (1977), Methylphenidate in hyperkinetic children: Differences in dose effects on learning and social behavior. *Science*, 198:1274–1276.

Thurber, S. & Walker, C.E. (1983), Medication and hyperactivity: A meta-analysis. *J. Gen. Psychol.*, 108:79–86.

Trites, R.L. (1988), Conners' Teacher Rating Scale: Reliability, validity and normative data. In: *Attention Deficit Disorder, vol. 3: New Research in Attention, Treatment, and Psychopharmacology,* ed., L.M. Bloomingdale. Oxford, England: Pergamon Press, Inc., pp. 159–160.

Trites, R.L., Blouin, A.G. & Laprade, K. (1982), Factor analysis of the Conners Teacher Rating Scale based on a large normative sample. *J. Consult. Clin. Psychol.*, 50:615–623.

Trites, R.L., Dugas, E., Lynch, G. & Ferguson, H.B. (1979), Prevalence of hyperactivity. *J. Pediatr. Psychol.*, 4:179–188.

Ullmann, R.K., Sleator, E.K. & Sprague, R.L. (1985), A change in mind: The Conners Abbreviated Rating Scales reconsidered. *J. Abnorm. Child Psychol.*, 13:553–565.

Wainright, A. (1996), *Conners' Rating Scales: 30 Years of Research.* Toronto: Multi-Health Systems.

Ward, M.F., Wender, P.H. & Reimherr, F.W. (1993), The Wender Utah Rating Scale: An aid in the retrospective diagnosis of childhood attention deficit hyperactivity disorder. *Am. J. Psychiatry*, 150:885–890.

Wender, P.H. (1971), *Minimal Brain Dysfunction in Children*. New York: John Wiley & Sons, Inc.

Zelko, F.A. (1991), Comparison of parent-completed behavior rating scales: Differentiating boys with ADD from psychiatric and normal controls. *J. Dev. Behav. Pediatr.*, 12:31–37.

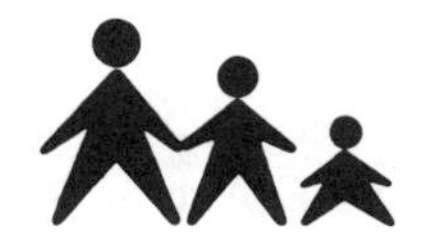

Methylphenidate Versus Amphetamine: A Comparative Review

L. EUGENE ARNOLD

Methylphenidate (MPH, Ritalin) and amphetamine (AMP), especially the latter's dextrorotary isomer dextroamphetamine (DEX, Dexedrine), and a proprietary mixture of three fourths dextroamphetamine and one fourth levoamphetamine (Adderall), are, respectively, the most commonly used and second most commonly used drugs for treatment of attention deficit hyperactivity disorder (ADHD). Although they are more similar than different in their pharmacodynamics and clinical effects, there are subtle differences that can be important at the level of the individual patient, if not in group data. This chapter reviews animal and human data to enable a better understanding of the differences and their potential clinical application. In addition to the author's knowledge of the literature, a computerized literature search through Medline and Psychoinfo was done for the years 1984–1996.

Although the subjective effects of MPH and AMP are similar (Heishman & Henningfield, 1991), the neurochemical effects of the two stimulants are distinct (Little, 1993), with different mechanisms of action (Glavin, 1985). MPH is a "pure uptake inhibitor" (Heron et al., 1994) without other presynaptic activity, whereas AMP has additional presynaptic activity (Hess et al., 1996), releasing dopamine (DA) and norepinephrine (NE) from the presynaptic neuron (e.g., During et al., 1992). Also, AMP has a slightly longer plasma half-life (4–6 hours) than MPH (2–3 hours) (e.g., Barkley et al., 1993). A significant proportion of AMP is directly excreted in the urine (especially acidic urine), whereas MPH is completely metabolized to inactive molecules (Barkley et al., 1993). AMP but not MPH lowers plasma and urinary 3-methoxy-4-hydroxyphenylglycol (MHPG) and NE turnover, whereas MPH but not AMP increases plasma NE (Elia et al., 1990). Presumably resulting from the subtle differences in mechanism of action, there are also behavioral and drug interaction differences in laboratory paradigms and individual patient variation in clinical response. These are reviewed and described below.

ANIMAL COMPARISONS

Table 1 summarizes 15 reports of animal research since 1984 that showed clear differences between MPH and AMP. Differences may have shown up in other laboratory studies but were not reported clearly enough to suit the purposes of this review. Of the 92 articles reviewed, most did not report any differences in the effects of the two drugs. In fact, most laboratory studies that included both drugs were not focused on comparing them but included them as probes to study some other issue; the differences found were in many cases unexpected. Many of the differences were significant at levels better than 0.05, making a type I error unlikely despite the low proportion of studies finding differences—except for

Ohio State University, Columbus, Ohio.

TABLE 1. SOME ANIMAL RESEARCH COMPARING METHYLPHENIDATE (MPH) AND AMPHETAMINE (AMP)

Reference	*Isomer*[1]	*Effects Studied*	*Findings*
Moss et al. (1984)	dl	Behavioral	Tetrahydrocannabinol pretreatment doubled AMP-induced gnawing without affecting AMP locomotor activity, but suppressed MPH-induced locomotor activity without affecting MPH-induced gnawing.
Mithani et al. (1986)	dl	Behavioral	Haloperidol pretreatment blocked place preferences induced by AMP, but not those induced by MPH.
Rosen et al. (1986)	dl	Behavioral	Under high-AMP dose discriminative stimulus training, MPH, but not AMP, generalization gradient was different for lead-exposed and control rats.
Svensson et al. (1986)	dextro	Behavioral	Reserpine pretreatment completely prevented MPH-induced, but not AMP-induced, locomotor hyperactivity.
Holtzman (1986)	dextro	Behavioral	In rat discrimination experiments, MPH generalized completely, but AMP only partially, with caffeine.
Sershen et al. (1988)	dl	Behavioral	Metaphit, a phencyclidine analog, antagonized the locomotor stimulation induced by MPH, but not that induced by AMP.
Zetterstrom et al. (1988)	dl	Biochemical	AMP, but not MPH, decreases striatal extracellular 3,4-dihydroxyphenylacetic acid (DOPAC), a metabolite of DA.[2]
Logan et al. (1988)	dextro	Behavioral	In BALB/cB7J mice, AMP up to 10 mg/kg short-term had no effect or inhibited locomotor activity (LA); MPH 10–32 mg/kg short-term stimulated LA. After 21 days of AMP 10 mg/kg, 3.2 mg/kg stimulated LA (no longer inhibited), and MPH no effect in doses that had acutely stimulated.
Zaczek et al. (1989)	citation of dl	Biochemical	MPH (and pemoline) did not induce the decrease in brain monoamine markers found with methamphetamine and previously with AMP.
Finn et al. (1990)	dextro	Behavioral	Pretreatment with reserpine or alpha-methyl-para-tyrosine attenuated the increase of locomotion induced by AMP or caffeine, but not that by MPH.
Nomikos et al. (1990)	dextro	Biochemical	Tetrodotoxin, which blocks voltage-dependent Na^+ channels, prevented MPH-induced, but not AMP-induced, increase in extracellular DA.

(*continued*)

TABLE 1. *(continued)* SOME ANIMAL RESEARCH COMPARING METHYLPHENIDATE (MPH) AND AMPHETAMINE (AMP)

Reference	*Isomer*[1]	*Effects Studied*	*Findings*
During et al. (1992)	dl	Biochemical	MPH released DA and neurotensin cosynchronously from rat prefrontal cortex; but with AMP, neurotensin release lagged behind DA release.
McNamara et al. (1993)	dl	Behavioral	Long-term administration of AMP sensitizes; long-term MPH develops tolerance. (Repeated doses of AMP over 7-day period augment the usual response of increased activity; repeated MPH decreases the subsequent responses.)
Jones & Holtzman (1994)	dextro & levo	Behavioral	Naloxone attenuated gross (though not fine) HA[3] induced by both amphetamine isomers, but not HA induced by MPH.
Heron et al. (1994)	dextro	Biochemical	MPH binds slowly to DA neuronal carrier; AMP interacts rapidly with DA neuronal carrier.
Wall et al. (1995)	dl	Biochemical	AMP caused efflux of DA & NE[4] across respective transporters in cell culture; MPH did not. Both inhibited influx.
Hess et al. (1996)	dl	Behavioral	AMP reduced activity in naturally HA Coloboma mice, increased in controls; MPH increased activity in both.

[1]Isomer = the form of amphetamine (AMP) that was compared to methylphenidate (MPH); dextro = d-amphetamine; levo = l-amphetamine; dl = racemic amphetamine.
[2]DA = dopamine.
[3]HA = hyperactivity.
[4]NE = norepinephrine.

the case of an apparent contradiction. Whereas Svensson et al. (1986) found that reserpine pretreatment prevented MPH-induced but not AMP-induced locomotor hyperactivity, Finn et al. (1990) found almost the reverse: Reserpine pretreatment attenuated locomotor hyperactivity induced by AMP, but not that induced by MPH. The apparent contradiction is not explained by species difference, because both investigators used rats. However, they could have been different strains (not specified). Another possible difference in technique was that Svensson et al., used habituated animals.

If reserpine pretreatment does indeed differentially modify the effects of the two stimulants, this could have implications for polypharmacy with a stimulant and one of the newer, atypical neuroleptics with serotonin activity, and possibly even with a stimulant and a serotonin-reuptake inhibiting antidepressant. This, of course, assumes extrapolation from rats to humans—not always a valid exercise. Other possible differential drug interactions are suggested by the literature on animal studies. One arises from the fact (Mithani et al., 1986) that haloperidol blocked place preferences that were induced by AMP but not those induced by MPH. (The combination of haloperidol and a stimulant is sometimes used in treatment of comorbid Tourette's syndrome and ADHD, or comorbid bipolar disorder and ADHD.) To my knowledge, there are no controlled studies comparing the clinical effects of the two stimulants in the presence of haloperidol or other neuroleptics.

It is not clear what we should make of the finding by Hess et al. (1996) in naturally hyperactive Coloboma mice, in which AMP reduced, but MPH increased, activity. Because MPH decreases activity in most naturally hyperactive humans, the mice must have been hyperactive through a different mechanism than most humans. Study of that difference might illuminate not only the mechanisms of stimulant action but also pathogenetic mechanisms and subtypes of ADHD. It is conceivable, of course, that the hyperactive Coloboma mice have the same pathogenetic mechanism as the minority of hyperactive humans who respond to AMP but not MPH.

HUMAN COMPARISONS OTHER THAN ADHD CLINICAL TRIALS

Table 2 summarizes the six reports found comparing MPH and AMP in human studies other than ADHD clinical trials. Interestingly, Little (1993) reported the same situation in treating depression, as noted see below with treatment of ADHD: two thirds efficacy for either drug, with only partial overlap of efficacy and no way of predicting which will be better for a given patient.

CONTROLLED COMPARISONS IN TREATMENT OF ADHD

Table 3 summarizes the seven controlled crossover comparisons found. Uncontrolled or noncrossover comparisons of MPH and AMP are not tabulated. Three of the latter are worth noting. Millichap and Fowler (1967) reviewed the available literature, consisting of one-drug studies in different samples, some not well controlled. After averaging the response rate across studies for each drug (with response defined differently from study to study, even using different instruments), they found a higher mean response rate for MPH and concluded that it is "the drug of choice." Arnold and Knopp (1973) pointed out the this conclusion was not based on any controlled direct comparison of MPH and AMP in the same sample, but it persists to the present as clinical belief in some circles despite the fact that the only one of the subsequent controlled crossover comparisons in Table 3 that supports it is the one in comorbid Tourette's syndrome. Weiss et al. (1971) compared the results of chlorpromazine, MPH, and d-AMP from three different samples studied in three different years. They believed that MPH was slightly more efficacious with about the same side effects. Conners (1972) came closer to a valid comparison, studying both stimulants in the same sample, but unfortunately with a parallel pretest–posttest design so that individual subject variables were not well controlled. He found MPH to show an advantage on the arithmetic and similarities subtests of the Wechsler Intelligence Scale for Children, but not on other subtests, tests, or scales in a reasonable assessment battery.

In examining Table 3, we need to remember that most group mean differences between the stimulants are not significant because of the small samples, so that we are essentially studying nonsignificant subtle trends. Within this constraint, it seems appropriate to note some themes. The most obvious is that no study shows congruence in response at the individual subject level. That is, every study has some subjects who responded to one drug but not the other. In most studies, this is a two-way street: some respond better to MPH, others better to AMP.

Another noteworthy theme is that every crossover study except the one in comorbid Tourette's syndrome shows a slight (nonsignificant) advantage for AMP in the number of individuals judged responsive or in the number judged to have a better response than to the other active condition(s). The references do not use strictly comparable reporting methods: For example, Winsberg et al. (1974) and Elia et al. (1991) report response or nonresponse in a binary fashion, while Arnold et al. (1978) and Pelham et al. (1990) report which is better or clinically preferable for maintenance even where both are efficacious. Castellanos et al. (1992) reported only those better with AMP and not those better with MPH, presumably 35 or less, since there were at least two nonresponders in that sample (reported by Elia et al. in the first 48 subjects). Nevertheless, because both drugs are reported the

TABLE 2. SOME HUMAN COMPARISONS OF METHYLPHENIDATE AND AMPHETAMINE OTHER THAN ADHD CLINICAL TRIALS

Reference	*Isomer*[1]	*Type of Study*	*Finding*
Lieberman et al. (1987)	dl, dextro?	Clinical (review)	In challenges with schizophrenic patients, MPH appears to have greater psychotogenic potency than AMP.
Little (1988)[2]	dl, dextro	Clinical (review)	In depression, 85% of AMP responders but only 43% of AMP nonresponders improve with antidepressant Tx; MPH responders and nonresponders improve equally.
Elia et al. (1990)	dextro	Biochemical	AMP but not MPH lowered plasma/urinary MHPG, norepinephrine turnover; MPH but not AMP raised plasma norepinephrine.
Little (1993)	dextro	Clinical	Depressed inpatients improved acutely after AMP or MPH, but only 5/18 showed equal improvement to both; 7 responded only to AMP, 5 only to MPH. Which was better was unpredictable, with no drug-specific target symptoms.
Little et al. (1993)	dl	Biochemical, postmortem	MPH binds more strongly, but AMP more weakly, than cocaine or bupropion to binding sites of [125I]RTI-55, a cocaine congener.
Matochik et al. (1994)	dextro	Biochemical	MPH changed metabolism in 2 of 60 brain regions sampled by PET; AMP did not change metabolism in any region (adult subjects with ADHD). With randomly assigned noncrossover Tx, CGI = 2.1 for MPH, 1.9 for AMP (lower score better but not significantly different); Conners change scores = 11.6 and 9.1 for MPH, 10.6 and 7.3 for AMP (NS). On 2 other scales, MPH significantly improved 11/60 feelings/symptoms, AMP 19/60, only 7 in common. Ratings nonblind.

CGI = clinical global impression; Tx = treatment.

[1]Isomer = the form of amphetamine (AMP) that was compared with methylphenidate (MPH); dextro = d-amphetamine; levo = l-amphetamine; dl = racemic amphetamine; NS = not significant.

[2]The Little (1988) review was challenged by Gwirtsman and Guze (1989), who argued that MPH response predicted antidepressant response to an adrenergic tricyclic antidepressant (TCA), whereas MPH nonresponse predicted response to a serotonergic TCA.

TABLE 3. CONTROLLED CROSSOVER COMPARISONS OF METHYLPHENIDATE (MPH) AND D-AMPHETAMINE (AMP) IN ADHD AND ITS HISTORICAL PRECURSORS[1]

Reference	No. & Sex	Age	MPH Dose	AMP Dose	Better Response	Other Findings	Side Effects
Winsberg et al. (1974)	15 M, 3 F	8.5 5–10	≤30 BID	≤20 BID	0 MPH 3 AMP 11 both 4 neither	AMP > MPH by E.S.[2] = 0.45 on aggressivity, 0.14 on inattentiveness, 0.41 on hyperactivity (all NS)	Same frequency, 6 subjects. Insomnia only AMP, GI only MPH, apathy more MPH
Arnold et al. (1978)	22 M, 7 F	8 5–12	38 mg 10–60/day	19 mg 5–30/day	10 MPH 12 AMP 1 caffeine 2 MPH-AMP tie 1 AMP-caffeine tie 3 none	Good or excellent response on 9-point blind rating in 10 subjects with MPH, 17 with AMP. MPH > AMP on DP[3] short attn item with E.S. 0.32. AMP > MPH with E.S.: CTRS[4] = 0.16; CTRS HA[4] = 0.13; CTRS aggr = 0.25; CTRS LOH[4] = 0.21; DT[3] = 0.11; DT inattn = 0.14; DT irrit = 0.19; DT expl = 0.15; DP var = 0.28; PBC[5] = 0.15; PBC aggr = 0.16; PBC inattn = 0.15; PBC HA = 0.18; PBC sociop = 0.18; PBC dep = 0.13; Target symptoms = 0.18 (NS)	MPH more stomachaches (E.S. = 0.17) and diastolic BP rise (0.10). AMP more appetite (E.S. = 0.10) and sleep (0.11) disturbance, wt loss. (all NS). AMP significantly less stomachaches than placebo.
Vyborova et al. (1984)	25 M, 3 F	6–14	38 mg/day	38 mg/day	9 better with AMP[6]	MPH better on mean global score.[6] MPH preferentially helped children with visuomotor disorders; AMP, those without.	
Pelham et al. (1990)	22 M	8–13	20 mg/day	10 SR q A.M.	5 MPH 6 AMP 4 pem[7] 7 none	AMP > MPH with E.S.: following rules 0.25, noncompliance 0.35, neg verbalization 0.24, CTRS[4] 0.33, counselor rating 0.12, %DRC[8] 0.14 (all NS); AMP less within-S variability (more consistent response)	MPH more crabby, tearful, muscle aches, dry mouth, twitches. AMP more whiny, drowsy, sad, withdrawn, jittery, stomachaches, nausea and vomiting, headaches, insomnia, anorexia (all NS).
Borcherding et al. (1990) (Elia sample)	45 M	6–12	12.5–45 BID	5–22.5 BID	See below	Abnormal movements (tics) and perseverative-compulsive behaviors (OC) on only 1 drug per patient (usually)	AMP more OC; MPH more co-occurence of abnormal movement & OC.
Elia et al. (1991)	48 M	8.6 6–12	12.5–45 BID	5–22.5 BID	4 MPH 8 AMP 34 both 2 neither	On C-GAS, 9 MPH & 5 AMP worse or same. MPH > AMP calming motor activity, CPT. AMP blood level higher, more variable & prolonged.	5 subjects had SE with MPH, 3 with AMP, 32 with both. AMP more meticulousness, anorexia; MPH more nervous habits, unhappy.

Castellanos et al. (1992) (Expanded Elia sample)	72 (incl. Elia 48)	6–12	12.5–45 BID	5–22.5 BID	35/72 better with AMP	11 of 13 subjects within IQ > 120, but only 24/59 with low IQ, responded better to AMP. Correlation IQ with improvement 0.39 for AMP, 0.06 for MPH.	Not reported.
Castellanos et al. (1997)	20 M	9.4 ± 2	12.5–45 BID	5–22.5 BID	11 MPH 6 AMP 3 neither	All comorbid with Tourette's disorder; at highest dose only, AMP but not MPH increased tic severity by 25% compared with placebo.	OC symptoms: 5 MPH, 1 AMP; appetite: 3 MPH, 4 AMP; insomnia: 1 MPH, 10 AMP.
Totals without Castellanos et al. (1992)	165				30 MPH 45 AMP		
Totals without either Vyborova et al. or Castellanos et al.	117				19 MPH 30 AMP 47 both 5 others 16 none		

Differences generally not statistically significant. Isomer was dextroamphetamine except in Vyborova et al. (1984).

CPT = continuous performance test; SE = side effects; C-GAS = Children's Global Assessment Scale; OC = obsessive compulsiveness; NS = not significant.

[1]Some studies were done prior to *DSM-III-R* introduction of the term ADHD, and used designations such as hyperkinetic/hyperkinesis or minimal brain dysfunction/damage (MBD).

[2]Effect Size = Cohen's d = difference of means/mean standard deviation. Only effect sizes of 0.10 or more are tabulated. For comparison, the effect size of the stimulant-placebo difference usually runs 1.0+ to 2.0 in ADHD studies. AMP > MPH means AMP better than MPH on the dependent variables listed.

[3]DP = Davids' Hyperkinetic Rating Scale by parent; DT = Davids' Hyperkinetic Scale by teacher. Davids' items: hyperactivity, short attention span (short attn), variability (varib), impulsiveness (imp), irritability (irrit), explosiveness (expl), poor schoolwork.

[4]CTRS = Conners Teacher Rating Scale. Factors: aggressive misconduct (aggr), daydreaming and inattention (inattn), hyperactivity (HA), lack of health (LOH).

[5]PBC = Parent Behavior Checklist by parent (similar to Conners' parent rating scale). Factors: unsocialized aggression (aggr), inattentive unproductiveness (inattn), sociopathy (sociop), withdrawal-depression (dep), somatic complaints.

[6]Vyborova et al. did not give number of MPH and AMP responders or scale data, merely stating that the number of responders to amphetaminil was higher than the number of responders to MPH by 1/3 of the sample, but that the AMP mean improvement in global score was lower by nearly half.

[7]Pelham et al. compared MPH 10 BID, MPH 20 SR/day, d-amphetamine spansule (SR) 10/day, and pemoline (pem) 56.25/day. For purpose of this comparison table, the results of the two MPH dosage forms are averaged.

[8]%DRC = % positive days on daily report card.

same way within a given study for each of the other six studies, it seems permissible to sum them up for comparison.

Summary of responders

Of the 165 subjects in the six nonduplicative studies (Winsberg et al., 1974; Arnold et al., 1978; Vyborova et al., 1984; Pelham et al., 1990; Elia et al., 1991; Castellanos et al., 1997), 45 responded better to AMP and 30 better to MPH. If we eliminate the study by Vyborova et al. (1984) because of the noncomparable dosing and the contradiction between response rate and mean global score, and eliminate the study by Castellanos et al. (1997) because of the focus on relatively rare comorbidity (Tourette's syndrome), the totals are 30 d-AMP and 19 MPH in the remaining four studies. If we add the 47 known double responders to each total, there were 77 (or more) d-AMP responders versus 66 (or more) MPH responders in these four studies, with 117 subjects and 16 nonresponders. This translates to a 66+% response rate for d-AMP and 56+% for MPH, with an 85% stimulant response rate if both are tried. These differences between MPH and d-AMP pooled rates of response are not statistically significant because of the small numbers.

Relative strengths

Beyond the global response, closer scrutiny of effects on specific symptoms suggests some subtle differences, some of which relate to comorbidity. Castellanos et al. (1997), of course, found MPH better in the presence of comorbid Tourette's syndrome. In several of the studies, AMP seemed to have a greater effect on such oppositional-defiant and conduct-disorder (ODD/CD) symptoms as aggression (with effect size (E.S.), Cohen's *d*, of 0.16, 0.25, and 0.45), irritability (E.S. 0.19), explosiveness (E.S. 0.15), noncompliance (E.S. 0.35), negative verbalization (E.S. 0.24), and rule-breaking (E.S. 0.25). These were nonsignificant, of course, at the sample sizes studied. In no study did MPH show a tendency of superiority on such symptoms. On the other hand, AMP did not show any impressive trend of advantage on inattention symptoms. For example, the study (Winsberg et al., 1974) that found an E.S. of 0.45 for AMP superiority on aggression found an E.S. of only 0.14 for AMP superiority on inattention. The study (Arnold et al., 1978) that found an E.S. of 0.25 for teacher rating of aggression found E.S. of only 0.02 and 0.14 for teacher ratings of inattention on two different scales. The advantage of MPH on the CPT reported by Elia et al. (1991) may be related to the report of Vyborova et al. (1984) that MPH preferentially helped patients with visuomotor disorders. If the suggestive trends noted here were upheld by further study, it could lead to a preference for MPH in ADHD comorbid with Tourette's syndrome or learning disorder (LD) and for AMP in ADHD comorbid with ODD/CD.

One of the few statistically significant differences reported was that AMP showed a more consistent response day-to-day, with less within-subject variability (Pelham, 1990). The significant association of AMP superiority with high IQ (Castellanos et al., 1992) was one of the more exciting differences found. It offered hope of a simple clinical predictor of which stimulant should be tried first in a given case. It also articulated neatly with the report of Vyborova et al. (1984) that MPH was better for children with visuomotor disorder and AMP better for those without; both findings could be accommodated by a hypothesis that AMP worked better for those without cognitive handicap and MPH better for those with cognitive handicap or low functional level. Unfortunately, this association with IQ was not replicated in a prospective study (F.X. Castellanos, personal communication, 1997 e-mail).

Side effects

Side effects were in general similar with both drugs. For example, Winsberg et al. (1974) reported that six of 18 subjects had side effects with each drug, whereas Elia et al. (1991) reported that 37 (of 48 subjects) had side effects with MPH and 35 with AMP. Within this context of similarity, there were some subtle trends and tendencies (most nonsignificant). Four studies (Arnold et al., 1978; Pelham et al., 1990; Elia et al., 1991; Castellanos et al., 1997), with 119 subjects, found more anorexia with AMP, compared to no study finding more anorexia with MPH. Two studies (Arnold et al., 1978; Winsberg et al., 1974), with 47 subjects, found more gastrointestinal (GI) complaints with MPH, compared to 1 study (Pelham et al., 1990), with 22 subjects, finding more GT complaints with AMP. Three studies (Elia et al., 1991; Pelham et al., 1990; Winsberg et al., 1974), with 88 subjects, found more apathy/tearfulness/unhappiness with MPH, compared to one study (Pelham et al., 1990), with 22 subjects, finding more sadness/withdrawal with AMP. Castellanos et al., (1997) found more exacerbation of tics with AMP than with MPH in patients comorbid for Tourette's disorder.

CLINICAL IMPLICATIONS AND DISCUSSION

Table 4 summarizes the relative advantages of MPH and AMP for treatment of ADHD, as suggested by the foregoing review and supplementary clinical experience. Many of the differences listed do not reach statistical significance. Although very similar in many ways, the two stimulants are in some ways complementary in patient responsiveness. The clearest lesson gleaned from the controlled studies is that the individual patient response profiles are noncongruent, and that nonresponse or intolerable side effects with one stimulant do not preclude a good response to the other. Interestingly, Little (1993) could have been talking about ADHD when he said this about MPH and AMP for depression: "Relatively few responded with equal improvement to both. . .symptomatic improvement is unpredictable and can only be determined by an empirical trial on an individual basis." Therefore, each should be tried before stimulant treatment is abandoned, and patients and parents should be forewarned of this.

While this review found no evidence to make MPH the drug of choice for ADHD, this does not detract from the fact that stimulants as a class constitute the drugs of choice. One can fill in where another fails, so that together they can help the vast majority of patients with ADHD. Possibly the response rate with trials of both MPH and AMP could be increased even further with a third stimulant: Pelham et al. (1990) reported that four of their 22 patients did best with pemoline. The advantage of trying both MPH and AMP has public policy implications: The bureaucratic Medicaid obstacles to AMP prescriptions in many states may be depriving some Medicaid ADHD children of their best treatment.

Beyond the basic principle of systematically trying a second stimulant if the first fails, there are some hints in Table 4 that might guide the choice of which stimulant to try first. For example, a child who already has a poor appetite might do better with MPH, while one prone to stomachaches might do better with AMP. If the child has a history of seizures and is not currently taking an anticonvulsant, AMP may be slightly safer. The type of comorbidity may be a consideration: A child with either Tourette's disorder or LD and no CD/ODD symptoms might try MPH first, while one with CD/ODD and no LD or Tourette's disorder might try AMP first. This is not to say that either stimulant would not help the other comorbidity or that either is guaranteed to help its favored comorbidity, but in the absence of any more compelling reason for choosing the first trial drug, why not follow the hint suggested by the literature review?

TABLE 4. RELATIVE ADVANTAGES OF METHYLPHENIDATE (MPH) AND AMPHETAMINE (AMP) FOR TREATMENT OF ADHD

Advantages of MPH	*Advantages of AMP*
Better CPT response[1]	More consistent response day-to-day[1]
Better with comorbid Tourette's disorder[1]	Higher proportion of patients with good/excellent response.[2]
Better with visuomotor disorder[3]	Better with comorbid conduct or oppositional/defiant[3]
Possibly better with comorbid learning disability[3]	May be better with high IQ[4]
Less anorexia[2]	Less depression/apathy[3]
Less weight loss[2]	Fewer stomachaches[3]
Less temporary growth suppression in low doses[3]	Safer when history of seizures;[3] slightly anticonvulsant in low doses[2]
Lower street value and abuse potential	Usually cheaper legally
More readily available to Medicaid patients	Variety of SR spansule strengths; SR seems more consistently efficacious than SR MPH
	Slightly longer half-life

Few of these reach statistical significance; most are tendencies noted in more than one report in the literature review.

CPT = continuous performance test; SR = sustained release.

[1]Statistically significant in a controlled study.

[2]Probable.

[3]Possible, suggested.

[4]Significant in post hoc analysis of controlled study but not replicated in prospective study.

This review has not addressed the issue of stereoisomers, which may also have subtle differential effects in individual patients. Five decades ago, Bradley (1950) noted that some hyperkinetic children responded better to racemic amphetamine whereas others responded better to the dextroisomer. MPH has four stereoisomers: the erythro and threo forms each have a dextro and a levo isomer. The commercially available MPH is a racemic (dl) mixture of the threo enantiomer. The most popular form of amphetamine is the dextroisomer (Dexedrine), which was used in most of the clinical studies in Table 3 and constitutes the basis for the comparison with MPH in Table 4. Arnold et al. (1973, 1976) found that levoamphetamine has clinical benefits in ADHD comparable with those of the dextro isomer and reported that a few patients responded to one isomer but not to the other. They also suspected some subtle tendencies for different side effects and even different clinical benefits by comorbidity. Adderall is 3/4 DEX and 1/4 levoamphetamine, with anecdotal (as yet undocumented) claims that a few children with ADHD respond better to this mix than to either straight DEX or MPH. On the assumption that stimulants as a class will continue to be the drugs of choice for treatment of ADHD, clinical science could benefit from more systematic controlled comparisons of the various isomers and combinations thereof of both these drugs. Such studies would require rather large samples to enable analysis of all the patient characteristics that might influence the choice of stimulant (e.g., age, gender, comorbidity, physical habitus).

SUMMARY

This chapter compared the two most common medications for ADHD using data from controlled studies. Medline and Psychinfo searches were done for 1984–1996 with the key words methylphenidate and amphetamine; these were supplemented with known prior literature. Of 92 animal studies found, 15 showed clear differences between the two drugs. Seven controlled crossover ADHD clinical trials and five other articles comparing the two drugs in humans were found. MPH is a pure reuptake inhibitor of catecholamines, especially dopamine; AMP also releases catecholamines. Laboratory animals showed differential interactions with other drugs and with behavioral paradigms. Human response profiles are noncongruent. An ADHD patient who does not respond to one stimulant should try the other. Of 117 patients in the four clearest crossover studies, 30 responded better to AMP, 19 to MPH, and 47 to both: an overall response rate of 85%. All crossovers except the one with comorbid Tourette's syndrome showed a nonsignificant tendency for AMP superiority in response rate. The summed data suggest suspected differences in side effects (AMP: more sleep and appetite loss, and exacerbation of tics in comorbid Tourette's syndrome; MPH: more stomachaches and depression/apathy) and effects on comorbid disorders (AMP: better for conduct/oppositional symptoms; MPH: better for Tourette's syndrome and possibly learning disorder). Most of the clinical differences are tendencies rather than being statistically significant.

REFERENCES

Arnold, L.E., Christopher, J., Huestis, R.D. & Smeltzer, D.J. (1978), Methylphenidate vs. dextroamphetamine vs. caffeine in minimal brain dysfunction. *Arch. Gen. Psychiatry*, 35:463–473.

Arnold, L.E., Huestis, R.D., Smeltzer, D.J., Scheib, J., Wemmer, D. & Colner, G. (1976), Levoamphetamine vs. Dextroamphetamine in minimal brain dysfunction. *Arch. Gen. Psychiatry*, 33:292–301.

Arnold, L.E., Kirilcuk, V., Corson, S.A. & Corson, E.O'L. (1973), Levoamphetamine and dextroamphetamine: Differential effect on aggression and hyperkinesis in children and dogs. *Am. J. Psychiatry*, 130:165–170.

Arnold, L.E. & Knopp, W. (1973), The making of a myth. *J.A.M.A.*, 223:1273–1274.

Barkley, R.A., DuPaul, G.J. & Costello, A. (1993), Stimulants. In: *Practitioner's Guide to Psychoactive Drugs for Children and Adolescents*, eds., J.S. Werry & M.G. Aman. New York: Plenum Medical Book Company, pp. 205–237.

Borcherding, B.G., Keysor, C.S., Rapoport, J.L., Elia, J. & Amass, J. (1990), Motor-vocal tics and compulsive behaviors on stimulant drugs: Is there a common vulnerability? *Psychiatry Res.*, 33:83–94.

Bradley, C. (1950), Benzedrine and dexedrine in the treatment of children's behavioral disorders. *Pediatrics*, 5:24–36.

Castellanos, F.X., Giedd, J.N., Elia, J., Marsh, W.L., Ritchie, G.F., Hamburger, S.D. & Rapoport, J.L. (1997), Controlled stimulant treatment of ADHD and comorbid Tourette's syndrome: Effects of stimulant and dose. *J. Am. Acad. Child Adolesc. Psychiatry*, 36: 589–596.

Castellanos, F.X., Gulotta, C. & Rapoport, J. (1992), Superior intellectual functioning and stimulant drug response in ADHD. Poster at May 26–29, 1992 New Clinical Drug Evaluation Unit (NCDEU) meeting, Boca Raton, Florida.

Conners, C.K. (1972), Psychological effects of stimulant drugs in children with minimal brain dysfunction. *Pediatrics*, 49:702–709.

During, M.J., Bean, A.J. & Roth, R.H. (1992), Effects of CNS stimulants on the *in vivo* release of the colocalized neurotransmitters, dopamine and neurotensin, from rat prefrontal cortex. *Neuroscience Letters* 140(1):129–133.

Elia, J., Borcherding, B.G., Potter, W.Z., Mefford, I.N., Rapoport, J.L. & Keysor, C.S. (1990), Stimulant drug treatment of hyperactivity: Biochemical correlates. *Clin. Pharmacol. Ther.*, 48:57–66.

Elia, J., Borcherding, B.G., Rapoport, J.L. & Keysor, C.S. (1991), Methylphenidate and dextroamphetamine treatments of hyperactivity: Are there true nonresponders? *Psychiatry Res.*, 36:141–155.

Finn, I.B., Iuvone, P.M. & Holtzman, S.G. (1990), Depletion of catecholamines in the brain of rats differentially affects stimulation of locomotor activity by caffeine, d-amphetamine, and methylphenidate. *Neuropharmacology*, 29:625–631.

Glavin, G.B. (1985), Methylphenidate effects on activity-stress gastric lesions and regional brain noradrenaline metabolism in rats. *Pharmacol. Biochem. Behav.*, 23:379–383.

Gwirtsman, H.E. & Guze, B.H. (1989), Amphetamine, but not methylphenidate, predicts antidepressant response [letter]. *J. Clin. Psychopharmacol.*, 9:453–454.

Heishman, S.J. & Henningfield, J.E. (1991), Discriminative stimulus effects of d-amphetamine, methylphenidate, and diazepam in humans. *Psychopharmacology*, 103:436–442.

Heron, C., Costentin, J. & Bonnet, J.J. (1994), Evidence that pure uptake inhibitors including cocaine interact slowly with the dopamine neuronal carrier. *Eur. J. Pharmacol.*, 264:391–398.

Hess, E.J., Collins, K.A. & Wilson, M.C. (1996), Mouse model of hyperkinesis implicates SNAP-25 in behavioral regulation. *J. Neurosci.*, 16:3104–3111.

Holtzman, S.G. (1986), Discriminative stimulus properties of caffeine in the rat: Noradrenergic mediation. *J. Pharmacol. Exp. Ther.*, 239:706–714.

Jones, D.N. & Holtzman, S.G. (1994), Influence of naloxone upon motor activity induced by psychomotor stimulant drugs. *Psychopharmacology*, 114:215–224.

Lieberman, J.A., Kane, J.M. & Alvir, J. (1987), Provocative tests with psychostimulant drugs in schizophrenia. *Psychopharmacology*, 91:415–433.

Little, K.Y. (1988), Amphetamine, but not methylphenidate, predicts antidepressant efficacy [review]. *J. Clin. Psychopharmacol.*, 8:177–183.

Little, K.Y. (1993), d-Amphetamine versus methylphenidate effects in depressed inpatients. *J. Clin. Psychiatry*, 54:349–355.

Little, K.Y., Kirkman, J.A., Carroll, F.I., Breese, G.R. & Duncan, G.E. (1993), [1251]RTI-55 binding to cocaine-sensitive dopaminergic and serotonergic uptake sites in the human brain. *J. Neurochem.*, 61:1996–2006.

Logan, L., Seale, T.W., Cao, W. & Carney, J.M. (1988), Effects of chronic amphetamine in BALB/cBY mice, a strain that is not stimulated by acute administration of amphetamine. *Pharmacol. Biochem. Behav.*, 31:675–682.

Matochik, J.A., Liebenauer, L.L., King, A.C., Szymanski, H.V., Cohen, R.M. & Zametkin, A.J. (1994), Cerebral glucose metabolism in adults with attention-deficit/hyperactivity disorder after chronic stimulant treatment. *Am. J. Psychiatry*, 151:658–664.

McNamara, C.G., Davidson, E.S. & Schenck, S. (1993), A comparison of the motor-activating effects of acute and chronic exposure to amphetamine and methylphenidate. *Pharmacol. Biochem. Behav.*, 45:729–732.

Millichap, J.G. & Fowler, G.W. (1967), Treatment of "minimal brain dysfunction" syndromes. *Pediatr. Clin. North Am.*, 7:767–777.

Mithani, S., Martin-Iverson, M.T., Phillips, A.G. & Fibiger, H.C. (1986), The effects of haloperidol on amphetamine- and methylphenidate-induced conditioned place preferences and locomotor activity. *Psychopharmacology*, 90:247–252.

Moss, D.E., Koob, G.F., McMaster, S.B. & Janowsky, D.S. (1984), Comparative effects of tetrahydrocannabinol on psychostimulant-induced behavior. *Pharmacol. Biochem. Behav.*, 21:641–644.

Nomikos, G.G., Damsma, G. & Wenkstern, D. (1990), *In vivo* characterization of locally applied dopamine uptake inhibitors by striatal microdialysis. *Synapse*, 6:106–112.

Pelham, W.E., Greenslade, K.E., Vodde-Hamilton, M., Murphy, D.A., Greenstein, J.J., Gnagy, E.M., Guthrie, K.J., Hoover, M.D. & Dahl, R.E. (1990), Relative efficacy of long-acting stimulants on children with attention-deficit hyperactivity disorder: A comparison of standard methylphenidate, sustained-release methylphenidate, sustained-release dextroamphetamine, and pemoline. *Pediatrics*, 86:226–237.

Rosen, J.B., Young, A.M., Beuthin, F.C. & Louis-Ferdinand, R.T. (1986), Discriminative stimulus properties of amphetamine and other stimulants in lead-exposed and normal rats. *Pharmacol. Biochem. Behav.*, 24:211–115.

Sershen, H., Berger, P., Jacobson, A.E., Rice, K.C. & Reith, M.E. (1988), Metaphit prevents locomotor activation induced by various psychostimulants and interferes with the dopaminergic system in mice. *Neuropharmacology*, 27:23–30.

Svensson, K., Hohansson, A.M., Magnusson, T. & Carlsson, A. (1986), (+)-AJ 76 and (+)-UH 232: central stimulants acting as preferential dopamine autoreceptor antagonists. *Naun. Schmied. Arch. Pharmacol.*, 334:234–245.

Vyborova, L., Nahunek, K., Drtilkova, I., Balastikova, B. & Misurec, J. (1984), Intraindividual comparison of 21-day application of amphetamine and methylphenidate in hyperkinetic children. *Act. Nerv. Superior*, 26:268–269.

Wall, S.C., Gu, H. & Rudnick, G. (1995), Biogenic amine flux mediated by cloned transporters stably expressed in cultured cell lines: Amphetamine specificity for inhibition and efflux. *Molecular Pharmacol.*, 47:544–550.

Weiss, G., Minde, K. & Douglas, V. (1971), Comparison of the effects of chlorpromazine, dextroamphetamine, and methylphenidate on the behavior and intellectual functioning of hyperactive children. *Can. Med. J.*, 104:20–25.

Winsberg, B.G., Press, M., Bialer, I. & Kupietz, S. (1974), Dextroamphetamine and methylphenidate in the treatment of hyperactive/aggressive children. *Pediatrics*, 53: 236–241.

Zaczek, R., Battaglia, G., Contrera, J.F., Culp, S. & De Sousa, E.B. (1989), Methylphenidate and pemoline do not cause depletion of rat brain monoamine markers similar to that observed with methamphetamine. *Toxicol. Appl. Pharmacol.*, 100:227–233.

Zetterstrom, T., Sharp, T. & Collin, A.K. (1988), *In vivo* measurement of extracellular dopamine and DOPAC in rat striatum after various dopamine-releasing drugs: Implications for the origin of extracellular DOPAC. *Eur. J. Pharmacol.*, 148:327–334.

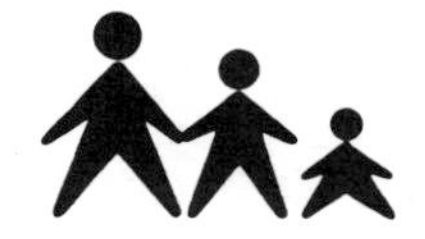

Treatment of Adult Attention Deficit Hyperactivity Disorder

THOMAS SPENCER,[1] JOSEPH BIEDERMAN,[1]
and TIMOTHY WILENS[2]

INTRODUCTION

In recent years, evidence has been accumulating that the syndrome of attention deficit hyperactivity disorder (ADHD) persists into adulthood in 10% to 60% of childhood-onset cases (Gittelman et al., 1985; Mannuzza et al., 1991b; Weiss et al., 1985). Considering current prevalence estimates that at least 5% of children may be affected with ADHD (Anderson et al., 1987; Bird et al., 1988), many adults may also have the disorder. Studies have consistently reported that the persistence of ADHD into adulthood is associated with high rates of academic failure (fewer years of education, poorer marks, and failed grades) and work failure (worse performance, impairment in task completion, lack of independent skills, and poor relationships with supervisors) (Klein and Mannuzza, 1989; Weiss et al., 1979) as well as high rates of psychiatric comorbidity including substance use disorders and antisocial personality (Klein and Mannuzza, 1989; 1991; Thorley, 1984; Weiss and Hechtman, 1986).

Over the last decade, the Pediatric Psychopharmacology Unit (PPU) of the Massachusetts General Hospital, Boston, has been involved in programmatic, multidisciplinary research that has contributed to the identification of adults with the diagnosis of ADHD using *Diagnostic and Statistical Manual of Mental Disorders* (*DSM*), *3rd edition*, *DSM-III-R*, and *DSM-IV* criteria (Biederman et al., 1986; 1990a; 1990b; 1991a; 1992; 1993b). The PPU work has focused on family-genetic risk factors, comorbidity, and novel pharmacotherapeutic approaches in ADHD patients of all ages.

RETROSPECTIVE DIAGNOSIS OF ADHD IN ADULTS

Although the adult diagnosis of ADHD may be somewhat controversial, the childhood diagnosis is not. We addressed the question whether retrospectively diagnosed adults, with a chief complaint of inattention or academic underachievement, shared clinical features with ADHD children. In our first study we examined 84 referred adults with a clinical diagnosis of childhood-onset, *DSM-III-R* ADHD confirmed by structured interview (Biederman et al., 1993b). Findings were compared with those from a preexisting sample of referred children with ADHD (n = 140), nonreferred ADHD adult relatives of those ADHD children (n = 43), and adult relatives of normal control children (n = 248). Subjects were evaluated with a comprehensive battery of psychiatric, cognitive, and psychosocial assessments.

---

[1]Pediatric Psychopharmacology Unit, Massachusetts General Hospital; and Department of Psychiatry, Harvard Medical School, Boston, Massachusetts.

[2]Pediatric and Adult Psychopharmacology Clinic, Massachusetts General Hospital; and Department of Psychiatry, Harvard Medical School, Boston, Massachusetts.

Referred and nonreferred adults with ADHD were similar to one another, but more disturbed and impaired than non-ADHD control subjects. The pattern of psychopathology, cognition, and functioning among the ADHD adults approximated the findings for ADHD children. These results from multiple nonoverlapping domains showed that referred and nonreferred ADHD adults had a pattern of demographic, psychosocial, psychiatric, and cognitive features that mirrored well-documented findings among ADHD children. These findings supported the validity of the diagnosis of ADHD in adults.

In both our clinical and research work with ADHD adults, we were struck by the relatively even gender distribution of ADHD in adulthood. This finding contrasts with the gender distribution in childhood, where ADHD is two to nine times more prevalent among boys than in girls. Thus, we attempted to determine whether ADHD was a valid clinical entity in adult female subjects and whether it was expressed differently in male and female adults. To this end we examined the clinical, cognitive, and functional characteristics of 128 referred adults with ADHD of both sexes (this sample included the 84 subjects discussed above) (Biederman et al., 1994). We found that referred men and women with ADHD were similar to one another but more disturbed and impaired than non-ADHD adult control subjects of the same gender. Compared to normal control women, ADHD women had higher rates of major depression, anxiety disorders, conduct disorder, school failure, and cognitive impairment. The pattern of psychopathologic, cognitive, and psychosocial findings among women with ADHD adults approximated the findings in men with ADHD subjects as well as observations of ADHD children of both genders. The consistency of these findings in both genders further supports the validity of the diagnosis of ADHD in adults.

Women with ADHD differed from their male counterparts in their significantly lower rates of having had conduct disorder in childhood. This finding is consistent with those reported in pediatric samples of girls with ADHD (Safer and Krager, 1988; Shaywitz and Shaywitz, 1987). Because conduct disorder is usually associated with severe disruptive behaviors, it is likely to lead to a parent- or teacher-initiated referral of the affected child. This may explain the overrepresentation of boys in pediatric samples and the more even gender representation in self-referred ADHD adults. Our results stress the viability and importance of identification of female subjects with ADHD.

FAMILY-GENETIC ASPECTS OF ADULT ADHD

Two family studies of adult ADHD suggest that the adult form of the disorder may be highly familial. Manshadi et al. (1983) studied the siblings of 22 alcoholic adult psychiatric patients who met the *DSM-III* criteria for ADD, residual type. The authors compared these patients with 20 patients matched for age and comorbid psychiatric diagnoses. Forty-one percent of the siblings of the adult ADHD probands were diagnosed with ADHD, compared with 0% of the non-ADHD comparison siblings.

We examined familial transmission in adult ADHD in the clinically referred sample discussed above. We interviewed 75 adults with ADHD about ADHD in their children (Biederman et al., 1995a). Diagnostic information on ADHD was derived from the ADHD module of the K-SADS supplemented with information regarding treatment for ADHD for the affected child, and school history including repeated grades, placement in special classes, and tutoring. Of the 84 children at risk, 48 (57%) met the criteria for ADHD. The rate of ADHD in children of ADHD adults was significantly higher than the previously reported rate of ADHD siblings of ADHD children (57% vs. 15%, $p < 0.001$). Of the 48 ADHD children of ADHD parents, 36 (75%) were treated for this disorder. These results suggest that the adult form of this disorder may have stronger familial etiologic risk factors than its pediatric form. The high familial loading of adult ADHD suggests that nonfamilial cases are more likely to go into remission during adolescence. This idea finds some support in a 4-year follow-up of ADHD children and adolescents (Biederman et al., 1996), which found that a family history of ADHD predicted persistence of the disorder during the follow-up period. If confirmed, then families selected via adult ADHD probands might be especially useful for testing genetic hypotheses about ADHD (Biederman et al., 1995a).

GENETIC

Segregation analyses of ADHD (Deutsch et al., 1990; Faraone et al., 1992) suggest that a single gene with incomplete penetrance is involved in the etiology of ADHD. A mathematical model of genetic transmission would be unlikely if reports were due to recall bias. Studies have implicated the dopamine D2 and D4 receptor genes and the dopamine transporter gene (Comings et al., 1991; Cook et al., 1995; LaHoste et al., 1996). These findings are consistent with genetic heterogeneity. We recently confirmed the association between D4 receptor genes and ADHD, examining triads that comprised an ADHD adult, the adult's spouse, and an ADHD child (Faraone et al., 1997). Because our triads were recruited through clinically referred ADHD adults, this further supports the validity of retrospectively diagnosing ADHD in adults.

NEUROBIOLOGY

Magnetic resonance imaging studies of the brain in childhood ADHD indicate that there are subtle anomalies in caudate (Castellanos et al., 1994, 1996; Hynd et al., 1993) and corpus callosum size and shape (Giedd et al., 1994; Semrud-Clikeman et al., 1994) or possible reductions in the right frontal area (Hynd et al., 1990) in ADHD. These data are consistent with a positron emission tomography (PET) study of adult ADHD and suggests that a neurobiologic link between childhood and adult ADHD may eventually be found (Zametkin et al., 1990). The subjects in this study were adult fathers of children diagnosed with ADHD. These adults had never before been diagnosed or treated. The investigators found reduced global and regional glucose metabolism in the premotor cortex and the superior prefrontal cortex—areas of the brain associated with control of attention and motor activity (Zametkin et al., 1990). While these findings have not been fully replicated in a similar PET scan study of adolescents (Zametkin et al., 1993), they are consistent with preliminary results of brain SPECT imaging in adolescents with ADHD (Amen et al., 1993).

SUBSTANCE ABUSE IN ADULTS WITH ADHD

Our group recently (Biederman et al., 1995b) evaluated the association between ADHD and psychoactive substance use disorders (PSUD: drug or alcohol abuse or dependence) in adults. We compared 120 referred ADHD adults to a preexisting sample of non-ADHD adults ($n = 248$). There was a significantly higher lifetime risk for PSUD in ADHD adults than in control subjects (52% vs. 27%, $p < 0.01$). Although ADHD adults and control subjects did not differ in the rate of alcohol use disorders, ADHD adults had significantly higher rates of drug and drug plus alcohol use disorders than control subjects. Childhood-onset conduct disorder and adult antisocial disorders conferred a significantly increased risk for PSUD independently of ADHD status. Mood and anxiety disorders increased the risk for PSUD in both ADHD adults and control subjects, but more demonstrably in control subjects. Although comorbidity increased the risk for PSUD in ADHD individuals, ADHD by itself was also a significant risk factor for PSUD in ADHD adults. There were no differences in the preferred drugs of abuse between ADHD adults and control subjects. In both ADHD adults and control subjects with a drug use disorder, marijuana was the most common drug of abuse (68% in ADHD adults and 72% in control subjects), followed distantly by cocaine and stimulants. Thus, these results refute the commonly held view that ADHD individuals abuse stimulants preferentially.

NEUROPSYCHOLOGIC STUDIES

Cognitive deficits, particularly impairments in attention and executive functions, are hypothesized to be a core part of ADHD (Douglas, 1972). This pattern of deficits is similar to that found in adults with frontal lobe damage and thus has generally supported the hypothesis that ADHD may be a brain disorder primarily affecting the frontal cortex or the regions projecting to the frontal cortex (Gorenstein et al., 1989; Shue and Douglas, 1992). In our studies of adult ADHD, we found significantly higher rates of repeated grades, tutoring, placement in special classes, and reading disability in ADHD adults than non-ADHD subjects (Biederman et al., 1993b). These ADHD adults also had lower scores on subscales of the Wide Range Achievement Test (arithmetic and reading scores) and the Wechsler Adult Intelligence Scale-Revised (vocabulary, block design, digit symbol, and estimated "freedom-from distractibility" IQ). In a recent study of the neuropsychology of unmedicated ADHD adults, we found significant and clinically meaningful deficits on the California Verbal Learning Test (CVLT) and the auditory continuous performance test (ACPT) (Seidman, 1995). These are consistent with the well-established deficits in verbal learning and attention for ADHD children. However, our results also show that the deficits seen in adults are not as pervasive as those seen in ADHD children. In our child and adolescent sample, we found ADHD to be associated with deficits on the Wechsler Intelligence Scale for Children (Faraone et al., 1993) the Stroop, Wisconsin Card Sorting, and Rey-Osterrieth Complex Figure tests (Seidman et al., 1995a, 1995b).

Our data cannot determine whether these differences between children and adults reflect developmental changes or differences in referral patterns for adult and child disorders. Nevertheless, the adult data show that ADHD adults have neuropsychologic features that are consistent with the diagnosis of ADHD. Because these data are collected with individually administered tests, they do not share method variance with structured, self-report clinical interviews. Thus, they provide converging evidence for the face validity of adult ADHD.

THE VALIDITY OF ADHD IN ADULTS

Concerns have been raised regarding the validity of the diagnosis of ADHD in adults. The validity of a clinical diagnostic entity requires documentation of its characteristic signs and symptoms (descriptive validity), evidence for a specific course, outcome, and treatment response (predictive validity), as well as evidence regarding etiology and pathophysiology (concurrent validity). To examine these issues, a systematic search was conducted of the psychiatric and psychologic literature for empirical studies dealing with adult ADHD with childhood onset (Spencer et al., 1994). The review of the literature identified 56 studies published since 1969. There were 32 case-controlled retrospective studies, 11 family-genetic studies, and 13 prospective follow-up studies of six cohorts. In all, they provided information on over 1,700 adults with a history of ADHD; in 663 of them, ADHD persisted into adulthood.

Evidence for descriptive validity comes from studies of adult patients who had ADHD in childhood. These studies document clinical features in adults that correspond to the syndrome of ADHD in children. These adults, who are impulsive, inattentive, and restless, have the clinical "look and feel" of ADHD children. Like their child counterparts, many adults with ADHD suffer from antisocial, depressive, and anxiety disorders. They also show evidence of occupational failure and intellectual performance deficits. Moreover, longitudinal follow-up studies show that children with documented cases of ADHD often continue to express the ADHD syndrome as adults. Such studies provide support for the descriptive validity of adult ADHD. In addition, the literature shows that adult ADHD can be reliably diagnosed and that the diagnosis confers considerable power to forecast complications and treatment response (Gittelman et al., 1985; Greenfield et al., 1988; Klein and Mannuzza, 1989, 1991; Mannuzza et al., 1991a; Thorley, 1984; Weiss et al., 1979, 1985; Weiss and Hechtman, 1986). Further, there is mounting evidence for genetic transmission, specific treatment responses, and abnormalities in brain structure and function in affected individuals (Biederman et al., 1992; 1990a; 1991a; 1991b; 1987; 1986; Cantwell, 1972; 1975; Deutsch et al., 1990; Faraone et al., 1992, 1991; Faraone and Santangelo, 1992; Goodman and Stevenson, 1989a; 1989b; Lopez, 1965; Manshadi et al., 1983; Morrison, 1980; Morrison and Stewart, 1971; 1973; Schachar and Wachsmuth, 1990; Stewart et al., 1980; Welner et al., 1977; Zametkin et al., 1990). The available literature provides converging evidence that adult ADHD is a valid clinical diagnosis.

THE PREVALENCE OF ADHD IN ADULTS

Assuming that the population rate of ADHD in children is 3.3% and that only 10% of such children have clinically significant symptoms in adulthood, Shaffer computed the rate of adult ADHD to be about 0.3% (Shaffer, 1994). However, this estimate is likely to be low for several reasons. Epidemiologic studies find the prevalence of childhood ADHD to be as high as 5.7% (Anderson et al., 1987) and 6.3% (Szatmari et al., 1989). In addition, the estimate of 10% persistence into adulthood is also at the low end. This is based on the work of Mannuzza et al. (1993), who excluded hyperactive children whose primary reason for referral was aggressive behavior. Because hyperactive children with aggressive behavior are at greatest risk for continued ADHD in adulthood (Hechtman, 1992), 10% is likely to be an underestimate. Notably, other studies report that as many as two thirds of ADHD children will have disabling symptoms of ADHD in young adulthood (Hechtman, 1992). Thus, the prevalence of adult ADHD may be as high as 4%. If the population rate in childhood is only 5% and the persistence into adulthood is only 40%, the prevalence of adult ADHD would be 2%.

There are other reasons to believe that ADHD is not rare in adulthood. Family studies have estimated that an average of 3.8% of fathers and 2.4% of mothers of *non-ADHD* comparison subjects had childhood-onset ADHD. (Biederman et al., 1990a; Cantwell, 1972; Faraone et al., 1992; Morrison and Stewart, 1971). These data are consistent with a report by Murphy and Barkley (1996), who used self-report rating scales to diagnose ADHD in 720 adults applying for or renewing their drivers' licenses in Massachusetts. In this sample, 4.7% of adults met the *DSM-IV* criteria for ADHD. These ADHD subjects met full *DSM-IV* criteria currently and in childhood.

TREATMENT OF ADULT ADHD

Although there has been a rapid growth in stimulant prescriptions for adults, the use of methylphenidate (MPH) in adults remains controversial. Many clinicians who treat adults have scant familiarity in diagnosing ADHD and in using stimulants. To develop treatment guidelines for the stimulant treatment of adults, we reviewed the available literature of medication trials in ADHD, attentive to issues of psychiatric comorbidity, age, gender, and ethnic background (Spencer et al., 1996). The review showed stimulants to be the most established treatment for ADHD: >100 controlled studies with >5,000 children and adolescents have established their efficacy in about 70% of subjects. The literature clearly establishes that stimulants improve not only abnormal behaviors of ADHD, but also self esteem, cognition, and social and family functioning. However, efficacy varied with age and psychiatric comorbidities. In addition, the great majority of studies have focused on latency-age Caucasian boys, and little is known about other subgroups. Most of the existing studies are very brief: of not more than a few weeks at most, with very few long-term studies. A very limited literature exists for stimulants at other ages, for female subjects (Barkley, 1989; Pelham et al., 1989), and for ethnic minorities (Brown and Sexson, 1988).

A potential barrier to therapeutics is the increasing recognition that ADHD is a heterogeneous disorder with considerable comorbidity with conduct, mood, and anxiety disorders (Biederman et al., 1991c) and tic disorders (Comings and Comings, 1988). It is not clear whether these groups respond preferentially to different psychotropic agents. For example, an emerging literature suggests that anxious and depressed ADHD children respond more poorly to stimulants than non-comorbid ADHD children in their ADHD symptoms (DuPaul et al., 1994; Pliszka, 1989; Swanson et al., 1978; Taylor et al., 1987; Voelker et al., 1983). In addition, stimulants are thought to be anxiogenic and depressogenic; however, the effect of stimulants on the comorbid anxiety and depression symptoms was not assessed in any study. Although stimulants may be depressogenic, it is possible that demoralization and failure caused by ADHD may improve with stimulants by improving performance in the affected ADHD patient.

Despite the volume of juvenile ADHD research, little is known about the effectiveness of MPH and the prognostic value of psychiatric comorbidity for ADHD in adults. In contrast to >100 controlled studies evaluating the efficacy of stimulants in children and adolescents with ADHD, there are only six controlled studies assessing the efficacy of MPH in adults with ADHD (Gualtieri et al., 1985; Iaboni et al., 1996; Mattes et al., 1984; Spencer et al., 1995; Wender et al., 1985; Wood et al., 1976). Whereas the studies of MPH in children and adolescents consistently report robust effects in the improvement of symptoms of ADHD,

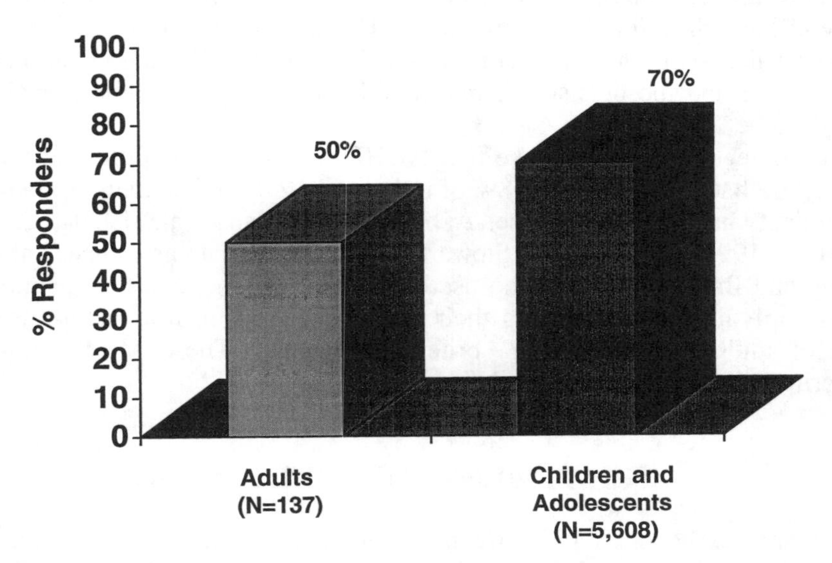

FIG. 1. Adult vs. child and adolescent controlled stimulant trials in ADHD.

equivocal results have been reported in the trials of MPH in adults with this disorder. Among the four early studies of MPH in adults with ADHD, the average rate of response was 50%, much lower than the 70% rate among children and adolescents (Spencer et al., 1996).

The reasons for the difference in stimulant response between children and adults with ADHD is unknown. Plausible reasons include insufficient dosing, uncertain diagnostic criteria, and lack of attention to issues of psychiatric comorbidity. For example, the estimated mean daily weight-corrected dose of MPH in the available studies of adult ADHD patients was 0.6 mg/kg/day. This dose is much lower than the 1 mg/kg/day commonly used in the treatment of children with this disorder (Wilens and Biederman, 1992). Thus, it is possible that more aggressive pharmacotherapy of adult patients could result in a more positive outcome than that reported in the literature. In addition, of four studies showing a poor or less than robust response to MPH, two used Utah criteria (Mattes et al., 1984; Wender et al., 1985), and one included patients without a clear history of childhood-onset symptoms (Wood et al., 1976). These latter studies did not examine psychiatric comorbidity as a predictor of treatment response.

Massachusetts General Hospital treatment trials of methylphenidate in adult ADHD

One investigation (Spencer et al., 1995) was a randomized, placebo-controlled crossover study of MPH in 23 adult patients with *DSM-III-R* ADHD. The aim of the study was to assess the efficacy of MPH in the treatment of ADHD symptoms and those of comorbid disorders by using standardized instruments for diagnosis; paying careful attention to comorbidity with separate assessment of ADHD, depressive, and anxiety symptoms; and administering a robust daily dose of ≤1.0 mg/kg.

Subjects were clinically referred adults with the diagnosis of *DSM-III-R* ADHD. They were ascertained from clinical referrals to the Adult and Pediatric Psychopharmacology Units of the Massachusetts General Hospital who met study inclusion criteria. Outpatients of either gender between 18 and 55 years of age were eligible for entry into the study if they met the *DSM-III-R* criteria for a diagnosis of childhood-onset ADHD as manifested in clinical evaluation and confirmed by structured interview.

Exclusion criteria included any clinically significant chronic medical condition (including serious hypertension defined as any values >100 mm Hg diastolic and 170 mm Hg systolic); clinically significant abnormal baseline laboratory values; a history of seizures, pregnancy or nursing; and a history of tics, mental retardation (IQ < 75), organic brain disorders, clinically

TABLE 1. DESCRIPTION OF SAMPLE (N = 23)

Mean age (± SEM) (range)	40 ± 2.1 (19–56)
Males	10 (43%)
Diagnosis[a]	
ADHD	23 (100%)
Mood disorder	6 (26%)
Anxiety disorder	9 (39%)
Antisocial personality	1 (4%)
Substance abuse	5 (22%)
No comorbid diagnosis	6 (26%)

[a]Patients can have more than one diagnosis.

Reprinted with permission from *Arch Gen Psychiatry* (1995), 52:438, ©1995 American Medical Association (Spencer et al., 1995).

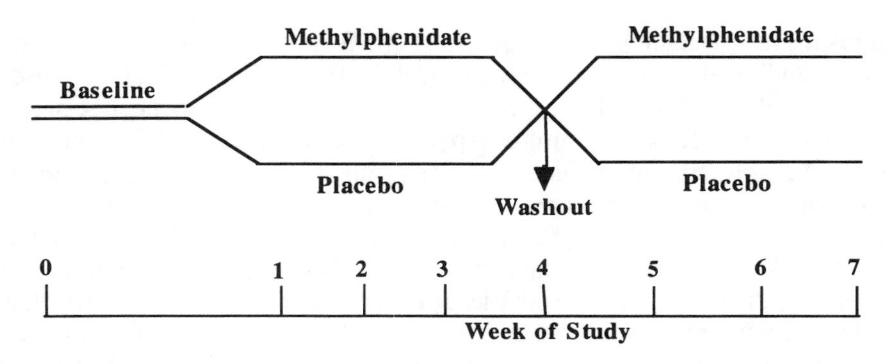

FIG. 2. Study design. Reprinted with permission from *Archives of General Psychiatry* (1995), 52:437, ©1995 American Medical Association (Spencer et al., 1995).

unstable psychiatric conditions (i.e., suicidal behaviors, psychosis), current (within the past 6 months) substance (drug or alcohol) abuse or dependence, or current use of psychotropics.

Each patient participated in a balanced 7-week, double-blind, placebo-controlled, crossover study design. The study consisted of two 3-week treatment periods with 1 week of washout in between. Medication (methylphenidate or placebo) was titrated from an initial dose of 0.5 mg/kg at week 1, to 0.75 mg/kg at week 2, to 1.0 mg/kg at week 3 as tolerated. Assessments were conducted weekly using several instruments. The Clinical Global Impression (CGI) Scale (National Institute of Mental Health, 1985) assessed overall severity and global improvement in each of the three domains of psychopathology (CGI-ADHD, CGI-anxiety, and CGI-depression). The ADHD Rating Scale (Barkley, 1990; DuPaul, 1990) assessed ADHD symptoms. The Hamilton Depression Scale (HAM-D) (Hamilton, 1960) and the Beck Depression Inventory (Beck et al., 1961) assessed depressive symptoms. The Hamilton Anxiety Scale (HAM-A) (Hamilton, 1959) assessed anxiety symptoms. Medication was administered three times daily.

Twenty-five subjects enrolled in the study, and of those, 23 (92%) completed it. The two subjects who dropped out, one man and one woman, were both taking MPH. One had an episode of chest pain in the third week of the trial while taking a dose of 1 mg/kg/day. Although dropped from the study, he elected to have further treatment with MPH after consultation with his internist. The second patient dropped out in the first week because of agitation, irritability, and general unease. Because these two dropout cases did not complete the treatment protocol, they are not included in the data analysis. Thus, the final sample consisted of 13 women and 10 men who ranged in age from 19 to 56 years (mean ± SEM = 40 ± 2 years). All met full criteria for a *DSM-III-R* diagnosis of ADHD with at least eight of 14 symptoms (*DSM-III-R*) and an onset of the clinical picture in childhood by the age of 7 years. In all cases, the disorder was continuous until the time of assessment and was associated with significant distress and disability. Only one subject had been diagnosed in childhood with ADHD, and none had been previously treated. As depicted in Table 1, 74% (n = 17) of ADHD subjects had at least one past comorbid psychiatric disorder. For 59% (n = 13) of the sample, the comorbid disorder was current. The average number of comorbid diagnoses was 2.6 ± 0.3 per subjects. Baseline ratings of depression (HAM-D = 5.6 ± 1.1 and Beck 8.6 ± 1.6) and anxiety (HAM-A = 5.7 ± 1.0) symptoms were relatively low. According to standard cutoff points for moderate severity on ratings of depression (HAM-D >16; Beck Depression Inventory >19) and anxiety (HAM-A >21), only 9% of subjects had scores of depression or anxiety above those cutoff points.

MPH treatment was more effective than placebo after the first week of treatment, and improvement was increasingly robust in subsequent weeks with increases in daily doses (Figure 3). Analysis of the ADHD Rating Scale (transformed) data by multivariate analy-

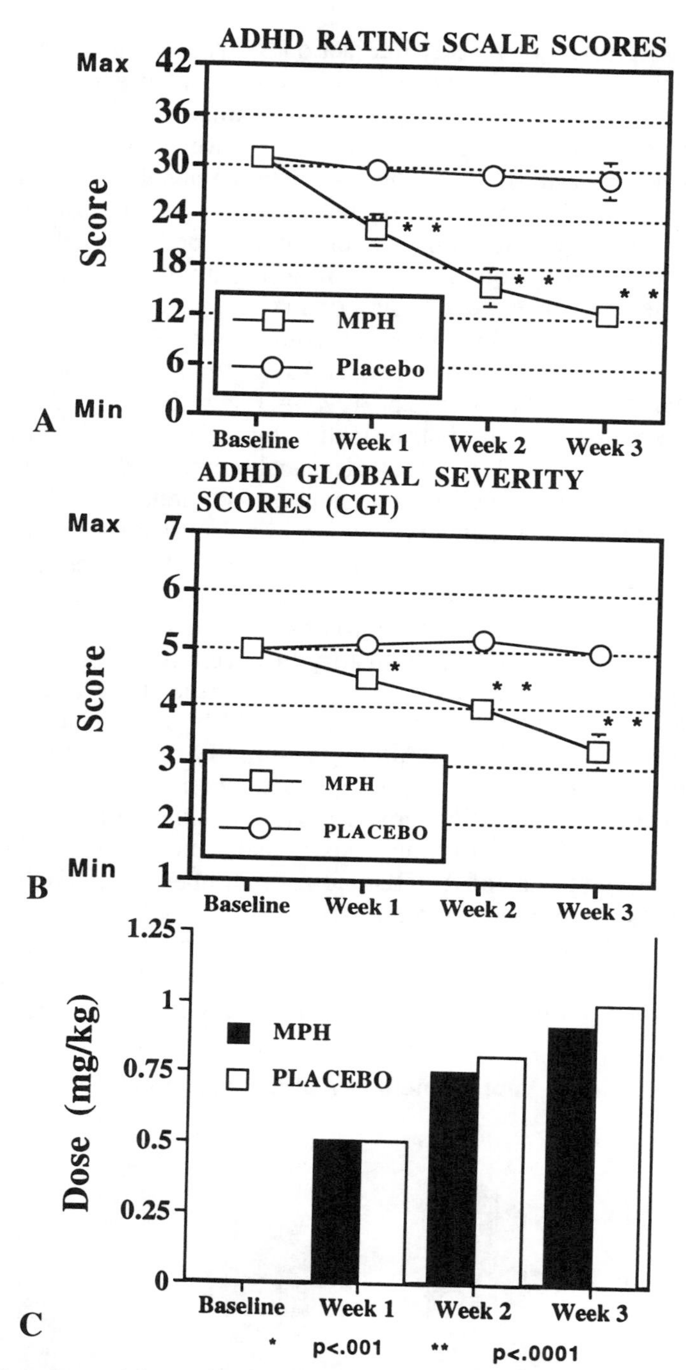

FIG. 3. ADHD rating scale and global severity scores by week and dose. Reprinted with permission from *Archives of General Psychiatry* (1995), 52:439, ©1995 American Medical Association (Spencer et al., 1995).

sis of variance (MANOVA) showed highly significant effects for ADHD symptoms for the effects of drug (MPH or placebo; $F[1,22] = 36$, $p = 0.0001$), time (weeks 0, 1, 2, 3; $F[3,20] = 11$, $p = 0.0002$) and the drug by time interaction ($F[3,20] = 12$, $p = 0.0001$). In addition, the MANOVA for ADHD symptoms found no significant order effect (MPH first vs. placebo first), no significant two-way interaction between drug and MPH order, and no significant three-way interaction between drug, weeks, and order. Our analyses of the ADHD severity score produced a similar pattern of results.

In contrast to the significant findings for ADHD, none were found for depression or anxiety by any of the study measures. To further evaluate the absolute rate of improvement in this sample, we analyzed end of treatment results using our preestablished definition of improvement defined as a subject attaining a score of 2 or better (much or very much improved) on the CGI and a reduction of at least 30% in individual rating scales. Because of the scarcity of subjects with current depression or anxiety, we could not evaluate the impact of treatment on these domains by this method of comparison. Seventy-eight percent (18/23) of patients had meaningful improvement in ADHD symptoms while taking MPH, compared to only 4% (1/23) taking placebo ($\chi^2 = 25.91$, $df = 1$, $p < 0.0001$). These results did not change when data were analyzed after stratification by order of randomization (MPH first, placebo second: $\chi^2 = 17.14$, $df = 1$, $p < 0.0001$; placebo first, MPH second: $\chi^2 = 9.21$, $df = 1$, $p = 0.0039$). To evaluate the effects of treatment on individual ADHD symptoms as well as clusters of ADHD symptoms (inattentive, hyper, impulsive), data on these variables were also examined. This analysis showed highly significant differences between MPH and placebo for reduction of each of the 14 symptoms of ADHD ($p < 0.001$ in all cases).

Results were also evaluated after stratification by sociodemographic characteristics, history of comorbidity (lifetime), and family history of psychopathology to examine the role of these factors as potential confounds in accounting for the study findings. These analyses showed that equally robust responses to MPH could be established after stratification of subjects by these variables (Table 2). Although similarly robust responses to MPH were observed in subjects with and without major depression, conduct disorder, or substance use disorders, we lacked adequate statistical power to fully evaluate the impact of treatment on these subgroups (Table 2). Correlation analysis revealed no meaningful associations between improvement of symptoms of ADHD and age, number of ADHD symptoms, severity scores, and ratings of depression or anxiety ($r \leq 0.30$ in all cases).

Treatment was generally well tolerated; only three subjects (13%) were unable to tolerate the target dose of 1.0 mg/kg. Although the rates of subjective adverse effects did not differ in MPH and placebo, they were more pronounced with active medication. The most

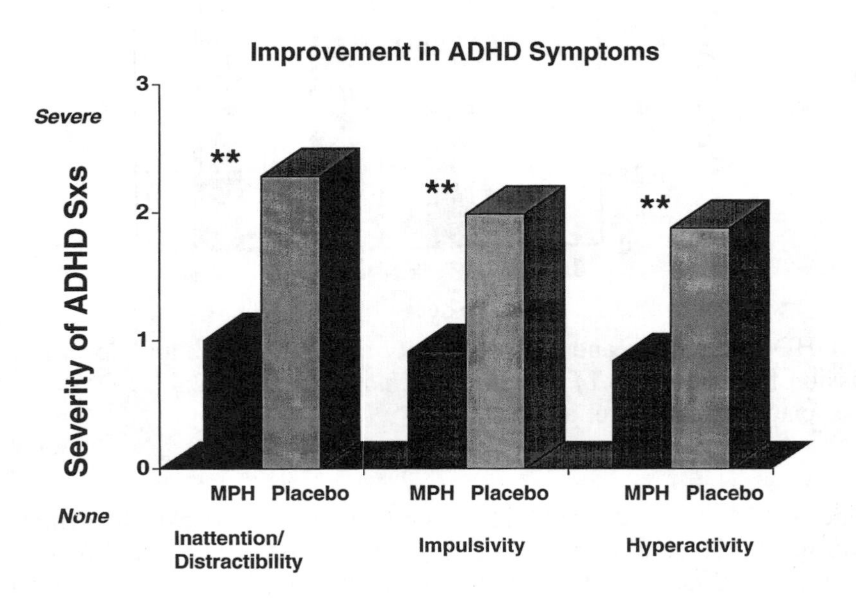

FIG. 4. Controlled study of methylphenidate in adult ADHD.

Table 2. Improvement Stratified by Gender and Comorbidity

		MPH	Placebo
Stratification	*N*	%	%
Gender			
Male	10	80*	10
Female	13	77**	0
Comorbid disorders			
+Major depression	6	67	0
−Major depression	16	82**	6
+Multiple (≥2) anxiety disorders	9	67*	0
−Multiple (≥2) anxiety disorders	13	86**	7
+Conduct disorder	3	67	33
−Conduct disorder	19	80**	0
+Substance abuse	5	60	0
−Substance abuse	17	83**	6
+Learning disability	8	100**	0
−Learning disability	14	71**	0

*$p \leq 0.01$
**$p \leq 0.0001$ by χ^2 analysis
Reprinted with permission from *Archives of General Psychiatry* (1995), 52:441, ©1995 American Medical Association (Spencer et al., 1995).

common adverse effects were loss of appetite, insomnia, and anxiety. Five subjects taking MPH, but no subject taking placebo, had the dose lowered because of side effects. Reasons for dose reduction included anxiety (n = 3), insomnia (n = 2), and euphoria (n = 1). While no meaningful changes in blood pressure were observed between MPH or placebo conditions (systolic, 123 ± 2.6 vs. 117 ± 1.7 mm Hg; diastolic 77 ± 2.0 vs. 75 ± 1.5 mm Hg), a small but statistically significant increase in heart rate (80 ± 2.4 vs. 76 ± 1.5 beats/minute) and decrease in weight (162.6 ± 7.6 vs. 165.2 ± 7.9 pounds) were observed with MPH but not with placebo. However, none of these findings were clinically significant, and no subject required altering the dose of medication as a consequence.

This study supported the hypothesis that robust MPH treatment (0.92 mg/kg/day) is efficacious in the treatment of ADHD symptoms and that the response in adults may be dose-dependent consistent with dose-dependent cognitive, behavioral, and academic improvement seen in children (Spencer et al., 1996). The overall response rate for ADHD symptoms was clinically and statistically higher during MPH treatment than during placebo (78% vs. 4%; $p < 0.0001$). Although this study did not have adequate power to examine the effects of comorbidity on outcome, MPH did not appear to relieve symptoms of depression or anxiety. Improvement in ADHD symptoms was independent of gender, psychiatric comorbidity with anxiety or moderate depression, or family history of psychiatric disorders.

Pemoline in the treatment of adult ADHD

Previous studies with the long-acting stimulant magnesium pemoline (Cylert) have been equivocal, with one very small open study not demonstrating efficacy (Wood et al., 1976) and one controlled study showing efficacy only when assessing those with childhood-onset disorder (Wender et al., 1981). However, in those studies, the dosing of pemoline was relatively low (<75 mg/day), the diagnosis was not always anchored in childhood, and the presence of comorbidity was not evaluated. We recently reported findings of an ongoing double-blind, placebo-controlled, crossover design study of the use of pemoline at doses of 3 mg/kg/day for adults with ADHD (Wilens et al., 1997).

We conducted a 10-week, double-blind, placebo-controlled, crossover design study of pemoline at a target daily dose of 3 mg/kg/day in 35 adult patients with *DSM-III*R and *DSM-IV* ADHD. As with the MPH study, we used standardized structured psychiatric instruments for diagnosis and separate assessments of ADHD, depressive, and anxiety symptoms. The study consisted of two 4-week treatment periods in which subjects received either placebo or pemoline, separated by a 2-week placebo washout phase. During the 4-week medication/placebo phases, pemoline or placebo was titrated up to 1 mg/kg/day in week 1 (~75 mg/day), to 2 mg/kg/day by week 2 (~150 mg), 3 mg/kg/day by week 3 (maximal dosing, ~225 mg), and dosed flexibly in week 4 (≤3 mg/kg) unless adverse effects emerged.

Of the 35 adults with ADHD who were randomized in the trial, 27 subjects (77%) completed the protocol. Treatment with pemoline in the final week of the active phase was best tolerated at doses substantially lower than the target dose of 3 mg/kg/day (mean ± SD, 2.2 mg/kg/day; 148 ± 95 mg). Pemoline was significantly better at reducing ADHD symptoms than was placebo ($Z = 2.4$, $p < 0.02$). Using a predefined 30% reduction in symptoms, 50% of pemoline-treated subjects and 17% of subjects in the placebo group were considered positive responders ($\chi^2 = 7.1, p = 0.008$). As in the MPH trial, the majority of ADHD subjects had at least one past comorbid psychiatric condition, with anxiety, mood, and substance use disorders most frequent. However, baseline ratings of depression and anxiety were relatively low. Response to pemoline was independent of dose, gender, or lifetime psychiatric comorbidity.

These results indicate that pemoline is moderately effective in the treatment of ADHD in adults. Although robust doses were targeted, most adults preferred more moderate dosing (120–160 mg/day). The current preliminary findings suggest that the magnitude of the anti-ADHD response with pemoline is less than that reported in ADHD adults receiving 1 mg/kg/day of MPH (~30% vs. 57% reduction in symptoms). Given the limited efficacy, tolerability, and concerns of hepatic dysfunction, pemoline should be considered second-line medication in ADHD adults.

Nonstimulant treatments for adult ADHD

Desipramine in the treatment of adult ADHD

Within the past two decades, the tricyclic antidepressants (TCAs) have been used increasingly as alternative or adjunctive treatments to the stimulants for ADHD in children and adolescents (Biederman et al., 1989; Donnelly et al., 1986; Garfinkel et al., 1983; Rapoport et al., 1974; Rapport et al., 1993; Wilens et al., 1993). The benefits of once-daily dosing, nonscheduled formulation, and reduced potential for abuse make these medications compelling to use in ADHD individuals, particularly adults. Moreover, TCAs may be additionally helpful for ADHD adults with concurrent anxiety and depressive symptoms (Biederman et al., 1993a), for which the TCAs have been extensively employed. We recently reported the results of a systematic, retrospective study in which robust doses of desipramine (DMI) or nortriptyline resulted in 68% of 37 adults manifesting a moderate improvement in their ADHD, which was sustained at 1 year (Wilens et al., 1995). However, in that nat-

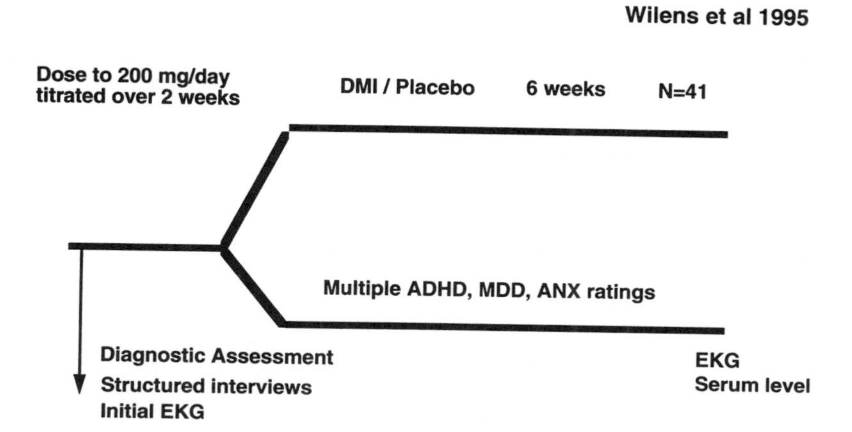

FIG. 5. Desipramine study in adult ADHD: double-blind, parallel design.

uralistic study, 84% of subjects were concurrently receiving other psychotropic medications, potentially confounding the response rate.

Thus, we conducted a randomized, 6-week, placebo-controlled, parallel design study of DMI in 48 adult patients with *DSM-III-R* ADHD using standardized instruments for diagnosis, and separate assessments of ADHD, depressive, and anxiety symptoms, at a target DMI dose of 200 mg/day (Wilens et al., 1996). Ascertainment, inclusion and exclusion criteria, and assessment technology were the same as in our MPH study (Spencer et al., 1995). The study consisted of one 6-week treatment period in which subjects received either placebo or DMI. They were rated on symptoms at baseline and subsequently at two-week intervals.

"Response" was defined as CGI improvement scale of 1 or 2 (very much or much improved) and 30% decrease in the ADHD total symptom scale between week 0 and week 6. The response rate at the end of the protocol was 68% for the DMI group and 0% for the placebo group ($\chi^2(1) = 22.0, p < 0.001$). We also tested for group differences using a random regression model that estimated a main effect of group (DMI vs. placebo), a main effect of week in study, and the interaction between the two. The model assumed a subject-specific residual that differed between subjects but was constant over time. We found a significant interaction between group and week showing a significant reduction in ADHD symptoms over the 6 weeks for DMI-treated but not placebo-treated patients ($z = 6.9, p < 0.001$).

Tomoxetine in the treatment of adult ADHD

Another potentially useful medication for the treatment of adult ADHD is the experimental compound tomoxetine, a novel cyclic compound, dissimilar in structure to other available antidepressants. It has a selective high affinity for noradrenergic function, and little affinity for other neurotransmitter systems and therefore fewer side effects than available antidepressants. Tomoxetine has been subject to extensive preclinical and clinical testing. Because of its high noradrenergic activity, its modest rate of side effects including limited cardiac effects, and the absence of abuse potential, tomoxetine offers potential benefit for the treatment of adults with ADHD.

We hypothesized that tomoxetine, in clinically meaningful doses, would be superior to

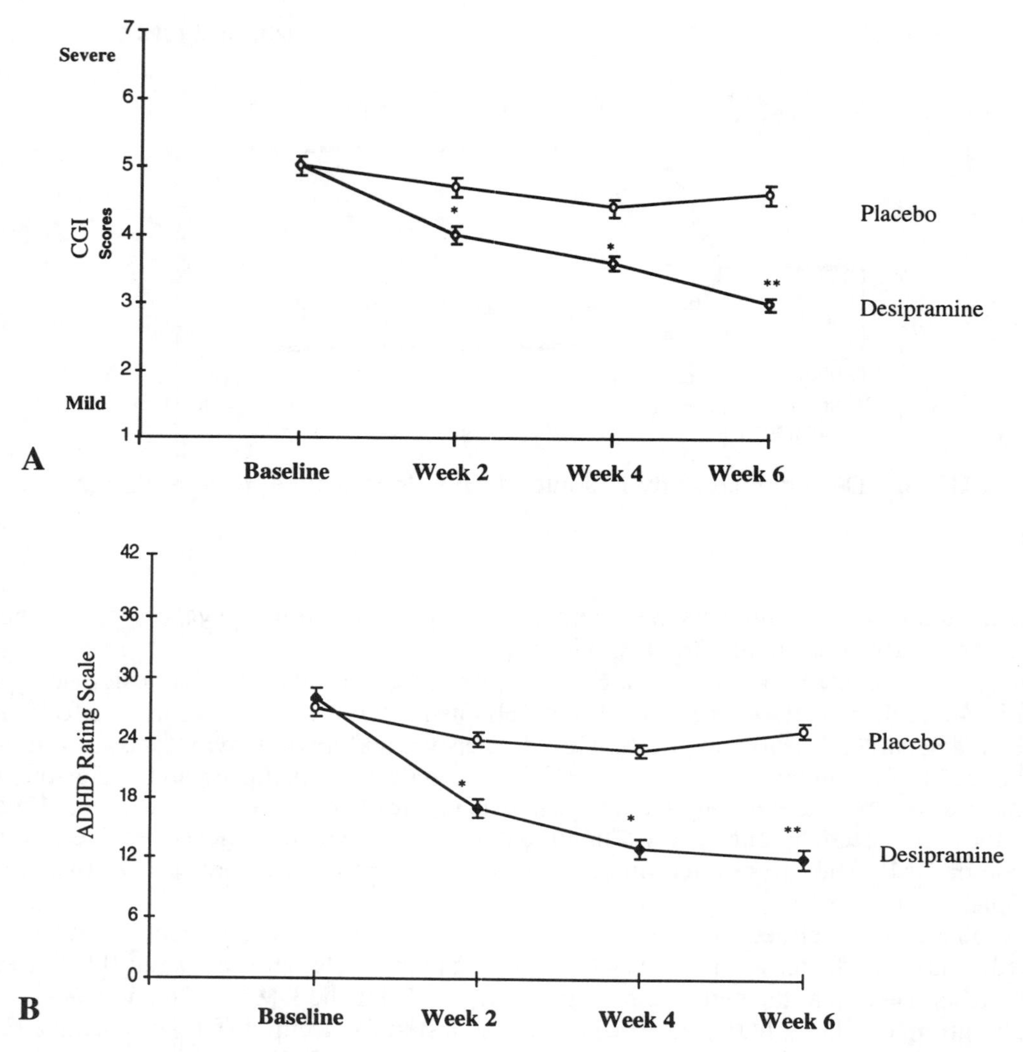

FIG. 6. **A:** Global severity score. **B:** ADHD rating scale.

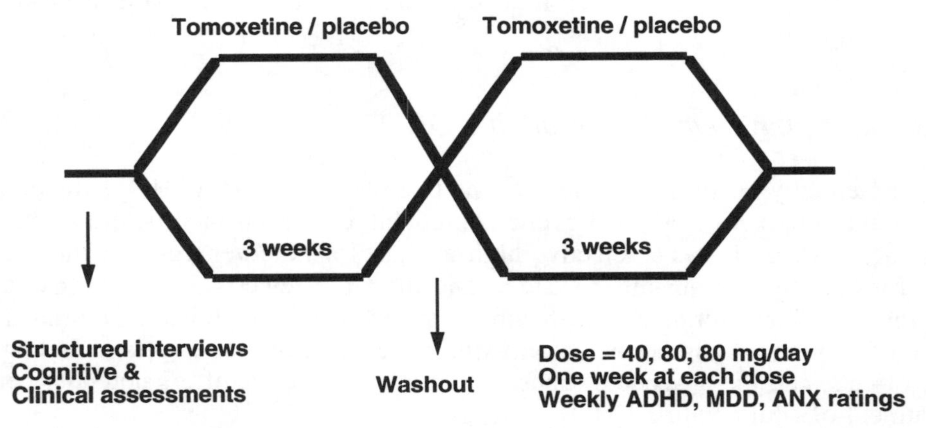

FIG. 7. Tomoxetine study in adult ADHD: double-blind, crossover design.

placebo in the treatment of adults with ADHD. To assess this, we conducted a double-blind placebo-controlled crossover study using the same design and assessment methodology as in the MPH study of adult ADHD (Spencer et al., 1998).

"Response" was defined as a 30% decrease in the ADHD total symptom scale between week 0 and week 3 (the CGI was not used in this study). Treatment with tomoxetine at an average oral daily dose of 76 mg/day was consistently more effective than placebo. The overall response rate for ADHD symptoms was clinically and statistically higher during tomoxetine treatment than during placebo (53% vs. 10.5%; $p < 0.05$). A random regression model found a highly significant drug by time interaction ($z = 3.4$, $p = 0.001$) in the reduction of ADHD symptoms that was robust enough to be detectable in a parallel-groups comparison during the first 3 weeks of the protocol ($z = 3.1$, $p = 0.002$). These effects showed improvements of ADHD symptoms over time for the tomoxetine group but not the placebo group.

We evaluated neuropsychologic outcome using a battery of tests that measure ADHD-relevant executive function domains, including (a) sustained attention, (b) response inhibition, (c) set shifting and categorization, (d) selective attention and visual scanning, and (e) organization and recall of visual construction. This neuropsychologic battery was administered three times, at baseline and after each arm of the study. Several cognitive tests used in our battery were significantly improved on tomoxetine vs. placebo treatment; these were the Stroop Color Word (52.1 ± 11 vs. 48.6 ± 13, $z = 2.6$, $n = 21$, $p < 0.05$) and Interference T-scores (53.9 ± 9 vs. 50.7 ± 10, $z = 2$, $p < 0.05$) with no evidence of cognitive deterioration on any test. Because these tests are thought to measure response inhibition, they suggest that tomoxetine treatment may improve inhibitory capacity. While we did not have sufficient power to fully examine potential medication-associated improvement in this sample, it is important that the demonstrated lack of cognitive deterioration in subjects receiving tomoxetine does not suggest a detrimental impact of tomoxetine on cognition.

This preliminary study showed that tomoxetine significantly improved ADHD symptoms and was well tolerated. Although preliminary, these promising initial results provide support for further studies of tomoxetine in the treatment of ADHD using a wide range of doses over an extended period of treatment.

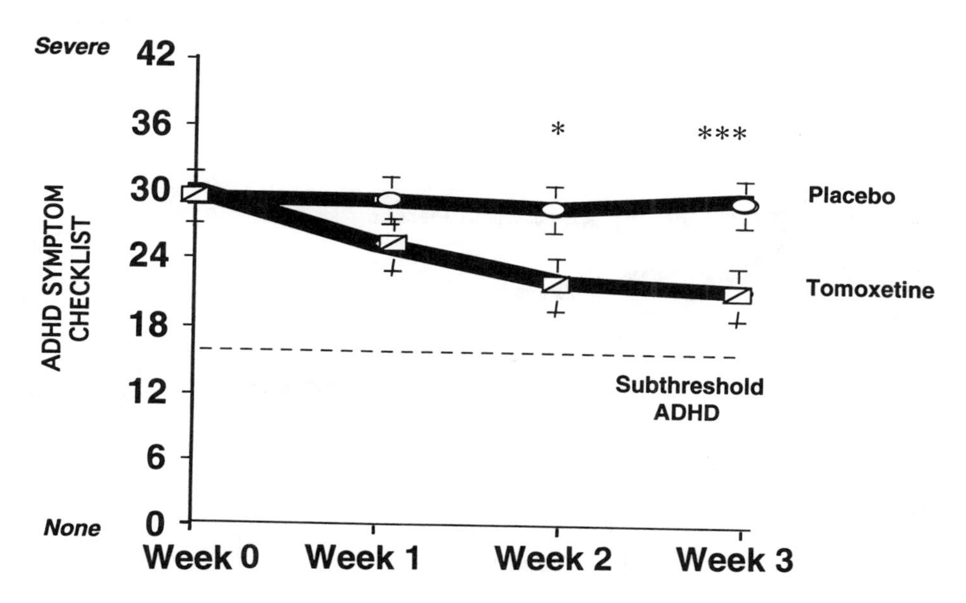

FIG. 8. Pilot tomoxetine study in adult ADHD (Spencer, et al., 1998).

Overview of methylphenidate, pemoline, desipramine, and tomoxetine in the treatment of adult ADHD

We compared and contrasted the four studies with each other to detect overall trends. For this comparison, response was defined as a 30% decrease in the ADHD total symptom scale, because the CGI was not used in the tomoxetine or the pemoline study. Using this liberal definition of response, an overall low placebo response of 15% was noted across the studies. While the magnitude of response to tomoxetine treatment (52%) and pemoline (50%) approximated the average improvement rate (54%) reported in previous studies of MPH in adult ADHD (Gualtieri et al., 1985; Mattes et al., 1984; Spencer et al., 1995; Wender et al., 1981; 1985; Wood et al., 1976), they were somewhat lower than the response rate observed in our prior, methodologically similar, trials of MPH (87%) and DMI (89%) (Spencer et al., 1995; Wilens et al., 1996) using similar definitions of response.

This suggests that tomoxetine and pemoline could have weaker effects in ADHD than other compounds. However, it is likely that the response to tomoxetine is an underestimate; tomoxetine may share a lagged response time with DMI, since they have a similar mechanism of action. The response to desipramine was similar (58%) by the end of week 2. Considering that a robust response rate of 89% was observed in the desipramine trial by the end of week 6, 4 weeks after reaching the target dose, the 3 weeks of tomoxetine treatment in the present study was probably insufficient for the full clinical effect of tomoxetine to unfold. Thus, to fully evaluate the role of tomoxetine in the treatment of ADHD, more information is needed with a longer study to establish the full efficacy of tomoxetine in the treatment of ADHD.

Across the four studies of MPH, pemoline, DMI, and tomoxetine, treatment response was not affected by gender or psychiatric comorbidity. The absence of meaningful associations between treatment response and psychiatric comorbidity indicates that response to pharmacotherapy was not due to the putative antidepressant or antianxiety effects of medication. In fact, there was a trend for stronger effects in non-comorbid cases than in those with psychiatric comorbidity. Moreover, in all four studies, baseline severity ratings of anxiety and depression were low, with little change over time; thus, medication-associated ADHD improvement was unlikely to be secondary to improvement in comorbid depression or anxiety and was not associated with worsening of anxiety or depression.

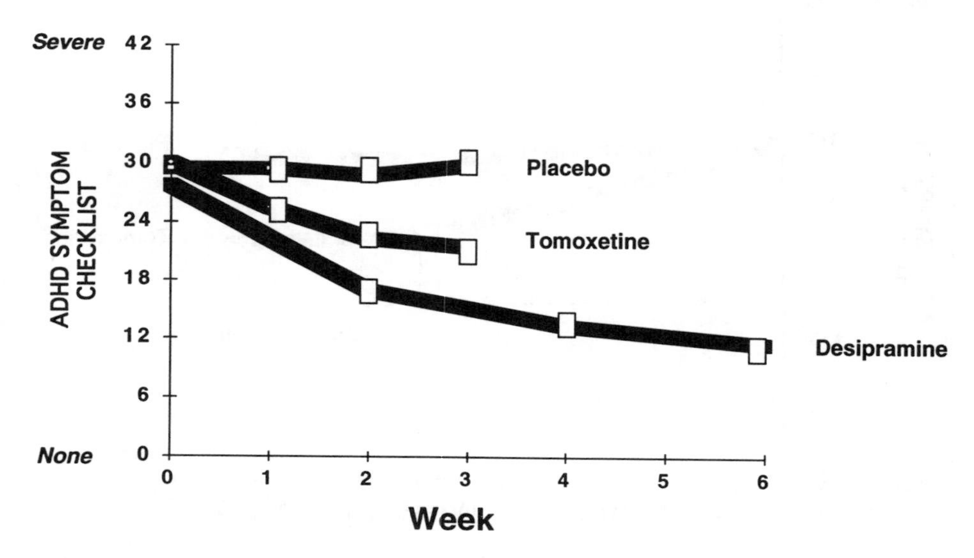

FIG. 9. Massachusetts General Hospital clinical trials in adult ADHD.

Future directions: A controlled trial of ABT-418 for attention deficit hyperactivity disorder in adults

Recent reports have suggested the potential usefulness of cholinergic agents for ADHD with improvement in working memory and neuropsychologic functioning associated with nicotine administration. To this end, we completed a controlled study to determine the anti-ADHD efficacy of ABT-418, a novel cholinergic activating agent with structural similarities to nicotine, in adults with ADHD. This was a double-blind, placebo-controlled, randomized, crossover trial, comparing a transdermal patch of ABT-418 (75 mg daily) to placebo in adults with *DSM-IV* ADHD. There were two 3-week treatment periods separated by 1 week of washout. We used standardized structured psychiatric instruments for diagnosis. To measure improvement, we used separate assessments of ADHD, depressive, and anxiety symptoms at baseline and at each weekly visit. Of the 33 subjects enrolled in the study (88% male), there were 29 completers (mean age ± SD, 40 ± 9 years). Overall, there was a modest reduction in the ADHD symptom checklist scores in adults treated with ABT-418 compared to placebo (by random regression, $p = 0.056$), which was more substantial in subjects with less severe ADHD ($p = 0.025$). Using a predetermined cutoff of >30% reduction in ADHD symptoms to denote response, 47% of subjects improved with ABT-418 compared to 22% taking placebo ($p = 0.19$); however, in subjects with less severe ADHD, a more robust effect of treatment was found (53% vs. 23%, $p = 0.044$). Similar trends were noted using the clinical global impression of improvement. There were no significant changes in anxiety or depression ratings throughout the study. ABT-418 was relatively well tolerated, with dizziness, skin irritation, gastrointestinal distress, and headaches most frequently reported. The results of this controlled investigation with the ABT-418 indicate that despite small numbers, there was a significant anti-ADHD effect, particularly in subjects with a less severe form of the disorder. Our results, coupled with other studies, suggest that cholinergic agents appear promising for the treatment of ADHD. Further controlled trials of ABT-418 using higher dosages and longer treatment are warranted.

CONCLUSION

Despite controversy regarding the validity of ADHD in adults, the clinical picture is highly reminiscent of childhood ADHD, with continued associated occupational failure and academic deficits. Similarly, many adults with ADHD suffer from antisocial, depressive, and anxiety disorders. Psychopharmacologic treatment trials show that the majority of adults with ADHD enjoy a robust response to the same stimulant and nonstimulant treatments as ADHD children. In addition, there is mounting evidence for underlying pathophysiology, genetic risk factors, and abnormalities in brain structure and function associated with this diagnosis. These findings provide compelling evidence that adult ADHD is a valid and meaningful clinical entity in adults. As in childhood ADHD, medication remains a key component of treatment for this older population.

REFERENCES

Amen, D., Paldi, J. & Thisted, R. (1993), Brain SPECT imaging. *Am. J. Psychiatry,* 32:1080–1081.

Anderson, J.C., Williams, S., McGee, R. & Silva, P.A. (1987), *DSM-III* disorders in preadolescent children: Prevalence in a large sample from the general population. *Arch. Gen. Psychiatry,* 44:69–76.

Barkley, R. (1989), Hyperactive girls and boys: Stimulant drug effects on mother–child interactions. *J. Child Psychol. Psychiatry,* 30:379–390.

Barkley, R.A. (1990), *Attention Deficit Hyperactivity Disorder: A Handbook for Diagnosis and Treatment.* New York: Guilford Press.

Beck, A., Ward, C. & Mendelson, M. (1961), An inventory for measuring depression. *Arch. Gen. Psychiatry,* 4:561–571.

Biederman, J., Baldessarini, R.J., Wright, V., Keenan, K. & Faraone, S. (1993a), A double-blind placebo controlled study of desipramine in the treatment of attention deficit disorder: III. Lack of impact of comorbidity and family history factors on clinical response. *J. Am. Acad. Child Adolesc. Psychiatry,* 32:199–204.

Biederman, J., Baldessarini, R.J., Wright, V., Knee, D. & Harmatz, J. (1989), A double-blind placebo controlled study of desipramine in the treatment of attention deficit disorder: I. Efficacy. *J. Am. Acad. Child Adolesc. Psychiatry,* 28:777–784.

Biederman, J., Faraone, S.V., Keenan, K., Benjamin, J., Krifcher, B., Moore, C., Sprich, S., Ugaglia, K., Jellinek, M.S., Steingard, R, Spencer, T., Norman, D., Kolodny, R., Kraus, I., Perrin, J., Keller, M.B. & Tsuang, M.T. (1992), Further evidence for family-genetic risk factors in attention deficit hyperactivity disorder (ADHD): Patterns of comorbidity in probands and relatives in psychiatrically and pediatrically referred samples. *Arch. Gen. Psychiatry,* 49:728–738.

Biederman, J., Faraone, S.V., Keenan, K., Knee, D. & Tsuang, M.T. (1990a), Family-genetic and psychosocial risk factors in *DSM-III* attention deficit disorder. *J. Am. Acad. Child Adolesc. Psychiatry,* 29:526–533.

Biederman, J., Faraone, S.V., Keenan, K., Steingard, R. & Tsuang, M.T. (1991a), Familial association between attention deficit disorder and anxiety disorders. *Am. J. Psychiatry,* 148:251–256.

Biederman, J., Faraone, S.V., Keenan, K. & Tsuang, M.T. (1991b), Evidence of familial association between attention deficit disorder and major affective disorders. *Arch. Gen. Psychiatry,* 48:633–642.

Biederman, J., Faraone, S.V., Knee, D. & Munir, K. (1990b), Retrospective assessment of *DSM-III* attention deficit disorder in non-referred individuals. *J. Clin. Psychiatry,* 51:102–107.

Biederman, J., Faraone, S.V., Mick, E., Spencer, T., Wilens, T., Kiely, K., Guite, J., Ablon, S., Reed, E.D. & Warburton, R. (1995a), High risk for attention deficit hyperactivity disorder among children of parents with childhood onset of the disorder: A pilot study. *Am. J. Psychiatry,* 152:431–435.

Biederman, J., Faraone, S.V., Milberger, S., Curtis, S., Chen, L., Marrs, A., Ouellette, C., Moore, P. & Spencer, T. (1996), Predictors of persistence and remission of ADHD: Results from a four year prospective follow-up study of ADHD children. *J. Am. Acad. Child Adolesc. Psychiatry,* 35:343–351.

Biederman, J., Faraone, S.V., Spencer, T., Wilens, T., Mick, E. & Lapey, K. (1994), Gender differences in a sample of adults with attention deficit hyperactivity disorder. *Psychiatry Res.,* 53:13–29.

Biederman, J., Faraone, S.V., Spencer, T., Wilens, T., Norman, D., Lapey, K., Mick, E., Krifcher Lehman, B. & Doyle, A. (1993b), Patterns of psychiatric comorbidity, cognition and psychosocial functioning in adults with attention deficit hyperactivity disorder. *Am. J. Psychiatry,* 150:1792–1798.

Biederman, J., Munir, K., Knee, D., Armentano, M., Autor, S., Waternaux, C. & Tsuang, M. (1987), High rate of affective disorders in probands with attention deficit disorder and in their relatives: A controlled family study. *Am. J. Psychiatry,* 144:330–333.

Biederman, J., Munir, K., Knee, D., Habelow, W., Armentano, M., Autor, S., Hoge, S.K. & Waternaux, C. (1986), A family study of patients with attention deficit disorder and normal controls. *J. Psychiatr. Res.,* 20:263–274.

Biederman, J., Newcorn, J. & Sprich, S. (1991c), Comorbidity of attention deficit hyperactivity disorder with conduct, depressive, anxiety, and other disorders. *Am. J. Psychiatry,* 148:564–577.

Biederman, J., Wilens, T., Mick, E., Milberger, S., Spencer, T., Faraone, S. (1995b), Psychoactive substance use disorder in adults with attention deficit hyperactivity disorder: Effects of ADHD and psychiatric comorbidity. *Am. J. Psychiatry,* 152:1652–1658.

Bird, H.R., Canino, G., Rubio-Stipec, M., Gould, M.S., Ribera, J., Sesman, M., Woodbury, M., Huertas-Goldman, S., Pagan, A., Sanchez-Lacay, A. & Moscoso, M. (1988), Estimates of the prevalence of childhood maladjustment in a community survey in Puerto Rico. *Arch. Gen. Psychiatry,* 45:1120–1126.

Brown, R.T. & Sexson, S.B. (1988), A controlled trial of methylphenidate in black adolescents. *Clin. Pediatr.,* 27:74–81.

Cantwell, D.P. (1972), Psychiatric illness in the families of hyperactive children. *Arch. Gen. Psychiatry,* 27:414–417.

Cantwell, D.P. (1975), Genetics of hyperactivity. *J. Child Psychol. Psychiatry,* 16:261–264.

Castellanos, F., Giedd, J., Eckburg, P., Marsh, W., Vaituzis, C., Kaysen, D., Hamburger, S. & Rapoport, J. (1994), Quantitative morphology of the caudate nucleus in attention deficit hyperactivity disorder. *Am. J. Psychiatry,* 151:1791–1796.

Castellanos, F., Giedd, J., Marsh, W., Hamburger, S., Vaituzis, A., Dickstein, D., Sarfatti, S., Vauss, Y., Snell, J., Rajapakse, J. & Rapoport, J. (1996), Quantitative brain magnetic resonance imaging in attention deficit hyperactivity disorder. *Arch. Gen. Psychiatry,* 53:607–616.

Comings, D.E. & Comings, B.G. (1988), Tourette's syndrome and attention deficit disorder. In: *Tourette's Syndrome and Tic Disorders: Clinical Understanding and Treatment,* eds., D.J. Cohen, R.D. Bruun & J.F. Leckman. New York: John Wiley & Sons, Inc., pp. 119–136.

Comings, D.E., Comings, B.G., Muhleman, D., Dietz, G., Shahbahrami, B., Tast, D., Knell, E., Kocsis, P., Baumgarten, R., Kovacs, B.W., Levy, D.L., Smith, M., Borison, R.L., Evans, D.D., Klein, D.N., MacMurray, J., Tosk, J.M., Sverd, J., Gysin, R. & Flanagan, S.D. (1991), The dopamine D2 receptor locus as a modifying gene in neuropsychiatric disorders. *J.A.M.A.*, 266:1793–1800.

Cook, E.H., Stein, M.A., Krasowski, M.D., Cox, N.J., Olkon, D.M., Kieffer, J.E. & Leventhal, B.L. (1995), Association of attention deficit disorder and the dopamine transporter gene. *Am. J. Hum. Genet.,* 56:993–998.

Deutsch, C.K., Matthysse, S., Swanson, J.M. & Farkas, L.G. (1990), Genetic latent structure analysis of dysmorphology in attention deficit disorder. *J. Am. Acad. Child Adolesc. Psychiatry,* 29:189–194.

Donnelly, M., Zametkin, A.J., Rapoport, J.L., Ismond, D.R., Weingartner, H., Lane, E., Oliver, J., Linnoila, M. & Potter, W.Z. (1986), Treatment of childhood hyperactivity with desipramine: plasma drug concentration, cardiovascular effects, plasma and urinary catecholamine levels, and clinical response. *Clin. Pharmacol. Ther.,* 39:72–81.

Douglas, V.I. (1972), Stop, look and listen: The problem of sustained attention and impulse control in hyperactive and normal children. *Can. J. Behav. Sci.,* 4:259–282.

DuPaul, G. (1990), The ADHD Rating Scale: normative data, reliability, and validity. Unpublished manuscript, University of Massachusetts Medical Center, Worcester, Massachusetts.

DuPaul, G., Barkley, R. & McMurray, M. (1994), Response of children with ADHD to methylphenidate: Interaction with internalizing symptoms. *J. Am. Acad. Child Adolesc. Psychiatry,* 33:894–903.

Faraone, S., Biederman, J., Chen, W.J., Krifcher, B., Keenan, K., Moore, C., Sprich, S. & Tsuang, M. (1992), Segregation analysis of attention deficit hyperactivity disorder: Evidence for single gene transmission. *Psychiatr. Genet.,* 2:257–275.

Faraone, S.V., Biederman, J., Keenan, K. & Tsuang, M.T. (1991), Separation of *DSM-III* attention deficit disorder and conduct disorder: Evidence from a family-genetic study of American child psychiatric patients. *Psychol., Med.,* 21:109–121.

Faraone, S.V., Biederman, J., Krifcher Lehman, B., Spencer, T., Norman, D., Seidman, L., Kraus, I., Perrin, J., Chen, W. & Tsuang, M.T. (1993), Intellectual performance and school failure in children with attention deficit hyperactivity disorder and in their siblings. *J. Abnorm. Psychol.,* 102:616–623.

Faraone, S.V., Biederman, J., Weiffenbach, B., Keith, T., Chu, M.P., Weaver, A., Spencer, T., Wilens, T., Frazier, J., Cleves, M., Sakai, J. & Cleves, M. (1997), The dopamine D4 gene 7-repeat allele is associated with attention deficit hyperactivity disorder in families ascertained through ADHD adults. Presented at the Scientific Proceedings of the American Academy of Child and Adolescent Psychiatrists, Toronto, Ontario, Canada.

Faraone, S.V. & Santangelo, S. (1992), Methods in genetic epidemiology. In: *Research Designs and Methods in Psychiatry,* eds., M. Fava & J.F. Rosenbaum. Amsterdam: Elsevier, pp. 93–118.

Garfinkel, B.D., Wender, P.H., Sloman, L. & O'Neill, I. (1983), Tricyclic antidepressant and methylphenidate treatment of attention deficit disorder in children. *J. Am. Acad. Child Adolesc. Psychiatry,* 22:343–348.

Giedd, J.N., Castellanos, F.X., Casey, B.J., Kozuch, P., King, A.C., Hamburger, S.D., Rapoport, J.L. (1994), Quantitative morphology of the corpus callosum in attention deficit hyperactivity disorder. *Am. J. Psychiatry,* 151:665–669.

Gittelman, R., Mannuzza, S., Shenker, R. & Bonagura, N. (1985), Hyperactive boys almost grown up: I. Psychiatric status. *Arch. Gen. Psychiatry,* 42:937–947.

Goodman, R. & Stevenson, J. (1989a), A twin study of hyperactivity: I. An examination of hyperactivity scores and categories derived from Rutter teacher and parent questionnaires. *J. Child Psychol. Psychiatry,* 30:671–689.

Goodman, R. & Stevenson, J. (1989b), A twin study of hyperactivity: II. The aetiological role of genes, family relationships and perinatal adversity. *J. Child Psychol. Psychiatry,* 30:691–709.

Gorenstein, E.E., Mammato, C.A. & Sandy, J.M. (1989), Performance of inattentive-overactive children on selected measures of prefrontal-type function. *J. Clin. Psychol.,* 45:620–632.

Greenfield, B., Hechtman, L. & Weiss, G. (1988), Two subgroups of hyperactives as adults: Correlations of outcome. *Can. J. Psychiatry,* 33:505–508.

Gualtieri, C.T., Ondrusek, M.G. & Finley, C. (1985), Attention deficit disorders in adults. *Clin. Neuropharmacol.,* 8:343–356.

Hamilton, M. (1959), The assessment of anxiety states by rating. *Br. J. Med. Psychol.,* 32:50–55.

Hamilton, M. (1960), A rating scale for depression. *J. Neurol. Neurosurg. Psychiatry,* 23:56–62.

Hechtman, L. (1992), Long-term outcome in attention-deficit hyperactivity disorder. *Psychiatr. Clin. North Am.,* 1:553–565.

Hynd, G.W., Hern, K.L., Novey, E.S., Eliopulis, D., Marshall, R., Gonzalez, J.J. & Voeller, K.K. (1993), Attention deficit-hyperactivity disorder and asymmetry of the caudate nucleus. *J. Child Neurol.,* 8:339–347.

Hynd, G.W., Semrud-Clikeman, M.S., Lorys, A.R., Novey, E.S. & Eliopulos, D. (1990), Brain morphology in developmental dyslexia and attention deficit/hyperactivity. *Arch. Neurol.,* 47:919–926.

Iaboni, F., Bouffard, R., Minde, K. & Hechtman, L. (1996), The efficacy of methylphenidate in treating adults with attention-deficit/hyperactivity disorder. Presented at the American Academy of Child and Adolescent Psychiatry, Philadelphia, Pennsylvania.

Klein, R.G. & Mannuzza, S. (1989), The long-term outcome of the attention deficit disorder/hyperkinetic syndrome. In: *Attention Deficit Disorder, Clinical and Basic Research,* eds., T. Sagvolden & T. Archer. Hillside, NJ: Erlbaum Assoc., pp. 71–91.

Klein, R.G. & Mannuzza, S. (1991), Long-term outcome of hyperactive children: A review. *J. Am. Acad. Child Adolesc. Psychiatry,* 30:383–387.

LaHoste, G.J., Swanson, J.M., Wigal, S.B., Glabe, C., Wigal, T., King, N. & Kennedy, J.L. (1996), Dopamine D4 receptor gene polymorphism is associated with attention deficit hyperactivity disorder. *Molec. Psychiatry,* 1:128–131.

Lopez, R.E. (1965), Hyperactivity in twins. *Can. Psychiat. Assoc. J.,* 10:421–426.

Mannuzza, S., Gittelman-Klein, R. & Addalli, K.A. (1991b), Young adult mental status of hyperactive boys and their brothers: A prospective follow-up study. *J. Am. Acad. Child Adolesc. Psychiatry,* 30:743–751.

Mannuzza S, Klein RG, Bessler A, Malloy P. & LaPadula, M. (1993), Adult outcome of hyperactive boys: Educational achievement, occupational rank and psychiatric status. *Arch. Gen. Psychiatry,* 50:565–576.

Mannuzza, S., Gittelman-Klein, R., Bonagura, N., Malloy, P., Giampino, T.L. & Addalli, K.A. (1991a), Hyperactive boys almost grown up: V. Replication of psychiatric status. *Arch. Gen. Psychiatry,* 48:77–83.

Manshadi, M., Lippmann, S., O'Daniel, R.G. & Blackman, A. (1983), Alcohol abuse and attention deficit disorder. *J. Clin. Psychiatry,* 44:379–380.

Mattes, J.A., Boswell, L. & Oliver, H. (1984), Methylphenidate effects on symptoms of attention deficit disorder in adults. *Arch. Gen. Psychiatry,* 41:1059–1063.

Morrison, J.R. (1980), Adult psychiatric disorders in parents of hyperactive children. *Am. J. Psychiatry,* 137:825–827.

Morrison, J.R. & Stewart, M.A. (1971), A family study of the hyperactive child syndrome. *Biol. Psychiatry,* 3:189–195.

Morrison, J.R. & Stewart, M.A. (1973), The psychiatric status of the legal families of adopted hyperactive children. *Arch. Gen. Psychiatry,* 28:888–891.

Murphy, K. & Barkley, R. (1996), Prevalence of *DSM-IV* symptoms of ADHD in adult licensed drivers: Implications for clinical diagnosis. *J. Attention Disorders,* 1: 147–161.

National Institute of Mental Health (1985), CGI (Clinical Global Impression) Scale—NIMH. *Psychopharmacology,* 21:839–844.

Pelham, W.E., Walker, J.L., Sturges, J. & Hoza, J. (1989), Comparative effects of methylphenidate on ADD girls and ADD boys. *J. Am. Acad. Child Adolesc. Psychiatry,* 28:773–776.

Pliszka, S.R (1989), Effect of anxiety on cognition, behavior, and stimulant response in ADHD. *J. Am. Acad. Child Adolesc. Psychiatry,* 28:882–887.

Rapoport, J.L., Quinn, P., Bradbard, G., Riddle, D. & Brooks, E. (1974), Imipramine and methylphenidate treatment of hyperactive boys: A double-blind comparison. *Arch. Gen. Psychiatry,* 30:789–793.

Rapport, M., Carlson, G., Kelly, K. & Pataki, C. (1993), Methylphenidate and desipramine in hospitalized children: I. Separate and combined effects on cognitive function. *J. Am. Acad. Child Adolesc. Psychiatry,* 32:333–342.

Safer, D.J. & Krager, J.M. (1988), A survey of medication treatment for hyperactive/inattentive students. *J.A.M.A.,* 260:2256–2258.

Schachar, R. & Wachsmuth R. (1990), Hyperactivity and parental psychopathology. *J. Child Psychol. Psychiatry,* 31:381–392.

Seidman, L. (1995), Neuropsychology of Adult ADHD. Presented at the Scientific Proceedings of the Annual Meeting of the American Academy of Child and Adolescent Psychiatry, New Orleans, Louisiana.

Seidman, L.J., Benedict, K., Biederman, J., Bernstein, J., Seiverd, K., Milberger, S., Norman, D., Mick, E. & Faraone, S. (1995a), Performance of ADHD children on the Rey-Osterrieth complex figure: A pilot neuropsychological study. *J. Child Psychol. Psychiatry,* 36:1459–1473.

Seidman, L.J., Biederman, J., Faraone, S., Milberger, S., Norman, D., Seiverd, K., Benedict, K., Guite, J., Mick, E. & Kiely, K. (1995b), Effects of family history and comorbidity on the neuropsychological performance of ADHD children: Preliminary findings. *J. Am. Acad. Child Adolesc. Psychiatry,* 34:1015–1024.

Semrud-Clikeman, M.S., Filipek, P.A., Biederman, J., Steingard, R., Kennedy, D., Renshaw, P. & Bekken, K. (1994), Attention-deficit hyperactivity disorder: Magnetic resonance imaging morphometric analysis of the corpus callosum. *J. Am. Acad. Child Adolesc. Psychiatry,* 33:875–881.

Shaffer, D. (1994), Attention deficit hyperactivity disorder in adults. *Am. J. Psychiatry,* 151:633–638.

Shaywitz, S.E. & Shaywitz, B.A. (1987), Attention deficit disorder: Current perspectives. *Pediatr. Neurol.,* 3:129–135.

Shue, K.L. & Douglas, V.I. (1992), Attention deficit hyperactivity disorder and the frontal lobe syndrome. *Brain Cognition,* 20:104–124.

Spencer, T., Biederman, J., Wilens, T. & Faraone, S. (1994), Is attention deficit hyperactivity disorder in adults a valid disorder? *Harv. Rev. Psychiatry,* 1:326–335.

Spencer, T., Biederman, J., Wilens, T., Prince, J., Hatch, M., Jones, J., Harding, M., Faraone, S. & Seidman, L. (1998), Effectiveness and tolerability of tomoxetine in adults with childhood onset ADHD. *Am. J. Psychiatry,* 155:693–695.

Spencer, T., Wilens, T.E., Biederman, J., Faraone, S.V., Ablon, S. & Lapey, K. (1995), A double-blind, crossover comparison of methylphenidate and placebo in adults with childhood-onset attention deficit hyperactivity. *Arch. Gen. Psychiatry,* 52:434–443.

Spencer, T.J., Biederman, J., Wilens, T., Harding, M., O'Donnell, D. & Griffin, S. (1996), Pharmacotherapy of ADHD across the lifecycle: A literature review. *J. Am. Acad. Child Adolesc. Psychiatry,* 35:409–432.

Stewart, M.A., deBlois, C.S. & Cummings, C. (1980), Psychiatric disorder in the parents of hyperactive boys and those with conduct disorder. *J. Child Psychol. Psychiatry,* 21:283–292.

Swanson, J., Kinsbourne, M., Roberts, W. & Zucker, K. (1978), Time-response analysis of the effect of stimulant medication on the learning ability of children referred for hyperactivity. *Pediatrics,* 61:21–24.

Szatmari, P., Offord, D.R. & Boyle, M.H. (1989), Ontario Child Health Study: Prevalence of attention deficit disorder with hyperactivity. *J. Child Psychol. Psychiatry Allied Disc.*, 30:219–230.

Taylor, E., Schachar, R., Thorley, G., Wieselberg, H.M., Everitt, B. & Rutter, M. (1987), Which boys respond to stimulant medication? A controlled trial of methylphenidate in boys with disruptive behaviour. *Psychol. Med.*, 17:121–143.

Thorley, G. (1984), Review of follow-up and follow-back studies of childhood hyperactivity. *Psychol. Bull.*, 96:116–132.

Voelker, S.L., Lachar, D. & Gdowski, L.L. (1983), The personality inventory for children and response to methylphenidate: Preliminary evidence for predictive validity. *J. Pediatr. Psychol.*, 8:161–169.

Weiss, G., Hechtman, L., Milroy, T. & Perlman, T. (1985), Psychiatric status of hyperactives as adults: A controlled prospective 15-year follow-up of 63 hyperactive children. *J. Am. Acad. Child Psychiatry*, 24:211–220.

Weiss, G., Hechtman, L., Perlman, T., Hopkins, J. & Wener, A. (1979), Hyperactives as young adults: A controlled prospective ten-year follow-up of 75 children. *Arch. Gen. Psychiatry*, 36:675–681.

Weiss, G. & Hechtman, L.T. (1986), *Hyperactive Children Grown Up*. New York: Guilford Press, pp. 84–141.

Welner, Z., Welner, A., Stewart, M., Palkes, H. & Wish, E. (1977), A controlled study of siblings of hyperactive children. *J. Nerv. Ment. Disorders*, 165:110–117.

Wender, P.H., Reimherr, F.W. & Wood, D.R. (1981), Attention deficit disorder ("minimal brain dysfunction") in adults: A replication study of diagnosis and drug treatment. *Arch. Gen. Psychiatry*, 38:449–456.

Wender, P.H., Reimherr, F.W., Wood, D.R. & Ward, M. (1985), A controlled study of methylphenidate in the treatment of attention deficit disorder, residual type, in adults. *Am. J. Psychiatry*, 142:547–552.

Wilens, T. & Biederman, J. (1992), The stimulants. *Psychiatr. Clin. North Am.*, 15(1):191–222.

Wilens, T., Frazier, J., Prince, J., Spencer, T., Bostic, J., Hatch, M., Abrantes, A., Sienna, M., Soriano, J., Millstein, R. & Biederman, J. (1997), A double blind comparison of pemoline in adults with ADHD. Presented at the Scientific Proceedings of the American Academy of Child and Adolescent Psychiatry, Toronto, Ontario, Canada.

Wilens, T.E., Biederman, J., Geist, D.E., Steingard, R. & Spencer, T. (1993), Nortriptyline in the treatment of attention deficit hyperactivity disorder: A chart review of 58 cases. *J. Am. Acad. Child Adolesc. Psychiatry*, 32:343–349.

Wilens, T.E., Biederman, J., Prince, J., Spencer, T.J., Faraone, S.V., Warburton, R., Schleifer, D., Harding, M., Linehan, C. & Geller, D. (1996), Six week, double blind, placebo controlled study of desipramine for adult attention deficit hyperactivity disorder. *Am. J. Psychiatry*, 153:1147–1153.

Wilens, T.E., Biederman, J.B., Mick, E. & Spencer, T. (1995), A systematic assessment of tricyclic antidepressants in the treatment of adult attention-deficit hyperactivity disorder *J. Nerv. Ment. Dis.*, 183:48–50.

Wood, D.R., Reimherr, F.W., Wender, P.H. & Johnson, G.E. (1976), Diagnosis and treatment of minimal brain dysfunction in adults: A preliminary report. *Arch. Gen. Psychiatry*, 33:1453–1460.

Zametkin, A., Liebenauer, L., Fitzgerald, G., Minkunas, D., Herscovitch, P., Yamada, E.

& Cohen, R. (1993), Brain metabolism in teenagers with attention-deficit hyperactivity disorder. *Arch. Gen. Psychiatry,* 50:333–340.

Zametkin, A.J., Nordahl, T.E., Gross, M., King, C., Semple, W.E., Rumsey, J., Hamburger, S. & Cohen, R.M. (1990), Cerebral glucose metabolism in adults with hyperactivity of childhood onset. *N. Engl. J. Med.,* 323:1361–1366.

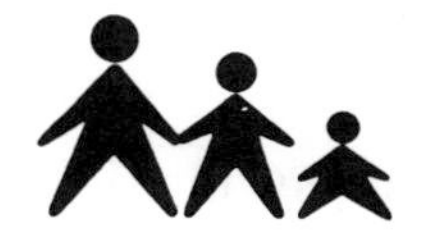

Psychostimulants in HIV-Infected Children and Adolescents: A Case Series

JENNIFER F. HAVENS[1] and E'METT O. McCASKILL[2]

INTRODUCTION

This case series describes the psychostimulant treatment of 12 HIV-infected children and adolescents, eight with attention deficit hyperactivity disorder (ADHD) and four with dementia related to HIV. In the ADHD sample, psychostimulant treatment showed good initial efficacy in all cases. Clinically significant side effects precluded maintenance treatment in three of the eight cases. In children with HIV-related dementia, psychostimulant treatment was effective in three of the four cases. Clinically significant side effects precluded maintenance treatment in one case. Adverse effects encountered included psychomotor agitation, visual hallucinations, and exacerbation of underlying seizure disorder.

To date, there have been 7692 reported cases of AIDS in children in the United States, 90% of them due to vertical transmission from an HIV-infected mother (Centers for Disease Control and Prevention, 1996). Recent findings on the efficacy of zidovudine in reducing the rate of transmission of HIV from mother to infant indicates a mechanism for minimizing the number of congenitally infected children (Connor et al., 1994). However, there is evidence that the women at highest risk for HIV infection (e.g., drug-using women) may be the most unlikely to access this important treatment advance (Wiznia et al., 1996).

Use of psychostimulants in the treatment of ADHD in HIV-infected children

The vast majority of HIV-infected children in the United States acquire HIV through vertical transmission from HIV-infected mothers, almost half of whom have their own injecting drug use as their risk factor for HIV infection. A significant number of the remainder have heterosexual contact with a drug-using man as their risk factor (CDC, 1996). Adults with substance abuse disorders have been shown to have increased rates of psychiatric comorbidity, particularly affective disorders and childhood histories of attention deficit hyperactivity disorder (Eyre et al., 1982; Haller et al., 1993; Rounsaville et al., 1982). Children born to drug-addicted adults are at increased risk for mental health problems, both because of the heritable nature of psychiatric disorders prevalent in adult substance abusers (Biederman et al., 1990; Goodman and Stevenson, 1989; Weissman et al., 1984) and because of exposure to abuse, neglect, and trauma associated with parental drug addiction (Kelley, 1992; Singer et al., 1992).

There have been several reports of the high prevalence of symptoms compatible with ADHD in HIV-infected children (Corsi et al., 1991; Hittleman et al., 1993). In one of the

[1]Pediatric Psychiatry, Babies' and Childrens' Hospital, and [2]The Special Needs Clinic, New York Presbyterian Hospital, New York, New York.

few studies focusing specifically on psychiatric disorder, Havens et al. (1994) reported that five out of 24 HIV-infected children (21%) met the criteria for pervasive ADHD. However, similar rates of ADHD were found in the matched control sample of noninfected children born to HIV-infected mothers and non–HIV-exposed children, suggesting that background factors in this population of HIV-exposed children (in particular, parental substance abuse) may be more relevant to psychiatric disorder than HIV infection itself.

The role of psychostimulants in the treatment of attention deficit hyperactivity disorder in children has been well established, with numerous studies demonstrating both their safety and their efficacy in the treatment of symptoms associated with hyperactivity, impulsivity, and attentional deficits (DuPaul and Barkley, 1990; Gittleman-Klein, 1987; Greenhill, 1991). To our knowledge, however, this is the first description of the use of psychostimulants in the management of ADHD in HIV-infected children and adolescents.

Use of psychostimulants in the treatment dementia related to HIV

Studies on neurologic functioning in HIV-infected children have described two relatively distinct neurodevelopmental patterns: static encephalopathy and progressive encephalopathy (Brouwers et al., 1991; Epstein et al., 1988). Static encephalopathy, characterized by nonprogressive deficits in cognitive, motor, and/or language function, is not directly attributable to HIV and is believed to be associated with the high-risk backgrounds of many HIV-infected children, which often include prenatal drug exposure, prematurity, and low birth weight (Diamond et al., 1987; Epstein et al., 1988; Mellins et al., 1994). Progressive encephalopathy is characterized by the loss of developmental milestones in young children and with declining IQ scores and increasing difficulties with language, attention, concentration, and memory in older children. This neurodevelopmental outcome, which corresponds to the AIDS dementia complex in adults, is most commonly diagnosed in late-stage illness and is a direct effect of HIV on the central nervous system.

There have been several reports of the use of psychostimulants in the management of attentional and affective symptoms in AIDS dementia in adults (Angrist et al., 1992; Fernandez and Levy, 1991; Holmes et al., 1989). A case study describes the use of clonidine in the treatment of behavioral symptoms in a preschool child with HIV encephalopathy (Cesena et al., 1995). In the current case series, we report on the use of stimulants in the management of HIV-related dementia in four children and adolescents.

METHOD

Subjects

The medical records of 12 HIV-infected children and adolescents receiving psychostimulant treatment in the Special Needs Clinic (a specialized child psychiatry program serving HIV-infected and affected children and their families) were reviewed. Eleven of the 12 children had acquired the virus through perinatal transmission; the route of infection was unknown in the twelfth child. All of the 12 children had been born to women with histories of substance abuse; only one of the children was in the custodial care of the mother at the time of treatment at the clinic. The children ranged in age from 4 to 14 years, with a mean age of 11. All of the children were Latino or African American; all were supported by public assistance or foster care supplements.

Table 1. Psychostimulant Treatment of HIV-Infected Children for Attention Deficit Hyperactivity Disorder (ADHD)

Patient	*Age/Sex*	*CDC Stage*	*Antiviral*	*Diagnosis*	*Stimulant Drug/Dose*	*Other Psychoactive Drugs*	*Clinical*	*Side Effects*	*Next Psychoactive Treatment*
D.B.	11/Male	Stage A	DDI/ZDU	ADHD Dev. Lan. Dis. Mild MR Full Scale IQ-67	MPH 20.0 bid, 1.2 mg/kg	None	Marked	None	
J.A.	10/Male	Stage A	ZDU	ADHD Dev. Lan. Dis. Full Scale IQ-78	MPH 10.0 bid, 0.8 mg/kg	None	Marked	None	
A.G.	13/Male	Stage C	ZDU	ADHD Dev. Lan. Dis. Enuresis SAD Full Scale IQ-89	MPH 10.0 mg bid, 0.65 mg/kg	None	Marked	None	
H.J.	14/Male	Stage C	ZDU/DDI	ADHD Full Scale IQ-84	Dextro- amphetamine 10 mg bid; 0.6 mg/kg	None	Marked	None	
C.P.	14/Male	Stage C	ZDU	ADHD Dysthymia Conduct Dis. Full Scale IQ-88	MPH 10.0 po bid, 0.4 mg/kg	None	Marked	None	
M.C.	4/Female	Stage A	ZDU	ADHD IQ-N/A	MPH 2.5 mg bid, 0.3 mg/kg	None	Moderate initial response	Visual Hallucinations leading to MPH discontinuation	Clonidine 0.5 mg bid

(continued)

Table 1. *(continued)* Psychostimulant Treatment of HIV-Infected Children for Attention Deficit Hyperactivity Disorder (ADHD)

Patient	*Age/Sex*	*CDC Stage*	*Antiviral*	*Diagnosis*	*Stimulant Drug/Dose*	*Other Psychoactive Drugs*	*Clinical*	*Side Effects*	*Next Psychoactive Treatment*
D.J.	11/Male	Stage C	ZDU/DDI	ADHD ODD Mild MR Encopresis Dev. Lan. Dis. Full-Scale IQ-69	MPH 10.0 bid; 0.55 mg/kg	None	Marked initial response	Agitation, irritability, social disinhibition	Thorazine 25 mg bid
N.P.	7/Female	Stage A	ZDU	ADHD Moderate MR Full Scale IQ-59 Seizure Disorder	MPH 10.0 bid; 1.0 mg/kg	Dilantin Diamox	Marked initial response	Exacerbation of underlying seizure disorder	Clonidine .05 mg bid and 0.1 mg qhs

CDC = Centers for Disease Control and Prevention; DDI = didanosine; ZDU = zinovudine; MPH = methylphenidate; ADHD = Attention Deficit Hyperactivity Disorder; ODD = Oppositional Defiant Disorder; MR = Mental Retardation; Dev. Lan. Dis. = Developmental Language Disorder; SAD = Separation Anxiety Disorder; IQ = Intelligence Quotient; N/A = Not Available.

Group I. Psychostimulant treatment for ADHD

Eight of the 12 children were treated with psychostimulants for ADHD. The ADHD diagnostic assessment followed the standard protocol in place in the Pediatric Psychiatry service at Columbia-Presbyterian Medical Center, which included intensive caregiver interviewing regarding child developmental and behavioral history, child interviewing and observations, and the collection of standard protocols from the classroom setting assessing ADHD and other symptomatology (Connor's Teachers Questionnaire). In addition, caregivers of six of the eight children underwent structured diagnostic interviewing with the Diagnostic Interview Schedule for Children, Version 2.1. At the time of admission, all eight children met the Diagnostic and Statistical Manual of Mental Disorders, 4th ed. criteria for ADHD with pervasive impairment in school, home, and peer settings. Their comorbid Axis I and Axis II diagnoses are shown in Table 1.

Group II. Psychostimulant treatment for dementia due to HIV disease

Four of the 12 children were treated with psychostimulants for HIV-related dementia. The diagnosis of HIV-related neuropsychiatric impairment was based on clinical interviewing with both children and their caregivers, with the following characteristic constellation of symptoms: memory impairment, attentional and concentrational difficulties, anhedonia, and fatigue. Caregivers reported motor slowing and oppositional behavior and resistance to activities of daily living. All four children were in advanced stages of HIV, illness with significant immunocompromise (see Table 2).

Psychostimulant treatment

Before stimulant treatment was given, consent was obtained from the appropriate custodial party (custodial parent or caregiver, or the Child Welfare Administration, for children in foster care). In addition, before medications were given, contact with the child's treating medical personnel was made to review current HIV medications and the psychiatric treatment plan.

Methylphenidate (MPH) was the initial psychostimulant agent in all cases. With the exception of the two preschool age children (M.C., T.B.) in the sample, the initial starting dose was 5–10 mg every morning or twice daily. Children's dosages were titrated upwards as clinically indicated, with the maintenance dosage ranging from 0.2 mg/kg to 1.2 mg/kg. In general, children treated for HIV-related dementia were initially given lower doses than medically healthier children being treated for ADHD. With one exception, all children maintained with psychostimulants were treated with MPH. One child showed a clinically superior response to dextroamphetamine and was maintained with this medication.

Antiretroviral therapy

All 12 children were maintained throughout psychostimulant treatment with antiretroviral treatment. The most common medication was zidovudine (ZDU), although didanosine (DDI) was also used, both as a single agent and in combination with ZDU (see Tables 1 and 2).

TABLE 2. PSYCHOSTIMULANT TREATMENT OF HIV-INFECTED CHILDREN FOR DEMENTIA RELATED TO HIV

Patient	*Age/Sex*	*CDC Stage*	*Antiviral*	*Diagnosis*	*Stimulant Drug/Dose*	*Clinical Effects*	*Side Effects*	*Clinical Global Stage Ratings*
V.M.	12/Male	Stage C	ZDU	Dementia due to HIV; Full Scale IQ-87	MPH/15.0 bid, 1.0 mg/kg	Self-report of increased energy and concentration	None	Moderate
P.B.	16/Male	Stage C	DDI	Dementia due to HIV; Full Scale IQ-74	MPH 5.0 mg bid, 0.2 mg/kg	Self-report of improvement in memory	None	Moderate
T.M.	11/Female	Stage C	DDI	Dementia due to HIV; Full Scale IQ-71	MPH/10.0 bid; 0.8 mg/kg	Self-report of increased energy	None	Moderate
T.B.	9/Male	Stage C	ZDU/DDI	Dementia due to HIV; Full Scale IQ-73	MPH/2.5; 0.1 mg/kg	Too active with Ritalin, stopped medication	Hypomanic response	Worse

CDC = Centers for Disease Control and Prevention; MPH = methylphenidate; ZDU = zinovudine; DDI = didanosine.

Assessments

Clinical response was assessed using the Efficacy Index of the Clinical Global Impressions (CGI) by the primary treating clinician. This index classifies therapeutic effect as unchanged, minimal (slight improvement), moderate (decided improvement) or marked (vast improvement).

RESULTS

Efficacy and adverse effects

Group I: Psychostimulant treatment for ADHD

All eight patients had either a moderate or a marked initial response to MPH. Three of the eight children developed adverse effects precluding maintenance treatment. The preschool child (M.C.) developed visual hallucinations and agitation within the first 2 weeks of receiving medication; another child (D.J.) developed irritability with increased peer conflict. The third child's (N.P.) seizure disorder was significantly exacerbated by stimulant treatment. Individual patient response is shown in Table 1.

Group II: Psychostimulant treatment for dementia due to HIV disease

Three of the four patients had a moderate response to MPH, with increased energy and improved attentional and concentrational abilities. One child (T.B.) developed hypomanic symptoms shortly after beginning to receive psychostimulants, including decreased sleep, excessive activity, and euphoric affect. Stimulant treatment was discontinued in this child. Individual patient response is shown in Table 2.

Length of treatment

Group I: Psychostimulant treatment for ADHD

The five children without adverse side effects have been maintained with long-term psychostimulant treatment, with all of them receiving stimulants for >2 years. The two children whose neuropsychiatric side effects precluded continued use (M.C., D.J.) developed them within the first 3 months of treatment. The child with seizure disorder (N.P.) was treated for 8 months before exacerbation of seizure activity precluded continued use.

Group II: Psychostimulant treatment for dementia due to HIV disease

The three children without adverse side effects have been maintained with long-term psychostimulant treatment. One child died of AIDS after a 12-month course of psychostimulant treatment; the two surviving children have been maintained with psychostimulants for 12–18 months. The child with adverse side effects developed them in the first month of treatment.

DISCUSSION

Eight of the 12 HIV-infected children and adolescents in our case series were safely and effectively treated with psychostimulants. For more than half of the HIV-infected children with ADHD, standard MPH doses were well tolerated in combination with maintenance antiretroviral agents. As has been reported in adults with HIV-related dementia, psychostimulants improved the quality of life for children struggling with the neurocognitive and behavioral effects of HIV progression.

Four of the 12 children experienced significant adverse side effects that precluded maintenance treatment. Two of them were of preschool age; one developed hallucinations, and the second manifested a hypomanic response to stimulants. A third school-age child manifested increased irritability and mood lability. These adverse effects warrant caution in the use of psychostimulants and speak to the complexity of differential diagnosis in this population.

The exacerbation of seizure disorder in the fourth child was predictable, given the tendency of MPH to lower the seizure threshold. Despite this risk, the level of behavioral symptomatology in this child mandated a clinical trial, which was conducted in close coordination with her treating neurologists.

In summary, two thirds of HIV-infected children tolerated psychostimulants with good efficacy. While the incidence of neuropsychiatric adverse effects argues for caution in the psychostimulant treatment of this population, such treatment should not be withheld when clinically indicated. Although the small number of patients and the open nature of the trial precludes any definitive conclusions, there was no evidence that psychostimulant dosage or antiretroviral medication had any clear relationship to clinical response or adverse side effects.

REFERENCES

Angrist, B., D'Hollosy, M., San Filipo, M., Satriano, J., Diamond, G., Simberkoff, M. & Weinreb, M. (1992), Central nervous system stimulants as symptomatic treatments for AIDS-related neuropsychiatric impairment. *J. Clin. Psychopharmacol.,* 12:268–273.

Biederman, J., Faraone, S., Keenan, K., Knee, D. & Tsuang, M.T. (1990), Family-genetic and psychosocial risk factors in *DSM-III* Attention Deficit Disorder. *J. Am. Acad. Child Adolesc. Psychiatry,* 29:526–533.

Brouwers, P., Belman, A.L. & Epstein, L.G. (1991), Central nervous system involvement manifestations and evaluation. In: *Pediatric AIDS: The Challenge of HIV Infection in Infants, Children and Adolescents,* eds., P. Pizzo & C. Wilfert. Baltimore: Williams & Wilkins, pp. 318–335.

Centers for Disease Control and Prevention (1996), *HIV/AIDS Surveillance Update,* 8:2.

Cesena, M., Douglas, L.O., Cebollero, A.M. & Steingard, R.J. (1995), Case study: Behavioral symptoms of pediatric HIV-1 encephalopathy successfully treated with clonidine. *J. Am. Acad. Child Adolesc. Psychiatry,* 34:302–306.

Connor, E.M., Spreling, R.S., Gelber, R., Kieslev, P., Scott, G., O'Sullivan, M.J., VanDyck, R., Bey, M., Shearer, W., Jacobson, R.L., Jimenez, E., O'Neill, E., Bazin, B., Delfraissy, J., Culnane, M., Coombs, R., Elkins, M., Moye, J., Stratton, P. & Balsey, J. (1994), Reduction of maternal–infant transmission of human immunodeficiency virus type 1 with zidovudine treatment. *N. Engl. J. Med.,* 331:1173–1180.

Corsi, A., Albizzati, A., Cervini, R., Grioni, A., Musetti, L. & Saccani, M. (1991), Hyperactive disturbance in the behavior of children with congenital HIV infection [abstr. W.D. 4280]. In: *Abstracts of the Seventh International AIDS Conference, vol. 2.* Florence, Italy, June 16–21.

Diamond, G.W., Kaufman, J., Belman, A.L., Cohen, L., Cohen, H.J., & Rubinstein, A. (1987), Characterization of cognitive functioning in a subgroup of children with congenital HIV infection. *Arch. Clin. Neuropsychol.,* 23:245–256.

DuPaul, G. & Barkley, R. (1990), Medication therapy. In: *Attention Deficit Hyperactivity Disorder: A Handbook for Diagnosis and Treatment,* ed. R.A. Barkley. New York: Guilford Press, pp. 573–612.

Epstein, L.G., Sharer, L.R. & Goudsmit, J. (1988), Neurological and neuropathological features of human immunodeficiency virus infection in children. *Ann. Neurol.,* 23: (suppl.) S19–S23.

Eyre, S.L., Rounsaville, B.J. & Kleber, H.D. (1982), History of childhood hyperactivity in a clinic population of opiate addicts. *J. Nerv. Ment. Dis.,* 170:522–529.

Fernandez, F. & Levy, J. (1991), Psychopharmacotherapy of psychiatric syndromes in asymptomatic and symptomatic HIV infection. *Psychiatr. Med.,* 9:377–394.

Gittleman-Klein, R. (1987), Pharmacotherapy in childhood hyperactivity: An update. In: *Psychopharmacology: The Third Generation of Progress,* ed., H.Y. Meltzer. New York: Raven Press, pp. 1215–1224.

Goodman, R. & Stevenson, J. (1989), A twin study of hyperactivity: II. The aetiological role of genes, family relationships, and perinatal adversity. *J. Child Psychol. Psychiatry,* 30:691–709.

Greenhill, L. (1991), Methylphenidate in the clinical office practice of child psychiatry. In: *Ritalin: Theory and Patient Management,* eds. L.L. Greenhill & B.B. Osman. Larchmont, New York: Mary Ann Liebert, Inc., pp. 97–118.

Haller, D.L., Knisely, J.S., Dawson, K.S. & Schnoll, S.H. (1993). Perinatal substance abusers: Psychological and social characteristics. *J. Nerv. Mental Dis.* 181:509–513.

Havens, J., Whitaker, A., Feldman, J. & Ehrhardt, A. (1994), Psychiatric morbidity in school-age children with congenital HIV-infection: A pilot study. *J. Dev. Behav. Pediatr.,* 15:S18–S25.

Hittleman, J., Nelson, N., Shah, V., Gong, J. & Peluso, F.S. (1993), Neurodevelopmental disabilities in infants born to HIV-infected mothers. *AIDS Reader,* July/August:126–132.

Holmes, V., Fernandez, F. & Levy, J.K. (1989), Psychostimulant response in AIDS-related complex patients. *J. Clin. Psychiatry,* 50:5–8.

Kelley, S. (1992), Parenting stress and child maltreatment in drug-exposed children. *Child Abuse Negl.,* 16:312–328.

Mellins, C.A., Levenson, R.L., Zawadzki, R., Kairam, R. & Weston, M. (1994), Effects of pediatric HIV infection and prenatal drug exposure on mental and psychomotor development. *J. Pediatr. Psychol.,* 19:617–628.

Rounsaville, B.J., Weissman, M.M., Kleber, H. & Wilber, C. (1982), Heterogeneity of psychiatric diagnosis in treated opiate addicts. *Arch. Gen. Psychiatry,* 39:161–166.

Singer, L., Farkas, K. & Kliegman, R. (1992), Childhood medical and behavioral consequences of maternal cocaine use. *J. Pediatr. Psychol.,* 17:389–406.

Weissman, M.M., Gershon, E.S., Kidd, K.K., Prusoff, B.A., Leckman, J.F., Dibble, E., Hamovit, J., Thompson, W.D., Pauls, D.L. & Guroff, J.J. (1984), Psychiatic disorders in the relatives of probands with affective disorders. *Arch. Gen. Psychiatry,* 41:13–21.

Wiznia, A.A., Crane, M., Lambert, G., Sansary, J., Harris, A. & Solomon, L. (1996), Zidovudine use to reduce perinatal HIV type 1 transmission in an urban medical center. *J.A.M.A.,* 275:19:1504–1507.

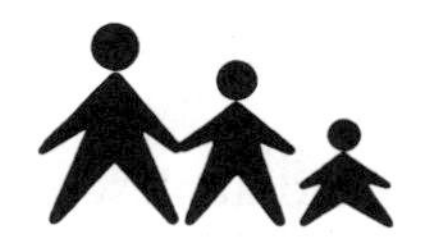

Coordinating Care in the Prescription and Use of Ritalin with Attention Deficit Hyperactivity Disorder Children/Adolescents

BETTY B. OSMAN

Attention deficit hyperactivity disorder (ADHD) is the most commonly diagnosed biobehavioral disorder of childhood today, affecting between 4% and 6% of school-age children and adolescents (American Psychiatric Association, 1994). This is an increase of more than 100% from 20 years ago, when the diagnosis was infrequently made. It is also recognized today that ADHD persists across the full span of development, from preschool to school age and adolescence, frequently continuing into adult life (Hechtman, 1992).

There has been a substantial body of research on the subject of ADHD in the last decade, and an explosion of books and articles for parents and educators. The basic parameters of the disorder, as well as its relation to other behavioral and cognitive conditions, continue to be debated nonetheless. The symptoms, though heterogeneous, are more readily recognized and treated today by parents and professionals in a variety of disciplines. Children with ADHD who previously would have gone unrecognized are now being helped, frequently with dramatic results, at least in part by stimulant medication.

The expression of ADHD symptoms varies within and among children, adversely affecting many areas of functioning: behavior at home, academic performance, and social appropriateness. The cardinal constructs of the disorder, defined in the *Diagnostic and Statistical Manual of Mental Disorders* (*DSM*) 4th ed. (American Psychiatric Association), are inattention, impulsivity, and, at times, hyperactivity to a degree that is excessive and inappropriate for the child's developmental stage, persists for more than 6 months, and has an onset before the age of 7. In addition, the behaviors associated with ADHD must be apparent across at least two settings, such as school and at home. Although the validity of this latter construct has been questioned, it remains a criterion for ADHD diagnosis.

Methylphenidate—or Ritalin, the trade name—has been prescribed for children and adolescents with attention deficit disorders for almost 40 years. Despite the controversy that continues to surround its use, the evidence of its efficacy in reducing the core symptoms of ADHD has been well documented in the literature as well as in clinical practice (Barkley, 1990; Spencer et al., 1995; Buitelaar et al., 1995; Greenhill and Osman, 1991). In addition to improving the core symptoms of ADHD, Ritalin also improves associated behaviors, including on-task behavior, academic performance, and social functioning. These appear to be cross situational, including home, clinic, and school settings (Wilens and Biederman, 1992; Greenhill, 1995). Although it is not a "cure," Ritalin is frequently the first line of treatment for children 6 years of age and older who have an ADHD diagnosis (Safer et al., 1996; Greenhill and Osman, 1991). It has been endorsed by the American Academy of Pediatrics (AAP) as an appropriate therapy, with the stipulation that evaluation, monitoring, and follow-up must be included in the regimen. In addition, a multimodal, individualized approach

Department of Behavioral Health, White Plains Hospital Center, White Plains, New York.

to the treatment of ADHD in children and adolescents has been strongly advocated (American Academy of Child and Adolescent Psychiatry, 1997; Silver, 1992; Swanson et al., 1998).

While this is not always common practice, an integrated interdisciplinary program is critical to the success of the treatment. The needs of youngsters with attention deficits and their families are wide-ranging and generally cannot be provided by a single individual or profession. The primary care physician may not have the knowledge, the resources, nor the time to oversee all aspects of pharmacotherapy, and parents as well as school personnel need to be consulted on an ongoing basis. Psychologists, social workers, school nurses, educators, speech and language therapists, and church and recreation leaders may all be called on to become involved in the progress of children for whom MPH is prescribed. Just as medical practitioners have expanded their knowledge and use of psychopharmacology with children (Safer et al., 1996; Vitiello, 1995), so do educators and clinicians monitoring the treatment need to have access to information about the drug, its side effects, and its influence on learning and behavior.

This chapter reviews the process of coordinating care for children and adolescents with attention deficits and discusses the role of each professional from assessment to termination of treatment. While physicians (pediatricians, psychiatrists, neurologists, and family practitioners) obviously play the most significant role in drug therapy (Wilens, 1995; Zito et al., 1997), other professionals can also be key in helping to determine whether the child is a candidate for medication as well as assuming responsibility for implementing the referral, assessment, and treatment phases of the therapy.

The behaviors associated with ADHD reflect a heterogeneous group of causes. For some youngsters, the primary determinants are of genetic origin or organically based, whereas for others, the cause may be psychogenic, e.g., reflecting anxiety or even a masked depression (Biederman et al., 1992). Mentally retarded, conduct-disordered, and learning-disabled children may also appear hyperactive or demonstrate deficits in attention. In addition, ADHD children frequently have other disorders along with their attentional deficits. Comorbidity is not uncommon (Shaywitz, 1991; Sverd, 1992; Tannock, 1994). An interdisciplinary perspective must therefore be maintained for an accurate differential diagnosis as well as appropriate treatment.

The development of an intersystem collaboration—that is, medical/psychologic, educational, family—is not easily achieved. The boundaries and diverse goals of each discipline may be constraints to interactive communication. The medical model typically focuses on cure, whereas the goals of education are the child's academic achievement and socialization. The family, on the other hand, is likely to be most concerned with issues of acceptance and the young person's self-esteem. For effective collaboration then, reciprocal role expectations must be established, and perspectives as well as information shared throughout the process of diagnosis and treatment.

REFERRAL

The majority of youngsters with ADHD are brought to the attention of the physician or mental health professional because of multiple difficulties in school and/or at home. Our experience at this hospital has been that the reasons most commonly given for referral of school-age children include inappropriate or disruptive behavior, temper tantrums, poor academic performance, and/or unsatisfactory social relationships with family, peers, and authority figures. Although there are accounts of children who are inattentive or hyperactive at home but not in school ("situational ADHD"), most ADHD children demonstrate these problems across settings. (This, in fact, is a criterion for designation.)

Parents frequently report that they "knew" something was amiss early in the child's life, even in infancy. Some precursors of ADHD observed in the first year of life may be irritability, excessive activity, poor sleeping, eating, and regulatory functions, and an aversion to being held or cuddled. By 3 years of age, more than half of all diagnosed ADHD children begin to manifest behavioral symptoms. Preschool children most likely to be referred to the family physician or pediatrician are those who are overly active, aggressive, and accident-prone because of their risk-taking behavior. If the child attends a day care or preschool program, the staff is likely to complain of inattention, hyperactivity, aggression, and noncompliant or oppositional behavior.

Some children, however, escape notice until elementary school, when, in all probability, it is the teacher or school psychologist who begins the referral process by alerting parents to the child's academic and social difficulties in school. The report of inappropriate behavior in class (disruptive or inattentive) and the lack of academic achievement frequently results in the recommendation to seek an evaluation and/or medical advice.

At that point, parents should, and generally do, turn to their pediatrician or family practitioner for guidance. Some physicians, knowledgeable about ADHD and the use of MPH, feel comfortable in assessing the situation in cooperation with the parents. Others, reluctant to be involved because of personal conviction or lack of experience with the drug, prefer to refer the family to specialists in neurology or psychiatry. With the realities of managed care today, however, referrals to specialists tend to be deferred when possible.

Before a trial of medication is considered, however, a multimodal evaluation is needed to ascertain the diagnosis and the advisability of recommending a psychostimulant. To make this determination, it is necessary to understand the past history as well as the present clinical picture. Comorbidity is frequently a problem in children and adolescents with the ADHD syndrome. As many as two thirds of elementary school–age children referred for clinical evaluation have at least one other diagnosable psychiatric disorder (Arnold and Jensen, 1995; Jensen et al., 1997; Nottelmann and Jensen, 1995), whereas other disorders may "mimic" ADHD, possibly contraindicating treatment with stimulants (Biederman et al., 1996).

ASSESSMENT

The decision to begin pharmacotherapy is rarely a simple one but rather is the outcome of a complex process of diagnostic assessment and evaluation. Several factors enter the equation: the physician's clinical judgment and understanding of the child, the family, and the school environment. Before prescribing a trial of medication as treatment, most physicians will also want to consult with—or refer to—nonmedical clinicians who routinely evaluate children and adolescents. Clinical child psychologists, school psychologists, and educational therapists are among the health care professionals who possess the necessary training, experience, and skills to conduct comprehensive assessments of ADHD.

The assessment and evaluation phase is perhaps the most important part of the treatment and generally follows numerous failed attempts to correct the problem by informal means at home as well as in school. Teachers tend to "wait and see" before referring a child to the child study team. Without a comprehensive diagnosis and examination of the child's entire situation, there can be no prescription for therapy. Given that the problems of children with ADHD often go beyond the disorder itself, any assessment must address not only the primary ADHD symptoms but other aspects of the child's behavioral, emotional, and social functioning as well. Equally important is the gathering of a detailed social history of the family to understand the context for the child's behaviors.

The first step in the evaluation process is a thorough physical examination by the pediatrician or family physician to affirm that the child is healthy and free of another condition or familial history that might weigh against the use of drug therapy (Copps, 1992). A referral for psychiatric evaluation would also be warranted if the youngster's behavior or mood deviates sufficiently from established norms. In addition to the physician or physicians involved, professionals in the mental health field and educators can contribute significantly to the diagnostic team. They are likely to have knowledge of the child and the dynamics of the family system, whereas the physician may have encountered only the mother/child dyad.

DIFFERENTIAL DIAGNOSIS

The diagnosis of ADHD is a clinical rather than a specific medical diagnosis. To date there are no laboratory tests that can be used to make a definitive diagnosis of the condition (Arnold and Jensen, 1995; Jensen et al., 1996; Barkley, 1990). Rather, ADHD is determined on the basis of family history, observation of the child, and behavioral symptoms presented to the clinician or physician. Although recent articles have reported that a type of brain scan, a "functional MRI," is being tested for the identification of children with ADHD (National Academy of Sciences, 1998), the technique is not yet available. Although some laboratory measures, such as the one developed by Gordon (1986), claim to distinguish subjects with ADHD from controls, to date computerized tests of attention and vigilance (CPTs), event-related potentials, and neuroimaging techniques have more promise in research than in clinical application (Barkley, 1990; Levy and Ward, 1995).

It is evident that to be constructive in treatment planning, a clinical evaluation for ADHD must be comprehensive and multidimensional. Parent, child, and teacher interviews; behavior rating scales; cognitive and academic evaluations; and, if indicated, medical tests should all be part of the protocol, along with a review of school and medical records. A pediatric examination or neurodevelopmental screening should be considered to rule out conditions that might produce ADHD-like symptoms.

Evaluation, whether with a primary care physician, psychiatrist, or psychologist, generally begins with information from parents. The initial parent interview consists of a detailed developmental medical and psychosocial history, because presenting symptoms, to be considered significant, must be inappropriate for the child's age and cognitive level. Whenever possible, both parents or caretakers should be present, as each may have a different view of the child and the presenting difficulties (Barkley, 1990). In our experience, fathers tend to see their children as being less hyperactive and "more normal" than mothers do. This may reflect the amount of time each parent spends with the child or, perhaps more important, a gender tolerance for active behavior. Barkley also found ADHD children to be more negative and noncompliant with their mothers than with their fathers. The mothers, in turn, were more negative and less responsive than fathers to the children's interactions.

Although sometimes criticized for its subjectivity and lack of reliability, the parent interview serves several purposes. First, it helps to establish a rapport between parent and professional that should result in greater cooperation and compliance with the treatment plan. Second, parents are the primary source of descriptive information about their child's behavior and developmental history. Finally, parents' perceptions and views of the child's problem, even if divergent, will help to focus and direct the assessment.

Some of the points to be covered in the interview include the following:

1. onset, duration, and severity of the problem.
2. history of previous diagnostic and treatment efforts.
3. medical history, including other prescribed medications.
4. evidence of depression or anxiety disorders in the child or family.
5. family history of tics or Tourette's syndrome.
6. any indication of a thought disorder or psychotic process.

7. the quality of the child's social relationships and interactions with parents, siblings, and playmates.
8. parental receptivity and willingness to comply with recommendations for treatment.

Answers in the affirmative to numbers 5 and 6 might contraindicate the use of Ritalin or any stimulant medication. Although some researchers have found tics associated with Tourette's syndrome to be exacerbated by MPH, the results are far from clear, and the advisability of using stimulants remains controversial (Sverd et al., 1992; Gadow, 1995; Konkol et al., 1990). Until more is known, it seems prudent to discuss the risks and benefits with the child and family. Should the physician choose to prescribe Ritalin for ADHD children with tics, relatively low dosages and careful monitoring should be implemented.

Because the academic and behavioral problems associated with ADHD tend to be most apparent in a school setting, school psychologists and educators have an obvious and critical role in helping to define the nature and extent of a child's problems. They also are likely to be viewed by parents as reliable sources of information and advice about their children. If speech/language, physical, or occupational therapists are or have been involved with the child, they too should be contacted, with written consent of the parents as mandated by law.

Psychoeducational assessment by a psychologist or team of clinicians and educators is necessary to appraise a youngster's attention deficits relative to other problems and their impact on cognitive functioning, academic performance, and social adjustment. Some of the instruments included in this kind of evaluation are a standardized intelligence test (usually the Wechsler Intelligence Scale for Children III [WISC III] or the preschool version, the Wechsler Preschool and Primary Scale of Intelligence-Revised [WPPSI-R]); drawings and copying forms (paper and pencil tasks); measures of academic skills and achievement; and tasks requiring attention, concentration, and memory. Projective techniques, such as story telling, may also be used if emotional factors seem relevant.

In the process of the evaluation, identifying the child's strengths and assets is equally important and useful in facilitating the treatment. Too often, psychologic evaluations highlight only the deficits and difficulties, discouraging all concerned.

Direct observation and a subsequent interview with the child who is the subject of concern are always part of the assessment phase (Hodges, 1993). The nature and content vary, of course, with the young person's age and developmental level and, of course, the situation. A child seen one-to-one in a clinician's office is likely to behave—and respond—differently from a child in the school environment. One-to-one the child may not appear to have ADHD at all, while the reported inattentiveness and/or hyperactivity may be variable, even within the school. An informal clinical observation of the classroom and a less structured situation, such as the lunchroom or playground, can provide important information about the child's behavior and the salient characteristics of the environment as well. Observation in different settings, therefore, is advisable whenever possible.

In talking with a child or adolescent, it is important to ascertain whether (s)he is aware that a problem exists and, if so, how it is perceived. Does he or she feel "different," unhappy at home or in school? And how does he or she feel about family and peer relationships? ADHD children frequently are unaware of the way others perceive them and the chaos they create in their environment. They tend to view themselves as innocent victims and others as the source of their problems.

The roles of the teacher and the special educator in the diagnostic process are crucial. Typically, the teacher is the first to recognize a problem based on classroom behavior and consults with a specialist within the school. Anecdotal records may be kept that can clarify the problem somewhat for parents and physicians, but such records are nonetheless subjective. Because individual differences among children are so great and because adults also differ in their perceptions of expected behavior, there may be little consistency among raters. Therefore, several perspectives and opinions within the school should be sought.

In the course of the evaluation, a variety of rating scales can be used to gather information from teachers, parents, and adolescents themselves. An example of a "broad-band" scale is the Child Behavior Check List (CBCL) (Achenbach, 1993), a standardized instrument assessing common dimensions of pathologic conditions in children, not only inattention and hyperactivity. Research has shown that the CBCL significantly discriminates ADHD from the control group and other psychiatric disorders of childhood (Mash and Johnson, 1983). The Youth Report (YRF) is a self-reporting scale similar to the CBCL that has been developed for children 11–18 years of age.

Among the most commonly used instruments are the Conners Rating Scales (CRS-R), revised in 1997 to include a range of problem behaviors. The long versions assess conduct problems, cognitive problems, anxiety, and social problems in addition to ADHD and hyperactivity. Shorter forms are designed more specifically for the diagnosis of ADHD, with norms for children 3–17. Used in combination, the parent and teacher rating scales yield information about the child's behavior from the perspective of adults who observe in a variety of settings (Conners, 1997). Other useful scales are the ActERs and the SNAP-IV (Swanson et al., 1995) and the Brown ADD scales (1996). A series of integrated scales (Yale Neuropsychoeducational Assessment Scales, YNPEAS [Shaywitz and Shaywitz, 1991; Shaywitz et al., 1992]) can also be used to systematically record historical events and clinical observations of the child and family.

Despite the obvious advantages of quantifiable data, no one instrument or source of data can provide sufficient information to enable the formulation of an accurate diagnosis. Although parent/physician/school-related instruments provide the framework for a diagnosis, the final determination is made when the clinician or diagnostic team has collected all the available information and determines that ADHD is present, whether or not there is a comorbid condition. The need for educational, medical, and/or psychosocial interventions is also determined as a result.

To summarize the foregoing, a comprehensive diagnostic approach for a child or adolescent with suspected ADHD should involve the following:

1. a comprehensive interview with parents or caretakers to obtain an inclusive developmental, medical, social, and educational history.
2. a medical examination to ascertain general health status and specific needs.
3. a developmentally appropriate interview with the child or adolescent to assess his/her understanding of the problem and possible solutions.
4. a clinical evaluation, including psychological assessment and evaluation.
5. appraisal of the child's academic skills and achievement.
6. the use of parent and teacher behavior rating scales.
7. appropriate adjunct assessments as indicated, e.g., speech/language, physical coordination.

TREATMENT PLAN

Finally, a meeting, sometimes labeled the "findings conference," of all who participated in the diagnostic process is needed to define problem areas and prescribe treatment methods. On completion of the evaluation, the diagnosis and its implications must then be interpreted to parents, the child, and school personnel. Parents have to be informed as explicitly as possible about the cause of attention deficit disorders and be reassured that their child's behaviors are not the result of parental mismanagement. Parents frequently tell us, "We must have done something wrong," not understanding that their child's problems stem from innate difficulties in neurophysiologic control.

In the findings conference, the recommendations for treatment are discussed. If pharmacologic therapy is proposed, the parents and the child need to understand why Ritalin is being prescribed and what it can be expected to accomplish. Although children cannot be given responsibility for their medical intervention, adolescents in particular need to take an active role in their treatment. They must be persuaded that there are benefits and be willing to comply with the regimen. At the same time, they must know that the medication will neither solve all their problems nor take control of their bodies or minds. Rather, the therapy should enable them to be more in charge of themselves. With Ritalin, young people can be helped to assume, rather than relinquish, responsibility for their actions.

The decision to recommend medication is based on several diverse factors in addition to the ADHD diagnosis: the physician's clinical judgment, based on knowledge of the family, young person, and school; and the symptoms that reflect the functional impairment. Consideration would also be given to the safety of the drug, the response rate, and side effects, as well as the patient's medical history. In making the decision, the risks of taking the drug must always be weighed against the consequences of not treating the disorder.

For most parents, the idea of giving a child medication is disturbing and even frightening. It is hard for the lay person to imagine that a drug can alter problem behaviors without being dangerous to the child's health. Parents should know that although there may be transient side effects initially, such as loss of appetite, sleep disturbance, and perhaps a mild stomachache (particularly if MPH is taken without food), there is no scientific evidence to date that children treated with appropriate doses suffer any long-term effects. However, more research is needed on the long-term effects of MPH (Spencer et al., 1996). On the other hand, MPH has been shown to be highly efficacious in reducing activity levels and improving attention in approximately 75% of ADHD children and adolescents (Quinn, 1997).

Parents may also have other concerns that they are reluctant to acknowledge. They need to be reassured that stimulant medication, titrated appropriately, will not sedate their children or turn them into "zombies." Although Ritalin is classified as a drug with the potential for abuse, studies have failed to find evidence of addiction in children or adolescents whose treatment with stimulants is carefully monitored. However, because ADHD children are characteristically sensitive to alterations in their environment, initiation of pharmacotherapy is recommended only after the child has had time to adjust to new surroundings, e.g., a new classroom at the beginning of the school year.

In the early weeks of the medication regimen, frequent contacts between professionals and the family should be standard practice. Once an effective and stable dose has been established, monitoring and follow-up can be tapered, except for regularly scheduled checkups. Medication may be used incorrectly or not taken at all for several reasons: the lack of perceived need for the drug by parents or child, reluctance of the child to comply (possibly because of unpleasant side effects), and/or family disorganization and/or carelessness.

For a physician to prescribe Ritalin or any drug and not provide appropriate follow-up is a disservice to parents and children. Yet, indications are that adequate monitoring is not always the rule. In a study of children in special education programs (Gadow, 1986), a quarter of the parents questioned felt that the physician did not devote enough time to "discussion of the medication, the child's condition, the therapeutic process, and treatment alternatives." In that study, contacts between parents and teachers were relatively common (63%), whereas communications between teachers and physicians were reported to be infrequent—only 16%. In addition to communicating with parents, it is imperative that teachers report to the physician or school nurse, completing requested rating scales or observation forms in a timely manner.

Although the importance of clinic and school involvement in pharmacotherapy is supported in theory, a disparity exists between what is considered an adequate standard for care and service delivery. It is noteworthy that although nonmedical clinicians and educators are called on to monitor children receiving medication, the amount of knowledge and training they receive in drug therapy is likely to be negligible or even nonexistent. Personal experiences such as reading, working with children, and the media are typical sources of their information. It is not uncommon for skepticism and misconceptions to result, based at least in part on less-than-scientific or sensational media reports. Ongoing contacts between physician, educator, clinician, and parents are unfortunately the exception rather than the rule, thereby compromising the efficacy of the treatment. The importance of communication and coordination of care during every phase of treatment cannot be overemphasized in the effort to maximize the therapeutic effects of MPH administration.

MONITORING

Once drug therapy has been implemented, a coordinated effort to monitor the effects of the drug is crucial; yet, this is probably the weakest link in the procedures followed in prescribing medication for children and teenagers. Despite its widespread use and strict guidelines for administration, Ritalin is still being inappropriately prescribed and improperly monitored in some instances. Articles in popular magazines have charged that Ritalin is being overprescribed and overused, as well as abused. Although this may be true to some extent, some researchers have found the drug to be *underprescribed* in some cases for children who need it to alleviate their symptoms (Jensen et al., 1999).

In response to irregular practices and the concern for children receiving medication, several states have passed legislation to regulate and restrict the prescribing of Ritalin. Because it is a Schedule II drug, only a one-month supply can be given, and the prescription must be renewed in writing. While this is cumbersome and time-consuming for parents as well as physicians, it does protect their children, and it makes regular contacts between physicians and parents during therapy more likely.

Close monitoring of the child's behavior by parents, physician, and school personnel, including observational measures and parent–teacher ratings, will signal when a child is benefiting from the treatment or appears to be responding adversely. Although most children benefit significantly from Ritalin, approximately 20%–30% may not respond or may have untoward side effects (Cantwell, 1996; Pelham, 1990). If not titrated correctly, the drug can have a negative effect on behavior (commonly lethargy), possibly to the point of impeding learning as well as social functioning (Gadow, 1992; Werry, 1988). Some children have also been reported to become "irritable" on the drug, with wider than usual "mood swings" (Gadow, 1992). Should these symptoms persist, a reduction of the dose or an alternative treatment should be considered.

Typically, the initial dosage prescribed is minimal (5 mg given once a day before school) (Greenhill, 1992; Spencer et al., 1996). If the drug is tolerated with no serious side effects, it is gradually increased until the therapeutic level is reached. Response to medication dosage cannot always be predicted, however. Some children are particularly sensitive to the effects of medication, requiring a lower-than-expected dose, whereas others need higher doses to control their symptoms. Increases, therefore, should always be made in small increments.

The relationship between dose and clinical response remains a source of controversy (Douglas, 1988; Solanto-Gardner, 1999; Spencer et al., 1996). An early study (Sprague and Sleator, 1977) found that at increased dosages, behavior was ameliorated but performance on cognitive tasks deteriorated. Recent studies have challenged this (Elia et al., 1991; Tannock et al., 1998), suggesting that both behavior and cognitive performance improve with stimulant treatment, even at higher doses. Response to medication is not diagnostic, however, as hyperactive and non-ADHD children have qualitatively similar behavioral and cognitive responses (Donnelly and Rapoport, 1985).

The scheduling of Ritalin administration also needs to be monitored collaboratively. Typically, Ritalin has been administered twice daily: at home in the morning before school, and at noon by the school nurse. Recently, however, a third (generally smaller) dose after school has been recommended (Swanson, et al., 1995; Stein et al., 1996; Barkley et al., 1991) to help the child through homework and/or to counter a rebound effect when the medication wears off. Parents are advised to keep a record or chart of their child's responsiveness in order to monitor indications of increased tolerance or adverse reactions to the medication.

One problem with giving medication at school is that as children get older they resent having to visit the nurse at lunchtime. In addition to the disruption in their schedule, many fear teasing or rejection by their peers. The understanding (and flexibility) of the nurse and parents may be key, but if the child is too resistant, little will be accomplished. A possible alternative is the Ritalin-SR (sustained release) preparation. Although it has the advantage of being given once per day, some clinicians find it to be somewhat less predictable and less effective than the standard preparation (Pelham et al., 1990).

The school nurse should communicate on a regular basis with the child's physician as well as with parents and the teacher. A youngster's frequent visits to the nurse with complaints of "not feeling well" could signify an adverse reaction to the medication or, just as likely, emotional stress related to school. It should be determined whether the nurse's office is a haven for an unhappy, frustrated student or whether the medication is causing a problem.

Whether to give Ritalin to children only on school days or on weekends too is another issue of concern to parents. The answer depends on the child's behavior at home and on whether an erratic schedule of the drug will be confusing to the child. Because some studies have shown that treatment with stimulants improves a child's social acceptance as well as school performance, it seems expedient to administer it throughout the week, although clearly there are exceptions. If the symptoms are not severe outside the school setting, a medication-free trial, or drug holiday, may be arranged for vacations and summer holidays. The purpose is to minimize side effects as well as to assess the effectiveness of the medication and the need to continue it. If all goes well, it may be suggested that the child return to school without the aid of the drug. Parents and the school must maintain contact, though, in the event that a resusmption of Ritalin is warranted. Some children and adolescents, of course, need to continue the medication all through the year, with camp directors assuming the monitoring during the summer.

In any case, ongoing periodic reassessment is necessary to document change or the lack thereof. At the very least, an annual assessment and review are needed to evaluate the progress, the value of continuing medication, and goals for the following year. Disagreement about the efficacy of treatment is a potential source of conflict between parents and the school that should be discussed on a continuing basis. Parents tend to wish for and sometimes expect "miracles" from Ritalin—that the child will somehow be changed.

Even when the treatment is successful, parents may not report dramatic behavioral changes at home, and children are not always aware of "feeling different." The effects at school, though, generally are more apparent. Teachers are likely to claim that the child is more organized and on task, more compliant to commands, and more responsive to and sociable with classmates (Schachar et al., 1986; Spencer et al., 1996). For children who do respond dramatically to the drug, significant improvement may be observed within a few hours to a day or two after therapy has begun. It is not uncommon for teachers to report changes in attention and social behavior even without prior notification that Ritalin has been administered.

Jennie, a beautiful little 8-year-old girl, is an example. She was diagnosed with "dyslexia" and "dysgraphia" in the 1st grade, and support services had been given each year at school.

Jennie was a polite and compliant child and had never been disruptive in class, but her academic progress had been slow. From the beginning of the school year, though, her teacher complained that she wasn't "paying attention," didn't complete assignments, and frequently put her head on the desk as if she were "tired" or "bored." In a meeting at school, the psychologist expressed concern about Jennie and suggested a medical consultation. Behavioral strategies were also recommended for implementation in the classroom.

On examination, Jennie's physician found her to be in good health but wondered about the possibility of ADHD. I was asked to see Jennie and subsequently concurred that she did meet the criteria for the diagnosis of ADHD–predominantly inattentive type. A trial of Ritalin was prescribed for Jennie, and Jennie's teacher was made aware of the plan but was not told when the Ritalin would be started.

Reports from school after the first day of medication were unequivocally enthusiastic. Jennie stayed alert during the entire reading lesson and wrote almost a page rather than the usual one sentence. Even her handwriting improved. Since then her progress has been dramatic, and today she feels "smarter," to quote her words.

As recent studies have shown, inattentiveness, even more than hyperactivity, is perhaps the cardinal symptom of ADHD and the one most associated with academic difficulties. It is also the symptom most evident in girls, who have been diagnosed in increasing numbers as clinicians become more aware of ADHD-I (Berry et al., 1985; Quinn, 1997). Girls tend not to be hyperactive but rather daydream and "tune out" in class, whereas boys are more likely to be impulsive and hyperactive (Gaub and Carlson, 1997). In addition, girls tend to internalize more and to experience symptoms of anxiety and depression more often than boys (Brown et al., 1991), who are more prone to acting-out behavior and conduct disorders (Hinshaw, 1992).

In addition to benefiting the child, Ritalin may have a secondary gain for teachers and parents. The quality of their interactions with the ADHD child are likely to improve as a consequence of the young person's change in behavior. At home as well as in school, the child is perceived as more manageable, more socially adept, and less disruptive, therefore gaining greater acceptance. At least one study (Schachar et al., 1986) found evidence of increased mother–child contact and decreased maternal criticism of children who responded well to MPH treatment. Although it is not always the case, we have also seen dramatic shifts in family systems following a successful trial of medication.

Parent–teacher communication is a mainstay of treatment during this period. In addition to receiving input from the teacher, parents need to be conscientious in informing teachers when medication is not taken or if other stresses and unusual events are occurring at home. Illness or death in the family, separation, divorce, and even vacations can be particularly difficult situations for hyperactive or ADHD children, affecting their responses to the medication. Noncompliance, including irregular administration of medication, is a potential problem for effective medical management. In our experience, this is less likely to occur when there is a sincere effort on the part of parents and professionals to work together in the interest of the child.

There are still many questions to be answered concerning the etiology, developmental course, outcome, and treatment of ADHD. Despite its effectiveness for most children and adolescents when used appropriately, Ritalin is not a panacea in the treatment of ADHD. Although there is general agreement about the beneficial effects of the drug for the short term, long-term gains remain less certain (Dulcan, 1990). It appears evident, then, that medication should not be used in isolation but rather as part of an integrated plan of therapeutic services. Studies have shown (Weiss and Hechtman, 1986) that with stimulant medication alone, a significant percentage of children with ADHD continue to demonstrate poor school performance, low self-esteem, and poor social relationship with peers. However, behavioral approaches and social skills training in conjunction with medication are promising (Pelham and Murphy, 1986).

Some young people may also need educational therapy, particularly if learning disabilities are involved. Regardless of the child's level of activity, academic skills need to be developed and remedicated. Typically, learning-disabled and ADHD youngsters work and perform best in a small group or one-on-one. Alternative treatments need to be considered, therefore, for use in conjunction with medication, or, in some instances, in lieu of pharmacotherapy.

Various nonmedical therapies have been used successfully for children with attentional problems (Ingersoll and Goldstein, 1993). They include behavior therapy and management, cognitive-behavioral therapy, and combined treatments for the child, as well as family therapy and parent management training. Teaching parents to use behavioral techniques and to cooperate with the school through regular communication can be highly effective. Other alternative treatments remain controversial and lack clear evidence of efficacy or substantial research to support their use (Ingersoll, 1993). They include the use of coffee (caffeine), (Rapoport et al., 1984), megavitamins (Cott, 1972), and special diets (Feingold, 1974; Mattes, 1983). Most of the studies comparing pharmacotherapy with contingency management strategies have found medication to be most effective (Gittelman-Klein et al., 1976), although a few have found the treatments to be equivalent (O'Leary and Pelham, 1978).

A relatively large body of research has been conducted using a combination of medical and behavioral intervention (Lalongo et al., 1993; Gadow, 1985; Gittelman-Klein, 1996; Pelham and Murphy, 1986; Satterfield et al., 1981). Although drug therapy has the best-documented record of success in treating ADHD children, studies suggest that a multifaceted approach consisting of education, behavioral interventions, parenting skills training, social skills training, and thrice-daily MPH dosing, is likely to result in more improvements in behavior and social, emotional, and academic functioning than does medication alone (Abikoff, 1991; Satterfield et al., 1981; Wender, 1987).

TERMINATION

How and when the decision is made to terminate medication has been less than systematically reported in the literature. Clinical reports suggest that therapeutic improvement or the lack thereof, may not, in fact, be the primary reason for ending drug therapy (Gadow, 1986). Frequently it is the parents, rather than the physician, who decide to terminate the drug. Lack of effectiveness of the medication, concerns about continuing medication, and rebound or side effects are cited as reasons for ceasing therapy. During adolescence, it may be the youngster who stops the medication, refusing to take it any longer. The typical teenager simply does not want to feel "different" (Sleator et al., 1981; Osman, 1997) or to acknowledge that he/she has a problem that requires a medical intervention. Then, too, as indicated earlier, many adolescents express the fear that subjugation to the pill means losing control over their own lives. They need to know that neither the problems they may be experiencing nor the medication they may be taking should allow them to disavow responsibility for their behavior.

On the positive side, most young people eventually do "outgrow" the need for drug therapy. Although the duration of treatment varies significantly from person to person, there does come a time when it may no longer be necessary. As in prescribing the drug initially, the decision to discontinue the therapy should be made by consensus of the family, the physician, and the school. Of course, older adolescents generally make their own decisions.

CONCLUSION

Children and adolescents with ADHD represent a diverse group with a broad range of needs. To appropriately serve them, clinical practice and care must be coordinated as well as individualized. Although the efficacy of MPH has been well researched and reported for this group, it is not a panacea for all youngsters. To determine the most appropriate form or forms of intervention, a multidisciplinary evaluation must be made of the child, the family, and the educational setting.

To implement recommendations for treatment, a plan for monitoring and evaluating the therapy or therapies is critical. With the physician in charge of prescription and titration of medical treatment, referral to—and communication with—other professionals are necessary for appropriate coordination of care. The interactions between family, school personnel, and physician actually are not different from those for children with other medical problems. The goal is to provide interventions that are realistic as well as beneficial to the child, the family, and the school.

REFERENCES

Abikoff, H. (1991), Interaction of Ritalin and multimodal therapy in the treatment of attention deficit-hyperactive behavioral disorders. In: *Ritalin: Theory and Patient Management*, eds. L.L. Greenhill and B.B. Osman. Larchmont, NY: Mary Ann Liebert, Inc., pp. 147–154.

Achenbach, T.M. (1993), *Empirically Based Taxonomy: How to Use Syndromes and Profile Types Derived from e 1991 CBCL.* Burlington, VT: University of Vermont, Department of Psychiatry, 4–18.

American Academy of Child and Adolescent Psychiatry (1997), Practice parameters for the assessment and treatment of children, adolescents and adults with attention-deficit/hyperactivity disorder. *J. Am. Acad. Child Adolesc. Psychiatry*, 36:855–1215.

American Psychiatric Association (1994), *Diagnostic and Statistical Manual of Mental Disorders, 4th ed. (DSM-IV).* Washington, DC: American Psychiatric Association.

Arnold, L.E. & Jensen, P.S. (1995), Attention deficit disorders. In: *Comprehensive Textbook of Psychiatry, 6th ed.*, eds., H. Kaplan & B. Sadock. Baltimore: Williams & Wilkins, pp. 2295–2310.

Baren, M. (1994), Managing ADHD. *Contemporary Pediatr.*, 11:29–48.

Barkley, R.A. (1990), *Attention Deficit Hyperactivity Disorder: A Handbook for Diagnosis and Treatment.* New York: Guilford Press.

Barkley, R.A., DuPaul, G.J. & McMurray, M.B. (1991), Attention deficit disorder with and without hyperactivity: Clinical response to three doses levels of methylphenidate. *Pediatrics*, 87:519–531.

Berry, C.A., Shaywitz, S.E. & Shaywitz, B.A. (1985), Girls with attention deficit disorder: A silent minority? A report on behavioral and cognitive characteristics. *Pediatrics*, 76:801–809.

Biederman, J., Faraone, S.V. & Lapey, K. (1992), Comorbidity of diagnosis in attention-deficit hyperactivity disorder. *Child Adolesc. Psychiatr. Clin. North Am.*,

Biederman, J., Faraone, S., Millberger, S., et al. (1996), A prospective four-year follow-up study of attention deficit hyperactivity and related disorders. *Arch. Gen. Psychiatry*, 53:437–446.

Brown, R.T., Bolden, K.A. & Clingerman, S.R. (1985), Pharmacotherapy in ADD adolescents with special attention to multimodality treatment. *Psychopharmacol. Bull.*, 21:192–211.

Brown, R.T., Madan-Swain, A. & Baldwin, K. (1991), Gender differences in a clinic referred sample of attention deficit disordered children. *Child Psychiatry Hum. Dev.*, 22:111–128.

Brown, T. (1996), *Brown Attention Deficit Disorder Scales: Manual.* San Antonio, TX: Psychological Corporation.

Buitelaar, J.K., Van der Gaag, R.J., Swab-Barneveld, H. & Kuiper, M. (1995), Prediction of clinical response to methylphenidate in children with attention-deficit hyperactivity disorder. *J. Am. Acad. Child Adolesc. Psychiatry*, 8:1025–1032.

Cantwell, D.P. (1996), Attention deficit disorder: A review of the past 10 years. *J. Am. Acad. Child Adolesc. Psychiatry*, 35:978–988.

Conners, K.C. (1997), Conner's Rating Scales—Revised. New York: Multi-Health Systems.

Copps, S. (1992), *The Attending Physician Attention Deficit Disorder: A Guide for Pediatrician and Family Physicians.* Atlanta, GA: SPI Press.

Cott, A. (1972), Megavitamins: The orthomolecular approach to behavioral disorders and learning disabilities. *Academic Therapy*, 7:245–258.

Donnelly, M. & Rapoport, J.L. (1986), Attention deficit disorders. In: *Diagnosis and Psychopharmacology of Children and Adolescent Disorders*, ed., T.M. Weiner. New York: John Wiley & Sons, Inc., pp. 178–197.

Douglas, V.I., Barr, R.G., Amin, K., O'Neill, M.E. & Britton, B.G. (1988), Dosage effects and individual responsitivity to methylphenidate in attention deficit disorder. *J. Child. Psychol. Psychiatry*, 29:453–475.

Dulcan, M.K. (1990), Using psychostimulants to treat behavioral disorders of children and adolescents with attention deficit disorder. *Psychiatr. Ann.,* 15:69–87.

Elia, J., Borcherding, B.G., Rapoport, J.L. & Keysor, C.S. (1991), Methylphenidate and dextroamphetamine treatments of hyperactivity: Are there true non-responders? *Psychiatr. Res.*, 36:141–155.

Feingold, B.F. (1974), *Why Your Child is Hyperactive.* New York: Random House.

Gadow, K.D. (1992), Pediatric psychopharmacology: A review of recent research. *J. Child Psychol. Psychiatry*, 33:153–195.

Gadow, K.D. (1985), Relative efficacy of pharmacological, behavioral and combination treatments for enhancing academic performance. *Clin. Psych. Rev.* 5:513–533.

Gadow, K.D. (1986), *Children on Medication, vol. 1,* Boston: College Hill Press, Inc., pp. 1–95.

Gadow, K.D., Nolan, E. et al. (1995), School observations of children with attention deficit disorder and comorbid tic disorder: Effects of methylphenidate treatment. *J. Dev. Behav. Ped.*, 16:167–176.

Gadow, K., Sverd, J., Nolan, E. & Ezor, S. (1995), Efficacy of methylphenidate for ADHD in children with tic disorder. *Arch. Gen. Psychiatry,* 52:444–455.

Gaub, M. & Carlson, L.L. (1997), Gender differences in ADHD: Meta-analysis and critical review. *J. Am. Acad. Child & Adolesc. Psychiatry*, 36:1036–1045.

Gittelman-Klein, B., Klein, D.F., Katz, S., Saraf, K. & Pollack, E. (1976). Comparative effects of methylphenidate and thorazine in hyperkinetic children: I. clinical results. *Arch. Gen. Psychiatry*, 33:1217–1231.

Gordon, M., McClure, F. & Post, E. (1986), *Interpretive Guide to the Gordon Diagnostic System*, DeWitt, NY: Gordon Systems.

Greenhill, L.L. (1995), Attention deficit/hyperactivity disorder: The stimulants. *Child Adolesc. Psychiatr. Clin.*, 4:123–168.

Greenhill, L.L. (1992), Pharmacotherapy: Stimulants. In: *Attention Deficit Hyperactivity Disorder*, ed. G. Weiss. Philadelphia: W.B. Saunders, pp. 411–447.

Greenhill, L.L. & Osman, B.B. (1991), *Ritalin: Theory and Patient Management.* Larchmont, NY: Mary Ann Liebert, Inc.

Hechtman, L. (1992), Long-term outcome in attention-deficit hyperactivity disorder. *Psychiatr. Clin. North Am.* 1:553–565.

Hinshaw, S.P., Heller, T. & McHale, J.P. (1992), Covert antisocial behavior in boys with attention deficit hyperactivity disorder, external validation and effects of methylphenidate. *J. Consult. Clin. Psychol.*, 60:274–281.

Hinshaw, S.P., Henker, B. & Whalen, C.K. (1984), Cognitive-behavioral and pharmacologic interventions for hyperactive boys: Comparative and combined effects. J. Consult. Clin. Psychol. 52:739–749.

Hodges, K. (1993), Structured interviews for assessing children. *J. Child. Psychol. Psychiatry*, 34:49–68.

Ingersoll, B.D. & Goldstein, S. (1993), *Attention Deficit Disorder and Learning Disabilities: Realities, Myths, and Controversial Treatments*. New York: Doubleday.

Jensen, P.S. (1999), Pediatric psychopharmacology in the United States: Issues and challenges in the diagnosis and treatment of Attention Deficit Hyperactivity Disorder. In eds. L.L. Greenhill & B.B. Osman *Ritalin: Theory and Practice, 2nd ed.*, Larchmont, New York: Mary Ann Liebert, Inc., pp. 1–3.

Jensen, P.S., Irwin, R.A.C. & Josephson, A.D. (1996), Data-gathering tools for real world clinical settings. *J. Am. Acad. Child Adolesc. Psychiatry*, 35:55–66.

Jensen, P.S., Kettle, L., Roper, M., Sloan, M., Dulcan, M., Hoverr, C., Bird, H. & Baumeister, J. (1999, in review), Suffer the restless children: Attention Deficit/Hyperactivity Disorder and its treatment in four U.S. communities.

Jensen, P.S., Martin, D. & Cantwell, D.P. (1997), Comorbidity of ADHD: implications for research, practice and DSM-V. *J. Am. Acad. Child & Adolesc. Psychiatry*, 36:1065–1079.

Konkol, R., Fischer, M. & Newby, R. (1990), Double-blind, placebo-controlled stimulant trial in children with Tourette's syndrome and ADHD [abstr]. *Am. Neurolog.* 28:424.

Lalongo, N.S., Horn, W.F., Pascoe, J.M., et al. (1993), The effects of a multimodal intervention with attention-deficit hyperactivity disorder children: A 9 month follow-up. *J. Am. Acad. Child Adolesc. Psychiatry*, 32:182–189.

Levy, F. & Ward, P.B. (1995), Neurometrics, dynamic brain imaging and attention deficit hyperactivity disorder. *J. Pediatr Child Health*, 31:279–283.

Mash, E.J., & Johnson, C. (1983), Parental perceptions of child behavior problems, parenting self-esteem, and mother's reported stress in younger and older hyperactive and normal children. *J. Consult. Clin. Psych.*, 51:86–99.

Mattes, J.A. (1983). The Feingold diet: A current reappraisal. *J. Learn. Disabil.*, 16:319–323.

National Academy of Sciences Proceedings. (Nov. 1998) Selective effects of methylphenidate in attention deficit hyperactivity disorder: A functional magnetic resonance study. 95: 14494–14499.

Nottelmann, E. & Jensen, P. (1995), Comorbidity of disorders in children and adolescents: Developmental perspectives. *Adv. Clin. Psychol.* 17:109–155.

O'Leary, S.G. & Pelham, W.E. (1978), Behavior therapy and withdrawal of stimulant medication with hyperactive children. *J. Pediatrics*, 61:211–217.

Osman, B.B. (1995), *No One to Play With: Social Problems of LD/ADD Children.* Novato, CA: Academic Therapy Publications.

Osman, B.B. (1997), *Learning Disabilities and ADHD: A Family Guide to Living and Learning Together*. New York: John Wiley & Sons, Inc.

Pelham, W.E., Jr., Carlson, C., Sams, S.E., Vallano, G., Dixon, J. & Hoza, B. (1993), Separate and combined effects of methylphenidate and behavior modification on boys with attention deficit-hyperactivity disorder in the classroom. *J. Consult. Clin. Psychol.*, 61:506–515.

Pelham, W.E., Jr., Greenslade, K.E., Vodde-Hamilton, M.A., Murphy, D.A., Greenstein, J.J., Gnagy, E.M. & Dahl, R.E. (1990), Relative efficacy of long-acting stimulants on children with attention deficit hyperactivity disorder: A comparison of standard methylphenadate, sustained-release methylphenidate, sustained-release dextroamphetamine, and pemoline. *Pediatrics*, 86:226–236.

Pelham, W.E., Jr. & Murphy, H.A. (1986), Behavioral and pharmacological treatment of attention deficit and conduct disorders. In: *Pharmacological and Behavioral Treatment: An Integrative Approach*, ed., Hersen, M. NY: John Wiley & Sons, Inc., pp. 108–148.

Pelham, W.E., Jr., Sturgess, J. & Hoza, J. (1987), The effects of sustained release 20 and 10 mg: Ritalin on cognitive and social behavior in children with attention deficit disorders. *Pediatrics*, 40:491–501.

Pliszka, S.R. (1989), Effect of anxiety on cognition, behavior, and stimulant response in ADHD. *J. Am. Acad. Child Adolesc. Psychiatry*, 28:882–887.

Polling, A., Gadow, K.D. & Cleary, J. (1991), *Drug Therapy for Behavior Disorders*, Elmsford, NY: Pergamon Press, Inc., pp. 90–108.

Quinn, P.O. (1997), *Attention Deficit Disorder: Diagnosis and Treatment from Infancy to Adulthood*. New York: Bruner/Mazel.

Rapaport, J.L., Berg, C.J., Ismond, D.R., Zahn, T.P. & Neims, A. (1984), Behavioral effects of caffeine in children. *Arch. Gen. Psychiatry*, 41:1073–1079.

Safer, D.J., Zito, J.M. & Fine, E. (1996), Increased methylphenidate use for attention deficit disorder in the '90s. *Pediatrics*, 98:1084–1088.

Satterfield, J.H., Satterfield, B.T. & Cantwell, D. (1981), Three year multimodality treatment study of 100 hyperactive boys. *J. Pediatr.*, 98:650–655.

Schachar, R., Hoppe, C. & Schell, A. (1995), Changes in family function and relationships in children who respond to methylphenidate. *J. Am. Acad. Child Adolesc. Psychiatry*, 26:728–732.

Schachar, R., Sanberg, S. & Rutter, M. (1986), Agreement between teachers' ratings and observations of hyperactivity, inattentiveness and defiance. *J. Abnorm. Psychol.*, 14:331–345.

Shaywitz, S.E., Holahan, J.M., Marchione, K.E., Sadler, A.E., & Shaywitz, B.A. (1992) The Yak Children's Inventory: Normative data and their implications for the diagnosis of attention deficit disorder in children. In: *Attention Deficit Disorder Comes of Age: Toward the Twenty-First Century*, eds., S. E. Shaywitz & B.A. Shaywitz. Austin, TX: PRO-ED, pp. 29–67.

Shaywitz, B.A. & Shaywitz, S.E. (1991), Comorbidity: A critical issue in attention deficit disorder. *J. Child Neurol.* 6 (suppl.):S13–S22.

Silver, L. (1992), *Attention-Deficit Hyperactivity Disorder: A Clinical Guide to Diagnosis and Treatment*. Washington, DC: American Psychiatric Press.

Sleator, E.K. & Ullmann, R.K. (1981), Can the physician diagnose hyperactivity in the office? *Pediatrics*, 67:13–17.

Solanto, M.V. (1999), Dose-response effects of Ritalin on cognitive self-regulation, learning and memory, and academic performance. In *Ritalin: Theory and Practice, 2nd ed.*, eds. L.L. Greenhill & B.B. Osman. Larchmont, NY: Mary Ann Liebert, Inc., pp. 219–235.

Spencer, T., Biederman, J., Wilens, T., Harding, M., O'Donnell, D. & Griffen, S. (1996), Pharmacotherapy of attention-deficit hyperactivity disorder across the life cycle. *J. Am. Acad. Child Adolesc. Psychiatry*, 35:409–432.

Spencer, T., Wilens, T. & Biederman, J. (1995), Psychotropic medication for children and adolescents. *Child Adolesc. Psychiatr. Clin. North Am.*, 1:97.

Sprague, R.L. & Sleator, E.K. (1977), Methylphenidate in hyperkinetic children: Differences in dose effects on learning and social behavior. *Science*, 198:1274.

Stein, M., Blondis, T.A., Schnitzler, E., O'Brien, T. Fishkin, J., Blackwell, B., Szumowski, E. & Roizen, N. (1996), Methylphenidate dosing: Twice daily versus three times daily. *Pediatrics*, 98:748–756.

Sverd, J., Gadow, K., Nolan, E., Spratkin, J. & Ezor, S. (1992), Methylphenidate in hyperactive boys with comorbid tic disorders. *Adv. Neurol.*, 58:271–282.

Swanson, J.M., Cantwell, D., Lerner, M., McBurnett, K. & Hanna, G. (1991), Effects of stimulant medication on learning in children with ADHD. *J. Learn. Disabil.*, 24:219–230.

Swanson, J.M., McBurnett, K., Christian, D.L. & Wigal, T. (1995), Stimulant medications and the treatment of children with ADHD. *Adv. Clin. Child Psychol.*, 17:265–322.

Swanson, J.M., Sergeant, S.A., Taylor, E., Sonega-Barke, E.J., Jensen, P.S. & Cantwell, D.P. (1998), Attention-deficit hyperactivity disorder and hyperkinetic disorder. *Lancet*, 355:429–433.

Tannock, R. (1994), Attention deficit disorders with anxiety disorders. In: *Subtypes of Attention Deficit Disorders in Children, Adolescents, and Adults*, ed., T.E. Brown. New York: American Psychiatric Press.

Tannock, R. (1998), ADHD: Advances in cognitive, neurobiological, and genetic research. *J. Child. Psychol. Psychiatry*, 39:65–99.

Ullmann, R. & Sleater, E. (1986), Responders, non-responders and placebo responders among children with ADD. *Clin. Pediatr.*, 25:594–599.

Vitiello, B. & Jensen, P.S. (1995), Psychopharmacology in children and adolescents: Current problems, future prospects: summary notes on the 1995 NIMH-FDA Conference. *J. Child Adolesc. Psychopharmacol.*, 5:5–7.

Weiss, G. & Hechtman, L.T., (1986), *Hyperactive Children Grown Up*. New York: Guilford Press, p. 186.

Wender, P.H. (1987), *The Hyperactive Child, Adolescent and Adult*. New York: Oxford University Press.

Werry, J. (1988), Imipramine and methylphenidate in hyperactive children. *J. Child Psychol. Psychiatry*, 21:27–35.

Wilens, T.E. & Biederman, J. (1992), The stimulants. *Pediatr Psychopharamcol.*, 15:191–222.

Wilens, T.E., Spencer, T., Biederman, J., Wozniak, J., & Connor, D. (1995), Combined psychotherapy: An emerging trend in pediatric psychopharmacology. *J. Am. Acad. Child Adolesc. Psychiatry*, 34:110–112.

Zito, J.M., dosReis, S.M., Safer, D.J., Zarin, D.M. & Riddle, M.A. (1997), Psychotropic treatment patterns for youth with attentional disorders based on United States physicians office visits [abstr.]. *Psychopharmacol. Bull.*, 33:608.

Section 5

Ritalin Effects in Children with Attention Deficit Hyperactivity Disorder

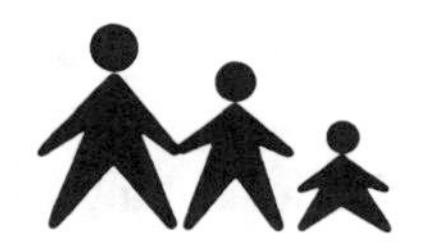

Prediction and Measurement of Individual Responses to Ritalin by Children and Adolescents with Attention Deficit Hyperactivity Disorder

WILLIAM E. PELHAM, JR.[1] and BRADLEY H. SMITH[2]

INTRODUCTION

The general conclusions and recommendations presented by Pelham and Milich (1991) in the first edition of this book remain unchanged; however, the current chapter includes several noteworthy revisions. Empirical research by independent investigators clearly support the findings and conclusions of Pelham and Milich (1991), but many important studies were not available when the first edition of this book was completed. Therefore, the literature review has been updated to include pertinent studies. Additionally, studies completed in the last several years have established that adolescents with attention deficit hyperactivity disorder (ADHD) have responses to Ritalin that are similar to those of children with ADHD (e.g., Smith et al., 1998a). In recognition of these research developments, we have expanded the focus of the chapter to include adolescents diagnosed with ADHD. Finally, research completed in the last few years has revealed some potential limitations of rating scales that were not discussed in the earlier chapter. These new findings are discussed in this new chapter, and we make a forceful argument for including direct measures of social behavior and academic performance when assessing individual responses of children and adolescents with ADHD to stimulant medication.

To make room for the additional material in this chapter, the experiment reported in the previous edition has been reduced to a summary. The case studies from the first edition are retained in their original form, except that additional information has been added to one of the cases. The additional information was generated when Andy, described later in Case 3, completed a medication assessment in a summer treatment program (STP) for adolescents. His case example therefore compares medication effects measured in comparable settings during childhood and adolescence.

THREE APPROACHES TO SELECTING A DOSE OF RITALIN

The key question facing most practitioners working with an ADHD patient is how to decide whether a psychostimulant should be included as a component of the child's or adolescent's treatment. Attempts to answer the question have varied, with three types of responses predominating. First, many professionals simply prescribe medication following traditional guidelines (e.g., start with a low dose and work upward), use minimal or no standard monitoring procedures to assess acute therapeutic effects, haphazardly assess the side

[1]Department of Psychology, State University of New York at Buffalo, Buffalo, New York.
[2]Department of Psychology, University of South Carolina, Columbia, South Carolina.

effects, and provide minimal monitoring of maintenance doses and compliance with treatment. Presumably, these professionals assume that the 70% positive response rate reported in the literature is sufficiently high, that the primary source of information (i.e., parents) will be dependable, that the dose-response curve will be linear, that potential adverse effects will be easily detected, and that compliance with medication will be nearly flawless.

Research in the past few years strongly suggests that the traditional approach to medication titration is inadequate. To begin with, open trials tend to overestimate medication efficacy (Greenberg et al., 1992). Second, dose-response curves appear to be asymptotic: as doses are increased the amount of incremental improvement decreases but the risk of clinically significant side effects increases (Smith et al., 1998a). Third, response to stimulant medication is complex, and one area of functioning may improve while another fails to improve or even deteriorates. Therefore, reliance primarily on a single source of information (e.g., parent report), as is common in the traditional approach, may fail to detect harmful effects. Fourth and finally, haphazard administration of medication can completely undermine the validity of a trial of stimulant medication, and compliance with stimulant prescriptions is very poor (e.g., Sherman and Hertzig, 1991). Thus, for several reasons, practitioners who rely on the traditional approach should seriously consider adopting alternative methods for selecting a dose of stimulant medication.

A second approach to deciding whether medication is useful has usually taken place in research settings and has involved attempting to find base-state measures that predict responses to medication. This approach assumes that a static measure made in the office or laboratory can identify individual characteristics of children or adolescents with ADHD that can be entered into an algorithm that will select which dose, if any, is appropriate for that individual. Indeed, early reviews suggested that ADHD children's response to stimulant medication could be predicted from base state information such as severity of the child's attention deficit (e.g., Hastings and Barkley, 1978). Further, clinical lore has long held that putative indices of organicity such as "soft" neurologic signs could be used to determine whether a child would respond to a stimulant. However, systematic research has failed to support this belief. No physiologic, neurologic, or psychologic measures of functioning have been identified that are reliable predictors of response to psychostimulants (Greenhill 1995, Spencer et al., 1996; see Solanto, 1984, and Zametkin and Rapoport, 1987, for reviews). It is the case that some individual characteristics (e.g., age) are correlated with response to medication, but the correlations are not large enough to facilitate clinical prediction (e.g., Taylor et al., 1987). Thus, agreement is becoming general that responses to stimulant medication by children and adolescents with ADHD cannot be predicted with accuracy from any baseline measure or individual characteristic. Until replicated, high-quality studies show otherwise, practitioners should not use base-state or individual differences measures to select doses of stimulant medication.

A third approach to deciding whether to medicate an ADHD child has become widely advocated in recent years. This approach involves conducting a brief, controlled trial to measure the child or adolescent's acute response to medication, and making a decision regarding a long-term regimen based on the results of the initial trial. The advantages of this tactic are obvious—systematic and controlled information regarding individual response is exactly what the clinician needs in order to decide whether to prescribe medication. However, this approach itself raises a series of questions. What procedures should be used to conduct such an assessment? What variables should be measured to evaluate a child's response? This latter question is a basic one that involves logic similar to that underlying the attempt to find base-state predictors of response; specifically, is there a single measure or are there a few easy-to-collect measures of response to medication that can adequately predict response on all important domains of functioning? These are important questions with both theoretical and practical implications.

With respect to the practical implications, for some time we have advocated employing comprehensive measures of stimulant effects in children and adolescents as part of a detailed initial assessment of treatment effectiveness (e.g., Pelham, 1982, 1986; Pelham and Hoza, 1987). The general design of these studies is a medication trial (i.e., no medication vs. one or more doses of medication), preferably with multiple replication of conditions in randomized order to control for order effects, random events, and the high degree of individual variability in behavior typically exhibited by children and adolescents with ADHD. The major refinements of this method are the choice of setting and measures employed.

One approach has involved measuring medication response on a large number of ecologically relevant variables on children and adolescents in a STP (Pelham and Hoza, 1987). The measures employed in the STP include direct measures of academic performance, percentage of time observed on-task in the classroom, observed frequencies of social behavior, computerized tests of learning and attention, and ratings completed by parents, STP counselors, and STP classroom teachers. This comprehensive approach has been recognized as a model treatment program (Pelham et al., 1996) and is the most comprehensive and scientifically dependable approach to measuring response to stimulant medication that has been used widely with children and adolescents with ADHD. A major limitation of the STP, however, is that it is difficult to implement because it requires a specialized setting and staff.

Several less intensive alternatives to the STP have been developed for outpatient assessments of response to stimulant medication. For example, some authors have suggested that a single measure of learning administered in the doctor's office is the best way to assess drug effects (e.g., Swanson et al., 1978, 1983). Still others have suggested that one or two measures taken in the doctor's office and/or a parent or teacher rating provide an adequate assessment (e.g., Barkley et al., 1988; Rapport et al., 1985; Sleator, 1986).

Protocols that use a limited number of easy-to-collect measures cost less and are easier to implement than drug evaluation protocols that are based on direct measures of social behavior or academic performance in the natural environment. However, lower cost does not necessarily mean that the measures are more cost effective. In order to be ecologically and clinically valid, measures must reliably predict drug response in the child or adolescent's natural environment. Unfortunately for the simplicity of measuring individual responses to stimulants, research indicates that measures that can be collected in the doctor's office have questionable ecologic validity. For example, traditional laboratory tasks, such as the Continuous Performance Task (CPT) and the Matching Familiar Figures Test (MFFT), account for minimal variance in parent and teacher ratings of inattention and overactivity (see Barkley, 1991 for a review). It is also disturbing that the computerized tests do not have any incremental validity for predicting direct measures of academic performance and social behavior beyond what is predicted by parent and teacher ratings of ADHD symptoms and related behaviors (Pelham and Milich, 1991). Furthermore, the magnitude of the correlations between computerized tests and ecologically valid measures diminishes with age, and many of the correlations become nonsignificant when age and IQ are partialed out of the relationship (Barkley, 1991). Therefore, computerized tests of inattention and impulsivity are not clinically valid measures of response to stimulants and should not be used to titrate doses of medication.

Although rating scales lack the scientific mystique of computerized tests, they appear to be better measures of response to stimulants than other measures routinely used in doctor's offices. Unfortunately, most of the research on the psychometric properties of rating scales has been in the context of diagnostic studies. For distinguishing between individuals with or without ADHD, rating scales developed for children with ADHD appear to have acceptable, if not good, ecologic validity (Atkins et al., 1985; Barkley, 1991). Research on ratings scales for adolescents is in its formative stages, and the scales for children may not be appropriate for adolescents (Conners, 1985). Moreover, very little research has addressed the validity of ratings used in the context of intensive studies of response to medication (e.g., with repeated measures and multiple crossovers of medication condition).

There are numerous methodological limitations to ratings, and most of these limitations have been discussed in detail elsewhere (e.g., Barkley, 1991). Research completed in our laboratory in the past few years sheds some new light on the validity of ratings and associated procedures for enhancing the validity of ratings. Moreover, this research has uncovered several limitations of ratings, of which many researchers and practitioners may not be aware.

For quite some time, researchers have commented that rating scales may generate different dose-response curves than direct measures of behaviors (e.g., Hinshaw, 1991; Pelham and Milich, 1991; Greenhill and Osman, 1991; Rapport et al., 1987). We recently completed a dose-response study of the effects of methylphenidate (MPH) treatment on adolescents with ADHD (Evans et al., in review; Smith et al., 1998a). In these studies, linear dose-response curves achieved the best fit on rating scales, and plateau-shaped curves achieved the best fit for observed frequency counts of behavior. The implications of this methodological phenomenon are striking. For example, if rating scales are used to measure impulsivity, a provider is likely to follow a linear dosing schedule and to give progressively higher doses until either a therapeutic effect is achieved or negative side effects preclude higher doses. On the other hand, if observed behavior frequencies are used with the expectation that there is a plateau-shaped dose-response curve, once the pivotal dose where the curve flattens has been exceeded, the practitioner should begin considering alternative treatments to Ritalin.

The differences in the dose-response curves for rating and frequency count measurement methods raise the possibility that exclusive reliance on rating scales and associated linear dose-response expectations can lead to excessively high doses of stimulants for children and adolescents with ADHD. The next logical question is this: "Which measurement method is more dependable, ratings or direct measures?" There are many well-known reasons to trust the validity of direct measures over ratings (see Barkley, 1991, for a review). Furthermore, recent research on children and adolescents with ADHD indicates that direct measures are superior to ratings when used to assess individual differences in response to medication.

In a placebo-controlled, double-blind, crossover study of the effects of Ritalin on the behavior and academic performance in STP and regular classroom settings, Pelham and colleagues uncovered a perplexing phenomenon. Initial teacher ratings placed the ADHD children in the pathologic range; however, with repeated completion of the rating instrument, the scores went well below baseline and into the normative range (Pelham et al., in review). The drift downward was so severe that after a few weeks of daily assessments, the teachers' ratings no longer differentiated between placebo and medication conditions (i.e., at least 0.3 mg/kg of Ritalin). In contrast, the levels of negative behavior as defined by objective criteria in daily report cards (DRC) remained steady on placebo days. More importantly, the DRC data distinguished between placebo and medication conditions throughout the study. Thus, exclusive reliance on rating scales may threaten the internal validity of medication assessments because ratings may show a spurious trend toward less pathologic scores. A possible clinical consequence of this measurement method effect is that in traditional medication titration (i.e., open trials starting with a low dose and moving to progressively higher doses), reliance on ratings can result in overdosing.

Another reason to include direct measures in medication evaluations is the potential for incremental improvements in predictions over rating data. Although parent and teacher ratings have proved to be pretty good predictors of long-term negative outcomes related to ADHD, direct measures may be even better. For example, data pertinent to this issue were generated by a follow-up study designed to examine the predictors of the onset and severity of substance use disorders among adolescents who were treated in the Pittsburgh STP when they were children. Preliminary analysis of these data (Molina, unpublished data) indicates that parent and teacher ratings on the Disruptive Behavior Disorders (DBD) scale (Pelham et al., 1992), explained only 5% to 8% of the variance in alcohol use. On the contrary, the observed behavioral measures (i.e., frequency of following activity rules, negative verbalizations, and noncompliance with adult requests) predicted between 10% and 26% of the variance in alcohol use. Furthermore, the observed behavior frequency measures were statistically significant predictors of alcohol use even when the DBD ratings were forced into the regression equation ahead of the behavior frequency measures. These findings further bolster our confidence in the use of direct measures of behavior.

It should be emphasized that rather than seeking the "single best measure" of response to treatment, we strongly endorse a multivariate approach to assessing stimulant treatment effects and side effects. Multivariate measurement strategies such as the Multitrait-Multimethod approach of Campbell and Fiske (1959) analyzed with modern statistical methods (see Figueredo et al., 1991) can control for many of the limitations and potential systematic biases encountered in studies that rely on a single measure. Moreover, evidence is mounting that response to stimulant medication is not a unitary phenomenon. For example, behavioral and academic domains may show different dose-response trends (Douglas et al., 1988; Hinshaw et al., 1989; Pelham and Milich, 1991; Pelham et al., 1987; Rapport et al., 1987; Rapport et al., 1994; Tannock et al., 1989). Furthermore, there are some indications that dosage effects may vary within these broadly defined domains, such as verbal compared with physical aggression (Hinshaw, 1991). Thus, we recommend using multiple measurement methods (e.g., ratings and direct measures), multiple informants (e.g., parents and teachers), multiple settings (e.g., structured activities and free play), and multiple domains of functioning (e.g., academic performance, inattention, and defiance). All four of these facets of measurement have been shown to affect putative responses of ADHD children to stimulant medication (Hinshaw, 1991; Pelham, 1993).

We also emphasize that demonstrating statistically significant change is not sufficient for documenting response to stimulant medication. In order to justify the use of stimulant medication, the changes must be clinically significant and should be indicative of functional improvements. One of the measures we use most often to measure clinically significant change is the DRC. This measure can be used to describe the percentage of individualized goals met across multiple measures, settings, and sources. Examples of this measure are given in the case studies. Other indications of clinically significant change include showing movement from a pathologic to normative range or using statistical indices of clinically meaningful change such as those described by Jacobson and Truax (1991). These latter two analyses of clinically meaningful change require data from normative control groups, which is often not available. Fortunately, the DRC approach can be used effectively without normative data, and the DRC method is therefore one of the most accessible for individualized assessments of response to medication. In a recent study, Pelham and colleagues found that the DRC measure was an extremely accurate predictor of mediation with response. For example, the odds ratio for a positive DRC was up to 5 times higher for medication (0.3 mg/kg MPH) versus placebo (Pelham et al, in review). Such findings can lead to very confident recommendations for continued treatment with stimulant medication.

A very large number of studies have compared drug-responder and drug-nonresponder groups of ADHD children on biochemical or electrophysiologic measures with the dual goals of discovering the underlying biologic basis for response to stimulants, as well as drawing subsequent inferences about the biologic nature of ADHD (see Zametkin and Rapoport, 1987, for a review). However, most of these studies have defined response to medication on a single measure, such as a learning task (e.g., Swanson et al., 1983) or a teacher rating scale (e.g., Shekim et al., 1982). If these single measures do not reflect a comprehensive response to medication on a full range of appropriate variables and therefore do not reflect the intended underlying neurobiologic variables, then the validity of results from such studies may be seriously compromised. It is likely that the univariate approach to measuring drug response has impaired progress in identifying physiologic markers of ADHD and other theoretical issues related to children and adolescents with ADHD.

Although this may not be an issue for clinical practice, researchers should be advised that analysis of group-level data fails to account for the highly idiosyncratic nature of individual medication response patterns shown by children and adolescents with ADHD (Pelham, 1993; Rapport et al., 1987; Rapport et al., 1994; Swanson et al., 1995). Consequently, stimulant response studies should assess group and individual differences in dose-response trends across multiple measures of functioning. In other words, research reports should include traditional group analyses (e.g., ANOVA) as well as individualized analyses that reflect case-by-case examinations of response to medication. It is possible to have a statistically significant effect of medication at a group level and have less than half of the sample of subjects show a positive response to stimulants.

To conclude this section, out of three widely used approaches to determining whether a child or adolescent with ADHD responds to stimulant medication, we strongly endorse using a brief, intensive assessment conducted in a naturalistic setting using a crossover design with multiple doses, multiple replications of each dose condition, and multiple objective (i.e., nonrating) measures of response. Although we have routinely used a placebo-control condition, recently completed studies employing a balanced-placebo design that crossed expectancy and medication conditions indicate that there is no placebo effect on the objectively recorded behavior or cognitive functioning of children with ADHD (Pelham et al., 1997). That is, boys with ADHD did not behave any differently on days when they were given a placebo and told it was a "real" pill than on days when they were accurately told that the placebo pill was "fake." It is not known whether there are placebo/expectancy effects of medication on parents and teachers, so it is worthwhile to keep individuals who are providing data about medication response blind to the medication condition.

A STUDY DEMONSTRATING THE IMPORTANCE OF DIRECT MEASURES

This section summarizes the study titled "Experiment 1" in the previous edition of this chaper (see Pelham and Milich, 1991, for a more detailed description of the study). The purpose of the experiment was to examine the concurrent and incremental validity of three easy-to-collect and commonly used measures of response to stimulant medication: (1) a continuous performance task (CPT); (2) a laboratory learning task; and (3) the Abbreviated Conners Teacher Rating Scale (ACTRS; Conners, 1973). CPTs have been perhaps the most frequently used laboratory task to measure medication effects in ADHD children, and they have proved to be highly sensitive to medication effects (see Pelham, 1986, for a review). Laboratory learning tasks have been advocated as more conservative measures of medication effects than CPTs (Swanson and Kinsbourne, 1979). The learning task most often used has been a paired-associate learning (PAL) task (e.g., Swanson et al., 1978, 1983). The task employed herein is a nonsense spelling task that provides information regarding medication effects comparable to that obtained with the PAL (e.g., Stephens et al., 1984). The ACTRS has been by far the mostly widely used measure of medication effects in ADHD children. It was originally developed to include items sensitive to drug effects, and it has proved to be highly sensitive to the effects of stimulant medication (see Gittelman and Kanner, 1986, for a review). What is more, the ACTRS is almost universally included when outpatient medication assessment protocols have been proposed.

The study was designed to determine whether the three selected measures, alone or in combination, could reliably predict drug response in a very comprehensive assessment that tapped several important domains of ADHD children's behavior and academic performance. The subjects were 26 boys diagnosed with ADHD who were enrolled in the 1985 STP at the Florida State University and who underwent a double-blind, placebo-controlled assessment of the effects of 0.3 mg/kg MPH given twice a day. In addition to problems with ADHD, 22 subjects were diagnosed as having an oppositional/defiant disorder (ODD) , five were diagnosed as having a conduct disorder, and 12 had a specific learning disability. None of the subjects was mentally retarded or had gross neurologic disorders. The mean IQ (WISC-R) for the group was 98.8 (SD = 14.6), and the mean reading achievement score (Woodcock-Johnson) was 85.9 (SD = 22.2). The mean age of the sample in months was 97.9 (SD = 17.7). The mean ACTRS score was 19.3 (SD = 4.26).

Direct measures of social behavior were gathered in the STP medication assessments (see Pelham and Hoza, 1987, for a detailed description). Briefly, as part of a behavior modification system, counselors recorded the frequencies with which numerous appropriate and inappropriate behaviors occurred daily. The following five categories were derived: (1) following rules, (2) positive peer behaviors (e.g., being a good sport), (3) noncompliance, (4) conduct problems (e.g., aggression), and (5) negative verbalizations (e.g., name-calling/ teasing). Teacher-recorded rates of on-task behavior and rule-following behavior were derived from a response-cost procedure. Furthermore, direct observations were made daily while children were in supervised, recreational periods. The percentages of time that individual children were engaged in positive, negative, or no interactions with their peers were recorded using a modification of the Reprogramming Environmental Contingencies for Effective Social Skills code (Walker et al., 1978).

Direct measures of academic performance were assessed with a timed arithmetic task and reading task, using materials selected as appropriate to each subject's instructional level. The number of arithmetic problems and reading questions attempted and the percentage completed correctly within the allotted time served as the dependent measures. Other daily academic tasks were also individualized according to each child's needs (e.g., language, spelling, additional reading, and arithmetic). Accuracy (percentage correct) and productivity (percentage of assigned seatwork completed) in these tasks were recorded daily.

Teacher ratings on the ACTRS were obtained for each child. Counselor ratings were gathered using a modification of the Revised Behavior Problem Checklist (Quay and Peterson, 1983) that included 35 items characteristic of ADHD and conduct disorders rated on a 7-point scale. Errors of commission and omission on a CPT were also recorded. A learning task in which children were required to learn how to spell a list of nonsense words was also administered once per condition (see Pelham et al., 1986, for a complete description).

In order to determine whether single measures predicted drug response, correlations were computed between two sets of variables: (1) drug effects (placebo score minus drug score) on the classroom teacher's ACTRS scores, errors on the nonsense spelling task, and errors of omission and commission on the CPT; and (2) drug effects (placebo score minus drug score) on the 17 other dependent measures gathered in the day treatment program. In addition to bivariate correlations, partial correlations were computed, with the effects of age and IQ controlled. The bivariate correlations were generally quite low, accounting occasionally for as much as 30% of the variance but usually no more than 10%. Further, after controlling for the effects of age and IQ, only nine of 68 partial correlations were significantly different from zero at the 0.05 level, with an additional eight showing a trend ($p <$ 0.10) toward significance. Many of the remaining 50 correlations (as well as some of the significant ones) were not even in the expected direction.

A differential pattern of change with the partial correlations is noteworthy. There was very little or no reduction in the bivariate correlations involving the nonsense spelling and

CPT. However, the reduction in the *r*s was dramatic for the ACTRS, with many significant correlations losing significance when the covariates were partialed out. We know from other research (Hoza, 1989) that the age covariate rather than the IQ accounts for this relationship. Younger ADHD boys tend to perform/behave worse than older ADHD boys, both in the laboratory and in school settings. When a sample includes a wide age range of children, an apparently large correlation between effects on two measures in which younger children perform more poorly is often a function of age rather than the drug effect per se. The differences between the bivariate and partial correlations between the ACTRS and the Daily Frequencies are very clear examples of such an effect.

Prediction was no better for correlations within domains than for correlations across behavioral domains. For example, the nonsense spelling task was as equally correlated with measures of social behavior, such as noncompliance and following rules in the classroom, as with academic measures, such as seatwork being completed and correct. The ACTRS showed a similar pattern, being equally correlated with measures of disruptive behavior and aca-demic performance. This is quite a surprising outcome. Swanson and colleagues (1991) have argued that tests of learning should be used to guard against adverse *cognitive* effects of stimulants. They have argued that laboratory tasks that tap learning are more highly correlated with academic classroom measures such as seatwork than with overt classroom behavior. We clearly did not obtain that outcome.

Clearly, none of the three single measures of drug response was sufficient when used alone to predict clinical response to medication on the 17 dependent measures. In order to determine whether the nonsense-spelling task, the ACTRS, and the CPT could be combined to improve prediction of the other dependent variables, multiple regressions were conducted for each criterion measure. Age and IQ were entered first, and the amount of additional variance (R^2 change) accounted for by the three predictor variables was measured. In only one of the 17 multiple regressions (following rules in the classroom) did the predictors account for a significant R^2 beyond the variance accounted for by age and IQ. Thus, combining the three variables failed to improve prediction of drug response across all the dependent measures.

In summary, a child's drug response on the ACTRS, a learning task, and a CPT task did not either singly or together reliably predict that child's response on 17 dependent measures of key behaviors gathered in a somewhat naturalistic setting across both classroom and recreational settings. These data show quite clearly that these three commonly recommended and commonly used single measures cannot alone or in combination be used to determine a child's responsivity to psychostimulant medication. Current recommendations for the use of these measures as the sole mechanisms of assessing stimulant response in short-term drug trials therefore lack credibility.

INDIVIDUALIZED MULTIVARIATE STUDIES OF RESPONSES TO STIMULANTS

It is our firm belief that the only adequate procedure for analyzing an ADHD child's response to psychostimulant medication for either clinical or research purposes is to conduct a comprehensive assessment that includes (1) the presenting symptoms (i.e., problems in daily life functioning) on which a change is desired in the patient, and (2) other domains in which a change of medication is unwanted (i.e., side effects). In addition, such an assessment should be conducted in as naturalistic a setting as possible so as to maximize the generalizability of the results to the child's natural setting.

The following case examples from assessments conducted in our STP illustrate how comprehensive assessments can be conducted and interpreted. They also illustrate the clear individual differences in children's responsiveness to stimulants—both across children within domains and within children across domains. As such, the examples provide further indications of the limited utility of some of the single measures of response discussed above.

Case examples

Case 1: Darryl

Darryl was an 11-year-old boy who was brought to the clinic by his mother because of academic difficulties, problems in peer relationships, and oppositional behavior. Darryl had long-standing diagnoses of ADHD and LD, and exhibited his problems in the school setting, even though his mother rated him as exhibiting more extreme symptoms of ADHD than did his teachers. A psychologic report from his school stated that Darryl had a short attention span, was easily distracted, demonstrated inconsistent work, and had few interactions with peers. Darryl had been taking SR-20 Ritalin, prescribed by his pediatrician, for 3 years before coming to the clinic, but he continued to exhibit the problems for which he was referred. During the 1988 STP, Darryl underwent a clinical medication assessment in the context of a protocol in which he received placebo twice daily, 10 mg MPH twice daily, SR-20 Ritalin every morning, 56.25 mg pemoline (Cylert) every morning and 10 mg Dexedrine Spansule every morning (see Pelham et al., 1990a, for a complete description of the protocol). On days on which he received long-acting forms of medication (the latter three), a noontime placebo was also administered. The dependent measures involved in Darryl's assessment were in most respects identical to those described above, with the few changes noted below.

The results of Darryl's medication assessment are shown in Table 1 and Figure 1. As indicated in Table 1, Darryl showed no response to medication on most dependent measures. For example, he demonstrated very high rates of rule following on placebo days, and these rates did not change with medication. He also had very low rates of negative behavior such as noncompliance, conduct problems, and negative verbalizations, and medication could not improve his behavior further. As might be expected from Darryl's low rates of negative behaviors, his counselors rated him very positively with placebo, and this rating did not change with medication. On one important measure of social functioning, positive peer interactions, Darryl showed a dramatic adverse effect of medication. He had a relatively low rate of positive peer interactions on placebo days, and this rate decreased markedly on medication days and was accompanied by concurrent increases in variability. As Table 1 indicates, Darryl was also considerably less likely to meet his daily report criteria with medication than with placebo, with the percentage of days that he received a positive report decreasing from 71% on placebo days to between 25% and 50% on active medication days. The criteria established for a positive daily report specifically targeted Darryl's primary presenting problems.

On measures of academic performance gathered in the classrooms, Darryl again showed either no response to medication or an adverse response. On placebo days, Darryl performed exceptionally well in seatwork completion and percentage of seatwork correct. In contrast, on each of the four medication conditions, he showed significant decreases in seatwork accuracy and/or completion. For example, his accuracy on 10-mg Ritalin days decreased by 5 standard deviations from his placebo level. Similarly, on days on which he received SR-20 Ritalin, he showed decreases of 0.5 and 1.5 standard deviations for seatwork completion and accuracy, respectively. Clearly, all four active medications had substantial adverse effects on productivity, accuracy, or both in Darryl's seatwork performance in the classroom.

Table 1. Results of the Clinical Medication Assessment for Case 1: Darryl

Variable Measured	*Placebo b.i.d. 7 Days*		*10 mg Methylphenidate b.i.d. 5 Days*		*SR-20 Ritalin q.A.M. 4 Days*		*56.25 mg Pemoline q.A.M. 5 Days*		*10 mg Dexedrine Spansule q.A.M. 4 Days*	
	Mean	*SD*	*Mean*	*SD*	*Mean*	*SD*	*Mean*	*SD*	*Mean*	*SD*
Recreational settings										
Daily frequencies										
Following rules (%)	86	3	83	6	85	7	83	4	87	2
Noncompliance	1.9	1.7	0.9	1.3	1.6	1.7	1.2	2.7	1.1	0.8
Positive peer interaction	70.3	13.7	41.8	20.4	52.4	12.8	53.4	25.0	58.2	26.3
Conduct problems	0.0	0.0	0.0	0.0	0.0	0.0	0.0	0.0	0.0	0.0
Negative verbalizations	0.7	0.5	0.8	1.0	0.5	0.6	0.8	0.8	0.5	1.0
Counselor rating (ACTRS)	1.7	0.6	1.7	0.6	1.7	0.6	1.7	0.6	1.0	0.0
Positive daily report card										
Days received (%)	71	49	20	45	50	58	40	55	75	50
Classroom setting										
Following rules (%)	99	4	100	0	100	0	98	4	98	5
Seatwork completion (%)	90	16	88	26	81	39	75	24	75	22
Seatwork correct (%)	96	4	75	8	89	14	96	4	85	22
Teacher rating (ACTRS)	1.7	2.9	0.0	0.0	0.0	0.0	0.3	0.6	0.7	1.2

ACTRS, Abbreviated Conners Teacher Rating Scale.

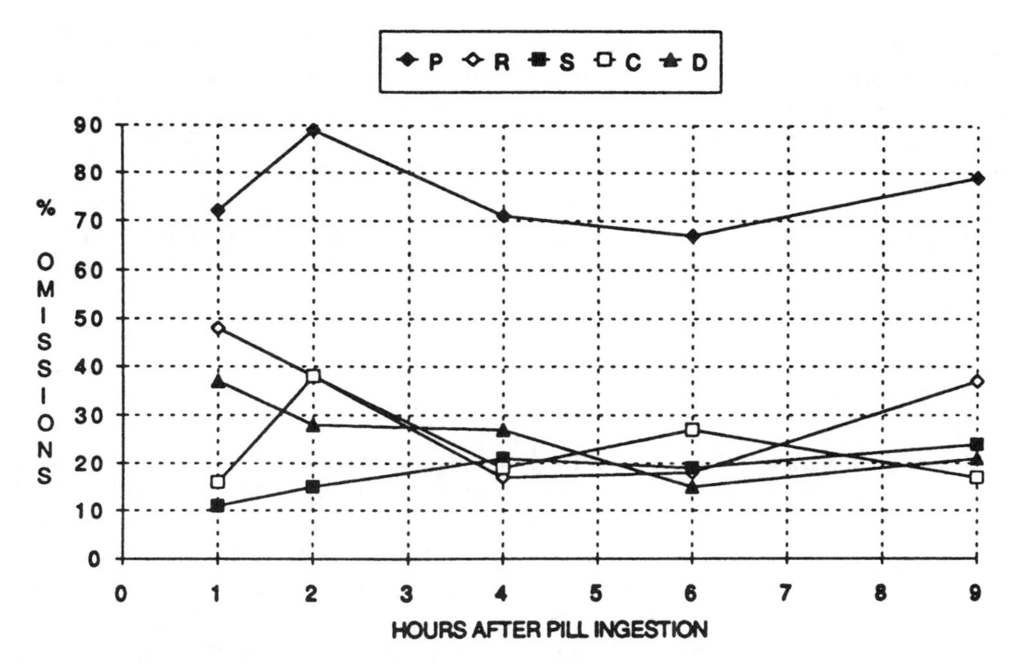

FIG. 1 Percentage errors of omission on the CPT task as a function of hours after pill ingestion. P = Placebo b.i.d; R = 10 mg methylphenidate b.i.d; S = Ritalin SR-20 q.A.M.; C = 56.25 mg pemoline q.A.M.; D = 10 mg Dexedrine Spansule q.A.M.

Darryl performed a CPT four times daily (60, 120, 240, 369, and 540 minutes after pill ingestion) on 1 day in each of the five medication conditions. The results are shown in Figure 1, which shows that his performance in all four active drug conditions was superior to that in the placebo condition. He demonstrated an overall decrease in the number of errors of omission made during the CPT, and the effects of medication maintained across times of the day. It is worth noting that the results of the CPT appear to be confounded with a practice effect, with his performance improving somewhat independently of medication each time he completed the task.

The numerous measures of side effects gathered during the STP reveal that Darryl was rated by counselors and teachers as consistently showing withdrawal and irritable behavior across all medications relative to placebo. Additionally, he had difficulty falling asleep on nights that he received Cylert or Dexedrine. Finally, Darryl showed a moderately adverse behavioral rebound in the evenings of days on which he had received 10 mg MPH twice daily. That is, his mother's ratings of his unmedicated evening behavior were worse on evenings when he had received 10 mg MPH during the day than on evenings when he had received a placebo during the day.

In summary, Darryl demonstrated a mixed response to the four stimulants evaluated. All medications appeared to improve his CPT performance, but on most measures of functioning in the STP, stimulants had little effect. Furthermore and most important, he became withdrawn and had profound decreases in positive social interactions and measures of academic performance with all four medications. Given that social interactions and academic performance were the two domains for which Darryl was referred for treatment, these were the dependent measures on which stimulant response had the greatest ecologic validity.

Thus, medication results on CPT omission errors did not reflect medication response on the social and academic symptoms for which Darryl was referred. Because of the adverse medication response on those measures and despite the beneficial response on the CPT, continued stimulant medication was *not* recommended as a component of Darryl's treatment plan. It is important to note that Darryl had been receiving Ritalin SR-20 for 3 years before this assessment. As in most cases in clinical practice, that administration was begun and continued without any systematic evaluation of the medication's effects. Darryl's case certainly both highlights the importance of using an assessment procedure when prescribing a stimulant and illustrates the importance of using multiple measures that reflect as closely as possible the child's presenting symptoms and are gathered in as naturalistic a setting as possible.

Case 2: Jerry

Jerry was an 8-year-old boy with a long history of severe behavior and learning problems. He showed a mixture of symptoms consistent with diagnoses of ADHD, ODD, and severe learning disabilities. In addition, some of his behaviors suggested a residual pervasive developmental disorder but did not clearly fit that diagnostic category. His main presenting problems, reported by both mother and teachers, were argumentativeness with adults, and fighting and teasing peers. Teacher ratings in particular reflected severe levels of these behaviors, particularly the disruptive and oppositional behaviors. He was described as frequently off-task in school, and his behavior was often disruptive in the classroom. He had been receiving special education for several years (full-time learning disability placement) and 0.9 mg/kg MPH three times daily for 2 years before treatment in the STP.

Jerry was evaluated during the 1989 STP on a protocol that included 7.5 mg Ritalin (0.3 mg/kg) twice daily for 6 days, 15 mg Ritalin (0.6 mg/kg) twice daily for 7 days, 22.5 mg Ritalin (0.9 mg/kg) twice daily for 6 days, and placebo twice daily for 6 days. Medication was administered in the morning and at noon in a random order, with medication varying over days. The dependent measures employed in Jerry's assessment were similar to those described in Case 1, with several additions: (1) a measure of on-task behavior in recreational settings (attention check) was implemented; (2) interrupting others was added as a point category; (3) independent observers coded on-task and disruptive behavior in the classroom setting; and (4) counselor ratings were gathered by use of the ACTRS. As with our other assessments, Jerry's medication assessment was conducted in the context of the behavioral treatment program that operated in all settings of the STP.

In general, Table 2 shows that Jerry continued to exhibit highly inappropriate behavior on placebo days in the behavioral treatment program. Consequently, there was substantial room for improvement with medication, and beneficial MPH effects were apparent on numerous measures. Jerry showed considerable improvement with medication on most measures of social behavior from the daily point system, with most of the improvement occurring on the 15-mg dose of Ritalin. For example, his rule following increased from 35% to 47% with the 7.7-mg dose, 65% with the 15-mg dose, and 68% with the 22.5-mg dose of medication. The 3% difference in following rules between the 15-mg and the 22.5-mg dose is not clinically meaningful, and therefore the lower of the two doses (i.e., 15 mg) was deemed to be appropriate. Thus, rather than selecting the highest dose the child can tolerate, we advocate selecting the dose that achieves maximal clinically meaningful improvement. Such improvement may reflect normalization of behavior or the dose beyond which no further incremental improvement occurs with higher doses.

Consistent with our multivariate approach to medication assessment, no single variable determines a dose recommendation. In Jerry's case, almost all the variables followed similar patterns that were seen with following activity rules. As shown in Table 2, peak improvement was obtained at the 15-mg dose for noncompliance, conduct problems, and neg-

TABLE 2. RESULTS OF THE CLINICAL MEDICATION ASSESSMENT FOR CASE 2: JERRY

	Placebo b.i.d. 6 Days		*7.5 mg Ritalin b.i.d.*[a] *6 Days*		*15 mg Ritalin b.i.d.*[b] *7 Days*		*22.5 mg Ritalin b.i.d.*[c] *6 Days*	
Variable Measured	*Mean*	*SD*	*Mean*	*SD*	*Mean*	*SD*	*Mean*	*SD*
Recreational settings								
Daily frequencies								
Following rules (%)	35.0	7.0	47	7	65	5	68	8
Noncompliance	25.6	7.0	18.3	6.7	7.8	6.3	8.9	6.1
Interrupting	0.4	0.1	0.5	0.1	0.7	0.0	0.7	0.1
Positive peer interaction	39.6	12.4	41.8	12.3	36.6	13.9	38.3	12.5
Conduct problems	4.2	3.6	1.3	1.2	0.6	0.5	1.8	3.5
Negative verbalizations	34.8	6.4	12.2	6.4	7.0	4.3	10.0	13.8
Attention check correct (%)	55.0	17.3	68.6	18.5	59.3	13.9	70.1	11.3
Counselor rating (ACTRS)	18.2	3.6	10.4	4.4	8.8	1.8	7.6	2.4
Positive daily report card								
Days received (%)	0	0	40	55	60	55	60	55
Classroom setting								
Following rules (%)	2	4	5	12	30	41	36	50
On-task behavior (%)	54	17	39	27	67	11	76	5
Disruptive behavior (%)	74	41	61	25	26	29	18	9
Seatwork completion (%)	67	34	75	27	58	21	61	20
Seatwork correct (%)	90	13	89	9	79	15	93	6
Teacher rating (ACTRS)	25.0	3.5	20.8	7.6	15.6	9.6	11.7	4.9

[a]0.3mg/kg. [b]0.6 mg/kg. [c]0.9 mg/kg.

ative verbalizations. In addition, Jerry's performance on his DRC, which reflected success in achieving individualized behavioral goals, was dramatically improved with medication (from 0 on placebo days to 60% on 15-mg days), and the effect peaked at 15 mg. In contrast, Jerry showed no medication effect on his positive peer interactions or the frequency with which he interrupted others' activities. Jerry's counselor ratings revealed a large effect of the lowest dose of MPH, with small incremental improvement with increasing dose beyond that.

Turning to the classroom setting, measures of classroom rule-following and observed disruptive behaviors improved dramatically with medication. These improvements were maximized with the 15-mg dose of MPH despite the fact that Jerry continued to disrupt his classroom even with the highest dose. Despite these improvements in disruptive behavior, Jerry showed high variability and little consistent effect of MPH on his seatwork completion and seatwork correct in the classroom. As might be expected given his improvements in observed disruption, Jerry's teacher's rating on the ACTRS also improved across all medication conditions, with a linear decrease of 4 or 5 points obtained with the addition of each 0.3 mg/kg MPH. The best rating with the concomitant lowest variability was obtained with the highest dose of MPH.

On measures of side effects taken during the STP, Jerry was observed to show some facial grimaces and tongue/lip movements, which were most apparent at 22.5 mg Ritalin and less apparent on 15-mg and lower doses. The reports were made primarily by the counselors who worked with Jerry throughout the day. His teachers did not report facial or mouth movements, and his mother reported them only to a slight degree. These movements dissipated when medication wore off, and the frequency and intensity of the tics decreased over the summer with continued 0.3 and 0.6 mg/kg dosages of medication, although they continued to occur at a high rate at the 0.9 mg/kg dose. No other side effects of medication were noted by teachers, counselors, or Jerry's mother.

Finally, on a CPT, valid data could not be obtained on placebo days because of Jerry's uncooperative behavior. On medication days, he showed consistent medication-related improvement, with omission rates of 50%, 44%, and 21%, and commission rates of 8, 36, and 15, with 0.3, 0.6, and 0.9 mg/kg MPH, respectively. As on his teacher's rating, Jerry clearly showed the greatest improvement on this task with the highest dose of medication.

In summary, the assessment showed that MPH had clear incremental effectiveness as an adjunctive treatment, but different dependent measures provided different information regarding which dose was best. As indicated by the daily frequency counts, the counselor ratings, observations in the classroom, and the DRC, the 0.6 mg/kg dose (15 mg twice daily) appeared to maximize response on most of the dependent measures. In addition, the facial tics were not nearly as pronounced with this dose as with the higher dose. However, both the ACTRS and the CPT documented putative additional improvement at the highest dose: 0.9 mg/kg. Had these two measures been relied on in an outpatient medication assessment, then the highest dose of medication would have been recommended *even though it did not produce incremental improvement on most measures* and even though it caused the greatest exacerbation of Jerry's facial tics, which were not noted by his teacher. It is important that before contact with our clinic, Jerry had undergone a "controlled" medication assessment at a local clinic. However, that assessment used *only* the ACTRS and a laboratory learning task to determine response to medication, with the result that Jerry had been receiving 0.9 mg/kg MPH three times daily for the 2 years before this assessment. On the basis of the STP medication evaluation, this 0.9 mg/kg dosage produced an unnecessarily high rate of side effects and had no clinical advantage compared with the 0.6 mg/kg dosage.

Case 3: Andy

Andy was a 9-year-old fourth-grader who was referred to the STP with extreme and longstanding symptoms of ADHD and ODD/conduct disorder. Parent and teacher ratings on standardized scales were consistent in describing Andy as having extreme symptoms of inattention, impulsivity, hyperactivity, oppositional behavior, and severe difficulties getting along with other children. His parents reported that Andy had shown these problems from an early age. In the school setting, teachers reported problems in his kindergarten year, and midway through the first grade year he was placed in a special education class because of his high rate of negative behavior. About this time, MPH was prescribed by his pediatrician. Despite these interventions, Andy's problems persisted. At the time of intake, he was receiving 10 mg twice daily on school days. Andy was evaluated on a protocol that included 8.75 mg MPH (0.3 mg/kg) twice daily, 17.5 mg MPH (0.6 mg/kg) twice daily, and placebo twice daily. Medication was administered twice daily in a random order, with medication varying over days with 9 or 10 days per condition. The dependent measures used in Andy's assessment were the same as described above for Case 2. The results of Andy's assessment are shown in Table 3.

As the table illustrates, Andy exhibited the behaviors for which he was referred in the STP setting, having relatively high rates of impulsive, disruptive, and oppositional behavior on placebo days. On days when he received MPH, he was substantially improved in both his behavior and his academic performance. Of particular interest for our purposes are the somewhat discrepant dose effects apparent in the recreational and classroom settings. On every measure in the classroom, Andy's improvement maximized at the 0.3 mg/kg

TABLE 3. RESULTS OF THE CLINICAL MEDICATION ASSESSMENT FOR CASE 3: ANDY

Dependent Variable	*Mean (SD) on Placebo Days in STP for Children*	*Mean (SD) on 0.3 mg/kg MPH Days in STP for Children*	*Mean (SD) on 0.6 mg/kg MPH Days in STP for Children*		*Mean (SD) on Placebo Days in STP for Adolescents*	*Mean (SD) on 10 mg MPH Days in STP for Adolescents*	*Mean (SD) on 20 mg MPH Days in STP for Adolescents*	*Mean (SD) on 30 mg MPH Days in STP for Adolescents*
Interrupting	16.1 (8.3)	5.0 (2.5)	2.3 (2.1)		16.8 (9.1)	9.8 (5.5)	7.5 (5.4)	4.4 (3.6)
Following activity rules[a]	48 (14)	67 (8)	70 (18)	Rule violations[b]	17.0 (6.4)	8.2 (5.2)	6.2 (1.3)	7.0 (5.2)
Teasing peers[c]	3.8 (2.5)	2.1 (1.2)	1.3 (1.0)		4.2 (3.7)	2.8 (1.2)	3.3 (4.8)	0.6 (0.6)
Noncompliance[d]	11.9 (6.5)	3.5 (2.5)	1.3 (1.1)		3.5 (4.8)	0.8 (0.8)	1.0 (0.9)	1.4 (2.1)
Minutes of time out[e]	21.0 (15)	5.7 (5.3)	0.0 (0.0)		41.0 (82.0)	3.3 (5.2)	7.0 (10.8)	0.0 (0.0)
Negative verbalizations[f]	17.6 (6.0)	6.4 (2.9)	3.0 (2.6)		58.7 (103)	13.0 (9.9)	11.7 (13.7)	5.2 (5.0)
Disruptive behavior[g]	14 (12)	4 (3)	6 (3)		12 (8)	11 (8)	5 (3)	2 (3)
On-task in the classroom[h]	60 (14)	79 (8)	79 (10)		74 (18)	71 (20)	84 (7)	56 (43)
% Work completed	45 (30)	68 (31)	70 (24)		12 (16)	93 (16)	58 (46)	92 (9)
% Classwork correct	91 (7)	95 (6)	98 (3)		36 (35)	84 (47)	88 (46)	72 (35)

[a]Follow activity rules is the percentage of time intervals the child did not break any program rules. Thus, higher percentages reflect better rule following.

[b]Rule violations is the frequency that the adolescent broke program rules during the entire day. Thus, lower freqencies reflect better rule following.

[c]Teasing peers in a daily frequency count of negative verbal behavior directed toward peers.

[d]Noncompliance is the daily frequency of failing to comply with a counselor's request within 10 seconds.

[e]Time outs were assigned for aggression, destruction of property, and repeated noncompliance. The duration of time outs was extended for continued misbehavior once a time out was assigned.

[f]Negative verbalization is the daily frequency of negative verbal behaviors including inappropriate complaining, verbal abuse to staff, and teasing peers.

[g]The variables disruptive behavior and on-task behavior reflect the daily average percentage of time intervals the subjects were observed exhibiting the behaviors in the classroom.

[h]On-task in the classroom is the percentage of intervals the student was observed to be engaged in appropriate classroom activities.

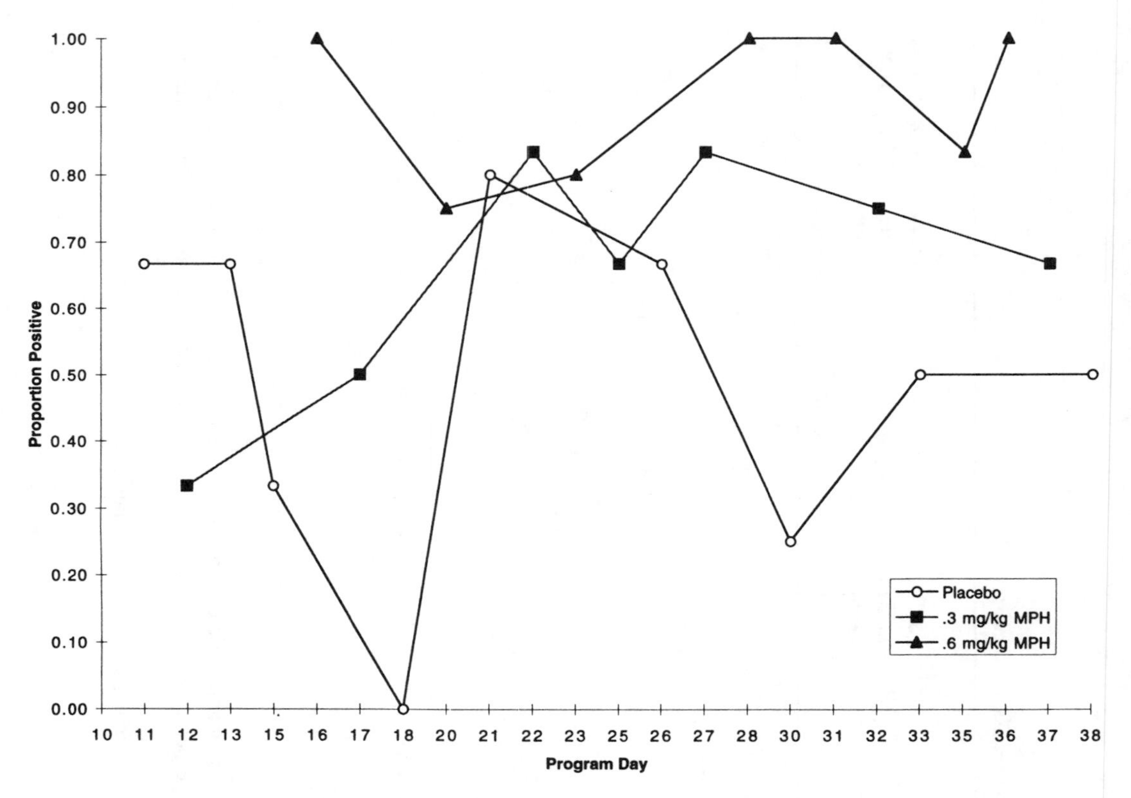

FIG. 2 Case 3: Andy's proportion of positive target behaviors on the daily report card as a function of day and medication condition.

dosage, affording no clinically meaningful improvement when the dosage was increased to 0.6 mg/kg. The same pattern was obtained on measures of impulsivity and inattention obtained in recreational settings (e.g., interruption and following rules). However, on measures that reflected oppositional behavior directed toward his peers (i.e., teasing) and counselors (e.g., noncompliance) Andy showed incremental improvement with the higher dosage of MPH.

The magnitude of this additional improvement is clearly illustrated by change in two measures: (1) the total of all the negative behaviors included in the daily frequency counts and (2) the percentage of goals reached on his DRC. Andy exhibited 47.7 inappropriate behaviors per day on placebo days, 16.2 on 0.3-mg/kg days, and 6.7 on 0.6-mg/kg days. Thus, although the bulk of the MPH effects on Andy's inappropriate behaviors in recreational settings came at the 0.3-mg/kg dosage, the higher dosage of MPH eliminated an additional 10 highly salient negative behaviors per day from Andy's interactions with peers and counselors. Similarly, the graph of the proportion of positive DRC targets achieved in the STP setting clearly demonstrates the incremental beneficial effect of 0.6 mg/kg versus 0.3 mg/kg and placebo (Figure 2). Andy's DRC targets included a variety of behavioral information with individualized goals, and, in order to provide individualized feedback designed to shape progressively better behavior, the DRC goals were refined or made more stringent on a weekly basis. The goals typically covered both social behavior and academic performance but focused on specific areas of difficulty. Performance on these goals was variable, and Figure 2 illustrates how the DRC data can be used to summarize data from multiple sources into a single useful summary measure.

In addition to the measures from the clinical medication assessment, Andy was tested individually on a CPT task six times—twice per medication condition—during the STP. He showed no clear pattern of MPH response, averaging 53% omission errors on placebo and 0.3-mg/kg days and 61% on days when he received 0.6 mg/kg. The overlap between his performance across testing days was great, with medication and placebo error rates virtually identical.

The ACTRS ratings completed by Andy's teachers and counselors were sensitive to medication effects and showed peak improvement at the low dose of MPH. This response pattern was similar to the academic measures and the direct measures of inattention and impulsivity. For example, the teacher's ACTRS ratings dropped dramatically from 22.2 on placebo days to 12.2 on 0.3 mg/kg-MPH days, but did not meaningfully decrease on 0.6-mg/kg days (i.e., the rating was 11.9).

When Andy came to the STP at age 9, he had been receiving MPH for 3 years, prescribed by his pediatrician at his school's request, and he had never had an evaluation of the medication's effectiveness. His physician had prescribed only 0.3 mg/kg/day despite the fact that Andy's behavior problems were sufficiently severe to have him maintained in a special education classroom. It is noteworthy that many of his continued problems occurred in unstructured settings when he was out of his special class placement, and many of them involved oppositional behavior and negative peer interactions. Our assessment revealed that a 0.6-mg/kg/day dose would likely provide incremental benefit for Andy in these important domains, even though it would not result in improvement on the ACTRS. Finally, the CPT did not reveal a beneficial medication effect for Andy.

Andy's behavior improved following his summer in the STP for children. However, his behavior seriously deteriorated in the year preceding his enrollment in the STP for adolescents. He continued to exhibit severe difficulties with peer relations and upset peers and staff at his school by making inappropriate sexual comments to his female classmates. His academic performance was acceptable (i.e., he was a B student); however, despite the fact that he was enrolled in a special education program for disruptive students, his continued participation in school was jeopardized by his high rate of disruptive and disrespectful behavior.

Following the STP, Andy had been referred to his pediatrician for medication management. When Andy's problems worsened, he was referred to a private psychiatrist, who prescribed 0.5 mg of clonidine three times daily, in conjunction with the 0.6 mg/kg/day of MPH. After an open trial with no objective measures of social behavior, on the basis of parent and school reports of no improvement, the psychiatrist discontinued the MPH and clonidine and began treating Andy with desipramine 35 mg twice daily and 25 mg at bedtime. The only information used by the physician to evaluate drug effects and side effects was unstructured parent and school reports. In sum, Andy's behavior was clearly out of control and getting worse, and the effects of potentially dangerous treatment with tricyclic antidepressants (Werry, 1995) and clonidine (Cantwell, et al., 1997) was being evaluated haphazardly.

Because of his continued problems with negative social behavior, Andy was referred to the STP for adolescents. Daily activities in the STP for adolescents were very similar to those in the children's STP but were adjusted to be developmentally appropriate. The dependent variables in the adolescent version of the STP had several noteworthy differences from the child program. First, measures of positive behaviors toward peers were not included because of developmental considerations and lack of success with these measures in previous studies of MPH treatment of adolescents with ADHD (e.g., Pelham et al., 1991). Second, academic work in the children's program was individualized and self-paced, as is typical in elementary school, whereas in the STP for adolescents, the format was similar to a junior high school setting (i.e., the students listened to lectures, took notes, studied notes, and were given exams; see Evans et al., 1994, for a description). Finally, many of the measures of behavior in the STP for children were modified in the STP for adolescents; as a consequence, many measures were not directly comparable across the two programs. For example, in the STP for children, rule following was measured by the percentage of fixed periods of time the child obeyed the program rules. In the STP for adolescents, rule following was measured by counting the frequency of rule violations. The measures presented in Table 3 are the measures that were most readily compared across the two programs. Smith et al. (1998a) provides more details about the adolescent program, and Smith et al., (1998b) provides a detailed comparison of the STP for children with the STP for adolescents.

The basic medication evaluation procedures for Andy were very similar in the STP for children and adolescents (i.e., a double-blind, placebo-controlled study with multiple replications of medication conditions rotated on a daily basis). However, there were two important differences. First, the medication assessment in the STP for adolescents had placebo and three different doses of MPH, but there were only two doses in Andy's medication evaluation in the STP for children. Second, instead of using mg/kg dosing, the adolescents were evaluated on a protocol that included 10 mg MPH, 20 mg MPH, 30 mg MPH, and placebo (see Rapport and Denney, 1997 for a discussion of this methodological consideration). In Andy's case, these doses translated to 0.26 mg/kg, 0.51 mg/kg, and 0.76 mg/kg. Thus, the doses were not directly comparable on a precise mg/kg basis. However, as can be seen in Table 3, the type of dosing did not change the dose-response pattern within domains of social behavior and academic performance across the two programs.

In the context of the STP for adolescents, Andy had severe problems with negative social behavior on placebo days. His poor academic performance on placebo days was largely due to his negative behavior, which resulted in frequent time outs from the classroom. Andy was very provocative to peers, and intensive behavioral intervention was necessary to prevent this behavior from inciting retaliatory aggression. The individualized behavior plan resulted in a 10-fold decrease in teasing peers from an average of about 10 a day to about one a day. Similarly, consistent implementation of time out for noncompliance and aggression led to a substantial reduction in these behaviors. However, his rate of teasing and noncompliance remained unacceptably high on placebo days. Moreover, the behavioral program did not substantially reduce Andy's inappropriately high rate of complaining and swearing.

Andy showed a generally positive response to medication, and the pattern of improvement across domains was similar to that observed in the children's program. More specifically, improvements in academic performance, inattention, and impulsivity peaked at the low to moderate doses, with minimal additional gain at higher doses. On the contrary, although improvements in oppositional and defiant behavior were evident at the low doses, additional clinically meaningful improvement was achieved with the highest dose. Andy's parents, counselors, and teachers did not report any prohibitive side effects. There was a slight loss of appetite and minor social withdrawal, sometimes with tearful affect, at the highest dose. Given the large amount of improvement in social behavior at the high dose, the cost/benefit (i.e., side effects vs. therapeutic gains) analysis favored the highest dose. Thus, we recommended that Andy take 30 mg of MPH in the morning and at noon. Because IOWA Conners ratings completed by his parents reflected improved behavior with low doses of MPH, we also recommended that a third dose of 15 mg be given at 4 P.M.

A final comment on Andy's medication assessments is in order. As can be seen from the large standard deviations, Andy's behavior was highly variable on placebo days and became less variable with higher doses of medication. Nevertheless, even on the highest doses, Andy exhibited a great degree of day-to-day variability on most measures. If the medication assessment procedures had not included multiple crossovers of conditions, the data could have been very difficult to interpret and therefore could have led to erroneous medication recommendations. It is noteworthy that the coefficient of variation (i.e., 100 times the standard deviation divided by the mean) is smaller for the STP for children than for adolescents. For example, the coefficient of variation for teasing peers when Andy was in the children's program was 66, 57, and 76 for the placebo, 0.3 mg/kg MPH, and 0.6 mg/kg MPH conditions, respectively. When Andy was in the STP for adolescents, the coefficients were 88, 42, 145, and 100 for placebo, 10 mg MPH, 20 mg MPH, and 30 mg MPH. A likely explanation for the higher coefficients of variation in the STP for adolescents is that there were fewer replications of medication conditions in the STP for adolescents (i.e., about 6) than in the STP for children (i.e., about 9). Thus, increasing the number of replications of medication conditions is likely to improve the precision of individual evaluations of response to stimulant treatment for children and adolescents with ADHD.

CONDUCTING A COMPREHENSIVE AND PRACTICAL OUTPATIENT MEDICATION ASSESSMENT

If widely used measures such as the ACTRS, CPT, and laboratory learning tasks do not necessarily provide the type of information to facilitate evaluation of individual responses to stimulant medication, where does this leave the practitioner? The question facing every clinician with an ADHD patient is how to decide whether a stimulant should be used and what the correct dose should be. The kinds of assessments that we conduct in the STP are clearly too complicated to be implemented in practice in most outpatient and/or school settings. However, the principles involved—assessing a wide range of ecologically valid measures of functioning in a natural setting, and emphasizing individual differences in response—can be followed in medication assessments that can be designed and conducted in less structured settings. What follows are guidelines for conducting outpatient medication assessments.

First, researchers, professional organizations, and pharmaceutical manufacturers are virtually unanimous in their agreement (1) *that stimulants should be used with ADHD children only after appropriate psychosocial and psychoeducational interventions have been conducted and are insufficient* and (2) *that stimulants should be used only in conjunction with these other interventions*. It has been clearly established that the appropriate psychosocial intervention for ADHD is a behavioral intervention, and that behavioral and psychostimulant interventions often have beneficial combined effects (Pelham, 1989; Pelham and Murphy, 1986). For that reason, the first step in determining whether to use medication with an ADHD child or adolescent is to establish a behavioral intervention first. After a sufficient period of parent training (i.e., Barkley, 1987) and classroom intervention (e.g., Pfiffner and O'Leary, 1993), if the child or adolescent has not shown maximal improvement, then the clinician should proceed with a medication assessment.

The major advantage of starting the behavioral intervention first is that the behavioral targets can serve as dependent measures in the medication assessmant. Although most home and school settings will not readily generate reliable frequency counts of behavior, it is possible to select objective behavioral goals that can be tracked in most settings. These goals can be incorporated into a daily report card, and the percentage of goals met can be a useful measure in stimulant medication assessments. For example, a teacher can record the percentage of school work completed and whether the child was reprimanded for teasing peers. Likewise, a parent can determine whether chores or homework have been completed by a predetermined deadline. DRC goals such as these are the foundation of the behavioral reinforcement system and provide clinically meaningful, face-valid information. DRC data have proved to be very sensitive to the effects of stimulant medication (Pelham, et al., in review). The DRC data should be given the greatest weight relative to ratings and other data in evaluation of the response to stimulant medication.

If the primary clinician is not a physician, then collaboration and clear communication between the clinician and a physician is critically important. The clinician should meet with the physician to discuss procedures for monitoring changes in dependent variables and tracking stimulant side effects. The child or adolescent should have a physical examination to rule out conditions that preclude an assessment with stimulants. The clinician and cooperating physician should select the type and doses of medication to be used. Our standard protocol includes placebo, 0.3 mg/kg methylphenidate twice daily, and 0.6 mg/kg methylphenidate twice daily (reduced to 0.15 and 0.3 mg/kg for low and high doses, respectively, for overweight children, for older and therefore heavier children, and for children who do not have behavior problems). Other preparations could be used for a variety of reasons. For example, a child may need a long-acting preparation because the school will not administer a midday dose (see Pelham et al., 1990a). If d-amphetamine is used, the dose recommended for MPH should be halved. If pemoline is used, the dose should be six times a single methylphenidate dose with A.M. administration only (Pelham et al., 1990a; Stephens et al., 1984).

Data supplied by parents and teachers could be biased if they are aware of the child or adolescent's medication status. Consequently, encapsulating pills may be necessary to keep parents, and in some cases teachers, blind to medication condition. If parents administer medication and provide ratings of behavior, then the pills should be encapsulated to disguise the active medication and placebo. Most local pharmacists are able to perform this function. The pills do not need to be encapsulated if most of the child's problems are at school and teachers do not see what pills the child is taking. It is unclear whether adolescents are influenced by an expectancy effect, so it may be worthwhile to blind the adolescents to medication status and possibly include an active placebo designed to mimic mild side effects (Fisher and Greenberg, 1993).

When determining the medication schedule, the clinician should ensure that times of the day during which the child or adolescent exhibits his or her target behaviors will overlap with peak medication times (for methylphenidate, between 60 and 180 minutes after ingestion). For example, if problems occur with peers in neighborhood recreational activities, then an after-school dose should be administered at least an hour before the child is allowed to go out and play in the neighborhood (Pelham et al., 1990b). Similarly, if a child works on his or her most difficult academic assignment immediately upon arrival at school, he or she must receive the morning dose sufficiently early to affect performance on that task (i.e., at least 60 minutes beforehand).

Although the most common recommendation is to vary medication condition weekly, we have found a great deal of difficulty interpreting data for individuals when using such schedules. The major problem is that events at school or home become confounded with medication condition, making it difficult to separate medication effects from other variables that influence the child's behavior at home and school. Because of their brief half-lives, stimulants can be varied daily. A daily manipulation of condition affords many alternations between drug and placebo conditions and distributes error associated with other events across drug conditions, therefore clarifying interpretation of medication effects for the individual.

Thus, a random schedule should be established in which medication condition changes daily, but the randomization should be limited to ensure that each dose is given at least once per week (e.g., week 1, P; 0.3, P, 0.6, 0.3). Each dose should be administered until stable data have been obtained and a pattern or lack thereof is clear (e.g., five times per condition). Thus, the entire assessment may take from 3 to 6 school weeks, depending on how many doses and drugs are evaluated. The pharmacist should package the medication in dated, individual envelopes according to the random order, and these should be given to the parents one week at a time.

The therapist should make certain that all adults involved with the child, as well as the child, know that the assessment is occurring. At the same time, everyone who will provide any information regarding the child's response should be kept blind to condition. Persons administering medication should keep precise records on the time medication was given and the reasons for missing any doses. Clinicians should examine the compliance data periodically and intervene to improve compliance, if necessary. The validity of the assessment depends on good compliance across medication conditions.

As discussed above, the dependent measures should include the DRC targets and other objective information from the school regarding child's major behavioral and academic problems. In addition, the IOWA Conners TRS should be completed daily by the teacher (Pelham et al., 1989), and teacher and parents should complete standard side effects rating scales daily. If a late afternoon or evening dose of medication is used, parents' ratings and records of objective behavior problems should be used (e.g., records of point charts for the ongoing behavioral interventions). Finally, parents, teachers, and other adults who interact with the child or adolescent while he or she is medicated should complete ratings of stimulant side effects.

After the assessment is completed, the clinician should break the blind, collate all the information gathered, compute means and standard deviations for dependent measures within each condition, and generate graphs of important target behaviors or summaries of target behaviors (e.g., the DRC proportion positive). Then, *giving most weight to the child's major problem areas*, the clinician should determine whether the *incremental* (*beyond* the ongoing behavioral intervention) improvement obtained with medication outweighs any side effects observed and, if so, the minimal dose that produces the desired change. Unfortunately, there are no clear-cut guidelines for deciding how much of an effect is sufficient to recommend medication. We generally consider the salience of the child's problematic behaviors and where in regard to a "normal" range of functioning he or she falls with medication. For example, given that disturbed peer relations are a hallmark of ADHD and one of the best predictors of long-range maladjustment (Milich and Landau, 1989; Pelham and Bender, 1982), it would be prudent to give improvement in peer interactions more weight than a teacher rating of inattention in deciding which dose to recommend for a child having problems with relationships with peers (see Case 3 above).

CONCLUSION

Research leaves little doubt that ADHD is a chronic condition that most often requires long-term treatment (Barkley et al., 1990; Hart et al., 1995; Biederman et al., 1996). Unfortunately, it has become equally well accepted that long-term pharmacotherapy with a stimulant, as the medications have been prescribed over the past several decades, is not an adequate long-term intervention (Weiss and Hechtman, 1993). Although the multivariate well-controlled crossover studies recommended in this chapter might appear at first glance to be unnecessarily complex, they appear essential to an accurate determination of a child's stimulant responsiveness. It is certainly reasonable to speculate that the failure of previous studies to demonstrate long-term beneficial effects of stimulants may stem from the failure to properly evaluate responses to medication. For example, children and adolescents who are given high doses may experience unnecessary side effects and stop taking the medication. Children and adolescents who are undermedicated will not fully benefit from the medication and suffer worse long-term outcomes. Widespread utilization of the rigorous medication assessments we have discussed should yield a better outcome for long-term stimulant regimens. Given that most medicated ADHD children will continue their medication and other components of treatment for many years (Safer and Krager, 1994), the initial short-term investment of time and effort expended to evaluate medication response should have clear long-term benefits.

REFERENCES

Atkins, M.S., Pelham, W.E. & Licht, M. (1985), A comparison of objective classroom measures and teacher ratings of attention deficit disorder. *J. Abnorm. Child Psychology*, 13:155–167.

Barkley, R.A. (1987), *Defiant Children: A Clinician's Manual for Parent Training*. New York: Guilford Press.

Barkley, R.A. (1991), The ecological validity of laboratory and analogue assessment methods of ADHD symptoms. *J. Abnorm. Child Psychology*, 19:149–178.

Barkley, R.A., Fischer, M., Edelbrock, C.S., & Smallish, L. (1990), The adolescent outcome of hyperactive children diagnosed by research criteria: I. An 8-year prospective follow-up study. *J. Am. Acad. Child Adolesc. Psychiatry,* 29:546–557.

Barkley, R.A., Fischer, M., Newby, R.F. & Breen, M.J. (1988), Development of a multimethod clinical protocol for assessing stimulant drug response in ADD children. *J. Clin. Child Psychol.* 17:14–24.

Beiderman, J., Faraone, S.V., Milberger, S., Curtis, S., Chen, L., Marrs, A., Ouellette, C., Moore, P. & Spencer, T.J. (1996), Predictors of persistence and remission of ADHD into adolescence: Results from a four-year prospective follow-up study. *J. Am. Acad. Child Adolesc. Psychiatry,* 35:343–351.

Campbell, D.T., & Fiske, D.W. (1959), Convergent and discriminant validation by the multitrait-multimethod matrix. *Psychol. Bull.,* 56:81–105.

Cantwell, D.P., Swanson, J. & Connor, D.F. (1997). Case Study: Adverse response to clonidine. *J. Am. Acad. Child Adoles. Psychiatry*, 36:539–544.

Conners, C.K. (1973), Conners parent and teacher questionnaire. *Psychopharmacology Bulletin Special Issue: Pharmacotherapy of Children* (Publication No. HSM 73-9002). Washington DC: NIMH.

Conners, C.K. (1985), Issues in the study of adolescent ADD-H/hyperactivity. *Psychopharmacol. Bull.,* 21:243–250.

Douglas, V.I., Barr, R.G., Amin, K., O'Neill, M.E., & Britton, B.G. (1988), Dosage effects and individual responsivity to methylphenidate in attention deficit disorder. *J. Child Psychol. Psychiatry*, 29:453–476.

Evans, S.W., Pelham, W.E., Smith, B.H., Bukstein, O., Gnagy, E.M., Greiner, A.R., Altenderfer, L., & Baron-Myak, C. (in review), Dose-response effects of methylphenidate on ecologically-valid measures of academic performance and classroom behavior in ADHD adolescents.

Evans, S.E., Pelham, W.E., Jr. & Grudburg, M.V. (1994), The efficacy of note taking to improve behavior and comprehension of adolescents with attention-deficit hyperactivity disorder. *Exceptionality,* 5:1–17.

Figueredo, A.J., Ferketich, S.L., & Knapp, T.R. (1991), More on the MTMM: The role of confirmatory factor analysis. *Res. Nurs. Health,* 14:387–391.

Fisher, S. & Greenberg, R.P. (1993), How sound is the double-blind design for evaluating psychotropic drugs? *J. Nerv. Men. Dis.* 181:345–350.

Gittelman, R. & Kanner, A. (1986), Psychopharmacotherapy. In: *Psychopathological Disorders of Childhood, 3rd ed.,* eds. H. Quay & J. Werry. New York: John Wiley & Sons, Inc., pp. 455–495.

Greenberg, R.P., Bornstein, R.F., Greenberg, M.D., & Fisher, S. (1992), A meta-analysis of antidepressant outcome under "blinder" conditions. *J. Consult. Clin. Psychol.* 60:664–669.

Greenhill, L.L. (1995), Attention-deficit hyperactivity disorder: The stimulants. *Child & Adoles. Psychiatric Clin. North Am.* 4:123–168.

Greenhill, L.L. & Osman, B.B., eds. (1991), *Ritalin: Theory and Patient Management.* Larchmont, NY: Mary Ann Liebert, Inc.

Hastings, J.E. & Barkley, R.A. (1978), A review of psychophysiological research with hyperactive children. *J. Abnorm. Child Psychol.* 6:413–448.

Hart, E.L., Lahey, B.B., Loeber, R., Appelgate, B. & Frick, P.J. (1995), Developmental change in attention-deficit hyperactivity disorder in boys: A four-year longitudinal study. *J. Abnorm. Child Psychol.* 23:729–749.

Hinshaw, S. (1991), Stimulant medication and the treatment of aggression in children with attentional deficits. *J. Clin. Child Psychol.* 20:301–312.

Hinshaw, S.P., Henker, B. et al. (1989), Aggressive, prosocial, and nonsocial behavior in hyperactive boys: Dose effects of methylphenidate in naturalistic settings. *J. Consult. Clin. Psychol.* 57:636–643.

Hoza, J. (1989), *Response to Stimulant Medication Among Children with Attention Deficit Hyperactivity Disorder.* Unpublished doctoral dissertation, Florida State University.

Jacobson, N.S. & Truax, P. (1991), Clinical significance: A statistical approach to defining meaningful change in psychotherapy research. *J. Consult. Clin. Psychol.* 59:12–19.

Milich, R. & Landau, S. (1989), The role of social status variables in differentiating subgroups of hyperactive children. In: *Attention Deficit Disorders IV: Current Concepts and Emerging Trends in Attentional and Behavioral Disorders of Childhood,* eds., J. Swanson & L. Bloomingdale. London: Pergamon, pp. 1–16.

Molina, B.S.G. The role of ADHD in the development of alcohol use and abuse. Unpublished data, University of Pittsburgh.

Pelham, W.E. (1982), Childhood hyperactivity: Diagnosis, etiology, nature and treatment. In: *Behavioral Medicine and Clinical Psychology: Overlapping Disciplines,* eds., R. Gatchel, A. Baum & J. Singer. Hillsdale, NJ: Lawrence Erlbaum Associates.

Pelham, W.E. (1986), The effects of stimulant drugs on learning and achievement in hyperactive and learning-disabled children. In: *Psychological and Educational Perspectives on Learning Disabilities,* eds., J.K. Torgesen & B. Wong. New York: Academic Press, pp. 259–295.

Pelham, W.E. (1989), Behavior therapy, behavioral assessment, and psychostimulant medication in treatment of attention deficit disorders: An interactive approach. In: *Attention Deficit Disorders IV: Current Concepts and Emerging Trends in Attentional and Behavioral Disorders of Childhood,* eds., J. Swanson & L. Bloomingdale. London: Pergamon, pp. 169–195.

Pelham, W.E., Jr. (1993), Pharmacotherapy for children with attention-deficit hyperactivity disorder. *School Psychol. Rev.* 22:199–227.

Pelham, W.E., & Bender, M.E., (1982), Peer relationships in hyperactive children: Description and treatment. In: *Advances in Learning and Behavioral Disabilities, vol. 1,* eds., K. Gadow & I. Bialer. Greenwich, CT: JAI Press, pp. 366–436.

Pelham, W.E., Jr., Griener, A., Gnagy, E.M., Hoza, B., Martin, L., Sams, S. & Wilson, T. (1996), Intensive treatment for ADHD: A model summer treatment program. In: *Model*

Programs in Child and Family Mental Health, ed., M.C. Robers. Mahwah, NJ: Lawrence Erlbaum Associates, pp. 193–214.

Pelham, W.E., Jr., Gnagy, E.M., Greenslade, K.E. & Milich, R. (1992), Teacher ratings of *DSM-III-R* symptoms of disruptive behavior disorders. *J. Am. Acad. Child Adolesc. Psychiatry,* 31:210–218.

Pelham, W.E., Greenslade, K.E., Vodde-Hamiliton, M.A., Murphy, D.A., Greenstein, J.J., Gnagy, E.M. & Dahl, R.E. (1990a), Relative efficacy of long-acting CNS stimulants on children with attention deficit-hyperactivity disorder: A comparison of standard methylphenidate, sustained-release methylphenidate, sustained-release dextroamphetamine, and pemoline. *Pediatrics,* 86:226–237.

Pelham, W.E. & Hoza, J. (1987), Behavioral assessment of psychostimulant effects on ADD children in a summer day treatment program. In: *Advances in Behavioral Assessment of Children and Families, vol. 3*, ed., R. Prinz. Greenwich, CT: JAI Press, pp. 3–33.

Pelham, W.E., Hoza, B. et al. (1997), Effects of methylphenidate and expectancy on ADHD children's performance, self evaluations, persistence, and attributions on a cognitive task. *Exper. Clin. Psychopharm.* 5:3–13.

Pelham, W.E., Jr., Hoza, B., Pillow, D.R., Gnagy, E.M., Kipp, H.L., Greiner, A.R., Trane, S.T., Greenhouse, J.T., Wolfson, L. & Fitzpatrick, E. *Effects of Methylphenidate and Expectency on Children with ADHD: Behavior, Academic Performance, and Attributions in a Summer Treatment Program and Regular Classroom Settings.* (In review).

Pelham, W.E., McBurnett, K., Harper, G., Milich, R., Clinton, J., Thiele, C. & Murphy, D.A. (1990b), Methylphenidate and baseball playing in ADD children: Who's on first? *J. Consult. Clin. Psychol.,* 58:130–133.

Pelham, W.E., Jr. & Milich, R. (1991), Individual differences in response to Ritalin in classwork and social behavior. *Ritalin: Theory and Patient Management,* eds. L. Greenhill & B.B. Osman. Larchmont, NY: Mary Ann Liebert, Inc., pp. 203–221.

Pelham, W.E., Milich, R., Murphy, D.A. & Murphy, H.A. (1989), Normative data on the IOWA Conners teacher rating scale. *J. Clin. Child Psychol.,* 18:259–262.

Pelham, W.E., Milich, R. & Walker, J. (1986), The effects on continuous and partial reinforcement and methylphenidate on learning in children with attention deficit disorder. *J. Abnorm. Psychol.,* 95:319–325.

Pelham, W.E. & Murphy, H.A. (1986), Behavioral and pharmacological treatment of attention deficit and conduct disorders. In: *Pharmacological and Behavioral Treatment: An Integrative Approach,* ed., M. Hersen. New York: John Wiley & Sons, Inc., pp. 108–148.

Pelham, W.E., Sturges, J., Hoza, J., Schmidt, C., Bijlsma, J.J., Milich, R., & Moorer, S. (1987), Sustained release and standard methylphenidate effects on cognitive and social behavior in children with Attention Deficit Disorder. *Pediatrics,* 80:491–501.

Pelham, W.E., Vodde-Hamilton, M. et al. (1991), The effects of methylphenidate on ADHD adolescents in recreational, peer group, and classroom settings. *J. Clin. Child Psychol.* 20(3):293–300.

Pfiffner, L.J. & O'Leary, S.G. (1993), Educational placement and classroom management. In: *Attention Deficit Hyperactivity Disorders: A Handbook for Diagnosis and Treatment,* ed., R.A. Barkley, New York: Guilford Press, pp. 234–255.

Quay, H.C. & Peterson, D.R. (1983), Interim manual for the *Revised Behavior Problem Checklist.* Box 248074, University of Miami, Coral Gables, FL 33124.

Rapport, M.D., Stoner, G., DuPaul, G.J., Birmingham, B.K. & Tucker, S. (1985),

Methylphenidate in hyperactive children: Differential effects of dose on academic, learning, and social behavior. *J. Abnorm. Child Psychol.,* 13:227–244.

Rapport, M.D. & Denney, C. (1997), Titrating methylphenidate in children with attention-deficit/hyperactivity disorder: Is body mass predictive of clinical response? *J. Am. Acad. Child Adoles. Psychiatry,* 36:523–530.

Rapport, M.D., Denney, C., DuPaul, G.J. & Gardner, M.J. (1994), Attention deficit disorder and methylphenidate: Normalization rates, clinical effectiveness, and response prediction in 76 children. *J. Am. Acad. Child Adolesc. Psychiatry,* 33:882–893.

Rapport, M.D., Jones, J.T., DuPaul, G.J., Kelly, K.L., Gardner, M.J., Tucker, S.B., & Shea, M.S. (1987), ADD and methylphenidate: Group and single-subject analyses of dose effects on attention in clinic and classroom settings. *J. of Clin. Child Psychol.* 16(4): 329–338.

Safer, D.J. & Krager, J.M. (1994), The increased rate of stimulant treatment for hyperactive/inattentive students in secondary school. *Pediatrics,* 94:462–464.

Shekim, W.O., Dekirmenjian, H., Javaid, J., Bulund, D.B. & Davis, J.M. (1982), Dopamine-norepinephrine interaction in hyperactive boys treated with d-amphetamine. *J. Pediatrics,* 100:830–834.

Sherman, M., & Hertzig, M.E. (1991), Prescribing practices of Ritalin: The Suffolk County, New York study. In: *Ritalin: Theory and Patient Management,* eds., L.L. Greenhill & B.B. Osman, Larchmont, NY: Mary Ann Liebert, Inc., pp. 187–193.

Sleator, E.K. (1986), Diagnosis. In: *Dialogues in Pediatric Management, vol. 1: Attention Deficit Disorder,* eds., E. Sleator & W. Pelham. Norwalk, CT: Appleton-Century-Crofts, pp. 11–43.

Smith, B.H., Pelham, W.E., Evans, S., Gnagy, E., Molina, B., Bukstein, O., Greiner, A., Myak, C., Presnell, M., & Willoughby, M. (1998a), Dosage effects of methylphenidate on the social behavior of adolescents diagnosed with attention deficit hyperactivity disorder. *Exper. Clin. Psychopharm.* 6:1–18.

Smith, B.H., Pelham, W.E., Gnagy, E., Yudell, R.S. (1998b), Equivalent effects of stimulant treatment for attention-deficit hyperactivity disorder during childhood and adolescence. *J. Amer. Acad. Child Adoles. Psychiatry,* 37:1–8.

Solanto, M.V. (1984), Neuropharmacological basis of stimulant drug action in attention deficit with hyperactivity: A review and synthesis. *Psychol. Bull.,* 95:387–409.

Spencer, T., Biederman, J., Wilens, T., Harding, M., O'Donnell, D., & Griffin, S. (1996), Pharmacotherapy of ADHD across the life cycle. *J. Amer. Acad. Child Adoles. Psychiatry,* 4:409–432.

Stephens, R., Pelham, W.E. & Skinner, R. (1984), The state-dependent and main effects of pemoline and methylphenidate on paired-associates learning and spelling in hyperactive children. *J. Consult. Clin. Psychol.,* 52:104–113.

Swanson, J.M., Cantwell, D., Lerner, M., McBurnett, K., Hanna, G. (1991), Effects of stimulant medication on learning in children with ADHD. *J. Learn. Disab.,* 24:219–230.

Swanson, J. & Kinsbourne, M. (1979), The cognitive effects of stimulant drugs on hyperactive (inattentive) children. In: *Attention and the Development of Cognitive Skills,* eds., G. Hale & M. Lewis. New York: Plenum Press, pp. 249–274.

Swanson, J., Kinsbourne, M., Roberts, W. & Zucker, K. (1978), Time-response analysis of the effect of stimulant medication on the learning ability of children referred for hyperactivity. *Pediatrics,* 61:21–29.

Swanson, J.M., McBurnett, K., Christian, D.L. & Wigal, T. (1995), Stimulant medications and the treatment of children with ADHD. In: *Advances in Clinical Child Psychology,* eds., T.H. Ollendick & R.J. Prinz. New York: Plenum Press, pp. 265–322.

Swanson, J.M., Sandman, E., Deutsch, C. & Baren, M. (1983), Methylphenidate (Ritalin) given with or before breakfast: Part I. Behavioral, cognitive, and electrophysiological effects. *Pediatrics,* 72:49–55.

Tannock, R., Schachar, R.J., Carr, R.P., Chajczyk, D. & Logan, G.D. (1989), Effects of methylphenidate on inhibitory control in hyperactive children. *J. Abnorm. Child. Psychol.*, 17:473–492.

Taylor, E., Schachar, R., Thorley, G., Wieselberg, H.M., Everitt, B. & Rutter, M. (1987), Which boys respond to stimulant medication? A controlled trial of methylphenidate in boys with disruptive behavior. *Psychol. Med.*, 17:121–143.

Walker, H.M., Street, A., Garrett, B., Crossen, J., Hops, H. & Greenwood, C.R. (1978), *RECESS: Reprogramming Environmental Contingencies for Effective Social Skills.* Eugene, OR: Center at Oregon for Research in the Behavioral Education of the Handicapped.

Weiss, G. & Hechtman, L. (1993), *Hyperactive Children Grown Up.* New York: Guilford Press.

Werry, J.S. (1995), Resolved: Cardiac arrhythmias make desipramine an unacceptable choice in children. *J. Am. Acad. Child Adoles. Psychiatry*, 34:1239–1241.

Zametkin, A.J. & Rapport, J.L. (1987), Neurobiology of attention deficit disorder with hyperactivity: Where have we come in 50 years? *J. Am. Acad. Child Adolesc. Psychiatry,* 26:5:676–686.

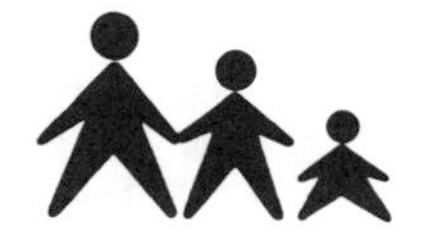

Dose-Response Effects of Ritalin on Cognitive Self-Regulation, Learning and Memory, and Academic Performance

MARY V. SOLANTO

A major concern for clinicians prescribing Ritalin is the determination of the appropriate dose. Ritalin is most often used to improve classroom behavior, academic performance, and social functioning; yet, research and clinical experience have raised the possibility that the dosage that maximizes improvement in one of these domains may not be optimal for another.

The possibility of differential dose-response curves for behavior and cognition was first suggested in a much-publicized report by Sprague and Sleator (1977), which revealed a disparity between the Ritalin dosage that maximally improved behavior as rated by teachers (1.0 mg/kg) and the dosage that optimized performance on a measure of information processing (0.3 mg/kg) (Figure 1). These data suggested that a Ritalin dosage that maximally improved the child's behavior in the classroom might have no effect or might even impair the ability to learn and retain academic material. Since the report by Sprague and Sleator, numerous studies have systematically examined the effects of varying Ritalin dosage on classroom and laboratory measures of impulsivity, learning, memory, and academic performance. By observing the simultaneous effects of different dosages on cognitive and behavioral tasks, researchers have been able to address the issue of disparities in dose-response curves for the variables. Furthermore, several careful dose-response studies have addressed the more specific question whether stimulants might exert *adverse* effects on cognition by inducing overt or covert cognitive constriction perseveration or "overfocusing" (Solanto, 1984).

This chapter evaluates the results of these studies of dosage effects on cognitive and behavioral functions and considers their implications for clinical practice, as well as for future research, including the delineation of treatment-relevant subtypes of attention deficit hyperactivity disorder (ADHD) and the understanding of central mechanisms of stimulant drug action.

DOSE-RESPONSE RELATIONSHIPS ON COGNITIVE MEASURES

For a full appreciation of the results of studies of the effects of Ritalin on cognitive function, it is necessary to have an understanding of dose-response relationships. A dose-response *curve* is obtained when dose of drug is plotted on the x axis and the magnitude of a particular response (e.g., activity level) at that dose is plotted on the y axis. Dose-response curves may assume various shapes, which can be described mathematically. When the dose-

Division of Child and Adolescent Psychiatry, Mount Sinai Medical Center, New York, New York.

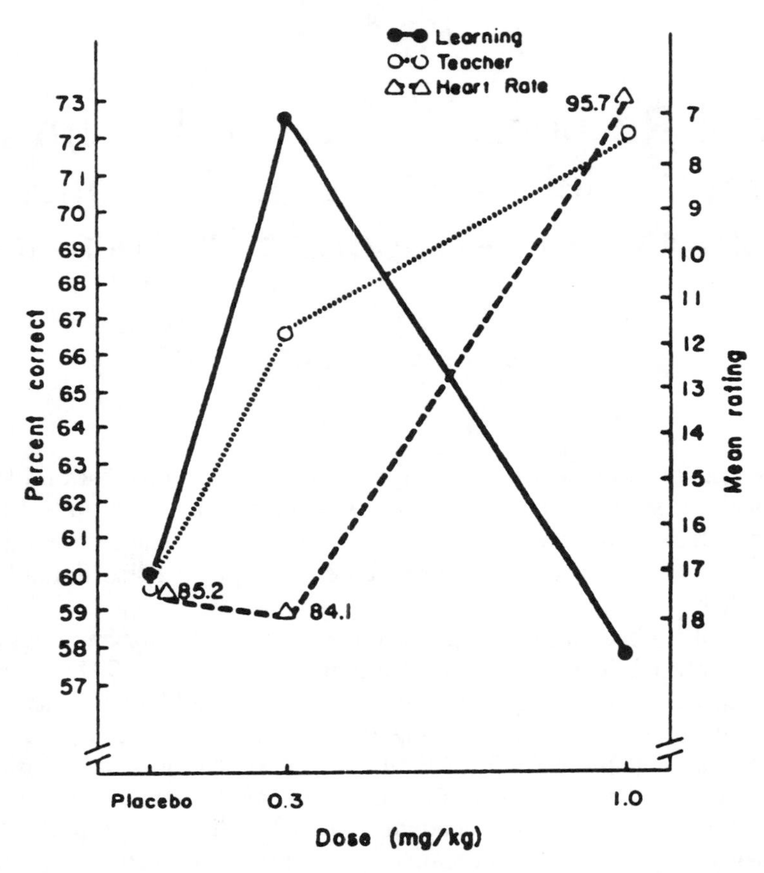

FIG. 1. Three different dose–response curves produced by three different target behaviors. The learning curve is the same as the accuracy curve from matrix 15 of the laboratory learning task. The teacher curve represents social behavior as rated by the teacher, who used a scale on which the numbers become smaller as the child improves. The heart rate curve indicates the number of beats per minute. From Sprague and Sleator (1977).

response curve assumes the form of a straight line, the slope is a constant number, and the curve is described as *linear* (Figure 2). In this instance, an increase in dosage will yield a stronger response. Curves that assume a form other than a straight line are described as *curvilinear*. Among them are the *quadratic* curve, in which there is *one* change in direction, and the *cubic* curve, in which there are *two* changes in direction of the curve. In its extreme form, the quadratic curve may resemble the inverted-U depicted in Figure 3. In this instance, there is clearly an optimal dosage above *and* below which the clinical response falls off. In another form (Figure 4), the quadratic curve may reach a peak beyond which there is leveling off of response with increasing dosage. In the cubic curve, shown in Figure 5, there may be more than one optimal dosage.

When statistical analysis of group data yields a significant effect of dosage, the data can be probed further by a *trend analysis* to determine the shape of the curve. The finding of a significant *linear* component means that at least part of the curve assumes the form of a straight line. If there is, in addition, a significant *quadratic* component, then the curve will have a form resembling, at least in part, those shown in Figures 3 or 4, in which increasing doses do *not* yield proportionate increases in clinical response. If *only* the linear component is significant, the curve will most closely resemble a straight line. Posthoc tests are

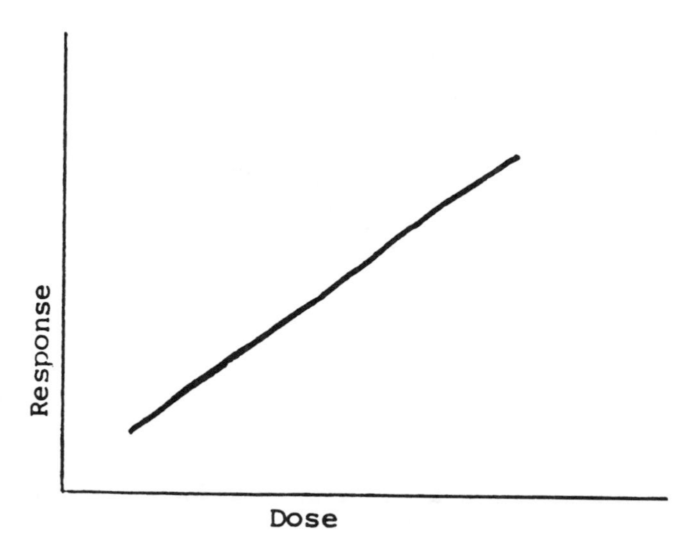

FIG. 2. Linear dose-response curve.

necessary to ascertain whether any two specific doses yield a significantly different response.

It is important to note that although the averaged data for the group in any study may yield curves such as those described above, this does not indicate that the response of any individual child will be predicted by the same curve. As will be discussed more fully, research in the field of stimulant drug response has revealed great variability between subjects in dosage effects on cognition and behavior.

COGNITIVE IMPULSIVITY

Children with ADHD display impulsivity in the cognitive sphere as well as in the behavioral realm. These children may be prone to select an answer or jump to a conclusion

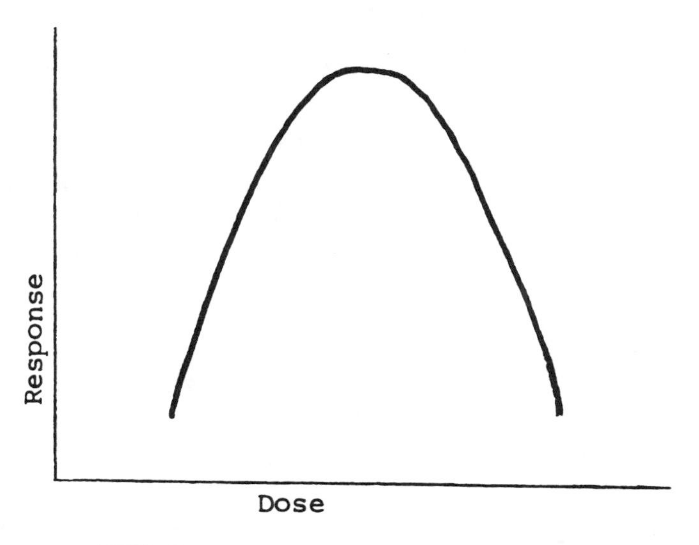

FIG. 3. Quadratic dose-response curve.

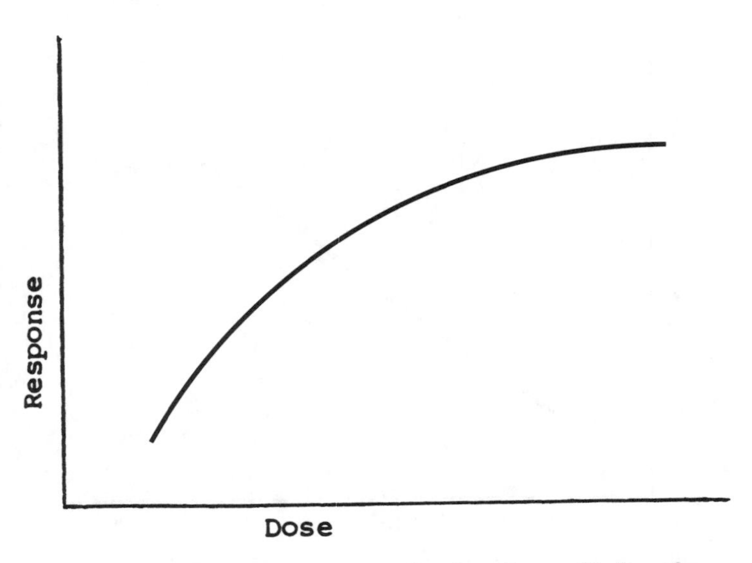

FIG. 4. Quadratic dose-response curve illustrating leveling-off of performance with higher doses.

without sufficient consideration of alternatives, they may fail to correct an obviously inaccurate response or they may fail to withhold or inhibit a response to an irrelevant or inappropriate stimulus.

The continuous performance test (CPT) has been used to measure impulsivity as well as attention in children with ADHD. On this task, visual stimuli are presented to the subject, who is told to respond only when a predesignated target stimulus appears. Failures to detect the target are errors of omission and have been traditionally considered to index attention. "False alarms," or responses to nontarget stimuli, are errors of commission and are considered to index impulsivity. A recent meta-analysis showed that methylphenidate significantly enhanced the ability of children with ADHD to respond differentially to target and nontarget stimuli (Losier et al., 1996). However, only a few studies have systemati-

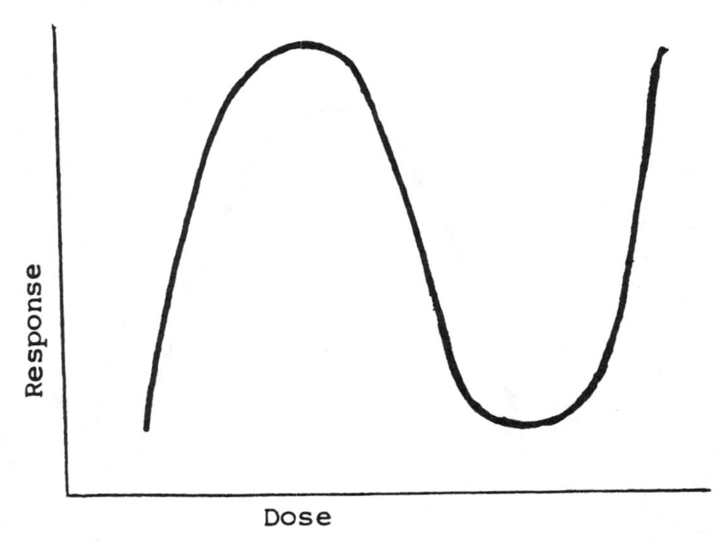

FIG. 5. Quadratic dose-response curve illustrating leveling-off in performance with increasing dose.

cally examined the effects of dosage on CPT performance. Low to moderate fixed doses of 5–15 mg (Rapport et al., 1986) or weight-based doses of 0.3–0.6 mg/kg (Barkley et al., 1989) were equally effective in reducing omission errors. In a subsequent study by Rapport et al. (1987), which expanded the dose range to 20 mg, only the 10- and 15-mg doses were significantly better than placebo; a small but nonsignificant *increase* in errors at 20 mg compared with 15 mg produced a significant quadratic effect. Conners (1996) more recently also reported a significant quadratic effect of dosage on CPT reaction time in a mixed sample of 25 adults and children (median age, 15 years) such that reaction time was significantly *worse* at 15 mg than at 10 mg. Effects on CPT commission errors have been inconsistent. In one study there was a linear effect of dosage and a significant decrease in errors only at the highest dose of 15 mg (Rapport et al., 1986), whereas in another there was equal reduction following low (0.3 mg/kg) and moderate (0.6 mg/kg) Ritalin doses (Barkley et al., 1989).

The Matching Familiar Figures Test (MFFT) and, more recently, the Stopping Task have also been widely used as measures of impulsivity in studies of ADHD. On each item of the MFFT, the child is presented with a stimulus picture of a familiar object (e.g., a house) and then must choose, from among six very similar response pictures, the single item that is identical with the stimulus figure in every detail. The most successful strategy involves systematic comparison between each response figure and the stimulus figure. Several studies that have investigated dosages ≤15 mg (Rapport et al., 1985a), 20 mg (Rapport et al., 1988), and 0.6 mg/kg (Douglas et al., 1988; Sebrechts et al., 1986) have quite clearly demonstrated *linear* improvement in performance (reduction in errors) on the MFFT with increasing dosage. Furthermore, the linear dose-response curves for MFFT performance paralleled the curves for observations of on-task behavior, teacher ratings of self-control, and academic efficiency (percentage of academic seatwork assignments completed correctly), with no significant differences in slope among these measures (Rapport et al., 1988).

The results of studies that have examined the effects of doses as high as 1.0 mg/kg on the MFFT have been conflicting, however. Brown and Sleator (1979) reported that performance was a *quadratic* function of dosage such that whereas the 0.3 mg/kg dosage reduced errors on the task, the 1.0-mg/kg dosage was no more effective than placebo. Tannock and her colleagues observed no effect of Ritalin on MFFT errors but did report that 0.3 and 1.0 mg/kg were equally effective in increasing latency to response on the task (Tannock et al., 1989a).

The MFFT has been criticized with respect to its reliability and validity as a measure of impulsivity (Block et al., 1974; Milich and Kramer, 1985). The Stop Signal Task (SST), introduced as a measure of inhibitory control in children with ADHD in 1990 (Schachar and Logan, 1990), assesses the individual's ability to inhibit a prepared motor response. On this task, the individual is instructed to respond as quickly as possible to each of a series of visual stimuli (X or O), presented singly on a computer screen, by pressing one of two designated response keys. On some trials, randomly determined, the visual stimulus is preceded by a tone, which is the signal to the subject to refrain from responding to the stimulus on that trial. In a comparison of two Ritalin doses, Tannock et al. (1989b) reported that 1.0 mg/kg was significantly more effective than 0.3 mg/kg in increasing the speed of the stopping process (reducing stop signal reaction time) in children with ADHD. Tannock et al. (1995b) subsequently compared three doses of Ritalin (0.3, 0.6, and 0.9 mg/kg) with respect to effects on performance on a "change task," a measure of cognitive switching requiring that the subject not only inhibit a response to the visual stimulus on stop signal trials but also shift to executing a different secondary response on those trials. Results revealed significant quadratic as well as linear effects of dose on stop signal reaction time (SSRT); posthoc tests showed that SSRT was maximally improved at the moderate 0.6 mg/kg dose, with lesser and equivalent improvements at the 0.3 and 0.9 mg/kg doses. In addition, there was a disjunction in the curves for effects on SSRT and observed motor activity, such that the latter was maximally improved at the highest dose. Reaction time for response reengagement (Change-RT) showed an overall effect of drug but no between-dosage differences. These results suggest that inhibitory control, at least when tested in a more complex paradigm involving a shift to a secondary task, may be optimized at a lower dose than that which minimizes overt motor activity. It would be interesting to ascertain if quadratic effects of dose are also found on the more simple Stopping Task measure of inhibitory control.

LEARNING AND MEMORY

Research on stimulant drug effects has attempted to identify and develop laboratory measures of learning and memory that might reflect or predict drug effects on children's ability to learn and retain academic material. The paired-associate learning test has been the most widely examined in this regard in children with ADHD. On paired-associate learning tests (PALTs), the individual is required to learn an association between each of a list of words, numbers, pictures, or symbols (the stimulus) with another word, number, picture, or symbol (the response).

Research by Swanson and colleagues (1978) first suggested that a PALT might be useful in distinguishing favorable from adverse responders to Ritalin. These authors used a version of the task, in which the child was told to associate a given animal picture with a particular "zoo" (North, South, East, West). Ritalin dosage was begun at 5 mg and incremented by 5 mg until the child exhibited either a 25% reduction in errors (a favorable response) or a 25% increase in errors (an adverse response). Using this method, the researchers classified 69.8% of their 53 subjects as favorable responders and the remainder as adverse responders. Subsequent research, however, has failed to validate the PALT as an index of Ritalin responsiveness on academic, behavioral, or other cognitive measures. Furthermore, studies have been notably inconsistent with respect to both overall drug effects and dosage effects of Ritalin on this task.

Gan and Cantwell (1982) examined the effects of three dosages of Ritalin (0.3, 0.5, and 1.0 mg/kg) in 20 attention deficit disorder with hyperactivity (ADDH) boys and reported that only the lowest dose was effective in improving performance on the PALT. Sebrechts and colleagues (1986) found no effect on the PALT of Ritalin dosages of 0.3 or 0.6 mg/kg.

Rapport and colleagues (1985b) assessed 12 children using the PALT, observations of on-task behavior, academic performance (percent completion and percent accuracy for academic seatwork) and teacher behavior ratings on the Abbreviated Conners Teacher Rating Scale (ACTRS) following placebo, and following fixed Ritalin doses of 5, 10, and 15 mg (corresponding to mean dosages of 0.22, 0.43, and 0.65 mg/kg, respectively). Effects of dosage (beginning with baseline and placebo levels) were significant for all dependent measures *except* the PALT. On the PALT, significant positive drug effects were obtained only when the *best* of each subject's responses on drug was selected and compared with baseline and placebo performance. The two subjects who were nonresponders on the PALT did improve on academic and behavioral measures, providing no support for the predictive validity of the measure. In a subsequent study by this same group (Rapport et al., 1989), more robust effects of dose (5, 10, 15, 20 mg) on the PALT were found, and the degree of effectiveness was a function of the subjects' prior mastery of the task. For those with no prior experience with the task, effects of all higher doses significantly increased PALT performance relative to placebo or 5 mg. For a group with partial mastery of the task, only the 20-mg dose reduced errors compared with placebo. Ritalin had no significant effect on those with prior mastery of the task.

In their 1988 study, described previously, Douglas et al. used a PALT consisting of arbitrarily associated word pairs, which were administered in three trials. Although there were no significant effects of Ritalin on overall performance, examination of individual trials revealed that on the second and third trials, only the 0.3 mg/kg dosage, and not the lower (0.15 mg/kg) or higher (0.6 mg/kg) dosages were effective in increasing the number of word pairs learned. The authors suggested that this may be evidence of a negative effect of a higher dose of Ritalin on a complex cognitive task. However, the subjects' response to Ritalin on the PALT was not related to their response to the drug on academic performance, on other laboratory measures of cognition, or behavior ratings by teachers or examiners. Marked intersubject variability in dose-response curves for learning, impulsivity, and other behavioral measures was clearly evident in the studies by both the Douglas and Rapport groups.

Kupietz et al. (1988) used a novel PALT in which a six-item list of beginning Chinese vocabulary words was paired with their English equivalents. They reported no significant effects of Ritalin (0.3, 0.5, and 0.7 mg/kg) in children with ADDH, although in a previous study with nine adults (Kupietz, 1980) a Ritalin dose of 5 mg, but not one of 10 mg, was effective in reducing errors on this same task. Another set of conflicting findings were those of Peeke et al. (1984), who reported that a Ritalin dosage of 10 mg (0.25–0.30 mg/kg) but not one of 21 mg (0.5–0.6 mg/kg) improved recognition and delayed recall on a verbal learning task in a study of nine ADD children, regardless of the type of the word encoding induced on the task (structural, acoustic, or semantic).

The inconsistent findings concerning the PALT admit several possible explanations, which require exploration in future research. The first is that Ritalin is only minimally effective in facilitating learning of new information; the improvement consistently seen on measures of academic productivity and accuracy may reflect drug effects on concentration and effort rather than on acquisition of new skills. A second possibly is that, as maintained by Swanson et al. (1991), there are definable subgroups of consistent positive and negative responders on the PALT, as well as on other cognitive outcome measures, whose results are obscured in the group data. The study of mastery by Rapport et al., (1989) suggests that the subjects' baseline task performance may be one variable that determines dose-responsiveness. The possible existence of subgroups with distinct dose-response curves on measures of learning or other domains of outcome is considered further in the discussion.

A third possibility is that Ritalin enhances dimensions or types of learning and/or memory that are not assessed by the PALT. Some support for this interpretation comes from a study by Evans and colleagues (1986) of the effects of three Ritalin doses (0.2, 0.4, and 0.6 mg/kg) on the Buschke Selective Reminding Test (SRT), which requires the subject to learn a list of unrelated words. Whereas both the SRT and the PALT are scored for immediate recall (e.g., the total number of items recalled on a given trial), only the SRT is scored for "long-term" storage (i.e. the total number of items recalled on *two* consecutive trials) and "long-term" retrieval (i.e., recall, on a given trial, of items in long-term storage). Evans et al. (1986) reported no significant effects of Ritalin on immediate retention (i.e. number of words recalled on the first trial, total number of words recalled across trials, or slope of words recalled across trials) on the SRT. By contrast, there were significant linear dose-response effects for the long-term storage and retrieval variables. It is relevant to note in this context that significant linear effects of Ritalin (0.3, 0.6, and 0.9 mg/kg) on *working memory* were reported by Tannock et al. (1995a) in nonanxious ADHD children.

The Stimulus Equivalence Paradigm (SEP) may have potential as a sensitive laboratory measure of cognitive response to Ritalin. This task encompasses both easy and complex types of associative learning as well as separate assessments of acquisition and recall. It consists of an acquisition phase in which the child learns simple "symmetric" associations between visual stimuli (e.g., A–B and A–C, where A, B, and C are distinct visual patterns), followed by a learning/recall phase in which these trained symmetric associations are tested for recall and more complex untrained "transitive" associations are assessed (e.g., the association between B and C through their common association with A). Vyse and Rapport (1989) compared the effects of fixed Ritalin dosages (5, 10, 15, and 20 mg) simultaneously on the SEP and on observations of on-task behavior, and academic efficiency. They reported pronounced linear effects of dosage on observed on-task behavior, as well as academic efficiency, and more moderate linear effects on the SEP. Whereas performance on the classroom measures was significantly enhanced by doses starting at 10 mg, performance on the SEP differed significantly from placebo only at the 20-mg dosage for the acquisiton score, and only at 15 and 20 mg for the learning/recall phase. The results of these studies suggest, as did the SRT study, that Ritalin may have more pronounced effects on recall than on acquisition. Furthermore, contrary to the postulation of Sprague and Sleator (1977), the results are also consistent with the possibility that *higher* doses of Ritalin may be required to enhance learning on complex cognitive tasks relative to those that improve overt behavior.

Some support for the latter interpretation is also provided in the recent report by O'Toole et al. (1997), who studied the effects of high (0.8 mg/kg) and low (0.3 mg/kg) Ritalin dosages on easy and hard versions of a nonverbal learning task. They reported that the high dosage was superior to the low dosage both in enhancing recall on the easy task and in enhancing both acquisition and recall on the hard version. It is important to emphasize that in this, as in all the previous studies described, there was considerable variability *between* subjects in the dose that optimized performance on a given measure, as well as considerable variability *within* individual subjects with respect to optimal dose across the different outcome measures.

COGNITIVE CONSTRICTION

Cognitive constriction may be conceptualized as a narrowing of attentional focus, such that stimuli that are "peripheral" in space, time, or meaning to the subject are relatively ignored. Although increased attentional focus is an obvious therapeutic benefit of Ritalin in children with ADHD, excessive narrowing of attentional focus may impair cognitive performance on certain types of tasks, because either the subject disregards relevant peripheral cues or becomes unable to shift perceptual set or strategy to meet changing situational demands (Robbins and Sahakian, 1979; Solanto, 1984). This reduction in cognitive flexibility may be manifested as perseveration of a (maladaptive or inaccurate) response, obsessive preoccupation with one activity, or repetitiveness in verbal or nonverbal communications. The possibility that such effects may be induced in children by stimulant drug treatment is consistent with cognitive research in humans demonstrating that an increase in physiologic arousal narrows the attentional focus (Wachtel, 1967). Furthermore, it is well known from pharmacologic research in animals that at high doses stimulants produce repetitive, non–goal-oriented "stereotypic" motor behaviors, with a concomitant narrowing in the range of behaviors (Solanto, 1984).

The Wisconsin Card Sorting Test (WCST) is a well-developed measure of cognitive flexibility. Performance on the WCST has been shown to be sensitive to lesions of the frontal lobe (Robinson et al., 1980), the brain region that mediates the executive functions of self-monitoring, self-correction, planning, and judgment, and which is strongly implicated as the site of the central dysfunction in ADHD (Barkley, 1997). This task requires the subject to sort cards that vary in three conceptual categories: color, shape, and number. Subjects are given accuracy feedback after each sort, but not explicitly told the correct sorting principle (e.g., color). After a criterion number of correct sorts, the sorting principle is changed without warning. Number of category shifts successfully achieved, and number of perseverative responses (sorts to the previously reinforced category) are recorded. Dyme and colleagues (1982) first examined the effect of a high dose of a Ritalin (1.0 mg/kg) on the WCST in a placebo crossover pilot study of five children with ADHD and found an increase in perseverative responses with the drug in three subjects.

Tannock and Schachar (1992) more thoroughly examined the effects of placebo and low (0.3 mg/kg) and high (1.0 mg/kg) Ritalin dosages on the WCST in 23 children with ADDH (*DSM-III*), who were each assessed twice under each of the three conditions. Subjects were also observed and coded during testing for other behavioral manifestations of constriction, such as repetitive tidying or aligning of cards, movement stereotypies, and topic perseveration. Group results showed a significant dose-related *increase* in WCST perseverative errors on the first drug administration, but a significant *decrease* in such errors on the second drug administration. Analysis of individual results revealed that 63% of children were more perseverative following 1.0 mg/kg than placebo, and 28% made more perseverative errors at 0.3 mg/kg compared with placebo. Coded perseverative behaviors increased during *both* drug sessions; severity but not frequency of these behaviors was dose-related. There were no systematic differences in diagnostic characteristics such as pervasiveness of ADDH or comorbid diagnoses between subjects with a drug-induced increase in number of perseverative or constrictive responses and those without.

An increase in perseverative errors following the first but not the second drug administration suggests at least two possible explanations. The first is that increased constriction is a concomitant of initial exposure to Ritalin which rapidly exhibits physiologic tolerance; however, the findings that prior treatment with stimulants did not predict perseverative responding on the WCST, and that other constrictive behaviors appeared to be increased during *both* assessments at each drug dosage, constitute arguments against this interpretation. Another possibility is that positive practice effects on this task, for which there are no alternative forms and which is sensitive to the development of insight, militated against the emergence of negative effects on performance at the second administration. The absence of significant differences in task performance on repeated placebo testing does not support this interpretation. It may nonetheless be possible, as the authors suggest, that Ritalin uniquely impairs the development of insight or strategy during the acquisition phase of novel and complex tasks.

Another approach to the assessment of cognitive flexibility emerges from the literature on intellectual function that differentiates *convergent* from *divergent* thinking (Guilford, 1956; Guilford, 1967). On measures of the former, such as the traditional IQ test, there is only one predesignated correct answer, whereas on the latter, represented in measurements of creativity, there are multiple correct answers. Tests of "spontaneous flexibility" that represent one type of divergent thinking (Guilford, 1967) were developed for use in a creativity test battery (Wallach and Kogan, 1965). Solanto and Wender (1989) selected two tests from this battery for use in their investigation of stimulant-induced constriction of cognitive function in children with ADHD: the Alternate Uses Test, on which the subject is asked to generate as many uses as possible for common objects (e.g., a brick or button), and the Instances Test, in which the subject must generate as many exemplars as possible of verbally specified class concepts (e.g., *round* things). Both tests are scored for the total number of responses. The Alternate Uses Test is scored in addition for the number of conceptual classes or categories of use represented among the responses.

Nineteen subjects were tested weekly in a repeated measures design following three placebo administrations and three Ritalin dosages (0.3, 0.6, and 1.0 mg/kg) in random order. Ritalin was found to significantly *increase* total responses and number of unique classes of responses on the Alternate Uses Test, which just compensated for a *decrease* in output across successive days of placebo testing, possibly caused by loss of interest or motivation. A similar result, approaching statistical significance, was obtained on the Instances test. No differences were found at baseline on the tasks between the ADDH group and a matched group of normal control subjects.

Although the group data did not reveal an adverse effect of Ritalin on the tasks, it was possible to identify a subgroup of eight children who did appear to manifest a form of cognitive perseveration. These children produced significantly more responses while receiving the drug without a commensurate increase in the number of classes represented among the responses; thus, they appeared to perseverate within response class. In addition, there was a decrease in lucidity of some individual responses as well as a decrease in the cohesion of the spontaneous speech produced by some of the children during the free play period. These observations were made following the 0.6 mg/kg dosage as well as the 1.0 mg/kg dosage. Systematic comparison of the "constrictive" responders with the remaining subjects revealed no differences in age, comorbid diagnoses, absolute dose of drug administered, or IQ on the Peabody Picture Vocabulary Test. However, the constrictive subgroup obtained better baseline scores on measures of learning (PALT) and vigilance (Children's Checking Task) as well as on the arithmetic subtest of the Wide Range Achievement Test. This subgroup also had lower baseline scores on the hyperactivity and inattentiveness factors of the Teacher Child Behavior Checklist. These findings may be consistent with studies that have suggested that ADHD children with less severe inattentiveness and hyperactivity show less improvement with drug treatment (Buitelaar et al., 1995; Taylor et al., 1987).

Using a nonverbal (figural) measure of creativity (the Torrance Tests of Creative Thinking), Funk et al. (1993) found no effect of their prescribed dosage of Ritalin on task performance of the ADHD group. There were also no differences at baseline between normal and ADHD children.

Perhaps the most comprehensive study in this area is that by Douglas and colleagues (1995), who utilized a battery of tests sensitive to cognitive flexibility-constriction, including the Alternate Uses and Instances Tests and the WCST, as well as the Reitan Trailmaking Test, and a Contingency Naming Task, which assessed rapid naming and memory retrieval skills as well as the ability to apply complex rules and to reverse them on cue. Seventeen children with ADHD were each tested twice following 0.3, 0.6, and 0.9 mg/kg doses of Ritalin; scores for the two assessments for each measure were averaged. There was significant linear improvement in performance on all measures except the Instances Test, and marginally significant linear improvement on the Reitan Trailmaking. Analysis of individual responses *failed* to identify a subgroup of children with an adverse response across measures following Ritalin administration. Furthermore, in contrast to the results of Tannock and Schachar (1992), the percentage of children making increased perseverative responses on the WCST did not exceed chance levels following either the first or second administrations of the highest Ritalin dosage.

The findings of these studies have generally not only failed to yield evidence of cognitive constriction as a function of Ritalin dosage, but have revealed *positive* drug effects on measures of divergent thinking that are suggestive of improvement in cognitive self-regulatory operations, particularly the executive functions of planning, inhibitory self-control, and deployment of effort (Douglas et al., 1995). Discrepancies among results, however, leave unresolved the potential existence of an adversely responding subgroup.

ACADEMIC PERFORMANCE

Given ample evidence that Ritalin improves attention and self-control in the classroom, it is perplexing that longitudinal follow-up studies have failed to demonstrate improvement in long-term academic outcome for stimulant-treated children with respect to grades, dropout rates, or highest level of education achieved (Weiss and Hechtman, 1986). Several studies have examined the effects of Ritalin on ability to perform academic work in the classroom. Typically, these studies either have used standard problem sets given to teachers for children to complete during the usual seatwork time (Douglas et al., 1988) or have collected the problem sets in language arts and arithmetic customarily used in the child's classroom and scored them for completion and accuracy rates to generate an Academic Efficiency Score (AES) (Rapport et al., 1985b).

Early studies examined the effects of doses ranging up to 0.6 mg/kg, with conflicting results. Pelham et al. (1985) reported a significant linear and marginal quadratic effect of doses of 0.15, 0.3, and 0.6 mg/kg on completion and accuracy rates for arithmetic problems; the results indicated a leveling-off in performance between 0.3 and 0.6 mg/kg. By contrast, the percentage of reading problems completed correctly improved linearly between 0.3 and 0.6 mg/kg and paralleled the increase in on-task behavior with increasing dosage.

In studies of 12 and 14 children, respectively, Rapport and colleagues examined the effects of placebo and fixed doses of 5, 10, and 15 mg on the AES. In the first study (Rapport et al., 1985b), there was a significant linear but nonsignificant quadratic effect of dose up to 15 mg (equivalent to a mean dosage of 0.65 mg/kg). The percentage of academic problems completed was significantly enhanced compared with placebo only at the 15-mg dose. Percentage accuracy was significantly and equivalently enhanced at all three medication doses. In the second study (Rapport et al., 1986), both linear and quadratic effects were significant, and there were no differences among doses for completion or accuracy rates. Ceiling effects may account for the leveling off observed in the latter study, since the subjects were performing in the 70% to 80% range at placebo, compared with 60% to 70% in the first study.

In order to avoid possible ceiling effects, Douglas et al. (1988) administered an arithmetic problem set of 60 items to their 19 subjects. Perhaps because of this precaution, these authors reported a linear increase in output and number correct, which extended to the 0.6 mg/kg dosage; furthermore, posthoc tests showed that the 0.6 mg/kg dosage was significantly more effective than either the 0.15- or the 0.3-mg/kg dosages when the task was administered in the classroom.

More recent studies have extended the dosage range to 20 mg. Rapport et al. (1988) reported pronounced linear but nonsignificant quadratic effects of placebo and fixed doses of 5, 10, 15, and 20 mg. The highest dose was not significantly better than either the 10-mg or the 15-mg doses in posthoc tests of the group data of 26 subjects. Analysis of individual data, however, revealed that an equal percentage (36%) of subjects responded optimally at the 15-mg and 20-mg doses.

Using the same set of fixed doses, Rapport and colleagues also reported a leveling off in group mean AES at 10 mg, with no further improvement (Vyse and Rapport, 1989) or smaller increments (Rapport et al., 1987) generated by the 15-mg and 20-mg doses. Linear and quadratic effects were significant for AES in both studies. Observed on-task behavior paralleled the changes in AES in both studies. These findings contrasted with the rate of correct responses per minute on the SEP complex learning task, which, as noted, was maximally improved at the highest dose (Vyse and Rapport, 1989).

Tannock and colleagues (1989b) found that high (1.0 mg/kg) and low (0.3 mg/kg) doses of Ritalin were equally effective in enhancing performance on simple arithmetic tasks; an intermediate dose was not examined.

As was true for measures of learning, impulsivity, teacher ratings, and on-task behavior, there was striking intersubject variability in dose-response curves for academic performance in these studies (Rapport et al., 1986; Rapport et al., 1985b; Rapport et al., 1988; Vyse and Rapport, 1989), with some children showing maximal improvement at the highest dosages and others performing best at low or moderate dosages. Furthermore, *intra*subject variability was apparent across measures—that is, individual children exhibited different response curves for different domains of behavior. Given subject heterogeneity, therefore, it is perhaps not surprising that the relatively small samples cited above generated different group trends for the effects of increasing dosage on academic performance.

The largest and more recent study of Ritalin effects on classroom functioning may prove to be the most informative. Rapport et al. (1994) administered placebo and fixed doses of 5, 10, 15, and 20 mg to 76 children and examined simultaneous effects on AES, observed percentage on-task behavior, and teacher ratings of behavior on the ACTRS. Results for all measures yielded highly significant linear *and* quadratic effects of dose. For the composite AES, as well as for ACTRS ratings, the 10-, 15-, and 20-mg doses were each superior to placebo and to the 5-mg dose, but not significantly different among themselves. For observed on-task behavior, however, the 20-mg dose conferred a significant advantage over all lower doses.

Classification of each subject's response on each measure at each dose with respect to whether or not it was "normalized" provided important insights into the clinical magnitude of the response. For observed on-task behavior and ACTRS scores, increasing rates of normalized scores were seen with doses up to 20 mg. However, the maximum rate of normalization for AES scores was achieved at 10 mg with no further increase at higher doses. Overall rates of normalization, using the best score for each subject on each measure, were lower for AES (53%) than for ACTRS (94%) or observed attention (76%). Furthermore, clinically significant improvement in a child's AES was much more likely to be predictive of significant improvement in ACTRS and attention than was improvement in ACTRS or attention predictive of substantially improved AES; that is, whereas subjects who improved academically were very likely to have also improved in terms of observed behavior, the reverse was not true. Thus, the study appeared to have identified a subgroup of children who were significantly improved or normalized behaviorally but not academically. In interpreting these results, however, it is important to bear in mind that the AES assessed performance on practice problem sets on subject matter that children had already been taught and, presumably, at least partially mastered. Thus, the finding that AES was maximized at 10 mg for the group data cannot be generalized to *new* learning. Indeed, although drug effects on new learning have not been examined in the classroom setting, results on some laboratory tasks suggest that complex learning may be maximized at higher doses.

CONCLUSIONS AND IMPLICATIONS

A review of the literature does not support a simple distinction between dose-response curves for behavioral and cognitive functions. Studies of cognitive inhibition reveal clearly linear effects, paralleling teacher ratings of self-control and observed on-task behavior, following weight-based doses up to 0.6 mg/kg and fixed doses at least up to 15 mg. On a more complex task, which required inhibition followed by switching to a secondary response, however, there were quadratic effects such that performance decreased at a high dosage (0.9 mg/kg) compared with an intermediate (0.6 mg/kg) dosage. The effects of Ritalin on learning and memory are insufficiently explored, in part because of difficulties in task selection and differentiating effects on acquisition and memory. Studies to date, however, suggest that recall may be more sensitive than acquisition processes to stimulant effects, and that effects on complex learning and problem solving may require higher doses. A recent series of studies has quite clearly established that for most children with ADHD, drug-induced cognitive perseveration or constriction is at most a transient effect of Ritalin treatment. Finally, the results of studies of dose-response effects on academic problem set performance are conflicting, with some reports of linear dose-response relationships and others, including a large-scale study, revealing a leveling-off of drug response above 10 mg. It is worth noting that no study has revealed that high doses *impair* academic performance to placebo levels.

Clinical implications

Permeating these findings and moderating the implications of this research for clinical practice is evidence of substantial intersubject variability in dose-response within a given domain of functioning, as well as *intra*subject variability across domains. Patient characteristics or laboratory measures that predict the effects of dosage on behavioral or academic response have yet to be developed. These reports should underscore for the clinician the importance of monitoring multiple indices of efficacy during dosage titration, including academic and cognitive as well as behavioral measures, and prioritizing the results to be achieved so as to maximize improvement in the targeted area while minimizing adverse effects in others.

Research implications

Further investigation of differences among children in dose-response curves across multiple domains of behavioral and cognitive functioning holds the tantalizing potential of characterizing subgroups with distinct and predictable patterns of response to Ritalin. In order to identify such subgroups, several methodological issues must be addressed. First, all subjects in a study must be exposed to the full range of doses; given high intrasubject variability of response both within and across measures, it cannot be assumed that an adverse response at a given dose presages an adverse response at higher doses. Furthermore, each subject must be exposed to multiple administrations of each dosage in order to establish consistency of positive or adverse response. In addition, given the discrepancies between drug effects on laboratory measures of learning, and performance on academic tasks, it is particularly important to develop paradigms to assess the impact of Ritalin on *new* learning in the classroom setting.

Once adverse or otherwise distinctively responding subgroups have been reliably identified on ecologically meaningful measures, these subjects must be studied for diagnostic, neuropsychologic, or neurophysiologic characteristics that they may have in common. One possible basis for the distinctive response of children may be differential sensitivity of norepinephrine and dopamine receptors, both of which are stimulated by Ritalin and other psychostimulants (Solanto, 1998). Evolving research suggests that these catecholamines may mediate different effects of the stimulants on behavior and cognition. Abundant evidence from animal studies, for example, implicates norepinephrine effects at the prefrontal cortex on the ability to delay or switch a response (Arnsten, 1997). Limited clinical research comparing desipramine (which primarily affects norepinephrine) with Ritalin (which affects both catecholamines) on cognitive tasks suggests that norepinephrine may mediate Ritalin effects on higher-order problem-solving abilities, particularly when they require inhibitory control; dopamine appears to be more important in mediating Ritalin effects on basic attentional processes and vigilance (Rapport et al., 1993). Differential relative involvement and/or sensitivity of these systems in the pathophysiology of ADHD in different children may underly the differential response to stimulants and other drugs in different domains of response.

Another distinction that may have relevance for subtyping is that between presynaptic inhibitory, and postsynaptic excitatory, effects of stimulants on catecholamine neurotransmission. Animal studies reveal that these effects are clearly dose related (Solanto, 1998), with one study of ADHD children suggesting that Ritalin effects on impulsivity-hyperactivity may be presynaptically mediated (Solanto, 1986). Differential relative sensitivity of pre- and postsynaptic receptors in individual patients may thus constitute another basis for differential response to stimulants across domains.

Clearly, research in this area is in its infancy. Increasing knowledge of the neuropathology of ADHD (Castellanos et al., 1996) and the neuropsychopharmacologic mechanisms of stimulant drug action (Solanto, 1998), however, offer promise for identifying treatment-relevant subtypes of ADHD.

REFERENCES

Arnsten, A.F.T. (1997), Catecholamine regulation of the prefrontal cortex. *J. Psychopharmacol.*, 11:151–162.

Barkley, R.A. (1997), Behavioral inhibition, sustained attention, and executive functions: Constructing a unifying theory of ADHD. *Psychol. Bull.*, 121:65–94.

Barkley, R.A., McMurray, M.D., Edelbrock, C.S. & Robbins, B.A. (1989), The response of aggressive and nonaggressive ADHD children to two doses of methylphenidate. *J. Am. Acad. Child Adolesc. Psychiatry*, 28:873–881.

Block, J., Block, J.H. & Harrington, D.M. (1974), Some misgivings about the Matching Familiar Figures Test as a measure of reflection-impulsivity. *Dev. Psychol.*, 10:611–632.

Brown, R.T. & Sleator, E.K. (1979), Methylphenidate in hyperkinetic children: Differences in dose effects on impulsive behavior. *Pediatrics*, 64:408–411.

Buitelaar, J.K., Van der Gaag, J., Swaab-Barneveld, H. & Kuiper, M. (1995), Prediction of clinical response to methylphenidate in children with attention-deficit hyperactivity disorder. *J. Am. Acad. Child Adolesc. Psychiatry*, 34:1025–1032.

Castellanos, F.X., Giedd, J.N., Marsh, W.L., Hamburger, S.D., Vaituzis, A.C., Dickstein, D.P., Sarfatti, S.E., Vauss, Y.C., Snell, J.W., Lange, N., Kaysen, D., Krain, A.L., Ritchie, G.F., Rajapakse, J.C. & Rapoport, J.L. (1996), Quantitative brain magnetic imaging in attention-deficit hyperactivity disorder. *Arch. Gen. Psychiatry*, 53:607–616.

Conners, C.K. (1996), Clinical use of the Continuous Performance Test: Diagnostic utility and drug sensitivity. Presented at the American Academy of Child and Adolescent Psychiatry, Philadelphia, PA.

Douglas, V.I., Barr, R.G., Amin, K., O'Neill, M.E. & Britton, B.G. (1988), Dosage effects and individual responsivity to methylphenidate in attention deficit disorder. *J. Child Psychol. Psychiatry*, 29:453–475.

Douglas, V.I., Barr, R.G., Desilets, J. & Sherman, E. (1995), Do high doses of methylphenidate impair flexible thinking in attention-deficit hyperactivity disorder? *J. Am. Acad. Child Adolesc. Psychiatry*, 34:877–885.

Dyme, I.Z., Sahakian, B.J., Golinko, B.E., & Rabe, E.F. (1982), Perseveration induced by methylphenidate in children: Preliminary findings. *Prog. Neuropsychopharmacol. Biol. Psychiatry*, 6:269–273.

Evans, R.W., Gualtieri, C.T. & Amara, I. (1986), Methylphenidate and memory: Dissociated effects in hyperactive children. *Psychopharmacology*, 90:211–216.

Funk, J.B., Chessare, J.B., Weaver, M.T. & Exley, A.R. (1993), Attention deficit hyperactivity disorder, creativity and the effects of methylphenidate. *Pediatrics*, 91:816–819.

Gan, J. & Cantwell, D.P. (1982), Dosage effects of methylphenidate on paired associate learning: Positive/negative placebo responders. *J. Am. Acad. Child Adolesc. Psychiatry*, 21:237–242.

Guilford, J.P. (1956), The structure of intellect. *Psychol. Bull.*, 53:267–293.

Guilford, J.P. (1967), Some theoretical views of creativity. In: *Contemporary Approaches to Psychology*, eds. H. Nelson & W. Bevan, Princeton: Van Nostrand Reinhold.

Kupietz, S.S., Richardson, E., Gadow, K.D. & Winsberg, B.G. (1980), Effects of methylphenidate on learning a "beginning reading vocabulary" by normal adults. *Psychopharmacology,* 69:69–72.

Kupietz, S.S., Winsberg, B.G., Richardson, E., Maitinsky, S. & Mendell, N. (1988), Effects of methylphenidate dosage in hyperactive reading-disabled children: 1. Behavior and cognitive performance effects. *J. Am. Acad. Child Adolesc. Psychiatry,* 27:70–77.

Losier, B.J., McGrath, P.J. & Klein, R.M. (1996), Error patterns on the continuous performance test in nonmedicated and medicated samples of children with and without ADHD: A meta-analytic review. *J. Child Psychol. Psychiatry*, 37:971–987.

Milich, R. & Kramer, J. (1985), Reflections on impulsivity: An empirical investigation of impulsivity as a construct. In: *Advances in Learning and Behavioral Disabilities, vol. 3*, eds., K. Gadow & I. Bialer. Greenwich, CT: JAI Press.

O'Toole, K., Abramowitz, A., Morris, R. & Dulcan, M. (1997), Effects of methylphenidate on attention and nonverbal learning in children with attention-deficit hyperactivity disorder. *J. Am. Acad. Child Adolesc. Psychiatry*, 36:531–538.

Peeke, S., Halliday, R., Callaway, E., Prael, R. & Reus, V. (1984), Effects of two doses of methylphenidate on verbal information processing in hyperactive children. *J. Clin. Psychopharmacol.*, 4:82–88.

Pelham, W.E., Bender, M.E., Caddell, J., Booth, S. & Moorer, S.H. (1985), Methylphenidate and children with attention deficit disorder. *Arch. Gen. Psychiatry*, 42:948–952.

Rapport, M.D., Carlson, G.A., Kelly, K.L. & Pataki, C. (1993), Methylphenidate and desipramine in hospitalized children: I. Separate and combined effects on cognitive function. *J. Am. Acad. Child Adolesc. Psychiatry*, 32:333–342.

Rapport, M.D., Denney, C., DuPaul, G.J. & Gardner, M.J. (1994), Attention deficit disorder and methylphenidate: Normalization rates, clinical effectiveness, and response prediction in 76 children. *J. Am. Acad. Child Adolesc. Psychiatry*, 33:882–893.

Rapport, M.D., DuPaul, G.J., Stoner, G., Birmingham, B.K. & Masse, G. (1985a), Attention deficit disorder with hyperactivity: Differential effects of methylphenidate on impulsivity. *Pediatrics*, 76:938–943.

Rapport, M.D., DuPaul, G.J., Stoner, G. & Jones, J.T. (1986), Comparing classroom and clinic measures of attention deficit disorder: Differential idiosyncratic and dose-response effects of methylphenidate. *J. Consult. Clin. Psychol.*, 54:334–341.

Rapport, M.D., Jones, J.T., DuPaul, G.J., Kelly, K.L., Gardner, M.J., Tucker, S.B. & Shea, M.S. (1987), Attention deficit disorder and methylphenidate: Group and single-subject analyses of dose effects on attention in clinic and classroom settings. *J. Clin. Child Psychol.*, 16:329–338.

Rapport, M.D., Quinn, S.O., DuPaul, G.J., Quinn, E.P. & Kelly, K.L. (1989), Attention deficit disorder with hyperactivity and methylphenidate: The effects of dose and mastery level on children's learning performance. *J. Abnorm. Child Psychol.*, 17:669–689.

Rapport, M.D., Stoner, G., DuPaul, G.J., Birmingham, B.K. & Tucker, S. (1985b), Methylphenidate in hyperactive children: Differential effects of dose on academic, learning, and social behavior. *J. Abnorm. Child Psychol.*, 13:227–244.

Rapport, M.D., Stoner, G., DuPaul, G.J., Kelly, K.L., Tucker, S.B. & Schoeler, T. (1988),

Attention deficit disorder and methylphenidate: A multilevel analysis of dose-response effects on children's impulsivity across settings. *J. Am. Acad. Child Adolesc. Psychiatry*, 27:60–69.

Robbins, T.W. & Sahakian, B.J. (1979), "Paradoxical" effects of psychomotor stimulant drugs in hyperactive children from the standpoint of behavioural pharmacology. *Neuropharmacology*, 18:931–950.

Robinson, A.L., Heaton, R.K., Lehman, R.A.W. & Stilson, D.W. (1980), The utility of the Wisconsin Card Sorting Test in detecting and localizing frontal lobe lesions. *J. Consult. Clin. Psychol.*, 48:605–614.

Schachar, R. & Logan, G.D. (1990), Impulsivity and inhibitory control in normal development and childhood psychopathology. *Dev. Psychol.*, 26:710–720.

Sebrechts, M.M., Shaywitz, S.E., Shaywitz, B.A., Jatlow, P., Anderson, G.M. & Cohen, D.J. (1986), Components of attention, methylphenidate dosage, and blood levels in children with attention deficit disorder. *Pediatrics*, 77:222–228.

Solanto, M.V. (1984), Neuropharmacological basis of stimulant drug action in attention deficit disorder with hyperactivity: A review and synthesis. *Psychol. Bull.*, 95:387–409.

Solanto, M.V. (1986), Behavioral effects of low-dose methylphenidate in childhood attention deficit disorder: Implications for a mechanism of stimulant drug action. *J. Am. Acad. Child Adolesc. Psychiatry*, 25:96–101.

Solanto, M.V. (1998), Neuropsychopharmacological mechanisms of stimulant drug action in attention deficit/hyperactivity disorder: A review and integration. *Behav. Brain Res.*, 94:127–152.

Solanto, M.V. & Wender, E.H. (1989), Does methylphenidate constrict cognitive functioning? *J. Am. Acad. Child Adolesc. Psychiatry*, 26:897–902.

Sprague, R.L. & Sleator, E.K. (1977), Methylphenidate in hyperkinetic children: Differences in dose effects on learning and social behavior. *Science*, 198:1274–1276.

Swanson, J.M., Cantwell, D., Lerner, M., MacBurnett, K. & Hanna, G. (1991), Effects of stimulant medication on learning in children with ADHD. *J. Learn. Disabil.*, 24:219–230.

Swanson, J.M., Kinsbourne, M.K., Roberts, W. & Zucker, K. (1978), Time response analysis of the effect of stimulant medication on learning ability of children referred for hyperactivity. *Pediatrics*, 61:21–29.

Tannock, R., Ickowiz, A. & Schachar, R. (1995a), Differential effects of methylphenidate on working memory in ADHD children with and without comorbid anxiety. *J. Am. Acad. Child Adolesc. Psychiatry*, 34:886–896.

Tannock, R. & Schachar, R. (1992), Methylphenidate and cognitive perseveration in hyperactive children. *J. Am. Acad. Child Adolesc. Psychiatry*, 33:1217–1228.

Tannock, R., Schachar, R., Carr, R.P., Chajczyk, D. & Logan, G.D. (1989a), Effects of methylphenidate on inhibitory control in hyperactive children. *J. Abnorm. Child Psychol.*, 17:473–491.

Tannock, R., Schachar, R. & Logan, G.D. (1989b), Dose response effects of methylphenidate on academic performance and overt behavior in hyperactive children. *Pediatrics*, 84:648–657.

Tannock, R., Schachar, R. & Logan, G. (1995b), Methylphenidate and cognitive flexibility: Dissociated dose effects in hyperactive children. *J. Abnorm. Child Psychol.*, 23:235–266.

Taylor, E., Schachar, R., Thorley, G., Weiselberg, H.M., Everitt, B. & Rutter, M. (1987), Which boys respond to stimulant medication? A controlled trial of methylphenidate in boys with disruptive behaviour. *Psychol. Med.*, 17:121–143.

Vyse, S.A. & Rapport, M.D. (1989), The effect of methylphenidate in children with ADDH: The stimulus equivalence paradigm. *J. Consult. Clin. Psychol.*, 57:425–435.

Wachtel, P.L. (1967), Conceptions of broad and narrow attention. *Psychol. Bull.*, 68:417–429.

Wallach, M.A. & Kogan, N. (1965), *Modes of Thinking in Young Children*. New York: Holt, Rinehart, & Winston.

Weiss, G. & Hechtman, L. (1986), *Hyperactive Children Grown Up*. New York: Guilford Press.

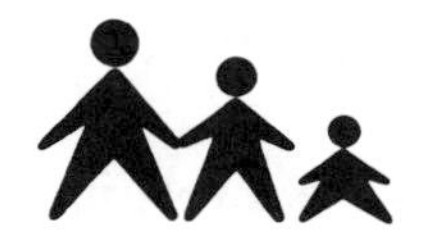

Ritalin Effects on Aggression and Antisocial Behavior

STEPHEN P. HINSHAW and STEVE S. LEE

A persisting belief in the field is that despite a wealth of evidence for the beneficial effects of methylphenidate (MPH, Ritalin) and other stimulants on inattentive, impulsive, hyperactive, noncompliant, and generally disruptive behavior patterns in children and adolescents with attention deficit hyperactivity disorder (ADHD), these medications are not helpful for aggressive and antisocial actions. For example, in describing the failure of stimulant interventions to effect long-term change in the outcomes of youth with ADHD, Milich and Loney (1979) claimed that the lack of efficacy of such medications for the secondary features of aggression, defiance, and negative affect was to blame. Ullmann and Sleator (1985) showed extremely modest effects of Ritalin on oppositional behavior patterns. Wilens and Biederman (1992) did not include conduct disordered behaviors in their review of stimulant medication; and in introducing their well-performed investigation of Ritalin benefits in home and school settings, Schachar et al. (1997) contended that Ritalin "has a limited impact on oppositional or aggressive behavior" (p. 754). Contentions from such well-respected investigators as these continue to be influential.

At the beginning of the current decade, we reviewed the extant evidence (Hinshaw, 1991) and concluded that stimulants do, in fact, yield statistically and even clinically significant effects on objectively measured and adult-rated aggression in children and adolescents with ADHD. The investigations reviewed at that time indicated that medication effects were strong for measures of naturalistically observed aggression but more equivocal for laboratory-based indexes of aggressive responding. Our purposes in the limited space available here are to (1) review the pertinent conceptual and methodological issues, (2) recount the major points made in Hinshaw (1991), (3) update research from the current decade, and (4) comment on the "disconnect" between the often dramatic effects of stimulants on aggressive behavior in short-term medication trials and the depressing failure of pharmacologic (or, indeed, any) treatments to bring about long-lasting effects on patterns of antisocial and delinquent behavior. We also discuss the specificity and ecologic validity of pharmacologic effects that are obtained and the crucial need to account for individual differences in appraising medication response.

At the outset, we highlight several important conclusions from recent, authoritative reviews (Connor and Steingard, 1996; Stoewe et al., 1995):

1. Nonspecific, "shotgun" approaches to the study of reducing child and adolescent aggression must yield to diagnosis-specific strategies (and ultimately to enhanced knowledge of etiology and pathophysiology).
2. The use of medication strategies for treating aggression never obviates the need for consideration of concurrent psychosocial interventions.

Department of Psychology, University of California at Berkeley, Berkeley, California.

3. Aggression occurs at above–base-rate levels in a wide array of psychiatric and neurologic conditions, such as psychosis, traumatic brain injury, seizure disorders, bipolar mood disorder, and pervasive developmental disorders (PDDs).
4. Medications other than stimulants have received the greatest support for effecting reductions in aggression for such domains (e.g., lithium for psychoses; neuroleptics, clomipramine, or clonidine for pervasive developmental disorders).
5. Empirical evidence for the aggression-reducing properties of stimulants has, in fact, emerged only for the diagnostic categories of ADHD and mild mental retardation, with some suggestive evidence for the aggressive aspects of pervasive developmental disorders.

Our coverage thus focuses on the treatment of aggression and antisocial behavior in ADHD and such frequently comorbid aggressive-spectrum disorders as oppositional defiant disorder (ODD) and conduct disorder (CD). We also consider whether Ritalin is a viable treatment for CD per se. For more general reviews of the neurobiology of aggression/antisocial behavior and for coverage of nonstimulant approaches, we refer the reader to the comprehensive reviews of Connor and Steingard (1996), Miczek et al. (1994), Stoewe et al. (1995), and Stoff et al. (1997).

KEY BACKGROUND ISSUES

Multidimensional nature of domain of interest

Aggressive behavior is not a unidimensional entity. As reviewed more extensively elsewhere (e.g., Hinshaw and Anderson, 1996; Hinshaw and Zupan, 1997), a variety of terms are in use to describe both the general and the specific types of actions that yield harm to others. *Externalizing* or *disruptive* behavior patterns refer to wide classes of impulsive, hyperactive, aggressive, and delinquent actions; more narrowly, *antisocial* behaviors refer to patterns of activity that clearly violate societal regulations and yield interpersonal harm. Within this latter category, behaviors can be classified as evidencing *overt* aggression (e.g., defiance, fights, bullying, verbal provocation) vs. *covert* antisocial behavior (e.g., cheating, lying, theft, property destruction, truancy). This distinction is important because overt vs. covert antisocial actions appear to have different heritabilities, family socialization influences, and predictive validities (Hinshaw and Anderson, 1996). It is noteworthy that *noncompliant* behavior patterns lie at the midpoint of the overt vs. covert bipolar dimension (Loeber and Schmaling, 1985).

Even within the realm of overt aggression, several clinically and theoretically important subcategorizations are salient. Aggressive actions can be (1) *physical* vs. *verbal,* (2) directed against *peers* vs. *adults,* (3) *proactive* (initiated, bullying) vs. *reactive* (retaliatory), or (4) *eruptive* vs. *hostile.* Unfortunately, because of low base rates, the results of the empiric investigations under review are not typically differentiated with respect to such subclassifications, but differential effects of medication on distinct subcategories of aggression and antisocial behavior could help to pinpoint the mechanisms of stimulant actions.

From a categorical perspective, the *Diagnostic and Statistical Manual of Mental Disorders, (DSM), 4th ed.* (American Psychiatric Association, 1994) lists two major disruptive behavior disorders: *ODD,* a pattern of negativistic, irritable, and noncompliant behaviors, and *CD,* a far more severe grouping of overt and covert antisocial behaviors such as cruelty to persons or animals, physical fighting, sexual assault, firesetting, property destruction, and serious status offenses. Although clear evidence exists that the domains of (1) attentional problems, impulsivity, and hyperactivity and (2) more explicitly aggressive and antisocial behavior patterns are at least partially independent (Hinshaw, 1987), comorbidity between ADHD and such disruptive behavior disorders is extensive, with rates approaching 50% (Biederman et al., 1991). Because associated aggressive features are so crucial in the long-term prognosis of children with ADHD (Barkley, 1996; Hinshaw et al., 1993), their successful treatment is essential for clinical management. Thus, in addition to examining the effects of Ritalin and other stimulants on dimensional measures of aggression and antisocial behavior, we also probe whether subgroups of ADHD children and adolescents with and without comorbid ODD or CD show similar or different responses to stimulant medications.

We note, in passing, that aggression and antisocial behavior are highly contextualized and that aggressive actions may be understandable or even warranted in some oppressive circumstances. Primary clinical concern must be directed to aggression that is unmodulated, destructive, cross sitational, and embedded in additional aspects of psychopathologic conditions (Richters and Cicchetti, 1993).

Measuring aggression and antisocial behavior

The predominant mode of assessment for externalizing behavior constitutes rating scales or questionnaires completed by adult informants, chiefly parents and teachers (Hinshaw and Nigg, 1999). Despite the ease and relative lack of expense of such instruments, their global nature (and the lack of training of the raters who complete them) can lead to a confounding of the domains of ADHD and aggression when these scales are used as diagnostic or outcome measures (e.g., Abikoff et al., 1993). For example, unless scales specifically designed to distinguish these domains are used, intercorrelations between ADHD-related and aggression-related clusters will be quite high (Loney, 1987; Ullmann et al., 1985). Thus, as emphasized in Hinshaw (1991), treatment effects that pertain specifically to aggression and antisocial behavior—as opposed to reflecting a general reduction of inattentive, impulsive, or noncompliant behavior—may be impossible to discern when rating scales are the primary outcome measure. In a similar vein, Hinshaw et al. (1995) found extremely high correlations between domains of overt aggression and covert antisocial actions with the use of staff or parent ratings (with *r*s ranging from 0.7 to 0.9), whereas objective observations of behaviors in each category yielded intercorrelations below $r = 0.3$. In our review, we therefore prioritize specific behavior observations, in which nonbiased observers make discrete recordings of objectively defined categories of ongoing social interaction.

Aspects of medication response: specificity, dose relationships

As emphasized by Miczek (1987), the specificity of effects of pharmacologic agents on aggressive behavior is of paramount importance. Specific antiaggression effects are those that reduce aggressive behavior without compromising general social functioning. That is, a given medication could suppress aggression while rendering the organism nonfunctional, cognitively impaired, or even comatose, but such effects are obviously neither clinically beneficial nor theoretically enlightening. Investigators of pharmacologic approaches to managing aggression must include measures of social approach, adaptive functioning, and (in school settings) learning and achievement to ensure that medication "successes" regarding aggression do not come at the expense of compromised cognitive or behavioral functioning. Multidomain and multimethod assessment procedures are therefore strongly desirable.

Sophisticated investigations in the field must consider a range of dosages of Ritalin or other stimulants in order to plot dose-response curves (Greenhill et al., 1996). Yet, examination of dose-response curves that are averaged across a given sample is not sufficient, as the mean may mask huge variation in dose response across individual participants (Hinshaw et al., 1989b; Rapport et al., 1988). As we highlight below, analyses that incorporate not only parametric analyses of dosage effects across a sample but also descriptions of individual patterns of dose response should become standard practice (Smith et al., 1998).

PRELIMINARY FINDINGS

Despite the lingering consensus that stimulant medications are not helpful for aggressive behavior, the initial publications on the efficacy of stimulant medications for behavior-disordered youth revealed antiaggression effects (e.g., Bradley, 1937). Yet, the diagnostic makeup of such samples was indeterminate, and outcome measures were quite global. Likewise, several trials performed in the 1960s and 1970s showed that MPH or dextroamphetamine reduced aggressive responding in delinquent or other aggressive populations (see reviews of Stewart et al., 1990), but these studies often failed to provide specific diagnostic indicators of the children or adolescents under investigation.

Investigations from recent years with more rigorous subject-selection criteria and improved, double-blind, placebo-controlled evaluation methods have yielded clear evidence that Ritalin and other stimulants effect reductions in the aggressive social behavior of children with ADHD in classroom or play yard settings (e.g., Gadow et al., 1990; Hinshaw et al., 1989b; Murphy et al., 1992; Pelham et al., 1991; see review of Hinshaw, 1991). When such investigations have included normal comparison participants, stimulant effects on aggression in children with ADHD have yielded evidence for normalization—that is, medicated children's rates of aggression are indistinguishable from those of normal youngsters (e.g., Hinshaw et al., 1989b). In contrast, when stimulant effects have been explored with respect to indices of laboratory or playroom aggression, the effects have been far less pronounced, have required relatively high dosages, or have been revealed only for subgroups of the sample (see Amery et al., 1984; Hinshaw et al., 1984; Hinshaw et al., 1989a; Pelham and Bender, 1982; Pelham et al., 1991). The disparity between the naturalistic investigations and those performed in laboratory or playroom settings may be related to the types of planful, retaliatory aggression featured in the latter, which appear to require rather strong dosage levels of stimulants. In addition, across a wide array of outcome measures (not limited to aggressive behavior per se), aggressive and nonaggressive subgroups of children and adolescents with ADHD have tended to show rather similar profiles of stimulant response (e.g., Hinshaw et al., 1989b; Klorman et al., 1988; Klorman et al., 1990). In all, whereas conclusions from Hinshaw (1991) apparently dispelled the misconception that stimulant medications fail to ameliorate maladaptive, aggressive behavior patterns, conclusions were limited to relatively short-term investigations of acute medication response and, for the most part, failed to adequately document dose-response profiles or individual response patterns.

Several unresolved issues and questions are apparent: (1) Can stimulants reduce covert antisocial behavior patterns as well as overt aggression? (2) Which subtypes of aggression and antisocial behavior are most likely to be influenced by medication? (3) Which dosage ranges are optimal for ameliorating aggressive behavior? (4) How strong are individual differences in stimulant responsiveness? (5) Can we understand better the differences between short-term efficacy and the apparent failure of medications to influence long-term change? In reviewing published findings from the current decade, we cite several key investigations but highlight that solid research on this topic is hardly a growth industry. Mounting objective observational studies is time-consuming and costly; and a host of logistic, financial, and ethical issues complicates the issue of examining experimentally manipulated medication use over lengthy time periods. In short, many key issues in the field are still unresolved.

INVESTIGATIONS FROM THE 1990s

Covert antisocial behavior

The clandestine nature and low base rates of such antisocial behaviors as stealing and property destruction have hampered experimental investigations of medication effects in this domain. Indeed, Hoza (1989) studied the impact of stimulants on counselor observations of overt and covert antisocial behaviors displayed by children attending a summer treatment program (STP) but found that extremely low base rates of the covert actions precluded detection of medication effects. With a different strategy, Hinshaw et al. (1992) devised a laboratory probe of ADHD boys' tendencies to steal, cheat, and deface property. In this paradigm, children worked individually and without adult supervision on a worksheet that contained two insoluble problems. The experimenter had "accidentally" left the answer key in the room; near the study area had been placed two dollar bills and 75 cents in change, desirable matchbox cars, and baseball cards, and a marker (which some boys used to deface property). Objective counts of stealing and property destruction were made at the end of the session; successful completion of the insoluble problems constituted evidence for cheating.[1] As detailed in Hinshaw et al. (1995), these measures of covert activity were reliable and valid; they predicted parent, teacher, and staff ratings of similar covert actions and showed clear divergence from objective measures of overt aggression.

Using a counterbalanced, crossover design across 2 days, Hinshaw et al. (1992) found that 0.3 mg/kg of Ritalin significantly decreased rates of stealing and property destruction, with evidence for normalization (i.e., medicated levels of these behaviors did not diverge from those of normal comparison boys). This finding constituted the first objective, empirical evidence for stimulant benefits in this domain. The medication led to significant *increases* in cheating behavior, however, presumably because of pharmacologic enhancement of achievement motivation. We point out that stealing and property destruction are clearly the more serious antisocial actions—for example, they are clear precursors of later delinquency—whereas cheating characterizes a large percentage of comparison youth and is often associated with school success. We comment subsequently on the likelihood that Ritalin and other stimulants can be considered preventive of this important class of behaviors or of delinquency in general.

Laboratory aggression

Casat et al. (1995) investigated laboratory aggression in a sample of six boys with ADHD who also had subclinical- or clinical-range scores on the Child Behavior Checklist Aggression scale (Achenbach, 1991). In a placebo-controlled, double-blind, dose-response trial of MPH (0.3 and 0.6 mg/kg), these investigators examined rates of aggressive responding

[1]With initial samples, our research team videotaped participants from behind a one-way mirror to detect covert behaviors, but checks of the room's permanent products (or lack thereof) at the end of the session provided wholly reliable counts of the behaviors of interest, avoiding disclosure issues surrounding the hidden videotaping.

as the boys played a computer game. Points could be earned for continuous play, but a fictitious peer occasionally took away the participant's points. The outcome measure of aggression was the boy's reciprocal aggression toward the peer, evidenced by pressing a button to subtract his points. (Note that such reciprocal aggression can be viewed as either retaliatory or proactive, in that hitting the "point subtraction" button not only penalized the peer but also protected the participant's own points for a fixed interval.) A linear dose-response curve regarding reduced aggressive responding was found, with only the higher dose yielding an effect significantly different from that of placebo. Thus, as in Hinshaw et al. (1984), Murphy et al. (1992), or Pelham et al. (1991), this study did not reveal evidence for relatively low weight-adjusted dosages of MPH on laboratory aggression but did yield significant findings at 0.6 mg/kg (see Hinshaw et al., 1989a). However, low statistical power with only six participants may have precluded the opportunity to find effects for the low dosage level; analysis of individual participant dose-response curves was not performed.

It is tempting to conclude (see Hinshaw, 1991) that at least moderate Ritalin dosages may be required to yield significant impact on laboratory indexes of aggression. Examination of individual dosage response curves, however, is more informative than examination of averaged dose-response across a sample. In addition, further clarification of medication effects on proactive/instrumental vs. reactive/retaliatory aggression from laboratory paradigms would be theoretically illuminating (see, for example, Atkins and Stoff, 1993). Finally, as discussed in Hinshaw (1991), a continuing research need is establishing the generalizability of such laboratory measures of aggressive responding to naturalistic indicators.

Naturalistic aggression

Public school settings

In an investigation continuing the examination of Ritalin on objectively observed aggressive responding in public-school classroom and lunchroom settings (see Gadow et al., 1990), Gadow et al. (1992) examined medication effects on the reciprocal responses of the peers of the ADHD children. With a sample of 11 boys with ADHD (who were also screened to include high levels of baseline aggression) as well as nondiagnosed peers in the classroom or lunch area, these investigators performed a double-blind, placebo-controlled trial of 0.3 and 0.6 mg/kg of Ritalin. As shown in Gadow et al. (1990), Ritalin yielded statistically and clinically significant benefits for the aggressive ADHD participants. The effects were specific, in that rates of appropriate social interaction did not decline (and in fact slightly increased) with active medication.

Extending these findings, Gadow et al. (1992) provided evidence for normalization of rates of aggressive responding in the classroom, in that levels of aggression for the aggressive ADHD participants receiving active medication were comparable with those of normal classmates. For some observational measures, however, rates of aggression with medication were reduced to levels *below* those of the peer group, leading to suspicion of overmedication or of behavioral toxicity. Clearly, it is essential to monitor individual differences in stimulant response on aggression. Furthermore, in the classroom (but not the lunchroom, where peer rates of disruption and aggression were slightly but nonsignificantly increased when the target sample was medicated), classmates' levels of nonphysical aggression were significantly reduced as a function of the target children's active medication. Thus, at least some evidence was found for reciprocal effects of stimulant medication on the aggressive responses of peers. Given the small sample size, the relatively low magnitude of the reciprocal effects, and the variable results across settings and outcome measures, replication is in order.

Summer treatment settings

In intensive STPs for children with ADHD and other disruptive behavior disorders (see Pelham and Hoza, 1996), Pelham et al. (1993), Bukstein and Kolko (1998), and Smith et al. (1998) have provided sophisticated analyses of stimulant effects on aggressive behavior in naturalistic classroom, playground, and small-group settings. In these reports, Ritalin has yielded significant aggression-reducing benefits that appear specific and of at least moderate effect size. Our analysis of key findings provides a window on such important topics as comparative effects with psychosocial intervention (Pelham et al., 1993), efficacy for aggressive, low-income youth (Bukstein and Kolko, 1998), and individual-level dose response effects in adolescents (Smith et al., 1998).

Ritalin vs. psychosocial treatment

In a study focusing on comparative effects of Ritalin and systematic behavior modification contingencies in a summer treatment program, Pelham et al. (1993) examined a wide range of outcome measures that included staff ratings of aggression as well as observed disruptive behavior. As with other outcome measures, the stimulant medication (double-blind, placebo-controlled comparison of 0.3- and 0.6-mg/kg dosages of Ritalin) produced larger effect sizes regarding such externalizing behavior than did the systematic behavioral contingencies, with little evidence for incremental effects of the combination of the two approaches. Regarding specificity, it is noteworthy that the medication also produced significant enhancement of academic performance in the same children (whereas the behavioral contingencies did not). We return to this report when we address stimulant effects on aggressive vs. nonaggressive subgroups of ADHD children (see below).

Effects on aggressive, low-SES youth

In the context of a summer program designed for children with ODD or CD diagnoses, Bukstein and Kolko (1998) examined 0.3 and 0.6 mg/kg of Ritalin in 18 inner-city, low-socioeconomic status (SES) youth (mean age of 9 years) who met the criteria for ADHD and who simultaneously displayed high levels of aggression based on preprogram ratings from parents and teachers. Most of the sample (83%) was of African-American ethnic heritage. First, regarding staff ratings of defiance, verbal aggression, and physical aggression, both the low and moderate dosage levels yielded significant benefit compared with placebo. The use of time-outs for behavioral control were also reduced with both dosages. For daily progress notes regarding physical aggression, however, only the 0.6 mg/kg dosage yielded significant improvement. Following Pelham et al. (1993), Bukstein and Kolko (1998) calculated individual effect sizes for each child by subtracting placebo levels of behavioral outcomes from medicated levels, dividing by the individual subject's placebo-level standard deviation. A majority of the participants showed effect sizes for aggressive outcomes of at least 0.5—usually held to be a moderate effect size—with some tendency for the children to yield greater improvement at the larger dose.

Crucially, however, a medication trial conducted in the home settings of the participants following the summer program each day (and on weekends) failed to reveal evidence of behavioral improvement for any outcome measure. As discussed by Bukstein and Kolko (1998), whether this striking difference in medication response between settings was related to poor medication compliance by families or to the general lack of structure of the households—in contrast to the high levels of structure in the summer program setting—is indeterminate. Nonetheless, this disparity should provide considerable caution regarding the hope for clinically significant aggression-reducing properties of stimulants in the home settings of aggressive children in impoverished households and neighborhoods (for similar conclusions within a middle-class sample, see Schachar et al., 1997).

Individual differences in adolescent medication response

In an exemplary investigation that shows the importance of examining diverse methods of analyzing data from medication trials, Smith et al. (1998) examined the stimulant response of 49 adolescents with ADHD who attended one of several STPs at the University of Pittsburgh. The overwhelming majority were male and Caucasian, with a wide diversity of socioeconomic backgrounds. Fixed dosage levels of 10/10/5 mg, 20/20/10 mg, and 30/30/15 mg MPH were investigated in contrast to placebo, in a daily, counterbalanced, double-blind trial. Objective counselor observations and ratings constituted the outcome measures, which included several categories relevant to overt and covert antisocial behavior. As in Hoza (1989), however, the category of covert conduct problems had extremely low placebo base rates.

Several key findings emerged. First, there were strong overall effects of medication (compared with placebo), demonstrating clearly that aggressive behavior patterns are amenable to significant and specific improvement with stimulant medication in adolescents with ADHD. Indeed, three fourths of the sample showed significant benefit. Second, for staff rating scale measures, overall medication effects tended to be linear, whereas observational categories of negative social interaction and aggression typically revealed a "plateau" effect of the lowest dosage level. That is, for these observational measures, at the group level the largest changes occurred between placebo and the lowest (10/10/5 mg) dosage levels, with improvements sharply declining in magnitude as dosages increased. Smith et al. (1998) thus characterized stimulant effects on aggression as "asymptotic."

Third, in a set of analyses intended to demonstrate "threshold" and "continuing gains" effects for individual participants, Smith et al. (1998) found that (1) thresholds were reached at relatively low dosages for most participants and that (2) once an adolescent reached at least a moderate effect size (compared with placebo) at a given dosage level, chances were roughly equal that increased dosage levels would yield deterioration vs. further improvement. In addition, the high doses were more likely to induce side effects (although few were prohibitive). Yet, certain adolescents did not show significant benefit regarding aggression until higher doses were used, revealing the strongly idiosyncratic nature of stimulant responsiveness.

In all, the multilevel analytic strategy of Smith et al. (1998) is vastly more informative than sole presentation of averaged group data. The aggression-reducing properties of Ritalin are highly individualized; yet, for most adolescents, moving to moderate or high dosage levels did not promote incremental benefit. Multilevel individualized analyses of medication response are essential (see also Rapport et al., 1988).

Summary

The results of the above-cited investigations reveal clearly that Ritalin reduces aggressive behavior in naturalistic summer programs with (1) specificity and (2) moderate to large effect sizes. Stimulant effects are larger than those emanating from systematic contingency management; they pertain to low–SES, aggressive youth with comorbid ADHD and also apply to adolescents with significant aggression as well. Analysis of individual response patterns is far more revealing than examination of averaged medication effects; Smith et al. (1998) suggest strongly that for most youths, sufficient benefits can be attained without resorting to unduly high dosage levels. Finally, medication effects appear far stronger in the context of structured programs (which also employ behavioral contingencies) than in home settings, in which medication compliance and general lack of structure may temper gains.

Aggressive vs. nonaggressive subgroups of children with ADHD

Supplementing their examination of the comparative and combined effects of Ritalin and systematic contingency management procedures in an STP (see above), Pelham et al. (1993) subdivided their ADHD samples of 31 children into those with (n = 15) and without (n = 16) comorbid diagnoses of CD. For most outcome measures of externalizing behavior, diagnostic subgroup status did not interact with medication dosage levels; when it did, the pattern of effects was that the CD-ADHD subsample had higher rates of baseline aggression, which (when medicated) improved to levels comparable with those of the non-CD subgroup. In other words, interactions were ordinal, with no evidence for qualitatively different medication response patterns for the comorbid subgroup.

Klorman et al. (1994) reached a similar conclusion with a large sample of children with clinical or subclinical ADHD (n = 107) who were examined with respect to parent and teacher ratings of externalizing behavior, laboratory measures of attentional functioning, and evoked potentials. The sample was subgrouped into those with and without comorbid aggression/oppositionality, on the basis of teacher ratings on the IOWA Conners scale; an additional group of subclinically hyperactive children was also examined. Ritalin dosages were gradually increased to a level of 0.3 mg/kg per dose. As for subgroup differences, whereas the medication vs. placebo effects on adult-rated aggression were numerically larger in the aggressive subgroup than in the ADHD-only or the subclinical group, this difference was attributed largely to "floor" effects in the latter subgroups (i.e., baseline levels of aggression were quite low). For other measures, including the cognitive (Sternberg) task, all groups showed comparable benefits. As stated by Klorman et al. (1994), "the clinical advantages of methylphenidate extend to aggressive/oppositional and mild or situational ADD" (p. 218).

The results of Matier et al. (1992) are somewhat harder to interpret, in that (1) only a single, 5-mg dose of Ritalin served as the pharmacologic variable and (2) the study did not include clinical measures of social behavior or aggression. In order to examine the effects of a low Ritalin dose on the cognitive performance of aggressive and nonaggressive children with ADHD, Matier et al. formed subgroups on the basis of persistent physical aggression; dependent measures constituted scores of inattention and impulsivity gleaned from continuous performance testing and of hyperactivity from actigraphy during the testing. Whereas both subgroups showed decreases in inattention while medicated (and whereas neither changed significantly with respect to impulsivity), only the nonaggressive group showed reduced motor overactivity with active medication. Matier, et al. conclude that hyperactivity may emanate from different sources in aggressive vs. nonaggressive subtypes. Yet, restriction to a single low dose limits clinical generalizability. Overall, research from the current decade continues to show that aggressive and nonaggressive subgroups of children with ADHD show similar patterns of dose response to stimulant medications (although reductions in aggression are far larger in high-aggressive subgroups).

Conduct disorder

Whether Ritalin and other stimulants show positive effects for youths with primary diagnoses of CD has been quite difficult to ascertain, for two key reasons: (1) Extant investigations have often failed to disentangle CD from the ADHD symptomatology that frequently accompanies severe conduct problems, and (2) outcome measures have focused on adult ratings rather than observed behavior. The predominant view has been that stimulants play no role in the treatment of CD (see literature review of Klein et al., 1997).

Kaplan et al. (1990) studied the stimulant responses of nine youths with aggressive CD in both inpatient and outpatient settings. In the double-blind trial (of a fixed dosage of 30 mg Ritalin) in which six of the youth participated, significant reductions in staff- or teacher-rated aggression were noted. All the adolescents, however, met the diagnostic criteria for ADHD from *DSM-III* criteria (American Psychiatric Association, 1980).

On the other hand, studying hospitalized adolescents with CD (n = 18), Brown, et al. (1991) noted that only seven displayed comorbid ADHD. Outcome measures for the double-blind trial of twice-daily dosages of placebo as well as 10, 15, and 20 mg of Ritalin included academic tasks, a cognitive measure of impulsivity, and the Conners Teacher Rating Scale. At the highest dosage level, significant effects were found for the Conduct factor of the rating instrument; improvements in academic tasks were found at lower dosage levels as well. A differential response of the CD + ADHD subgroup vs. the CD-only youth on cognitive and academic performance reported by Brown, et al. is tempered by the extremely small sample sizes. The authors were careful to note that the results should not be interpreted as indicating clinical significance regarding the medication findings for CD teenagers, because (1) results pertained only to an inpatient setting and selected measures and (2) the potential for abuse of stimulants in severely CD adolescents may be strong.

Finally, in a major recent investigation, Klein et al. (1997) examined the effects of stimulant treatment on youth with CD diagnoses. In the course of recruiting and selecting the sample (age range 6–15 years), however, they found that 69% of the youth (overall n = 83) met the criteria for comorbid ADHD. Active medication vs. placebo status was assigned randomly for a 5-week period, with the medicated participants receiving, on average, just over 40 mg of MPH per day.

Highly significant effects of active medication were found for parent and teacher ratings of conduct problems, ranging from overt assault and serious rule violations to covert antisocial behaviors (lying, property destruction), as well as for classroom observations of defiant and aggressive behaviors. Specificity was observed, in that academic performance was also rated as improved with medication. Importantly, statistical control of initial ADHD symptoms did not reduce the strong impact of medication on either global ratings of improvement or conduct disorder symptoms per se. Thus, the benefits of MPH on serious conduct problems were independent of medication effects on inattention, impulsivity, or hyperactivity. These important findings are tempered by (1) the difficulty, in a clinical trial, of obtaining a "pure" CD sample and (2) the lack of full normalization of CD-related behaviors with stimulants, despite clearly significant benefits.

SUMMARY

Space limitations dictate that we list key conclusions numerically:

1. Considerable evidence converges on the conclusion that Ritalin and other stimulants yield clear but short-term reductions in aggression and antisocial behavior, in children with ADHD and with CD, that are typically specific and of moderate to strong magni-

tude. Yet, full normalization of CD has been harder to establish, largely because of the extensive comorbidity between ADHD and CD in clinical samples.[2]

2. Effects are strongest in the context of structured STPs, in which regular behavioral contingencies are simultaneously in place. Benefits are also apparent, however, in school settings (Gadow et al., 1992; Klein et al., 1997). Laboratory indicators of retaliatory aggression tend to show stimulant-related gain only at moderate to high dosage levels.
3. The covert antisocial behaviors of stealing and property destruction are also reduced with stimulant medication in laboratory settings (Hinshaw et al., 1992) and in the natural environment (Klein et al., 1997).
4. Large individual differences in the aggression-reducing properties of stimulants are apparent. The exemplary investigation of Smith et al. (1998) demonstrates that examination of averaged data regarding dose-response curves fails to tell the complete story regarding individual response to treatment.
5. The rather strong gains demonstrated in structured environments with objective observational systems stand in marked contrast to the nonsignificant benefits yielded, in some reports, when parents provide ratings of aggression and general social functioning at home (Bukstein and Kolko, 1998; Schachar et al., 1997). Findings are mixed, however, in that other investigations reveal clear effects on parent ratings (Klein et al., 1997).

This last point requires additional discussion. First, it bears on the "efficacy" and "effectiveness" distinction in clinical trials methodology (Clarke, 1995; Hoagwood et al., 1995). The former is concerned primarily with internal validity, requiring homogeneous samples, tight experimental control, and rigorous adherence to fixed treatment protocols; the latter pertains to assessing treatment effects in the "real world," with heterogeneous samples marked by diagnostic comorbidity, delivery of treatment in the natural environment, and participant selection of desired interventions. As our medication trials move from laboratories and controlled summer research programs to the vagaries of the homes and neighborhoods that house aggressive, hyperactive children, such variables as medication noncompliance, ongoing bias in parents' perceptions of their offspring, and general lack of environmental structure may combine to diminish significant pharmacologic benefits (for parallels in the treatment of bipolar disorder with lithium, see Maj et al., 1989).

Second, the types of aggression and antisocial behavior that are most troublesome to society emanate from the relatively small group of youngsters with early-onset aggression, who commonly display comorbid ADHD and verbal learning deficits and who tend to come from families with multiple psychiatric disorders in biologic relatives (Hinshaw and Anderson, 1996; Moffitt, 1993). Indeed, such youth with such early-onset patterns account for well over half of the violent behavior occurring in society (Hinshaw and Anderson, 1996). Violence-ridden neighborhoods, poverty, harsh and inconsistent parenting, and deviant peer networks characterize the environments of such youths. For families of such youths, the typical treatments offered by clinics are rarely sought and seldom implemented in consistent fashion. Thus, if a stimulant regimen is prescribed, regular dosing is unlikely, and any positive medication effects must be measured against familial, neighborhood, and school-related factors that are hardly auspicious. Thus, consideration of the positive benefits of Ritalin and the stimulants on aggressive and antisocial behavior patterns must take into account the extremely problematic blend of intraindividual, environmental, and cultural risk

[2]It is conceivable that stimulant medications reduce aggression that is impulsive and poorly modulated but that because of their positive effects on planful behavior, they might increase predatory, premeditated aggression. Data do not appear available in this regard.

factors within which serious, early-onset antisocial behavior patterns are embedded. Despite the promise of these medications for treating aggressive behavior and even CD, clinical realities dictate a far broader perspective on the difficulties inherent in fully treating serious antisocial behavior in our society.

ACKNOWLEDGMENT

Supported in part by National Institute of Mental Health grants R01-MH45064 and U01-MH50461, awarded to Stephen P. Hinshaw.

REFERENCES

Abikoff, H., Courtney, M., Pelham, W. & Koplewicz, H. (1993), Detection bias in teacher ratings of attention-deficit hyperactivity disorder and oppositional defiant disorder. *J. Abnorm. Child Psychol.,* 21:519–533.

Achenbach. T.M. (1991), *Manual for the Child Behavior Checklist/4–18 and 1991 Profile.* Burlington, Vermont: University of Vermont Department of Psychology.

American Psychiatric Association. (1980), *Diagnostic and Statistical Manual of Mental Disorders, 3rd ed.* Washington, DC: American Psychiatric Association.

American Psychiatric Association. (1994). *Diagnostic and Statistical Manual of Mental Disorders, 4th ed.* Washington, DC: American Psychiatric Association.

Amery, B., Minichiello, M.D. & Brown, G.L. (1984), Aggression in hyperactive boys: Response to d-amphetamine. *J. Am. Acad. Child Adolesc. Psychiatry,* 23:291–294.

Atkins, M.S. & Stoff, D.M. (1993), Instrumental and hostile aggression in childhood disruptive behavior disorders. *J. Abnorm. Child Psychol.,* 21:165–178.

Barkley, R.A. (1996), Attention-deficit hyperactivity disorder. In: *Child Psychopathology,* eds., E.J. Mash & R.A. Barkley. New York: Guilford Press, pp. 63–112.

Biederman, J., Newcorn, J. & Sprich, S. (1991), Comorbidity of attention deficit hyperactivity disorder with conduct, depressive, anxiety, and other disorders. *Am. J. Psychiatry,* 148:564–577.

Bradley, C. (1937), The behavior of children receiving benzedrine. *Am. J. Psychiatry,* 94:577–585.

Brown, R.T., Jaffe, S.L., Silverstein, J. & Magee, H. (1991), Methylphenidate and hospitalized adolescents with conduct disorder: Dose effects on classroom behavior, academic performance, and impulsivity. *J. Youth Adolesc.,* 20:501–518.

Bukstein, O.G. & Kolko, D.J. (1998), The effects of methylphenidate on aggressive, urban children with attention deficit hyperactivity disorder. *J. Clin. Psychol.,* 27:340–351.

Casat, C.D., Pearson, D.A., Van Davelaar, M.J. & Cherek, D. (1995), Methylphenidate effects on a laboratory aggression measure in children with ADHD. *Psychopharmacol. Bull.,* 31:353–356.

Clarke, G.N. (1995), Improving the transition from basic efficacy research to effectiveness studies: Methodological issues and procedures. *J. Consult. Clin. Psychol.,* 63:718–725.

Connor, D.F. & Steingard, R.J. (1996), A clinical approach to the pharmacotherapy of aggression in children and adolescents. In: *Understanding Aggressive Behavior in Children,* eds., C. Ferris & T. Grisso. *Annals of the New York Academy of Sciences,* 794:290–307.

Gadow, K.D., Nolan, E.E., Sverd, J., Sprafkin, J. & Paolicelli, L. (1990), Methylphenidate in aggressive-hyperactive boys: I. Effects on peer aggression in public school settings. *J. Am. Acad. Child Adolesc. Psychiatry,* 29:710–718.

Gadow, K.D., Paolicelli, L.M., Nolan, E.E., Schwartz, J., Sprafkin, J. & Sverd, J. (1992), Methylphenidate in aggressive hyperactive boys: II. Indirect effects of medication treatment on peer behavior. *J. Child Adolesc. Psychopharmacol.,* 2:49–61.

Greenhill, L.L., Abikoff, H.B., Arnold, L.E., Cantwell, D.P., Conners, C.K., Elliott, G., Hechtman, L., Hinshaw, S.P., Hoza, B., Jensen, P.S., March, J., Newcorn, J., Pelham, W.E., Severe, J.B., Swanson, J.M., Vitiello, B. & Wells, K. (1996), Medication treatment strategies in the MTA Study: Relevance to clinicians and researchers. *J. Am. Acad. Child Adolesc. Psychiatry,* 35:1304–1313.

Hinshaw, S.P. (1987), On the distinction between attentional deficits/hyperactivity and conduct problems/aggression in child psychopathology. *Psychol. Bull.,* 101:443–463.

Hinshaw, S.P. (1991), Stimulant medication and the treatment of aggression in children with attentional deficits. *J. Clin. Child Psychol.,* 20:301–312.

Hinshaw, S.P. & Anderson, C.A. (1996), Oppositional defiant and conduct disorders. In: *Child Psychopathology,* eds., E.J. Mash & R.A. Barkley. New York: Guilford Press, pp. 108–149.

Hinshaw, S.P., Buhrmester, D. & Heller, T. (1989a), Anger control in response to verbal provocation: Effects of stimulant medication for boys with ADHD. *J. Abnorm. Child Psychol.,* 17:393–407.

Hinshaw, S.P., Heller, T. & McHale, J.P. (1992), Covert antisocial behavior in boys with attention deficit hyperactivity disorder: External validation and effects of methylphenidate. *J. Consult. Clin. Psychol.,* 60:274–281.

Hinshaw, S.P., Henker, B. & Whalen, C.K. (1984), Self-control in hyperactive boys in anger-inducing situations: Comparative effects of cognitive-behavioral training and of methylphenidate. *J. Abnorm. Child Psychol.,* 12:55–77.

Hinshaw, S.P., Henker, B., Whalen, C.K., Erhardt, D. & Dunnington, R.E. (1989b), Aggressive, prosocial, and nonsocial behavior in hyperactive boys: Dose effects of methylphenidate in naturalistic settings. *J. Consult. Clin. Psychol.,* 57:636–643.

Hinshaw, S.P., Lahey, B.B. & Hart, E.L. (1993), Issues of taxonomy and comorbidity in the development of conduct disorder. *Dev. Psychopathol.,* 5:31–49.

Hinshaw, S.P. & Nigg, J.T. (1999), Behavior rating scales in the assessment of disruptive behavior disorders in childhood. In: *Assessment in Child and Adolescent Psychopathology,* eds., D. Shaffer, J. Richters & C.P. Lucas, New York: Guilford Press.

Hinshaw, S.P., Simmel, C. & Heller, T. (1995), Multimethod assessment of covert antisocial behavior in children: Laboratory observations, adult ratings, and child self-report. *Psychol. Assess.,* 7:209–219.

Hinshaw, S.P. & Zupan, B.A. (1997), Assessment of antisocial behavior in children and adolescents. In: *Handbook of Antisocial Behavior,* eds., D.M. Stoff, J. Breiling & J.D. Maser. New York: John Wiley & Sons, Inc., pp. 36–50.

Hoagwood, K., Hibbs, E., Brent, D. & Jensen, P. (1995), Introduction to the special section: Efficacy and effectiveness in studies of child and adolescent psychotherapy. *J. Consul. Clin. Psychol.,* 63:683–687.

Hoza, J. (1989), *Response to Stimulant Medication Among Children with Attention Deficit Hyperactivity Disorder.* Unpublished dissertation, Department of Psychology, Florida State University.

Kaplan, S.L., Busner, J., Kupietz, S., Wasserman, E. & Segal, B. (1990), Effects of methylphenidate on adolescents with aggressive conduct disorder and ADHD: A preliminary report. *J. Am. Acad. Child Adolesc. Psychiatry,* 29:719–723.

Klein, R.G., Abikoff, H., Klass, E., Ganeles, D., Seese, L.M. & Pollack, S. (1997), Clinical efficacy of methylphenidate in conduct disorder with and without attention deficit hyperactivity disorder. *Arch. Gen. Psychiatry,* 54:1073–1080.

Klorman, R., Brumaghim, J.T., Fitzpatrick, P.A. & Borgstedt, A.D. (1990), Clinical effects of a controlled trial of methylphenidate on adolescents with attention deficit disorder. *J. Am. Acad. Child Adolesc. Psychiatry,* 29:702–709.

Klorman, R., Brumaghim, J.T., Fitzpatrick, P.A., Borgstedt, A.D. & Strauss, J. (1994), Clinical and cognitive effects of methylphenidate on children with attention deficit disorder as a function of aggression/oppositionality and age. *J. Abnorm. Psychol.,* 103:206–221.

Loeber, R. & Schmaling, K. (1985), Empirical evidence for overt and covert patterns of antisocial conduct problems: A meta-analysis. *J. Abnorm. Child Psychol.,* 13:337–352.

Loney, J. (1987), Hyperactivity and aggression in the diagnosis of attention deficit disorder. In: *Advances in Clinical Child Psychology, vol. 10,* eds., B.B. Lahey & A.E. Kazdin. New York: Plenum Press, pp. 99–135.

Maj, M., Priozzi R. & Kemali, D. (1989), Long-term outcome of lithium prophylaxis in patients initially classified as complete responders. *Psychopharmacology,* 98:535–538.

Matier, K., Halperin, J.M., Sharma, V., Newcorn, J.H. & Sathaye, N. (1992), Methylphenidate response in aggressive and nonaggressive ADHD children: Distinctions in laboratory measures of symptoms. *J. Am. Ac. Child Adolesc. Psychiatry,* 31:219–225.

Miczek, K.A. (1987), The psychopharmacology of aggression. In: *Handbook of Psychopharmacology: New Directions in Behavioral Pharmacology,* eds., L.L. Iversen, S.D. Iversen & S.H. Snyder. New York: Plenum Press, pp. 183–328.

Miczek, K.A., Haney, M., Tidey, J., Vivian, J. & Weerts, E. (1994), Neurochemistry and pharmacotherapeutic management of aggression and violence. In: *Understanding and Preventing Violence, vol. 2: Biobehavioral Influences,* eds., A.J. Reiss, K.A. Miczek & J.A. Roth. Washington, DC: National Academy Press, pp. 245–514.

Milich, R. & Loney, J. (1979), The role of hyperactive and aggressive symptomatology in predicting adolescent outcome among hyperactive children. *J. Pediatr. Psychol.,* 4:93–112.

Moffitt, T.E. (1993), Adolescence-limited and life-course-persistent antisocial behavior: A developmental taxonomy. *Psychol. Rev.,* 100:674–701.

Murphy, D.A., Pelham, W.E. & Lang, A. (1992), Aggression in boys with attention-deficit hyperactivity disorder: Methylphenidate effects on naturalistically observed aggression, response to provocation, and social information processing. *J. Abnorm. Child Psychol.,* 20:451–466.

Pelham, W.E. & Bender, M.E. (1982), Peer relationships in hyperactive children: Description and treatment. In: *Advances in Learning and Behavioral Disabilities,* eds., K. Gadow & I. Bialer. vol. 1, Greenwich, CT: JAI Press, pp. 365–436.

Pelham, W.E., Carlson, C., Sams, S.E., Dixon, M.J. & Hoza, B. (1993), Separate and combined effects of methylphenidate and behavior modification on boys with attention-deficit hyperactivity disorder in the classroom. *J. Consult. Clin. Psychol.,* 61:506–515.

Pelham, W.E. & Hoza, B. (1996), Intensive treatment: A summer treatment program for children with ADHD. In: *Psychosocial Treatments for Child and Adolescent Disorders: Empirically Based Strategies for Clinical Practice,* eds., E.D. Hibbs & P.S. Jensen. Washington, DC: American Psychological Association, pp. 311–340.

Pelham, W.E., Milich, R., Cummings, E.M., Murphy, D.A., Schaughency, E.A. & Greiner, A. (1991), Effects of background anger and methylphenidate on emotional arousal and aggressive responding in attention deficit/hyperactivity disordered boys with and without concurrent aggression. *J. Abnorm. Child Psychol.,* 19:407–426.

Rapport, M.D., Stoner, G., DuPaul, G.J., Kelly, K.L., Tucker, S.B. & Schoeler, T. (1988),

Attention deficit disorder and methylphenidate: A multilevel analysis of dose-response effects on children's impulsivity across settings. *J. Am. Acad. Child Adolesc. Psychiatry,* 27:60–69.

Richters, J.E. & Cicchetti, D. (1993), Mark Twain meets *DSM-III-R*: Conduct disorder, development, and the concept of harmful dysfunction. *Dev. Psychopathol.,* 5:5–29.

Schachar, R.J., Tannock, R., Cunningham, C. & Corkum, P.V. (1997), Behavioral, situational, and temporal effects of treatment of ADHD with methylphenidate. *J. Am. Acad. Child Adolesc. Psychiatry,* 36:754–763.

Smith, B.H., Pelham, W.E., Evans, S., Gnagy, E., Molina, B., Bukstein, O., Greiner, A. & Willoughby, M. (1998), Dosage effects of methylphenidate on the social behavior of adolescents diagnosed with attention-deficit hyperactivity disorder. *Exper. Clin. Psychopharm.,* 6:187–204.

Stewart, J.T., Myers, W.C., Burket, R.C. & Lyles, W.B. (1990), A review of the pharmacotherapy of aggression in children and adolescents. *J. Am. Acad. Child Adolesc. Psychiatry,* 29:269–277.

Stoff, D.M., Breiling, J. & Maser, J.D., eds. (1997), *Handbook of Antisocial Behavior.* New York: John Wiley and Sons, Inc.

Stoewe, J.K., Kruesi, M.J.P. & Lelio, D.F. (1995), Psychopharmacology of aggressive states and features of conduct disorder. *Child Adolesc. Psychiatr. Clin. North Am.,* 4:359–379.

Ullmann, R.K. & Sleator, E.K. (1985), Attention deficit disorder with or without hyperactivity: Which behaviors are helped by stimulants? *Clin. Pediatr.,* 24:547–551.

Ullmann, R.K. & Sleator, E.K. & Sprague, R.L. (1985), A change of mind: The Conners Abbreviated Rating Scales reconsidered. *J. Abnorm. Child Psychol.* 13:553–565.

Wilens, T.E. & Biederman, J. (1992), The stimulants. *Psychiatr. Clin. North Am.,* 15:191–222.

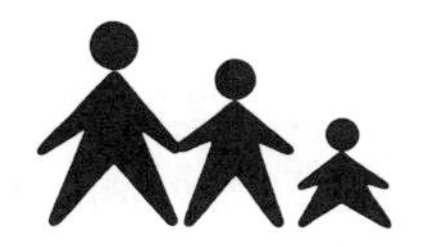

Methylphenidate Treatment of *DSM-IV* Types of Attention Deficit Hyperactivity Disorder

KEITH McBURNETT

The effectiveness of methylphenidate (MPH, Ritalin) for attention deficit hyperactivity disorder (ADHD) is one of the best-established instances of treatment success in managing child behavioral health problems. However, most of the evidence for Ritalin's effectiveness comes from studies of children who would today most likely fit the *Diagnostic and Statistical Manual of Mental Disorders (DSM), 4th ed.* (American Psychiatric Association, 1994) subcategory of ADHD, combined type (ADHD-C). This chapter surveys the data and theoretical issues bearing on the use of Ritalin for the other subtypes. The topics include: (1) history, derivation, validity, and correlates of *DSM-IV* types; (2) a review of the small amount of research literature on Ritalin treatment of different types of ADHD (because this literature is incomplete, we also discuss several theoretical questions that bear on prediction of response to Ritalin across types); (3) we ask are there correlates of *DSM-IV* types that might imply differential response; and (4), finally, we offer tentative conclusions about what recommendations for clinical practice can be drawn based on what is known about ADHD types?

HISTORY AND DERIVATION OF DSM-IV ADHD TYPES

Each edition of the *DSM* has categorized ADHD differently. The best explanation for this confusing state of affairs is that the committees that drafted each edition had available only the research findings, case reports, and personal clinical experience that existed at the time. The historical context of *DSM-IV* ADHD is described in greater detail elsewhere (McBurnett, 1996), but a brief summary here is appropriate. *DSM-II* (American Psychiatric Association, 1968), the first edition to cover child disorders, provided only a clinical description of hyperkinetic reaction of childhood (or adolescence). *DSM-III* (American Psychiatric Association, 1980) provided three lists of symptoms (inattention, hyperactivity, and impulsivity). If a child had at least a minimum number of symptoms from each of these groups, the correct *DSM-III* category was attention deficit disorder with hyperactivity (ADD-H). If a child had at least the minimum number of inattention and impulsive symptoms, but fewer than the threshold specified for hyperactivity, the *DSM-III* diagnosis was attention deficit disorder without hyperactivity (ADD-WO). Members of the *DSM-III-R* (American Psychiatric Association, 1987) committee were not convinced that there were significant numbers of children with ADD-WO or that it was a meaningful distinction, and they substituted a single list of symptoms, with a single cutpoint, for diagnosing ADHD in *DSM-III-R*. The *DSM-IV* committee, informed by targeted literature reviews (Biederman et al., 1997; Lahey and Carlson, 1991; McBurnett, 1997) and field tests of proposed changes to the diagnostic criteria (Frick et al., 1994; Lahey et al., 1994; McBurnett et al., 1993; Waldman

Department of Psychiatry, University of Chicago, Chicago, Illinois.

et al., 1995), decided that (1) the *DSM-III-R* system was flawed in specifying a single symptom list and only one major type of ADHD, but (2) *DSM-III* was flawed in specifying three symptom lists and in requiring impulsivity as a criterion for ADD-WO. Key to the *DSM-IV* reorganization was the overwhelming evidence that ADHD symptoms consist of an inattentive factor and a hyperactive-impulsive factor. The *DSM-IV* now requires that at least six out of a list of nine symptoms of inattention be present, and/or six out of a list of nine hyperactive-impulsive symptoms be present, in order to meet one of the cutpoint criteria (the threshold for number of symptoms) for the ADHD diagnosis.

Within limits, it is fair to draw comparisons to pre-*DSM-IV* types of ADHD. The predominantly inattentive (ADHD-I) type is similar to *DSM-III-R* ADD-WO, although the impulsivity requirement for that diagnosis may partially confound its association with characteristics of hyperactivity-impulsivity. ADHD-I is also similar to undifferentiated ADHD in *DSM-III-R*. However, the lack of specific diagnostic criteria in *DSM-III-R* undifferentiated ADHD makes this diagnosis more like an NOS label ("not otherwise specified"), a qualifier being increasingly used in the *DSM* system to apply to cases that for a variety of reasons do not meet all of the criteria for a diagnosis. Some researchers dealt with this specification problem by adding research diagnostic criteria to undifferentiated ADHD—for example, the criterion that significant levels of hyperactivity-impulsivity *not* be present (Kuperman et al., 1996). The combined type (ADHD-C) is similar to *DSM-III* ADD-H and to *DSM-III-R* ADHD. The predominantly hyperactive-impulsive type (ADHD-HI), however, was previously undescribed in the clinical literature, except for indications from two studies that such cases could be found in community samples (Bauermeister et al., 1992; Newcorn et al., 1989).

VALIDITY OF ADHD TYPES: ASSOCIATED IMPAIRMENT AND COMORBIDITY

Functional impairment can be measured as a broad, global construct, such as with the clinician's judgment of overall functioning level, or it can be measured according to more narrow domains, such as homework problems. The way that functional impairment is distributed across ADHD types can also occur in (1) a general fashion (impairment that is common to all types), or in (2) more specific associations with the underlying dimensions of inattention or hyperactivity-impulsivity, or in (3) even more specific associations with one single type of *DSM-IV* ADHD. The unique pattern of impairment that accompanies each type establishes its discriminant validity and provides important clues for its predictive validity for stimulant response.

Type-specific impairment

If a given characteristic were associated with only one type of ADHD, the association would be type-specific rather than dimension-specific. One such hypothesis was that internalizing comorbidity would be associated specifically with the ADHD-I type (e.g., Eiraldi et al., 1997). Several studies with *DSM-III* diagnoses found that anxiety was associated more strongly with ADD-WO than with ADHD-H, even though both diagnoses had elevated levels of inattention. However, comparisons of ADHD types as defined by *DSM-IV* have not replicated the reported association of anxiety with the inattentive-only type (ADHD-I). These negative findings have potentially important implications for MPH treatment because of the suggestion that anxiety predicts lower rates of response and shifting of the dose-response curve to the left (better response at low doses).[1] The previous edition of this chapter cautioned that anxiety might limit the response to MPH in children with ADD-WO. As we note below, there is no longer a basis for assuming that children with ADHD-I are generally more anxious than other children with ADHD and therefore will not respond to MPH as well as other children with ADHD.

Another form of type-specific impairment reported for *DSM-III* ADD-WO has received preliminary support in a study of *DSM-IV* types. Some *DSM-III* studies found that daydreaming, forgetfulness, appearing sluggish or drowsy, etc., constituted a factor of "sluggish cognitive tempo" and were associated with ADD-WO (Lahey and Carlson, 1991). The only post-*DSM-IV* study to examine this issue identified a similar unique factor constituted by symptoms of "often forgets," "often daydreams," and "is often sluggish or drowsy." For purely descriptive reasons, this factor was termed alertness/orientation problems in that study (McBurnett et al., 1998b), but essentially it overlaps with Lahey's construct of sluggish cognitive tempo. This factor was associated primarily with ADHD-I. These findings suggest that ADHD-I is a fundamentally different kind of disorder from the other types, differing not only by low quantity of hyperactivity but also on qualitative aspects of cognitive/attentional symptomatology.

Dimension-specific impairment

If a given characteristic were associated with both types of ADHD that exceed the cutoff for the same symptom group, the association would be dimension-specific rather than type-specific. Dimension specificity is probably the most logically coherent way to organize the empiric associations of impairment and ADHD types. Table 1 presents a graphic summary of the general association of dimension-specific impairment across types.

Pre-*DSM-IV* data suggested that the two latent factors of ADHD symptoms were associated with specific forms of impairment and comorbidity (see the *DSM-IV Sourcebook* reviews cited above). Inattention, and/or the *DSM-III* subtype of ADD-WO, were associated with academic impairment and anxiety. Hyperactivity, and/or the *DSM-III* subtype of ADD-H, were associated with active dislike by peers, behavioral noncompliance, and other externalizing comorbidities such as oppositional, aggressive, or conduct problems. From this earlier literature, it is reasonable to predict that *DSM-IV* ADHD types that are defined by high and low levels of these symptom groups would show the same relationships with specific measures of impairment and comorbid disorders. (At the same time, it must be kept in mind that high levels of either symptom group are associated with *global* measures of functional impairment and appear to negatively affect peer *liking*).

Post-*DSM-IV* research has tended to confirm associations found with earlier *DSM* types (Baumgaertel et al., 1995; Faraone et al., 1998; Gaub and Carlson, 1997; Paternite et al., 1996; Wolraich et al., 1996). Dimension-specific distribution of impairment was reported in the Field Trials (Lahey et al., 1994) and even more clearly in a cross validation (McBurnett et al., 1998c). This principle also was supported in a review of a dozen studies involving *DSM-IV* types (McBurnett et al., 1998a): academic impairment tended to aggregate in ADHD-C and ADHD-I, and behavioral disturbance aggregated in ADHD-C and ADHD-HI. However, there is a consistent tendency for ADHD-C to show greater severity

[1]We can only speculate about the reasons that anxiety was associated with *DSM-III* ADHD-WO in some earlier studies, but not with *DSM-IV* ADHD-I in more recent studies. Perhaps the requirement of impulsivity without hyperactivity in *DSM-III* ADD-WO overselected for anxiety problems in that group, or perhaps adult informants did not discriminate well between impulsivity and anxiety symptoms.

Table 1. Distribution of Dimension-Specific Impairment Across Types

Type	*Hyperactivity-Impulsivity*	*Impaired Social Behavior*	*Inattention*	*Learning Problems*
ADHD-I			Cutoff met	Present
ADHD-HI	Cutoff met	Present		
ADHD-C	Cutoff met	Present	Cutoff met	Present

overall, beyond what would be accounted for by its predicted association with both types of dimension-specific impairment. Only a few exceptions to the general rule of dimension-specific impairment have occurred, apparently related to methodological differences and power limitations. The relatively low rates of ADHD-HI are almost always a handicap to this research, resulting in inadequate power in some studies to test correlates of this diagnosis.

DEMOGRAPHICS AND PREVALENCE OF TYPES

Prevalence and proportion of types

The most common subtype in clinic-referred samples is ADHD-C, but the most common subtype in community samples is ADHD-I (McBurnett et al., 1998a). This suggests that children having the most impaired type (ADHD-C) are referred most often to clinics, even though ADHD-I is actually the most common form of ADHD in children. Not surprisingly, ADHD-HI is the least common form of ADHD in both community and clinic samples, except for preschool or very young school-age children, for whom ADHD-HI exceeds ADHD-I. The overall prevalence of *DSM-IV* ADHD (estimable only by community samples) appears higher than was indicated in previous studies of *DSM-III-R* ADHD (mean prevalence from four *DSM-IV* studies = 12.8%). The increase in prevalence appears to be due to higher rates of ADHD-I (mean 7% across studies). This increase in prevalence can be interpreted as a strength of *DSM-IV*, in that it appears to *correct* a problem of misplacement of inattentive-only children in the *DSM-III-R* category of undifferentiated ADD. By setting independent cutpoints for separate types, the *DSM-IV* typology can accommodate cases with unidimensional impairment in a way that *DSM-III-R* could not.

Age variation across types

The mean age of children across subtypes is consistently ordered across clinic samples: ADHD-HI is the youngest at the time of referral to clinics, and ADHD-I is the oldest. This is probably because hyperactivity-impulsivity becomes apparent to adults (and triggers referral in some fraction of the total population with either hyperactive type) during the preschool years, but inattention often becomes apparent only when children are challenged by the increasing demands of academic performance across the elementary grade range. The group with both kinds of symptoms represents a combination of those cases referred early on the basis of their hyperactivity, and cases referred later on the basis of their academic problems, resulting in an average referral age that is intermediate to the unidimensional groups (McBurnett et al., 1998c). The evidence that these age differences are products of referral bias is bolstered by the general lack of an age difference across types in community samples (McBurnett et al., 1998a). Concerns have been raised that some unknown percentage of children with ADHD-HI will have sufficient symptoms of inattention at later ages to qualify for the ADHD-C diagnosis. The data in our clinic study suggest otherwise: because the mean IQ of our young ADHD-H group was significantly higher than for the other groups, it is unlikely that many of our ADHD-H patients have the cognitive difficulties that could eventually manifest as high levels of inattention.

Although ADHD types differ in age, there is little evidence to recommend differences in MPH dosing as a function of age. Recent studies suggest that (1) children of younger ages benefit from MPH (Musten et al., 1997), and (2) the effective dose for a given child may be stable across ages (Smith et al., 1998).

Gender distribution across types

Boys are the predominant gender, and there is modest variation in the exact gender ratio across subtypes. The lowest ratio of boys to girls most often occurs for the ADHD-I subtype. The boy-to-girl ratio for ADHD-I and ADHD-HI appears to be similar in community and clinic samples, but for ADHD-C, the ratio of boys to girls is greater in clinic than community samples. This may reflect a referral bias reflecting special concerns about boys with ADHD-C, but it is clear from population-sampled studies that more boys than girls meet criteria for all types of ADHD.

DO DIFFERENCES AMONG ADHD TYPES IMPLY DIFFERENCES IN METHYLPHENIDATE MANAGEMENT?

To summarize up to this point: By definition, *DSM-IV* types differ by definition in levels of inattentive and hyperactive-impulsive symptoms. In terms of associated impairment, ADHD-C and ADHD-HI children have higher levels of aggression/oppositionality and peer problems than those with ADHD-I, and ADHD-C and ADHD-I children have more learning problems than those with ADHD-HI. No substantial evidence has demonstrated any differential association of anxiety with ADHD type. Do these type differences in inattention, hyperactivity, learning problems, and aggression/oppositionality tell us anything about response to MPH?

If the targets of MPH treatment in a given case are the specific impairments associated with these symptoms, then different measures of response may be appropriate for different types. This becomes especially important when multiple measures of response (e.g., different subscales on parent or teacher rating forms, cognitive tests, or measures of academic productivity) are used, because multiple measures frequently do not agree (Swanson et al., 1991). Knowledge of diagnostic subtype might also guide the clinician to focus on a certain domain of functioning when querying an adult informant about drug response or when selecting a target tailored to an individual case. Thus, the guidelines that can be recommended are that the cognitive and academic domains are most appropriate for evaluating MPH response in ADHD-I, and the social behavioral domains are most appropriate for evaluating response in ADHD-HI. How much to relay on either domain in cases of ADHD-C involves more complex issues, discussed in the following sections. Common sense dictates that these guidelines must be supplemented by the needs of the individual case.

Methylphenidate effects on learning problems

One of the complexities involved in comparing drug effects across domains is that functioning in different domains may respond at different doses. In particular, it has been reported that effortful new learning is optimally improved by lower doses than those required for optimal improvement of social behavior (Swanson et al., 1991). The dose-response curve for social behavior and for simple, low-effort cognitive performance is generally linear or curvilinear, reflecting continued improvement with increasing dose. However, a handful of studies have reported a quadratic (U-shaped or inverted U-shaped) dose-response curve for effortful new learning (e.g., Sprague and Sleator, 1977; Swanson and Kinsbourne, 1978). These studies suggest that optimal benefits on effortful learning may occur at low to moderate doses but that increasingly higher doses result in less improvement than lower doses. This phenomenon is *not* consistently reported across studies (Klein, 1991; Rapport and Kelley, 1991) and is therefore somewhat controversial. However, there is more agreement that performance on effortful cognitive tasks responds well to low to moderate doses (Swanson et al., 1991). Though more direct empiric research is needed on this problem, the implication is that children with ADHD-I may not require doses as high as those required by children with ADHD-HI and ADHD-C.

Methylphenidate effects on type-related comorbidities

There is increasing evidence that aggression is positively treated by stimulants, both as an indirect effect of reducing hyperactivity-impulsivity and as a direct effect of stimulants on aggression itself (Barkley et al., 1989; Gadow et al., 1990; Hinshaw et al., 1989; Kaplan et al., 1990; Klein et al., 1997; Klorman et al., 1994; Murphy et al., 1992; Pelham et al., 1985; Pelham et al., 1987). This suggests that the broad range of disruptive social behavior in ADHD-C and ADHD-HI responds well to MPH. Reductions in aggression/oppositionality may not occur until moderate to high doses are reached (e.g., Casat et al., 1995). However, given the highly impairing nature of these behavior problems and the relative lack of evidence for cognitive impairment from high doses (Douglas et al., 1995; Klein et al., 1997), high doses may be advisable for some children.

The reported absence of differences in anxiety across ADHD types causes us to rethink the implications of anxiety for dose differences. Whereas we previously recommended lower doses of MPH for ADD-WO because of its association with anxiety (McBurnett et al., 1991), this recommendation is not appropriately extended to ADHD-I. Instead, comorbid anxiety disorder should be considered on an individual case basis because of its association with poor response to methylphenidate (Buitelaar et al., 1995; DuPaul et al., 1994; Pliska, 1989; Tannock et al., 1995; Taylor et al., 1987; Zahn et al., 1975). It should be noted that research into comorbidities associated with ADHD types is in a preliminary stage, and later studies may alter these recommendations.

EMPIRIC FINDINGS OF METHYLPHENIDATE RESPONSE ACROSS TYPES OF ADHD

To date, no comparisons of response to MPH by children with *DSM-IV* ADHD types have been reported. Only a handful of studies have evaluated response in children with ADD-WO, and most of them are quite methodologically limited. In one of these studies (Ullman and Sleator, 1985), children with ADD-WO were grouped together with children with ADD-H. MPH improved teacher ratings of inattention and hyperactivity for the group. Children with ADD-WO made up 18% of the group, but because their results were pooled and not reported separately, no conclusions regarding response in ADD-WO can be drawn.

Famularo and Fenton (1987) conducted a multiple baseline study of MPH response in six girls and four boys, aged 7–12 years, who met the *DSM-III* criteria for ADD-WO but not for any other disorder. This study is particularly interesting because it used academic grades as the dependent variable. Dosages were individually determined by balancing clinical response with adverse effects. The doses ranged from 0.4 to 1.2 mg/kg/day in two doses, so apparently the highest single dose was 0.6 mg/kg. The children's grades in each of five subjects (science, reading, spelling, mathematics, and social studies) were obtained for three consecutive grading periods in the same school year. During the middle grading period, the children received the twice-daily MPH treatment. The children's grade average for the pretreatment grading period was 2.02. This increased to 2.84 during treatment and fell to 2.30 following discontinuation of MPH. The grade average during treatment was found to be significantly higher than the pre- and posttreatment grade averages. When grades were examined for individual children, eight of the 10 children showed grade improvement in at least three of the five subjects during treatment, compared with pretreatment baseline. Though not specifically reported, the data in this study show that five of the children showed a grade decline in at least three of the five subjects upon discontinuation of treatment. (Not included in the subject group were an additional three children whose parents requested continuation of MPH following grade improvement during the treatment period.) This study has numerous design and methodological limitations, such as the absence of a placebo condition and the fact that neither teachers nor parents were blind to treatment conditions. Nonetheless, the study does suggest that MPH may be beneficial for some ADD-WO children and that these benefits may be reflected in the ecologically critical outcome measure of school grades.

The best-designed study of methylphenidate in ADD/WO children to date was reported by Barkley et al. (1991). The study evaluated 23 ADHD and 17 ADD-WO children between the ages of 6 and 11 in a triple-blind, placebo-controlled, crossover (within-subject) design for response to twice-daily doses of 5, 10, and 15 mg MPH. The dependent measures included parent and teacher ratings, psychologic tests, and behavioral observations during an arithmetic task. For both the parent and teacher ratings, there were no significant drug condition by group interactions, indicating that the dose-related effects of MPH on behavior ratings did not significantly differ for ADD with and without hyperactivity. Likewise, there were no significant drug conditions for any of the psychologic measures or behavioral observations, again suggesting equivalent response of the diagnostic types to MPH.

Separate analyses of variance were not reported for the ADD-WO group alone (following the statistical convention for post-hoc analyses). There were positive main effects on behavior ratings for the combined group of ADD subtypes. There were no main effects of MPH on most of the psychologic tests. MPH did improve math accuracy but not the total number of problems worked. The drug also reduced omission (but not commission) errors on a continuous performance task. On most of the behavioral observation measures, MPH produced a significant improvement. There were no significant drug effects on ratings of the number or severity of side effects.

At the conclusion of the study, a psychologist and a pediatrician reviewed each individual case and made a clinical judgment regarding the optimal dosage, based on summaries of the dependent measures. Clear differences in the recommended dosage for clinical management resulted between the ADD-H and ADD-WO groups. In the ADD-WO group, 24% were judged to have no response, 35% were recommended for the low dose (5 mg twice daily), 29% were recommended for the moderate dose (10 mg twice daily), and 12% were recommended for the high dose (15 mg twice daily). In the ADD-H group, only 5% were determined to have no response, 24% were recommended for the low dose, 52% were recommended for the medium dose, and 19% were recommended for the high dose. These differences in recommended clinical management doses suggest that more ADD-WO children respond optimally to MPH at low to moderate doses, whereas in comparison, more children with ADD-H respond optimally to moderate to high doses. Additionally, it appears that a greater percentage of ADD-WO children do not show a positive response to any dose of MPH.

SUMMARY AND CONCLUSIONS

Given the relatively high prevalence of inattentive forms of ADHD, it is surprising that so few studies of MPH response in children with ADHD types have appeared. Quite possibly, the elimination of subtyping in *DSM-III-R* suppressed research activity involving subtypes of the disorder. Perhaps the reemergence of subtypes in *DSM-IV* will stimulate new research efforts in this area. Although more empirical studies are needed, some tentative conclusions can be offered. First, the discriminant validity of *DSM-IV* subtypes appears to be established by dimensionally specific forms of impairment: The two types defined by high levels of inattention are accompanied by academic impairment, and the two types defined by high levels of hyperactivity-impulsivity are accompanied by social behavioral impairment. The ADHD-I type may also be characterized by type-specific problems of alertness, orientation, and "sluggish cognitive tempo," but the evidence for this distinction is preliminary. *DSM-IV* types do not appear to differ appreciably on anxiety, based on the available evidence, but the two hyperactive types are accompanied by higher rates of other externalizing problems (aggression, oppositional-defiant behavior, etc.). If anxiety is present in an individual case, the clinician should be mindful that the likelihood of positive response to MPH is lessened, and should carefully monitor any changes in peer interactions, social withdrawal, and academic productivity. Second, the intended targets for methylphenidate may differ across *DSM-IV* ADHD types. The primary functional target in ADHD-I is likely to be academic functioning. Secondary targets may be any memory retrieval, alertness/orientation, and organizational problems that may be present. The primary functional targets in ADHD-HI and ADHD-C are more likely to be excessive motor activity, aggressive/oppositional behavior, and/or peer problems. As children with ADHD-I are relatively free of the aggressive and disruptive behavior problems that would be targeted in the other two types, low to moderate doses may effectively address their primary problems in academic functioning and organization.

Last, in the absence of dose-response studies comparing *DSM-IV* ADHD types, we are left to draw inferences from the few studies of *DSM-III* types. These studies suggest that MPH may be a useful treatment of ADHD-I. However, the percentage of nonresponders may be higher in ADHD-I, and the dosage that is optimal for clinical management may be lower. Specifically, this "best dosage" tends to be in the low to moderate range for most children with *DSM-III* ADD-WO, but a small percentage (12% in one study) of these children may respond best to a high dosage. The converse extrapolation of this *DSM-III* data is that a child with ADHD-I who fails to respond to a low to moderate dosage is highly likely (88%) to be a nonresponder or an adverse responder to MPH.

REFERENCES

American Psychiatric Association (1968), *Diagnostic and Statistical Manual of Mental Disorders, 2nd ed.* Washington, DC: American Psychiatric Association.

American Psychiatric Association (1980), *Diagnostic and Statistical Manual of Mental Disorders, 3rd ed.* Washington, DC: American Psychiatric Association.

American Psychiatric Association (1987), *Diagnostic and Statistical Manual of Mental Disorders, 3rd ed.-rev.* Washington, DC: American Psychiatric Association.

American Psychiatric Association (1994), *Diagnostic and Statistical Manual of Mental Disorders, 4th ed.* Washington, DC: American Psychiatric Association.

Barkley, R.A., DuPaul, G.J. & McMurray, M.B. (1991), Attention deficit disorder with and without hyperactivity: Clinical response to three dose levels of methylphenidate. *Pediatrics,* 87:519–531.

Barkley, R.A., McMurray, M.B., Edelbrock, C.S. & Robbins, K. (1989), The response of aggressive and nonaggressive ADHD children to two doses of methylphenidate. *J. Am. Acad. Child Adolesc. Psychiatry,* 28:873–881.

Bauermeister, J.J., Alegria, M., Bird, H.R., Rubio-Stipec, M. & Canino, G. (1992), Are attentional-hyperactivity deficits unidimensional or multidimensional syndromes? Empirical findings from a community survey. *J. Am. Acad. Child Adolesc. Psychiatry,* 31: 423–431.

Baumgaertel, A., Wolraich, M.L. & Dietrich, M. (1995), Comparison of diagnostic criteria for attention deficit disorders in a German elementary school sample. *J. Am. Acad. Child Adolesc. Psychiatry,* 34:629–638.

Biederman, J., Newcorn, J.H. & Sprich, S. (1997), Comorbidity of attention deficit/hyperactivity disorder. In: *DSM-IV Sourcebook, vol. 3,* eds., T.A. Widiger, A.J. Frances, H.A. Pincus, R. Ross, M.B. First & W. David. Washington, DC: American Psychiatric Association.

Buitelaar, J.K., Van der Gaag, R.J., Swaab-Barneveld, H. & Kuiper, M. (1995), Prediction of clinical response to methylphenidate in children with attention deficit/hyperactivity disorder. *J. Am. Acad. Child Adolesc. Psychiatry,* 34:1025–1032.

Casat, C.D., Pearson, D.A., Van Davelaar, M.J. & Cherek, D.R. (1995), Methylphenidate effects on a laboratory aggression measure in children with ADHD. *Psychopharmacol. Bull.,* 31:353–356.

Douglas, V.I., Barr, R.G., Desilets, J. & Sherman, E. (1995), Do high doses of stimulants impair flexible thinking in attention-deficit hyperactivity disorder? *J. Am. Acad. Child Adolesc. Psychiatry,* 34:877–885.

DuPaul, G.J., Barkley, R.A. & McMurray, M.B. (1994), Response of children with ADHD to methylphenidate: Interaction with internalizing symptoms. *J. Am. Acad. Child Adolesc. Psychiatry,* 33:894–903.

Eiraldi, R.B., Power, T.J., & Nezu, C.M. (1997), Patterns of comorbidity associated with subtypes of ADHD among 6- to 12-year-old children. *J. Am. Acad. Child Adolesc. Psychiatry,* 36:503–514.

Famularo, R. & Fenton, T. (1987), The effect of methylphenidate on school grades in children with attention deficit disorder without hyperactivity: A preliminary report. *J. Clin. Psychiatry,* 48:112–114.

Faraone, S.V., Biederman, J., Weber, W. & Russell, R.L. (1998), Psychiatric, neuropsychological, and psychosocial features of *DSM-IV* subtypes of attention deficit/hyperactivity disorder: Results from a clinically referred sample. *J. Am. Acad. Child Adolesc. Psychiatry,* 37:185–193.

Frick, P.J., Lahey, B.B., Applegate, B., Kerdyck, L., Ollendick, T., Hynd, G.W., Garfinkel, B., Greenhill, L., Biederman, J., Barkley, R.A., McBurnett, K., Newcorn, J. & Waldman, I. (1994), *DSM-IV* field trials for the disruptive behavior disorders: Symptom utility estimates. *J. Am. Acad. Child Adolesc. Psychiatry,* 33:529–539.

Gadow, K.D., Nolan, E.E., Sverd, J., Sprafkin, J. & Paolicelli, L. (1990), Methylphenidate in aggressive-hyperactive boys: I. Effects on peer aggression in public school settings. *J. Am. Acad. Child Adolesc. Psychiatry,* 29:710–718.

Gaub, M. & Carlson, C.L. (1997), Behavioral characteristics of *DSM-IV* ADHD subtypes in a school-based population. *J. Abnorm. Child Psychol.,* 25:103–111.

Hinshaw, S.P., Hencker, B., Whalen, C.K., Erhardt, D. & Dunnington, R.E., Jr. (1989), Aggressive, prosocial, and nonsocial behavior in hyperactive boys: Dose effects of methylphenidate in naturalistic settings. *J. Consult. Clin. Psychol.,* 57:636–643.

Kaplan, S.L., Busner, J., Kupietz, S., Wasserman, E. & Segal, B. (1990), Effects of methylphenidate on adolescents with aggressive conduct disorder and ADHD: A preliminary report. *J. Am. Acad. Child Adolesc. Psychiatry,* 29:719–723.

Klein, R.G. (1991), Effects of high methylphenidate doses on the cognitive performance of hyperactive children. *Bratisl. Lek. Listy,* 92:534–539.

Klein, R.G., Abikoff, H., Klass, E., Ganeles, D., Seese, L.M. & Pollack, S. (1997), Clinical efficacy of methylphenidate in conduct disorder with and without attention-deficit/hyperactivity disorder. *Arch. Gen. Psychiatry,* 54:1073–1080.

Klorman, R., Brumaghim, J.T., Fitzpatrick, P.A., Borgstedt, A.D. & Strauss, J. (1994), Clinical and cognitive effects of methylphenidate on children with attention deficit disorder as a function of aggression/oppositionality and age. *J. Abnorm. Psychol.,* 103: 206–221.

Kuperman, S., Johnson, B., Arndt, S., Lindgren, S. & Wolraich, M. (1996), Quantitative EEG differences in a nonclinical sample of children with ADHD and undifferentiated ADD. *J. Am. Acad. Child Adolesc. Psychiatry,* 35:1009–1017.

Lahey, B.B., Applegate, B., McBurnett, K., Biederman, J., Greenhill, L., Hynd, G.W., Barkley, R.A., Newcorn, J., Jensen, P., Richters, J., Garfinkel, B., Kerdyk, L., Frick, P.J., Ollendick, T., Perez, D., Hart, E.L., Waldman, I. & Shaffer, D. (1994), *DSM-IV* field trials for attention deficit hyperactivity disorder in children and adolescents. *Am. J. Psychiatry,* 151:1673–1685.

Lahey, B.B., & Carlson, C.L. (1991), Validity of the diagnostic category of attention deficit disorder without hyperactivity: A review of the literature. *J. Learning Disabil.,* 24:110–120.

McBurnett, K., (1996), Development of the *DSM-IV*: Validity and relevance for school psychologists. *School Psychol. Rev.,* 25:259–273.

McBurnett, K., (1997), Attention-deficit/hyperactivity disorder: Review of diagnostic issues. In: *DSM-IV Sourcebook, vol. 3*, eds., T.A. Widiger, A.J. Frances, H.A. Pincus, R. Ross, M. First & W. Davis. Washington, DC: American Psychiatric Association, pp. 111–114.

McBurnett, K., Lahey, B.B. & Pfiffner, L.J. (1993), Diagnosis of attention deficit disorders in DSM-IV: Scientific basis and implications for education. *Exceptional Children,* 60:108–117.

McBurnett, K., Lahey, B.B., & Swanson, J.M. (1991), Ritalin treatment in attention deficit disorder without hyperactivity. In: *Ritalin: Theory and Patient Management,* eds., L.L. Greenhill & B.B. Osman. Larchmont, NY: Mary Ann Liebert, Inc.

McBurnett, K., Pfiffner, L.J. & Ottolini, Y. (1998a), Types of ADHD. In: *ADHD,* ed., M.A. Stein. Chicago.

McBurnett, K., Pfiffner, L.J. & Ottolini, Y.L. (1998b), *Attention and Alertness/Orientation in Attention-Deficit Hyperactivity Disorder.* Chicago: University of Chicago Press.

McBurnett, K., Pfiffner, L.J., Willcutt, E., Tamm, L., Lerner, M. & Ottolini, Y.L. (1998c), *Experimental Cross-Validation of* DSM-IV *Field Trials.* Chicago: University of Chicago Press.

Murphy, D. A., Pelham, W.E. & Lang, A.R. (1992), Aggression in boys with attention-deficit/hyperactivity disorder: Methylphenidate effects on naturalistically observed aggression, response to provocation, and social information processing. *J. Child Abnorm. Psychol.,* 20:451–466.

Musten, L.M., Firestone, P., Pisterman, S., Bennett, S. & Mercer, J. (1997), Effects of methylphenidate on preschool children with ADHD: Cognitive and behavioral functions. *J. Am. Acad. Child Adolesc. Psychiatry,* 36:1407–1415.

Newcorn, J.H., Halperin, J.M., Healy, J.M., O'Brien, J.D., Pascualvaca, D.M., Wolf, L.E., Morganstein, A., Sharma, V. & Young, J.G. (1989), Are ADDH and ADHD the same or different? *J. Am. Acad. Child Adolesc. Psychiatry,* 28:734–738.

Paternite, C.E., Loney, J. & Roberts, M.A. (1996), A preliminary validation of subtypes of *DSM-IV* attention-deficit/hyperactivity disorder. *J. Attention Disorders,* 1:70–86.

Pelham, W.E., Jr., Bender, M.E., Caddell, J., Booth, S. & Moorer, S.A. (1985), Methylphenidate and children with attention deficit disorder: Dose effects on classroom academic and social behavior. *Arch. Gen. Psychiatry,* 42:948–952.

Pelham, W.E., Jr., Sturges, J., Hoza, J., Schmidt, C., Bijlsma, J.J., Milich, R. & Moorer, S. (1987). Sustained release and standard methylphenidate effects on cognitive and social behavior in children with attention deficit disorder. *Pediatrics,* 80:491–501.

Pliska, S.R. (1989), Effect of anxiety on cognition, behavior, and stimulant response in ADHD. *J. Am. Acad. Child Adolesc. Psychiatry,* 28:882–887.

Rapport, M.D. & Kelley, K.L. (1991), Psychostimulant effects on learning and cognitive function: Findings and implications for children with attention deficit/hyperactivity disorder. *Clin. Psychol. Rev.,* 11:61–92.

Smith, B.H., Pelham, W.E., Gnagy, E. & Yudell, R.S. (1998), Equivalent effects of stimulant treatment for attention-deficit/hyperactivity disorder during childhood and adolescence. *J. Am. Acad. Child Adolesc. Psychiatry,* 37:314–321.

Sprague, R.L. & Sleator, E.K. (1977), Methylphenidate in hyperkinetic children: Differences in dose effects on learning and social behavior. *Science,* 198:1274–1276.

Swanson, J.M., Cantwell, D., McBurnett, K. & Hanna, G. (1991), Effects of stimulant medication on learning in children with ADHD. *J. Learning Disabil.,* 24:219–230.

Swanson, J.M. & Kinsbourne, M. (1978), Should you use stimulants to treat the hyperactive child? *Mod. Med.,* 46:71–80.

Tannock, R., Ickowicz, A. & Schachar, R. (1995), Differential effects of methylphenidate on working memory in ADHD children with and without comorbid anxiety. *J. Am. Acad. Child Adolesc. Psychiatry,* 34:886–896.

Taylor, E., Shachar, R., Thorley, G., Wieselberg, H.M., Everitt, B. & Rutter, M. (1987), Which boys respond to stimulant medication? A controlled trial of methylphenidate in boys with disruptive behavior. *Psychol. Med.,* 17:121–143.

Ullman, R.K. & Sleator, E.K. (1985), Attention deficit disorder children with or without hyperactivity: Which behaviors are helped by stimulants? *Clin. Pediatr.,* 24:547–551.

Waldman, I.D., Lilienfield, S.O. & Lahey, B.B. (1995), Toward construct validity in the childhood disruptive behavior disorders: Classification and diagnosis in *DSM-IV* and beyond. In: *Advances in Child Clinical Psychology* Vol. 17, eds., T.H. Ollendick & R.J. Prinz. New York: Plenum Press, pp. 323–363.

Wolraich, M.L., Hannah, J.N., Pinnock, T.Y., Baumgaertel, A & Brown, J. (1996), Comparison of diagnostic criteria for attention-deficit/hyperactivity disorder in a county-wide sample. *J. Am. Acad. Child Adolesc. Psychiatry,* 35:319–324.

Zahn, T.P., Abate, F., Little, B.C. & Wender, P.H. (1975), Minimal brain dysfunction, stimulant drugs, and automatic nervous system activity. *Arch. Gen. Psychiatry,* 32:381–387.

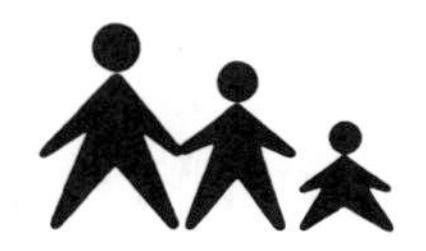

Methylphenidate: Effects on Language, Reading, and Auditory Processing

ROSEMARY TANNOCK

Language impairments, reading disorders, and auditory processing deficits are three interrelated neurodevelopmental impairments that frequently coexist with attention deficit hyperactivity disorder (ADHD). These coexisting difficulties arise in preschool years (McGee et al., 1991) but may be noticed first in the school setting. Also, these additional problems are often overlooked or interpreted (erroneously) as manifestations of inattentive, noncompliant, or disruptive behavior (e.g., "He simply won't listen when I'm talking to him—he just looks spacey and doesn't respond." "It's impossible to have a conversation with him—he interrupts us when we are talking, then flips from one topic to another, hesitates, mumbles and starts over again—we just don't know what he is trying to say." "Whenever it's time for reading, she doesn't even try, but just wastes time sharpening her pencil, twirling her hair, or fiddling with things in her desk."). These interrelated language-based problems are discernible in early childhood and without effective treatment tend to persist across the developmental span and impair academic, social, and occupational functioning. For example, they interfere with everyday activities at school, such as understanding teachers' instructions, reading instructions in workbooks, and copying correctly homework assignments written on boards. These additional problems also impair the individual's ability to understand and contribute to conversations, negotiate conflicts with parents or peers, participate effectively in games or other social activities, and recall and follow directions.

ADHD is most commonly treated with psychostimulant medication, particularly methylphenidate (MPH) (Safer et al., 1996). This is because psychostimulants are effective in ameliorating the core behavioral symptoms of ADHD, at least in the short term (Schachar et al., 1996). The majority of children with ADHD are prescribed stimulant medication by pediatricians or family physicians, and, in many cases, medication is the sole treatment received (Wolraich et al., 1990), despite strong recommendations for a multimodal approach (American Academy of Child and Adolescent Psychiatry, 1997). Accordingly, the issue of whether stimulants also ameliorate coexisting problems in language, reading, and auditory processing is of considerable clinical concern.

In this chapter, for ease of exposition, I discuss each of the three sets of problems separately. Thus, for each set, I first provide a brief overview of its defining characteristics, next comment on the rate of overlap with ADHD, and then review the empirical evidence for the effects of stimulant treatment on this aspect of function. In the final section, I invoke Baddeley's (1986, 1997) multicomponent model of working memory to account for the following: (1) the overlap among language, reading, auditory processing problems, and ADHD and (2) the limited effects of MPH on various aspects of language, reading, and auditory processing.

Brain and Behavior Research Program, The Hospital for Sick Children; and University of Toronto, Toronto, Ontario, Canada.

STIMULANT EFFECTS ON ORAL LANGUAGE AND LANGUAGE PROBLEMS IN ADHD

Language problems in ADHD

Communication disorder is an umbrella term that refers to an unexpected delay or deviance in the acquisition of speech or language or both, which cannot be explained in terms of mental or physical handicap, hearing loss, emotional disorder, or environmental deprivation (Bishop, 1992). A specific link between ADHD and communication disorders is indicated by several clinical and epidemiologic studies, with estimates of the overlap ranging from 15% to 75%, depending on the precise definitions of each disorder, the methods used to diagnose them, and the nature of the communication problems (reviewed by Baker and Cantwell, 1992; Tannock and Schachar, 1996). Traditionally, two broad categories of communication disorders are distinguished: *speech disorders* and *language disorders.*

Speech disorders refer to problems with the motor production of speech sounds, including problems with articulation (frequent and recurring mispronunciations of several speech sounds), dysfluency (pauses, hesitations, restarts, self-corrections, trail-offs) that interrupts the normal rhythm of speech, speech rate (too fast or too slow so that speech is rendered uninterpretable), or altered voice quality (abnormal pitch, loudness, nasality, hoarseness). In general, speech problems are less strongly related to ADHD and, when they do exist, tend to occur together with broader-band language problems (Beitchman et al., 1989; Cantwell and Baker, 1991).

By contrast, *language disorders* refer to problems with the conventional system of arbitrary signals and rules used for communication. Distinctions are made between *receptive* and *expressive* language disorders; both can be further classified in terms of which components of language are involved (e.g., phonological, lexical, semantic). Receptive language disorders may manifest as difficulties in following directions, understanding the meaning of words or sentence structure, and making inferences; typically, these difficulties are also accompanied by difficulties in expressive language. Expressive language disorders may be manifested by an extremely limited vocabulary, difficulties in word finding, use of immature or incorrect grammatical markers, difficulty with pronoun case marking or marking or maintaining tense, problems in ordering the words grammatically to convey a meaningful message, or omission of critical parts of sentences (e.g., "And the dog it runned down the uh . . . the thing—uh what's it called? And then he jumps and they felled into the water.").

Although problems in both receptive and expressive language have been reported in children with ADHD, expressive language appears to be particularly impaired (Baker and Cantwell, 1992; Beitchman et al., 1987; Oram et al., 1999). For example, in a recent study, we found that ~20% of children with ADHD had impairments in receptive language, 33% had expressive impairments, 30% had word retrieval problems, and 25% had impairments in phonological awareness (Oram et al., 1999). None of the language problems had been identified formally before this systematic evaluation. It is important to note that these children were not selected for language impairments: rather, they were referred *solely* for an evaluation of stimulant medication for treatment of the ADHD symptoms. One reason why these language problems had not been identified previously may be because they were obscured by the more salient behavioral symptoms (Cohen et al., 1993). These findings highlight the importance of including routine screening of language abilities in the assessment for ADHD.

More recently, another set of language-related problems have been recognized: *pragmatic language disorders,* the inappropriate use of language as a cognitive and social tool to convey information, to participate in the community, and to learn. These problems involve the application of language in social or learning situations and the use of language for problem solving and in expressing affect. They are not language specific because they do not necessarily involve phonological, lexical, or syntactic problems. Pragmatic disorders may manifest as a failure to understand or use social conventions, such as turn-taking and other conversational rules; the use of unusual prosodic features (e.g., intonation patterns); difficulties in using self-talk (private speech) during problem solving; or failure to modulate tone, volume, or gestural accompaniments when expressing affect.

Pragmatic deficits are evident in the majority of children with ADHD, even in those with adequate abilities in the basic systems of language—phonology, morphology, syntax, semantics (reviewed by Tannock and Schachar, 1996). Moreover, pragmatic deficits appear to be more strongly associated with ADHD than with learning disorders (Humphries et al., 1994). The high rate of pragmatic disorders in ADHD is not surprising, because the defining features of ADHD include difficulties in using language appropriately within social and learning contexts. For example, the *Diagnostic and Statistical Manual of Mental Disorders* (*DSM*), *4th ed.* proposes that in social situations: (1) inattention may be expressed as frequent shifts in conversation, not listening to others, or not keeping one's mind on conversations; (2) hyperactivity may be manifested as excessive talkativeness; and (3) impulsiveness may manifest itself as frequent and inappropriate initiation of conversation, excessive interruption of others, making comments out of turn, or blurting out answers before questions have been completed, so that "others may complain that they cannot get a word in edgewise" (American Psychiatric Association, 1994, p. 79).

Children with ADHD exhibit a wide range of pragmatic deficits. These communication problems include: (1) excessive talkativeness during spontaneous conversation, during task transitions, and in play settings (Barkley et al., 1983; Zentall, 1988); (2) marked problems in introducing, maintaining, and changing topics appropriately, as well as in negotiating turn-taking during conversation (Humphries et al., 1994; Ludlow et al., 1978; Zentall, et al., 1983); (3) difficulties adjusting language to the listener or specific context (Landau and Milich, 1988; Whalen et al., 1979; Zentall, 1988); (4) production deficits and dysfluencies when confronted with tasks such as story retelling or giving directions that require planning and organization of verbal responses (Hamlett et al., 1987; Milich and Lorch, 1994; Purvis and Tannock, 1997; Tannock et al., 1993; Zentall, 1988); and (5) lack of specificity, accuracy, and conciseness in the selection and use of words to convey information, resulting in ambiguity of intent or meaning (Purvis and Tannock, 1997; Tannock et al., 1996).

Stimulant effects on oral language and language problems

It is not uncommon to hear anecdotal reports from parents expressing their delight in the positive effects of stimulant medication on their children's language. Examples include "I am able to actually have a conversation with my son for the first time! He listens and stays on one topic," "Finally, I can follow what he is saying—his speech isn't so garbled and muddled as it used to be," "At last, we can communicate. He really has some good ideas and now I can follow what he is getting at." Also, many clinicians and researchers note that with medication, children appear to use more politeness markers (greetings, social markers or acknowledgements such as "please," "thank you," and "would you mind?") and to modulate the volume and tone of their speech. But these clinical anecdotes have yet to be confirmed by systematic analysis. There are very few controlled investigations of the impact of stimulant medication on children's oral language, and the limited data available are disappointing—few systematic effects have been found.

One of the first comprehensive investigations of stimulant effects on language consisted of a double-blind, placebo-controlled, crossover study to investigate the effects of the psychostimulant dextroamphetamine, on the oral language produced by 12 hyperactive boys and 12 normally developing boys (Ludlow et al., 1978). A series of structured language activities (e.g., picture description, story telling, communicative task) was used to elicit spoken language. None of these children had specific language impairments, but the hyperactive boys differed from the comparison group in their *use* of language (i.e., the hyperactive boys used less task-related speech and more disruptive speech) but not in linguistic complexity. Drug effects were minimal in both groups. In the normal comparison group, stimulant medication increased speech fluency (words per minute) and task-directed speech (story telling time). Anecdotal comments from the families indicated that these normal boys "talked incessantly and related every last detail of an event at the dinner table." (Ludlow et al., 1978). By contrast, stimulant medication did not have any impact on task-related speech or on disruptive speech; rather, it decreased the amount of off-task speech used by the hyperactive boys. Also of interest was the finding that the psychostimulant increased the use of complex sentences (sentences with embedded clauses) in both groups of boys (Ludlow et al., 1978). Constructions with embedded clauses require extra processing because they require the speaker to hold the semicompleted main phrase "on-line" in working memory while inserting the embedded clause, as in the following example: *"The frog, who was sitting on the lily pad, watched the boy carefully."*

Given the multiple statistical comparisons that were conducted, it is possible that this latter effect was simply a spurious finding; however, evidence of similar changes in our controlled studies of MPH (described below) suggest that this beneficial effect is robust.

Measures of language use have been included in a few studies examining the impact of stimulant medication on cognitive and social functioning. For example, some studies suggest that MPH may increase talkativeness in children with ADHD (e.g., Barkley, 1990; Creager and Van Riper, 1967). Because children with ADHD are often excessively and inappropriately talkative, these data suggest an adverse effect of stimulants on their use of language. By contrast, other studies report little or no effect of psychostimulants on the effectiveness, functional content, or dysfluency (false starts, rephrasings) of children's communication (Hamlett et al., 1987; Whalen et al., 1979). The few discernible effects were restricted to the quality or style of the children's language. It was less vigorous and intense, contained fewer exclamative comments, and was accompanied by mild dysphoria, suggesting a negative impact on the prosodic and affective quality of speech (Whalen et al., 1979).

My colleagues and I have also been investigating the effects of MPH on language in children with ADHD. We attempted to provide a more precise characterization of language abilities in children with ADHD and to determine the effects of this stimulant medication on critical aspects of language that are believed to be deficient in children with ADHD. The latter include social interaction (dialogue), narration/description (monologue), and self-regulation (self-talk, or private speech). One study consisted of a randomized, placebo-controlled, double-blind, crossover design to investigate dose effects of MPH (0.3, 0.6, 0.9 mg/kg) on the spontaneous language produced by two boys with ADHD during conversation with an adult (Tannock et al., 1995). A detailed analysis of two linguistic systems (speech function, cohesion) provided information about the boys' social language and cognitive processing. MPH produced both positive and negative changes in the socially appropriate uses of language in the children's conversation.

MPH produced several pronounced positive changes. They included increased conversational responsiveness, greater semantic continuity and linguistic complexity (indexed by increased use of conjunction, which is a linguistic device that explicitly signals the relation between contiguous clauses produced by the speaker), and increased cohesiveness within the children's turns at speaking (Tannock et al., 1995). These changes are consistent with the concept of cognitive focusing. With MPH, the children were more likely to extend their utterances through the use of conjunction rather than by simply stringing clauses without explicit signals that they were semantically related to one another. Moreover, an examination of the various type of conjunction revealed that stimulant medication increased children's use of more complicated conjunction (consequential conjunction, such as "because," "therefore") rather than the simplest forms (additives, such as "and," "and then"). The use of these types of conjunction places high demands on working memory, because the individual must hold the two ideas to be expressed on-line and in correct sequence while retrieving the appropriate conjunction from long-term memory and then inserting it after expressing the first part of the complex sentence. For example: *"The boy fell over the log because he wasn't looking where he was going."*

Recall that Ludlow et al. (1978) reported similar effects for dextroamphetamine: Children were more likely to use embedded sentences, which also make high demands on working memory.

Other stimulant-related changes suggested that the "focusing" effect of stimulant medication might also produce some negative effects on children's social construction of conversation, consistent with the concept of "cognitive overfocusing" (Kinsbourne, 1991; Robbins and Sahakian, 1979; Solanto, 1984; Tucker and Derryberry, 1990). For example, MPH increased the frequency of unclear referencing (i.e., unclear use of pronouns as in "*He* goes in the room and it . . . Uh . . . *the thing* . . . comes off and *they* come out again") so that the partner must make an inference or be left with an inadequate understanding of the text. Also, stimulant medication decreased the children's reference to the conversational partner and produced greater topic continuity to the extent that it resulted in socially unacceptable domination of the conversation (Tannock et al., 1995). In one of the children, this excessive perseverance on one or two topics occurred at the medium and high doses, which produced the greatest behavioral improvements.

Obviously, the case study approach does not permit general conclusions concerning the effects of stimulant medication on language in children with ADHD. Accordingly, we attempted to replicate and extend these findings in a larger sample (n = 48) of children with ADHD with and without comorbid language impairments, in whom we examined narrative abilities, conversation, and private speech (Benedetto-Nasho and Tannock, in press; Tannock, 1997). We included quantitative measures (number of utterances, words, different words) as well as measures of fluency (pauses, retracings with and without self-correction) and measures of the two linguistic systems examined in our previous case studies (cohesion, speech function).

Our preliminary analyses indicated that medication effects are sparse but specific in that the effects are restricted primarily to enhancing language used for self-regulation. For example, in the narrative task (story retelling), MPH increased the frequency with which the children stopped their retelling in midutterance and self-corrected before proceeding (e.g., "He went . . . *The dog* went . . *The boy and* the dog went into the field"). The psychostimulant had no impact on uncorrected retracings (e.g., "He went . . . he went . . . He went into the wood") or on the quantitative measures of cohesion. Moreover, in conversational interaction with an adult, MPH increased children's use of complex conjunctions (irrespective of the presence of concurrent language impairments), replicating our previous findings based on the two case studies (Tannock et al., 1999). These findings suggest that stimulant medication enables the child to exert more control over his or her use of language in terms of being better able to monitor and self-correct oral language and to be more precise in the manner with which temporal and causal relationships are marked for the listener.

Most striking, however, were the effects of MPH on the children's private speech (self-talk) used during a challenging arithmetic computation task (Benedetto-Nasho and Tannock, in press). Private speech, which refers to self-directed language for metaconscious control, follows a developmental path from externalized and audible speech for oneself accompanying or preceding action, ultimately to internalized or inner speech for regulating thought and action. MPH decreased children's use of the more immature, externalized form of self-talk and increased their use of the more mature internalized form, which was associated with focused attention and motor quiescence. Moreover, MPH decreased children's use of finger counting (which we conceptualized as another immature manifestation of self-talk) and increased arithmetic productivity. Our findings confirm those of a previous uncontrolled study of stimulant effects of self-talk in children with ADHD (Berk and Potts, 1991).

In summary, stimulant medication prescribed for the treatment of ADHD symptoms may improve some aspects of pragmatic dysfunction, perhaps mediated by its beneficial effects on working memory and other higher-order cognitive functions. By contrast, there is no compelling evidence to date that it has any systematic impact on deficits in the basic subsystems of language (phonology, syntax, semantics). Co-occurring deficits in the basic language systems will require specific intervention using techniques developed in the field of speech-language pathology.

STIMULANT EFFECTS ON READING AND READING DISORDERS IN ADHD

Reading problems in ADHD

The term *developmental reading disorder* or *dyslexia* refers to unexpected difficulty in learning to read despite intact sensory and intellectual abilities and sufficient educational opportunities. Reading skills are multidimensional, with various components contributing to word identification, reading fluency, and text comprehension.

The most reliable index of reading disorder (RD) is the failure to develop accurate, rapid, context-free word identification skills (e.g., Shaywitz et al., 1996). In the majority of cases, the cause of word identification failure is an underlying deficit in specific language-based skills, called *phonological processing* (for recent reviews, see Adams, 1990; Shaywitz et al., 1996; Vandervelden and Siegel, 1996; Wagner et al., 1994; Wolf, 1991). Phonological processing involves auditory skills that afford the ability to recognize, differentiate, and manipulate phonemes, which are single speech sounds in words. It is a multidimensional construct that may include several latent abilities, including: (1) auditory analysis and synthesis of phonemes, which refers to the ability to segment whole words into constituent units—phonemes—and to blend isolated phonemes to form whole words, respectively; (2) retrieval of phonological codes or pronunciations associated with letters, word segments, and whole words, from a long-term store; and (3) phonological coding of information in working memory for short-term storage during ongoing processing (for indepth reviews, see Adams, 1990; Wagner and Torgeson, 1987; Wagner et al, 1994; Wolf, 1991). Individuals with deficits in these abilities have no basis for segmenting orthographic (spelling) patterns corresponding to the sound units and either extracting rules for their synthesis or using them to decode by analogy (e.g., Lovett, 1992).

Another common deficit believed to be specific to RD involves a deficit in *rapid automatized naming* (Denckla and Rudel, 1976; Wolf, 1991). Naming speech is not a unitary entity. Rather, it is conceptualized as the surface behavioral manifestation of a complex and rapid integration of many cognitive, perceptual, and linguistic subprocesses (Wolf, 1997). According to one hypothesis, deficiencies in naming speed reflects inadequacies in a precise timing mechanism necessary to the development of orthographic codes and to their integration with phonological codes (Bowers and Wolf, 1993). Rapid naming, which demands fast oral production of names of visual stimuli (letters, digits, colors, objects), influences the development of word identification skills and may also influence reading comprehension, albeit to a lesser extent (Badian, 1993; Bowers, 1995; Felton and Brown, 1990; Meyer et al., 1998). Speed of naming is believed to be distinct from phonological processing (Bowers, 1995; Meyer et. al., 1998; Wolf, 1997). Individuals with deficits in both phonological awareness and visual naming speed (double deficit) have been found to be more impaired than individuals with weaknesses in only one domain (Wolf, 1997).

Adequate *language comprehension* and adequate word identification skills are both required for reading comprehension, but the roles of these two subskills change across the different stages of reading development (e.g., Vellutino et al., 1993). That is, word identification is central at the beginning reading stage, but once that subskill is adequate, language comprehension plays a central role in reading comprehension. Poor readers are typically deficient in listening comprehension and other aspects of receptive language (Vellutino et al., 1993).

Epidemiologic and clinical studies suggest a comorbidity rate between ADHD and RD of 15% to 30% when relatively stringent criteria are used for defining each of the separate disorders (e.g., Shaywitz et al., 1992; Semrud-Clikeman et al., 1992). It has been proposed that learning disorders (including RD) may be more commonly associated with attention deficit disorder without hyperactivity as defined by *DSM-III* (Barkley et al., 1990; Edelbrock et al., 1984; Hynd et al., 1991). However, data from recent investigations of the *DSM-IV* subtypes of ADHD do not support this proposition. Reading disorder has not been found to be more common in the Predominantly Inattentive Type (e.g., Faraone et al., 1998; Marshall et al., 1997; Morgan et al., 1996; Paternite et al., 1996).

ADHD children with RD appear to exhibit distinct neuropsychologic and neurochemical profiles compared with ADHD children who are average readers. Numerous neuropsychologic studies have demonstrated that children with ADHD+RD exhibit the same types of deficits in phonological processing and naming speed that are typically associated with RD (e.g., Felton et al., 1987; Korkman and Pesonen, 1994; Närhi and Ahonen, 1995, Pennington et al., 1993). These findings indicate that these children's reading problems cannot be attributed solely to the behavioral symptoms of ADHD. Also, children with ADHD+RD are likely to exhibit concomitant language impairments, including deficits in receptive and expressive abilities in semantic and syntactic components of language, as well as in narrative abilities (Purvis and Tannock, 1997; Tannock et al., 1996). Moreover, the comorbid group also exhibit the cognitive and neuropsychologic deficits associated with ADHD (i.e., deficits in sustained attention, inhibition, and executive control), although the findings are not always consistent (cf. Pennington et al., 1993; vs. Reader et al., 1994).

From a neurochemical perspective, preliminary evidence suggests that noradrenergic (NA) function may differentiate ADHD+RD from ADHD. Specifically, children with ADHD+RD have higher plasma levels of the NA-metabolite 3-methoxy-4-hydroxyphenylglycol (MHPG) than do normal readers with ADHD, but the two groups did not differ in plasma levels of the dopamine metabolite, homovanillic acid. Moreover, plasma MHPG levels were inversely related to academic achievement (reading, spelling, arithmetic) and verbal processing (verbal IQ) but were not related to parent or teacher ratings of behavior, visuospatial processing (performance IQ), or laboratory measures of inattention or impulsivity (Halperin et al., 1993, 1997). However, the studies did not include either a normal comparison group or a group with RD only. Thus, they could not determine whether children with ADHD+RD have unusually high MPHG levels, whether those with ADHD have unusually low MHPG levels, whether elevated MHPG levels are related to RD rather than to ADHD per se, or whether both ADHD groups differ from normal control subjects and children with RD. Moreover, plasma MHPG levels may not accurately reflect central mechanisms. Nonetheless, these findings are provocative. They have led to the speculation that ADHD+RD may be due to dysregulation (Pliszka et al., 1996) or overreactivity (Mefford and Potter, 1989) of the locus coeruleus, resulting in increased MHPG turnover, which in turn may cause disruption of the posterior attention system associated with early stages of information processing. Because the most effective medications for ADHD stimulate the α_2-adrenergic receptors (Shenker, 1992), these findings suggest that pharmacologic treatment may have differential effects on ADHD children with and without comorbid RD.

Finally, it is important to note that children with ADHD (including those without word identification or phonological processing problems) have deficits in rapid automatized naming, particularly naming speed for colors and objects (Carte et al., 1996; Martinussen et al., 1998; Nigg, et al., 1998; Tannock et al., 1996) and may also have deficits in listening comprehension (Milich and Lorch, 1994) and reading comprehension (Brock and Knapp, 1996). The recent evidence that deficits in naming speed are associated with ADHD per se challenge the current tenet that naming speed deficits are specific to RD (e.g., Wolf, 1991).

Stimulant effects on reading and reading disorders in ADHD

Numerous well-controlled medication trials have demonstrated that stimulants produce positive short-term effects on academic productivity (see Carlson and Bunner, 1993; Elia et al., 1993; Swanson et al., 1991 for reviews). In terms of productivity in reading, there is consistent evidence that when receiving stimulant medication, children with ADHD attempt and correctly complete more reading comprehension questions than at baseline or when receiving placebo (e.g., Balthazor et al., 1991; Elia et al., 1993; Forness et al., 1991; Pelham et al., 1985). These beneficial effects appear to be sustained with extended stimulant treatment, although the evidence is less robust than for short-term effects (Famularo and Fenton, 1987; Forness et. al., 1992; Kupietz et al., 1988). Also, the effects apply to long-acting preparations and other stimulants such as pemoline and dextroamphetamine (Elia et al., 1993; Pelham et al., 1990). Moreover, the positive effects of stimulants on the number of comprehension questions attempted and completed correctly have been reported to be comparable in ADHD children with and without comorbid RD, although the comorbid samples have been too small to enable firm conclusions to be drawn (Elia et al., 1993; Forness et al., 1992).

By contrast, there is no evidence that stimulants enhance the speed or accuracy of reading (Ballinger et al., 1984; Forness et al., 1991) or have any direct impact on phonological decoding per se (Balthazor et al., 1991; Richardson et al., 1988). Moreover, the impact of stimulant medication on reading comprehension itself (as opposed to productivity measures) is unclear, primarily because of lack of data: only three studies were identified that assessed reading comprehension directly (Ballinger et al., 1984; Brock and Knapp, 1996; Cherkes-Julkowski et al., 1995). One study suggests that MPH may ameliorate impairments in reading comprehension, but the study was uncontrolled, and the sample comprised children with predominantly inattentive symptoms of ADHD whose phonological processing skills were intact (Brock and Knapp, 1996). Another noted the superior reading comprehension of ADHD children who were receiving medication vs. those who were not receiving medication, but this was not a randomized controlled study, and therefore performance differences could not be attributed unequivocally to the effects of stimulant medication (Cherkes-Julkowski et al., 1995). The third study, which was a randomized, double-blind, placebo-controlled, crossover study of nine boys with ADHD+RD, failed to find any evidence of direct effects of MPH on reading comprehension, although the medication did enhance the children's speed of responding to a letter-matching task and a sentence-verification task (Ballinger et al., 1984).

On the other hand, there is some evidence that stimulant medication may enhance the verbal retrieval mechanisms involved in word recognition (Ballinger et al., 1984; Evans et al., 1986; Peeke et al., 1984; Richardson et al., 1988). Also, several recent controlled studies suggest that MPH may enhance naming speed and accuracy of contingency naming. For example, MPH was found to decrease errors for naming color and shape in verbal fluency and contingency naming tasks but had no impact on rule use in these tasks (Douglas et al., 1995). Also, in a recent study we investigated dose effects of MPH on phonological decoding (word attack skills), phonological awareness (auditory analysis skills), and naming speed (letter, digit, color naming) in 51 children with ADHD. Approximately 50% of the sample met the criteria for some form of comorbid language impairments, and 25% of these children also had RD (Oram et al., 1999). As expected, the group with comorbid language/reading problems was significantly more impaired than the ADHD-only group and a group of normal peers on all these measures. Also, the ADHD-only group was significantly slower in naming speed than was the normal comparison group, even though none of the ADHD group was impaired in reading or in oral language. MPH had no impact on phonological decoding or speed of naming digits or letters, but unexpectedly it did result in faster color naming speed (without any loss in accuracy), irrespective of the presence of concurrent language impairments or reading disorder.

The unexpectedly beneficial and apparently specific effects of MPH on color naming but not on letter or digit naming was replicated in our current study involving 45 children with ADHD (Martinussen et al., 1998). Approximately half of the sample met criteria for the Predominantly Inattentive Subtype, with the remaining children meeting the criteria for Combined Subtype. About one-third of the sample had comorbid RD, equally distributed between the subtypes. Children in both the ADHD and the ADHD+RD groups were significantly slower in naming speed (colors, digits, and letters) compared to normative data (e.g., Denckla and Rudel, 1974; Biddle, 1996). Also, both groups showed stimulant-related improvements in the speed of color naming, but there were no effects on naming digits or letters, or on phonological awareness. We also included a measure of executive function: inhibitory control, using the stop-signal paradigm (Logan 1994). As expected from our previous research (Tannock et al., 1989, 1995), MPH enhanced inhibitory control. There was no evidence that MPH had differential effects on the ADHD subtypes or on children with comorbid RD (Hoosen-Shakeel et al, 1998).

To summarize, the limited data available suggest that stimulant medication enhances academic productivity (completion of more reading comprehension questions) and some aspects of naming speed. By contrast, it does not have any immediate impact on phonological processing, the speed of reading, or reading comprehension per se.

STIMULANT EFFECTS ON AUDITORY PROCESSING AND CENTRAL AUDITORY PROCESSING DISORDER (CAPD) IN ADHD

Central auditory processing disorder in ADHD

Central auditory processing disorder (CAPD) is broadly defined as a deficit in processing audible signals that cannot be attributed to peripheral hearing impairments or intellectual impairments. It may be reflected by deficits in one or more of the following phenomena: sound localization and lateralization, auditory discrimination, auditory pattern recognition, recognition of the temporal aspects of audition, and decrease in auditory performance with competing or degraded acoustic signals (American Speech-Language Hearing Association, 1996). As a result, organizing and processing information presented via the auditory track is problematic, particularly in the presence of high levels of background noise. By contrast, information presented visually may be processed normally.

Children with CAPD are described as poor listeners, with short attention span to auditory information. They have problems following directions, particularly in settings that are noisy or have poor acoustics, and may order words and phrases incorrectly. A history of severe or recurrent otitis media is common among these children. CAPD may also involve poor phonological processing (James et al., 1994), distractibility, and inattention as well as possible difficulties in memory, reading, spelling, and written language (ASHA, 1992).

There is consistent evidence that children with ADHD are impaired in auditory processing, even in the absence of a formal diagnosis of CAPD (Cook et al., 1993; Gascon et al., 1986; Keith et al., 1989; Keith and Engineer, 1991; Ludlow et al., 1983; Pearson et al., 1991; Riccio et al., 1994). Preliminary studies suggest that the rate of comorbidity between ADHD and CAPD ranges from 45% to 75% (Cook et al., 1993; Keith et al., 1989; Riccio et al., 1994). Moreover, a high frequency of language impairments and language-based learning disabilities occur in children with ADHD, CAPD, and CAPD+ADHD, suggesting a common underlying factor (e.g., Gomez and Condon et al., 1999; Keith 1989; Riccio et al., 1994).

Stimulant effects on auditory processing in ADHD

The few studies to address the impact of stimulants on CAPD provide consistent evidence of beneficial effects on performance on measures of auditory vigilance and auditory processing in children with ADHD (Cook et al., 1993; Gascon et al., 1986; Keith and Engineer, 1991). Moreover, stimulant medication also improves the behavioral symptoms of ADHD in children meeting the diagnostic criteria for both ADHD and CAPD (Cook et al., 1993). The sensitivity of both ADHD and CAPD measures to stimulant therapy suggests a close relationship between these two disorders.

DISCUSSION AND IMPLICATIONS

The immediate (and often dramatic) beneficial effects of psychostimulants (particularly MPH) on the core behavioral symptoms of ADHD have been documented in an extensive number of well-controlled short-term trials (see reviews by Gadow, 1986; 1992; Jacobvitz et al., 1990; Rapport and Kelly, 1991; Schachar et al., 1996). Moreover, there is growing evidence that the salutory effects are maintained with longer-term treatment (e.g., Gillberg et al., 1997; Schachar et al., 1997). Also, stimulant medication enhances many aspects of cognitive functioning and improves the productivity (and sometimes accuracy) of academic work (see reviews by Carlson and Thomeer, 1991; Rapport and Kelly, 1991; Solanto, 1991).

By contrast, as evidenced from the preceding review, the effects of stimulant medication on the psychological processes underlying problems in language, reading, and auditory processing have received relatively little attention from researchers and are not well understood. Notwithstanding the dearth of well-controlled studies, the available data reveal limited and highly circumscribed effects, which stand in sharp contrast to the beneficial effects of stimulants on behavior and other aspects of cognitive function. Stimulant medication appears to have little or no impact on the basic systems of language, reading, or reading-related processes per se, but it does improve academic productivity and performance on tests of auditory processing. Moreover, stimulants may enhance some aspects of naming speed and verbal retrieval mechanisms, the use of oral language for self-regulation, and the quality or style of speaking.

How are we to account for the complex interrelationships between problems in language, reading, auditory processing, and ADHD and for the minimal effects of stimulants on language and reading? Previously, I had proposed that deficits in executive function underlie the problems both in pragmatic aspects of language functioning and in behavior regulation associated with ADHD (Tannock and Schachar, 1996). Executive function is a psychologic construct used to describe complex cognitive abilities thought to be mediated by the frontal lobes (e.g., Duncan, 1986; Goldman-Rakic, 1987; Shallice, 1982). These abilities, which guide action by internal representations or mental models, include the ability to prioritize, organize, and strategize, as well as control processes that allow an individual to initiate, sustain, inhibit, and shift thought and action (Duncan, 1986; Goldman-Rakic, 1987). Moreover, I had suggested that treatment of this common factor of executive dysfunction (e.g., with stimulant medication) should produce concomitant effects on pragmatic functioning and behavior (Tannock and Schachar, 1996). The findings from this review generally support that proposition, but they do not account for the minimal effects of stimulants on other aspects of language. Here, I extend my original thesis by invoking Baddeley's tripartite model of working memory (e.g., Baddeley, 1997; Baddeley et al., 1998; Gathercole, 1998) to account for interrelationships between problems in language, reading, auditory processing, and ADHD as well as the minimal effects of stimulants on language and reading abilities.

Working memory: an explanatory model

Working memory refers to the ability to hold in mind and process limited amounts of information. For example, it permits the dynamic on-line holding, processing, and relinquishing of units of information as you read and comprehend this line of text. According to a widely accepted model, working memory comprises three components: the central executive system, the phonological loop, and the visuospatial sketchpad (Baddeley, 1986, 1997). The central executive system performs a range of high-level functions that are not restricted to specific properties of information. These include regulatory and control activities to permit planning and control of action (the coordination of the flow of information through the working memory system, retrieval of information from long-term memory stores), specific strategic and computational processes (retrieval strategies, logical reasoning, mental arithmetic), and both storage and processing functions (Baddeley, 1997; Daneman and Carpenter, 1980; Just and Carpenter, 1992).

By contrast, the phonological loop and the visuospatial sketchpad are specialized for processing and manipulating limited amounts of information within highly specific domains. These "slave systems" are thought to keep the information on-line for subsequent processing by the central executive (Baddeley, 1997). The phonological loop is specialized for the retention of verbal information over short time periods; it comprises a phonological store, which holds information in terms of its sound-based or phonological qualities, and a rehearsal process, which serves to maintain decaying phonological representations in the phonological store. The visuospatial sketchpad is specialized for the retention of spatial and visual properties of limited amounts of information. It comprises a visual store in which the physical characteristics (shape, color) of objects and events can be represented, as well as a spatial mechanism that is used for planning movements.

Converging evidence from cognitive neuroscience supports the tripartite distinction between the three components of working memory. For example, the neural substrate of the phonological loop appears to involve the left-hemisphere regions of Broca's area, the perisylvian region, and the prefrontal cortex. By contrast, the functions of the visuospatial sketchpad appear to be mediated by parietal and prefrontal regions of the right hemisphere (Cohen et al., 1997; Courtney et al., 1998; Smith et al., 1996). The central executive may also be located in prefrontal areas (Cohen et al., 1997; D'Esposito et al., 1995).

An important conceptual advance in this model is the recent proposition that the phonological loop has evolved as a system to support language learning, particularly word acquisition and possibly syntax as well (Baddeley et al., 1998). Based on evidence that identifies direct links between the phonological loop capacity and word learning in normal populations and in a variety of patient populations, Baddeley and colleagues (1998) have proposed that the primary function of the phonological loop is to provide temporary storage of unfamiliar sound patterns while more permanent representations are being constructed.

What I am proposing here is that development of the distributed networks implicated in one or more of these components of the working memory system is highly susceptible to perturbations caused by genetic factors, environmental toxins, stress, perinatal events, etc. (Gallaburda, 1993). Disruptions of the neural networks underlying this working memory system would impair the rapid timing mechanisms involved in the on-line construction and integration of the temporary auditory, visual, and motoric representations. In turn, these temporal disturbances would result in a broad spectrum of cognitive processing deficits that would vary in modality, severity, and specificity, depending on the extent and onset of the disruption or damage and the availability of compensatory mechanisms. For example, disruptions of the phonological loop could result in specific deficits that are restricted primarily to this one system. Impairments may range from isolated phonological errors and limited vocabulary that are resolved by school entry, to more global impairments in phonological processing, receptive and expressive language impairments that manifest as reading and spelling difficulties, and continued language deficits that persist into adolescence and adulthood. This symptom profile might manifest as a severe reading disorder. Disruptions of the central executive might result in deficits in planning, organization, and inhibition, and manifest as ADHD. By contrast, more extensive disruptions, involving both the central executive and the phonological loop, might result in a broad range of deficits in planning, organization, inhibition, phonological processing, naming speed, reading comprehension, spelling, and oral language. This symptom profile might manifest as comorbid ADHD+RD.

This multicomponent model of working memory could also account for the limited effects of stimulant medication on the fundamental systems of language and reading processes, but enhancement of self-regulatory processes and auditory processing. I suggest that the specificity of effects arises because the impact of stimulants is restricted to the neural substrate of the central executive and has no effect on that of the phonological loop. Supportive evidence is provided by recent neuroimaging studies. Specifically, the therapeutic effects of MPH are mediated through its indirect activation of catecholamine receptors (particularly dopamine and norepinephrine) by increasing concentrations of the endogenous agonist in the synaptic cleft (Shenker, 1992). Recent imaging studies indicate that psychostimulants (MPH and dextroamphetamine) activate those neural networks involved in attentional and self-regulatory processing, such as the frontal cortex, subcortical structures, and cerebellum (Ernst et al., 1997; Volkow et al., 1997). Accordingly, stimulants should enhance effortful, controlled processing associated with the central executive, which are precisely the effects described in this review—improvements in the use of oral language for self-regulation and academic productivity. Also, this model might account for the selective impact of MPH on rapid naming of color, which requires semantic processing and selective attention (i.e., controlled, effortful processing), but no impact on naming speed of letters or digits that are processed more automatically (Carte et al., 1996; Wolf, 1991). Moreover, there is preliminary evidence that stimulant medication does not enhance rapid temporal processing, which refers to the ability to process rapid and brief auditory or visual information (Barkley et al., 1997). These findings might account for the lack of stimulant effects on phonological processing (rapid auditory analysis and synthesis of single speech sounds) that is mediated by the phonological loop.

Finally, the findings from a recent imaging study of the effects of stimulant medication (dextroamphetamine) on cerebral glucose metabolism in healthy adults during a continuous visual attention task with random auditory distractors provides an explanation for the beneficial pharmacologic effects on auditory processing (Ernst et al., 1997). The results indicated that normalized regional glucose metabolic rates of the temporal cortex were significantly *decreased* after dextroamphetamine, whereas subcortical, limbic, frontal, and cerebellar rates were increased. That is, activity was *inhibited* in the brain region involved in auditory and language processing. Also, subjects reported that they were able to ignore the auditory distractors more easily after stimulant medication. The pattern of findings suggests that stimulants improve signal-to-noise ratio in processing information. Thus, the subjects could more easily treat the auditory stimuli as background noise after receiving stimulant medication through more effective inhibition of the temporal neural activity subserving auditory processing.

Clinical and research implications

The core problems of ADHD (inattention, impulsivity, overactivity) are complicated with concurrent problems in language, reading, and auditory processing more often than might be expected by chance. But parents and teachers may focus on the more salient disruptive behavioral symptoms of ADHD and overlook the possibility of concurrent language-based problems. Thus, systematic assessment of language and reading should be a routine component of any assessment for ADHD. Because central auditory processing disorder has not yet been validated as a diagnostic entity that is distinct from language-based learning disabilities, routine assessment is not warranted at this time. However, clinicians should be aware that many of the difficulties experienced by children with ADHD could reflect problems with processing the language of instruction at school and the everyday language of social interaction.

The present review indicates that there is insufficient evidence to date that psychopharmacologic treatment of ADHD symptoms has any substantial impact on these additional language-based problems. Moreover, cognitive-behavioral modification techniques that aim to make a child explicitly aware of effective cognitive processes by using strategies such as self-talk and self-monitoring may not be effective for children with concurrent language impairments. Rather, coexisting language impairments require specific intervention using techniques from speech-language pathology. For school-age children, this will necessitate close collaboration between a speech-language pathologist and the classroom teacher. Likewise, reading disorders require specific intervention. Intervention programs that provide intense remedial reading instruction (e.g., 1 hour per day for a total of 35 hours of instruction) that focuses on the core deficits have been demonstrated to be effective in improving reading in children with severe reading disorders (e.g., Lovett et al., 1994). A randomized clinical trial is currently under way to determine the effectiveness of these programs for children with ADHD+RD as well as the need for adjunctive stimulant medication (Tannock, MRC Project Grant MT13366).

The clinician's role is to educate and consult with the parents, the child, and school personnel about the significance and implications of the coexisting language-related problems, and to constitute a collaborative alliance among the parents, the child, professionals within the school system, and community agencies. Also, the clinician should provide or coordinate treatment for the ADHD and any other coexisting psychiatric problems (e.g., anxiety, depression) as well as monitor the overall treatment plan and outcome.

From a research perspective, this review highlights the importance of delineating what underlies the coexisting problems of ADHD, language impairments, reading disorders, and auditory processing problems. Also, further research is needed to understand the impact of stimulant medication and other types of pharmacologic and psychologic (remedial) intervention on these interrelated problems. Future investigations that incorporate imaging techniques along with the behavioral and pharmacologic approaches are required for a better understanding of the brain-behavior relationships.

ACKNOWLEDGMENT

Supported in part by a Medical Research Council of Canada Scientist Salary Award and National Institute of Health project grant (HD31714).

REFERENCES

Adams, M.J. (1990), *Beginning to Read: Thinking and Learning About Print.* Cambridge, MA: MIT Press.

American Academy of Child and Adolescent Psychiatry (1997), Practice parameters for the assessment and treatment of children, adolescents, and adults with attention-deficit/hyperactivity disorder. *J. Am. Acad. Child Adolesc. Psychiatry,* 36(suppl.):85S–121S.

American Psychiatric Association (1987), *Diagnostic and Statistical Manual of Mental Disorders, 3rd ed.-rev. (DSM-III-R).* Washington, DC: American Psychiatric Association.

American Psychiatric Association (1994), *Diagnostic and Statistical Manual of Mental Disorders, 4th ed. (DSM-IV).* Washington, DC: American Psychiatric Association.

American Speech-Language-Hearing Association (1996), Central auditory processing: Current status of research and implications for clinical practice. *Am. J. Audiology,* 5:41–54.

Baddeley, A.D. (1986), *Working Memory.* Oxford: Oxford University Press.

Baddeley, A.D. (1997), *Human Memory: Theory and Practice, 2nd ed.* Boston: Allyn & Bacon.

Baddeley, A.D., Gathercole, S. & Papagano, C. (1998), The phonological loop as a language learning device. *Psychol. Rev.,* 105:158–173.

Badian, N.A. (1993), Phonemic awareness, naming, visual symbol processing, and reading. *Reading Writing,* 5:87–100.

Baker, L. & Cantwell, D.P. (1992), Attention deficit disorder and speech/language disorders. *Comprehensive Mental Health Care,* 2:3–16.

Ballinger, C.T., Varley, C.K. & Nolen, P.A. (1984), Effects of methylphenidate on reading in children with attention deficit disorder. *Am. J. Psychiatry,* 141:1590–1593.

Balthazor, M.J., Wagner, R.K. & Pelham, W.E. (1991), The specificity of effects of stimulant medication on classroom learning-related measures of cognitive processing for attention deficit disorder children. *J. Abnorm. Child Psychology,* 19:35–52.

Barkley, R.A. (1990), *Attention Deficit Hyperactivity Disorder: A Handbook for Diagnosis and Treatment.* New York: Guilford Press.

Barkley, R.A., Cunningham, C. & Karlsson, J. (1983), The speech of hyperactive children with their mothers: Comparisons with normal children and stimulant effects. *J. Learn. Disabil.,* 16:105–110.

Barkley, R.A., DuPaul, G.J. & McMurray, M.B. (1990), A comprehensive evaluation of attention deficit disorder with and without hyperactivity as defined by research criteria. *J. Consult. Clin. Psychol.,* 58:775–789.

Beitchman, J.H., Hood, J., Rochon, J. & Peterson, M. (1989), Empirical classification of speech/language impairment in children: II. Behavioral characteristics. *J. Am. Acad. Child Adolesc. Psychiatry,* 28:118–123.

Beitchman, J.H., Tuckett, M. & Batth, S. (1987), Language delay and hyperactivity in preschoolers: Evidence for a distinct group of hyperactives. *Can. J. Psychiatry,* 32:683–687.

Benedetto-Nasho, E., & Tannock, R. (in press), Math computation performance and error patterns of children with attention deficit hyperactivity disorder. *J Attention Dis.*

Berk, L. & Potts, M. (1991), Development and functional significance of private speech among attention-deficit hyperactivity disordered and normal boys. *J. Abnorm. Child Psychol.,* 19:357–377.

Biddle, K.R. (1996), *The Development of Visual Naming Speed and Verbal Fluency in Average and Impaired Readers: The Implications for Assessment, Intervention, and Theory.* Unpublished doctoral dissertation. Tufts University, Boston, MA.

Biederman, J., Newcorn, J. & Sprich, S. (1991), Comorbidity of attention deficit hyperactivity disorder with conduct, depressive, anxiety and other disorders. *Am. J. Psychiatry,* 148:564–577.

Bishop, D.V.M. (1992), The underlying nature of specific language impairment. *J. Child Psychol. Psychiatry,* 33:1–64.

Bowers, P.G. (1995), Tracing symbol naming speed's unique contributions to reading disabilities over time. *Reading Writing,* 7:189–216.

Bowers, P.G. & Wolf, M. (1993), Theoretical links among naming speed, precise timing mechanisms and orthographic skills in dyslexia. *Reading Writing,* 5, 69–85.

Brock, SE. & Knapp, PK. (1996), Reading comprehension abilities of children with Attention-Deficit/Hyperactivity Disorder. *J. Attention Disorders,* 1:173–185.

Cantwell, D.P. & Baker, L. (1987), Psychiatric symptomatology in language-impaired children: A comparison. *J. Child Neurology,* 2:128–133.

Cantwell, D.P. & Baker, L. (1991), *Psychiatric and Developmental Disorders in Children with Communication Disorder.* Washington DC: American Psychiatric Press.

Carlson, C.L. & Bunner, M.R. (1993), Effects of methylphenidate on the academic performance of children with attention-deficit hyperactivity disorder and learning disabilities. *School Psychol. Rev.,* 22:184–198.

Carlson, C.L. & Thomeer, M.L. (1991), Effects of Ritalin on arithmetic tasks. In: *Ritalin: Theory and Patient Management,* eds., L.L. Greenhill & B.B. Osman. Larchmont, NY: Mary Ann Liebert, Inc., pp. 195–202.

Carte, E.T., Nigg, J.T. & Hinshaw, S.P. (1996), Neuropsychological functioning, motor speed, and language processing in boys with and without ADHD. *J. Abnorm. Child Psychol.,* 24:481–498.

Cherkes-Julkowski, M., Stolzenberg, J., Hatzes, N. & Madaus, J. (1995), Methodological issues in assessing the relationships among ADD, medication effects and reading performance. *J. Learn. Disabil.,* 6:21–30.

Cohen, J.D., Peristein, W.M., Braver, T.S., Nystrom, L.E., Noll, D.C., Jonides, J. & Smith, E.E. (1997), Temporal dynamics of brain activation during a working memory task. *Nature,* 386:604–608.

Cohen, N., Davine, M., Horodezky, N., Lipsett, L. & Isaacson, L. (1993), Unsuspected language impairment in psychiatrically disturbed children: Prevalence and language and behavioral characteristics. *J. Am. Acad. Child Adolesc. Psychiatry,* 32:595–603.

Cook, J.R., Mausbach, T., Burd, L., Gascon, G.G., Slotnick, H.B., Patterson, B., Johnson, R.D., Hankey, B. & Reynolds, B.W. (1993), A preliminary study of the relationship between central auditory processing disorder and attention deficit disorder. *J. Psychiatry Neurosci.,* 18:130–137.

Courtney, S.M., Petit, L., Maisog, J.M., Ungerleider, L.G. & Haxby, J.V. (1998), An area specialized for spatial working memory in human frontal cortex. *Science,* 279:1347–1351.

Creager, P., & Van Riper, C. (1967), The effect of methylphenidate on the verbal productivity of children with cerebral dysfunction. *J. Speech Hearing Res.,* 10:623–628.

Daneman, M. & Carpenter, P.A. (1980), Individual differences in working memory and reading. *J. Verbal Learning Verbal Behav.,* 19:450–466.

Daneman, M. & Merrikle, P.M. (1996), Working memory and language comprehension: A meta-analysis. *Psychonom. Bull. Rev.,* 3:422–433.

Denckla, M. & Rudel, R.G. (1974), Rapid automatized naming of pictured objects, colors, letters and numbers by normal children. *Cortex,* 10:186–202.

Denckla, M. & Rudel, R.G. (1976), Rapid automatized naming (RAN): Dyslexia differentiated from other learning disabilities. *Neuropsychologia,* 14:471–479.

D'Esposito, M., Detre, J.A., Alsop, D.C., Shin, R.K., Atlas, S., & Grossman, M. (1995), The neural basis of the central executive system of working memory. *Nature,* 378: 279–281.

Douglas, V.I., Barr, R.G., Desilets, J. & Sherman, E. (1995), Do high doses of stimulants impair flexible thinking in attention-deficit hyperactivity disorder? *J. Am. Acad. Child Adolesc. Psychiatry,* 34:877–885.

Duncan, J. (1986), Disorganization of behavior after frontal lobe damage. *Cogn. Neuropsychol.,* 3:272–290.

Edelbrock, C., Costello, A.J. & Kessler, M.D. (1984), Empirical corroboration of attention deficit disorder. *J. Am. Acad. Child Adolesc. Psychiatry,* 23:285–290.

Elia, J., Welsh, P.A., Gulotta, C.S. & Rapoport, J.L. (1993), Classroom academic performance: Improvement with both methylphenidate and dextroamphetamine in ADHD boys. *J. Child Psychol. Psychiatry,* 34:785–804.

Ernst, M., Zametkin, A.J., Matochik, J., Schmidt, M., Hons, P.H., Liebenauer, L.L., Hardy, K.K. & Cohen, R.M. (1997), Intravenous dextroamphetamine and brain glucose metabolism. *Neuropsychopharmacology,* 17:391–401.

Evans, R.W., Gualtieri, C.T. & Amara, I. (1986), Methylphenidate and memory: Dissociated effects on hyperactive children. *Psychopharmacology,* 90:211–216.

Famularo, R. & Fenton, T. (1987), The effect of methylphenidate on school grades in children with attention deficit disorder without hyperactivity: A preliminary report. *J. Clin. Psychiatry,* 48:112–114.

Faraone, S.V., Biederman, J., Weber, W. & Russell, R.L. (1998), Psychiatric, neuropsychological and psychosocial features of *DSM-IV* subtypes of Attention-Deficit/Hyperactivity Disorder: Results from a clinically-referred sample. *J. Am. Acad. Child Adolesc. Psychiatry,* 37:185–193.

Felton, R.H. & Brown, I.S. (1990), Phonological processes as predictors of specific reading skills in children at risk for reading failure. *Reading Writing,* 2:39–59.

Felton, R.H., Wood, F.B., Brown, I.S., Campbell, S.K. & Harter, M.R. (1987), Separate verbal memory and naming deficits in attention deficit disorder and reading disability. *Brain Language,* 31:171–184.

Forness, S.R., Cantwell, D.P., Swanson, J.M., Hanna, G.L. & Youpa, D. (1991), Differential effects of stimulant medication on reading performance of hyperactive boys with and without conduct disorder. *J. Learn. Disabil.,* 24:304–310.

Forness, S.R., Swanson, J.M., Cantwell, D.P., Youpa, D. & Hanna, G.L. (1992), Stimulant medication and reading performance: Follow-up on sustained dose in ADHD boys with and without conduct disorders. *J. Learn. Disabil.,* 25:115–123.

Gadow, K. (1986), *Children on Medication, vol. I: Hyperactivity, Learning Disabilities, and Mental Retardation.* San Diego, CA, College-Hill Press.

Gadow, K. (1992), Pediatric psychopharmacology: A review of recent research. *J. Child Psychol. Psychiatry,* 33:153–195.

Gallaburda, A.M. (1993), Neuroanatomical basis of developmental dyslexia. *Behav. Neurol.,* 11:161–173.

Gascon, G.G., Johnson, R., & Burd, L. (1986), Central auditory processing and attention deficit disorders. *J. Child Neurol.,* 1:27–33.

Gathercole, S.E. (1998), The development of memory. *J. Child Psychol. Psychiatry,* 39:3–27.

Gillberg, C., Melander, H., von Knorring, A., Janols, L., Thernlund, G., Häglöff, B., Eidevall-Wallin, L., Gustafsson, P. & Kopp, S. (1997), Long-term stimulant treatment of children with attention-deficit hyperactivity disorder symptoms. *Arch. Gen. Psychiatry,* 54:857–864.

Goldman-Rakic, P.S. (1987), Development of cortical circuitry and cognitive function. *Child Dev.,* 58:601–622.

Gomez, R. & Condon, M. (1999), Central auditory ability in children with ADHD with and without learning disabilities. *J. Learning Disabil.,* 32:150–158.

Halperin, J.M., Newcorn, J.H., Koda, V.H., Pick, L., McKay, K.E. & Knott, P. (1997), Noradrenergic mechanisms in ADHD children with and without reading disabilities: A replication and extension. *J. Am. Acad. Child Adolesc. Psychiatry,* 36:1688–1697.

Halperin, J.M., Newcorn, J.H., Schwartz, S.T., McKay, K.E., Bedi, G. & Sharma, V. (1993), Plasma catecholamine metabolite levels in ADHD boys with and without reading disabilities. *J. Clin. Child Psychol.,* 22:219–225.

Hamlett, K.W., Pellegrini, D.S. & Connors, C.K. (1987), An investigation of executive processes in the problem solving of attention deficit disorder-hyperactive children. *J. Pediatr. Psychol.,* 12:227–240.

Hoosen-Shakeel, S., Ickowicz, A., Schachar, R. & Tannock, R. (1998), *The Effects of Methylphenidate on Children with Attention-Deficit/Hyperactivity Disorder.* Presented at the 24th Annual Harvey Stancer Research Day, University of Toronto, Department of Psychiatry, June 18.

Humphries, T., Koltun, H., Malone, M. & Roberts W. (1994), Teacher-identified oral language difficulties among boys with attention problems. *Dev. Behav. Pediatr.,* 15:92–98.

Hynd, G.W., Lorys, A.R., Semrud-Clikeman, M., Nieves, N., Huettner, M.I.S. & Lahey, B.J. (1991), Attention deficit disorder without hyperactivity: A distinct behavioral and neurocognitive syndrome. *J. Child Neurol.,* 6(Suppl):S37–S43.

Jacobvitz, D., Sroufe, L.A., Stewart, M. & Leffer, N. (1990), Treatment of attentional and hyperactivity problems in children with sympathomimetic drugs: A comprehensive review. *J. Am. Acad. Child Adolesc. Psychiatry,* 29:677–688.

James, D., van Steenbrugge, W. & Chiveralls, K. (1994), Underlying deficits in language-disordered children with central auditory processing difficulties. *Appl. Psycholinguistics,* 15:311–328.

Just, M.A. & Carpenter, P.A. (1992), A capacity theory of comprehension: Individual differences in working memory. *Psychol. Rev.,* 99:122–149.

Keith, R.W. & Engineer, P. (1991), Effects of methylphenidate on the auditory processing abilities of children with attention deficit-hyperactivity disorder. *J. Learning Disabil.,* 24:630–636.

Keith, R.W., Rudy, J., Donahue, P.A., & Katbamna, B. (1989), Comparison of SCAN results with other auditory and language measures in a clinical population. *Ear Hear.,* 10:383–386.

Kinsbourne, M. (1991), Overfocusing: An apparent subtype of attention deficit-hyperactivity disorder. In: *Pediatric Neurology: Behavior and Cognition of the Child with Brain Dysfunction,* eds., N. Amir, I. Rapin, D. Branski. Basel: S. Karger, pp. 18–35.

Korkman, M. & Pesonen, A.E. (1994), A comparison of neuropsychological test profiles of children with attention-deficit hyperactivity disorder and/or learning disorder. *J. Learning Disabil.,* 27:383–392.

Kupietz, S.S., Winsberg, B.G., Richardson, E., Maitinsky, S. & Mendell, N. (1988), Effects of methylphenidate dosage in hyperactive reading-disabled children: I. Behavior and cognitive performance effects. *J. Am. Acad. Child Adolesc. Psychiatry,* 27:70–77.

Landau, S. & Milich, R. (1988), Social communication patterns of attention-deficit-disordered boys. *J. Abnorm. Child Psychol.,* 16:69–81.

Logan, G.D. (1994), On the ability to inhibit thought and action: A user's guide to the stop signal paradigm. In: *Inhibitory Processes in Attention, Memory, and Language,* eds., D. Dagenbach, T.H. Carr. San Diego: Academic Press.

Lovett, M.W. (1992), Developmental dyslexia. In: *Handbook of Neuropsychology, vol 7: Child Neuropsychology,* eds., S.J. Segalowitz, & Rapin, I., F. Boller, J. Grafman. Amsterdam: Elsevier Science Publishers, pp 163–185.

Lovett, M.W., Borden, S.L., DeLuca, T., et al. (1994), Treating the core deficits of developmental dyslexia: Evidence of transfer-of-learning following strategy- and phonologically based reading training programs. *Dev. Psychol.,* 30:805–822.

Ludlow, C.L., Cudahy, E.A., Bassich, C., & Brown, G.L. (1983), Auditory processing skills of hyperactive, language impaired and reading disabled boys. In: *Central Auditory Processing Disorders: Problems of Speech, Language, and Learning,* eds., E.Z. Lasky, J. Katz. Baltimore: University Park Press, pp. 163–184.

Ludlow, C.L., Rapoport, J.L., Bassich, C.J., & Mikkelsen, E.G. (1978), Differential effects of dextroamphetamine on language performance in hyperactive and normal boys. In: *Treatment of Hyperactive and Learning Disordered Children,* eds., R.M. Knights, D.J. Bakker. Baltimore: University Park Press, pp. 185–205.

Marshall, R.M., Hynd, G.W., Handwerk, M.J. & Hall, J. (1997), Academic underachievement in ADHD subtypes. *J. Learning Disabil.,* 30:635–642.

Martinussen, R., Frijters, J., & Tannock, R. (1998), Naming speed and stimulant effects in ADHD. Presented at the annual meeting of the American Academy of Child and Adolescent Psychiatry, Anaheim, California, Oct. 27–Nov. 1.

Mefford, I.N. & Potter, W.A. (1989), A neuroanatomical and biochemical basis of attention deficit disorder with hyperactivity in children: A defect in tonic adrenaline mediated inhibition of locus coeruleus stimulation. *Med. Hypoth.,* 29:33–42.

Meyer, M.S., Wood, F.B., Hart, LA. & Felton, R.H. (1998), Selective predictive value of rapid automatized naming in poor readers. *J. Learning Disabil.,* 31:106–117.

McGee, R., Partridge, F., Williams, S., & Silva, P.A. (1991), A twelve year follow-up of preschool hyperactive children. *J. Am. Acad. Child Adolesc. Psychiatry,* 30:224–232.

Milich, R. & Lorch, E.P. (1994), Television viewing methodology to understand cognitive processing in ADHD children. *Adv. Clin. Child Psychol.,* 16:177–201.

Morgan, A.E., Hynd, G.W., Riccio, C.A., & Hall, J. (1996), Validity of *DSM-IV* ADHD predominantly inattentive and combined types: Relationship to previous *DSM* diagnoses/subtype differences *J. Am. Acad. Child Adolesc. Psychiatry,* 35:325–333.

Närhi, V. & Ahonen, T. (1995), Reading disability with or without attention deficit hyperactivity disorder: Do attentional problems make a difference? *Dev. Neuropsychol.,* 11:337–349.

Nigg, J.T., Hinshaw, S.P., Carte, E.T. & Treuting, J.J. (1998), Neuropsychological correlates of childhood attention deficit hyperactivity disorder: Explainable by comorbid disruptive behavior or reading problems? *J. Abnorm. Psychol.,* 107:468–480.

Oram, J., Fine, J., Okamoto, C. & Tannock, R. (1999), Assessing the language of children with Attention Deficit Hyperactivity Disorder. *Am. J. Speech-Language Dis.,* 8:72–80.

Paternite, C.E., Loney, J. & Roberts, M.A. (1996), A preliminary validation of subtypes of *DSM-IV* attention-deficit/hyperactivity disorder. *J. Attention Dis.,* 1:70–86.

Pearson, D.A., Lane, D.M. & Swanson, J.M. (1991), Auditory attention switching in hyperactive children. *J. Abnorm. Child Psychol.,* 19:479–492.

Peeke, S., Halliday, R., Callaway, E., Prael, R. & Reus, V. (1984), Effects of two doses of methylphenidate on verbal information processing in hyperactive children. *J. Clin. Psychopharmacol.,* 4:82–88.

Pelham, W.E., Bender, M.E., Caddell, J., Booth, S. & Moorer, S. (1985), The dose-response effects of methylphenidate on classroom academic and social behavior in children with attention deficit disorder. *Arch. Gen. Psychiatry,* 42:948–952.

Pelham, W.E., Greenslade, K.E., Vodde-Hamilton, M.A., Murphy, D.A., Greenstein, J.J., Gnagy, E.M. & Dahl, R.E. (1990), Relative efficacy of long-acting CNS stimulants on children with attention deficit-hyperactivity disorder: A comparison of standard methylphenidate, sustained-release methylphenidate, sustained-release dextroamphetamine, and pemoline. *Pediatrics,* 86:226–237.

Pennington, B.F., Groisser, D. & Welsh, M.C. (1993), Contrasting cognitive deficits in attention deficit hyperactivity disorder versus reading disability. *Devel. Psychol.,* 29:511–523.

Pliszka, S.R., McCracken, J.T. & Maas, J.W. (1996), Catecholamines in Attention-Deficit Hyperactivity Disorder: Current perspectives. *J. Am. Acad. Child Adolesc. Psychiatry,* 34:264–272.

Purvis, K. & Tannock, R. (1997), Language abilities in children with attention deficit hyperactivity disorder, reading disabilities, and normal controls. *J. Abnorm. Child Psychol.,* 25:133–144.

Rapport, M.D. & Kelly, K.L. (1991), Psychostimulant effects on learning and cognitive function: Findings and implications for children with attention deficit hyperactivity disorder. *Clin. Psychol. Rev.,* 11:61–92.

Reader, M.J., Harris, E.L., Schuerholz, L.J. & Denckla, M.B. (1994), Attention deficit hyperactivity disorder and executive dysfunction. *Dev. Neuropsychol.,* 10:493–512.

Riccio, C.A., Hynd, G.W., Cohen, M.J., Hall, J. & Molt, L. (1994), Comorbidity of central auditory processing disorder and attention-deficit hyperactivity disorder. *J. Am. Acad. Child Adolesc. Psychiatry,* 33:849–857.

Richardson, E., Kupietz, S.S., Winsberg, B.G., Maitinsky, S. & Mendell, N. (1988), Effects of methylphenidate dosage in hyperactive reading-disabled children: II. Reading achievement. *J. Am. Acad. Child Adolesc. Psychiatry,* 27:78–87.

Robbins, T. & Sahakian, B. (1979), Paradoxical effects of psychomotor stimulant drugs in hyperactive children from the standpoint of behavioral pharmacology. *Neuropharmacology,* 18:931–950.

Robbins, T., Sahakian, B., & Logan, G. (1995), Methylphenidate and cognitive flexibility: Dissociated dose effects in hyperactive children. *J. Abnorm. Child Psychol.,* 23:235–266.

Safer, D.J., Zito, J.M. & Fine, E.M. (1996), Increased methylphenidate usage for attention deficit disorder in the 1990s. *Pediatrics,* 98:1084–1088.

Schachar, R., Tannock, R. & Cunningham, C. (1996), Treatment of hyperactive disorders.

In: *Hyperactive Disorders,* ed., S. Sandberg. (Cambridge Monographs in Child and Adolescent Psychopathology), pp. 433–476.

Schachar, R., Tannock, R., Cunningham, C., & Corkum, P.V. (1997), Behavioral, situational, and temporal effects of treatment of ADHD with methylphenidate. *J. Am. Acad. Child Adolesc. Psychiatry,*

Semrud-Clikeman, M., Sprich-Buckminster, S., Krifcher, Lehman, B., Faraone, S.V. & Norman, D. (1992), Comorbidity between ADDH and learning disability: A review and report in a clinically referred sample. *J. Am. Acad. Child Adolesc. Psychiatry,* 31:439–448.

Shallice, T. (1982). Specific impairments in planning. *R. Soc. London,* B298:199–209.

Shaywitz, S.E., Escobar, M.D., Shaywitz, B.A., Fletcher, J.M. & Makuch, R. (1992), Evidence that dyslexia may represent the lower tail of a normal distribution of reading ability. *N. Engl. J. Med.,* 326:145–150.

Shaywitz, S.E., Fletcher, J.M. & Shaywitz, B.A. (1996), A conceptual model and definition of dyslexia: Findings emerging from the Connecticut Longitudinal Study. In: *Language, Learning, and Behavior Disorders: Developmental, Biological, and Clinical perspectives,* eds., J.H. Beitchman, N. Cohen, M.M. Konstantareas, R. Tannock. New York: Cambridge University Press, pp. 199–223.

Shenker, A. (1992), The mechanism of action of drugs used to treat attention-deficit hyperactivity disorder: Focus on catecholamine receptor pharmacology. *Adv. Pediatr.,* 39:337–382.

Smith, E.E., Jonides, J. & Koeppe, R.A. (1996), Dissociating verbal and spatial memory using PET. *Cerebral Cortex,* 6:11–20.

Solanto, M.V. (1984), Neuropharmacological basis of stimulant drug action in attention deficit disorder with hyperactivity: A review and synthesis. *Psychol. Bull.* 95:387–409.

Solanto, M.V. (1991), Dosage effects of Ritalin on cognition. In: *Ritalin: Theory and Patient Management,* eds. L.L. Greenhill & B.B. Osman. Larchmont, NY: Mary Ann Liebert, Inc., pp. 233–246.

Swanson, J.M., Cantwell, D., Lerner, M., McBurnett, K. & Hanna G. (1991), Effects of stimulant medication on learning in children with ADHD. *J. Learning Disabil.,* 24:219–230.

Tannock, R. Medical Research Council of Canada, Project Grant MT13366.

Tannock, R. (1997), ADHD: The challenge of characterizing everyday use of language. *Plenary address, International Systemic Functional Linguistics Congress,* July 23, Toronto, Canada.

Tannock, R., Fine, J., Heintz, T. & Schachar, R. (1995), A linguistic approach detects stimulant effects in two children with attention deficit hyperactivity disorder. *J. Child Adolesc. Psychopharmacol.,* 5:177–189.

Tannock, R., Fine, J.F., Oram, J. & Peets, K. (1999) Stimulant effects on oral language abilities in children with ADHD.

Tannock, R., Oram, J., Ickowicz, A. & Fine, J. (1996), *Language Skills of Children with Attention Deficit Hyperactivity Disorder: Proceedings of the 43rd Annual Meeting of the American Academy of Child and Adolescent Psychiatry,* Philadelphia, October 22–27.

Tannock, R., Purvis, K. & Schachar, R. (1993), Narrative abilities in children with attention deficit hyperactivity disorder and normal peers. *J. Abnorm. Child Psychol.,* 21:103–117.

Tannock, R., & Schachar, R. (1996), Executive dysfunction as an underlying mechanism of behavior and language problems in attention deficit hyperactivity disorder. In: *Language, Learning, and Behavior Disorders: Developmental, Biological, and Clinical Per-*

spectives, eds., J.H. Beitchman, N. Cohen, M.M. Konstantareas, R. Tannock. New York: Cambridge University Press, pp. 128–155.

Tannock, R., Schachar, R., Carr, R., Chajczyk, D. & Logan, G. (1989), Effects of methylphenidate on inhibitory control in hyperactive children. *J. Abnorm. Child Psychol.,* 17:473–491.

Tucker, D.M. & Derryberry, D. (1990), Motivated attention: Anxiety and the frontal executive functions. *Neuropsychiatry Neuropsychol. Behav. Neurol.,* 5:233–252.

Vandervelden, M.C. & Siegel, L.S. (1996), Phonological recording deficits and dyslexia: A developmental perspective. In: *Language, Learning, and Behavior Disorders: Developmental, Biological, and Clinical Perspectives,* eds., J.H. Beitchman, N. Cohen, M.M. Konstantareas, R. Tannock. New York: Cambridge University Press, pp. 224–226.

Vellutino, F.R., Scanlon, D.M. & Tanzman, M.S. (1993), Components of reading ability: Issues and problems operationalizing word identification, phonological coding, and orthographic coding. In: *Frames of Reference for the Assessment of Learning Disability: New Views on Measurement Issues,* ed., G.R. Lyon. Baltimore: Brookes Publishing, pp. 243–332.

Volkow, N.D., Wang, G.J., Fowler, J.S., Logan, J., Angrist, B., Hitzemann, R., Lieberman, J. & Pappas, N. (1997), Effects of methylphenidate on regional brain glucose metabolism in humans: Relationship to dopamine D2 receptors. *Am. J. Psychiatry,* 154:50–55.

Wagner, R.K. & Torgeson, J.K. (1987), The nature of phonological processing and its causal role in the acquisition of reading skills. *Psychol. Bull.,* 101:192–212.

Wagner, R.K., Torgeson, J.K., Rashotte, C.A. (1994), Development of reading-related phonological processing abilities: New evidence of bidirectional causality from a latent variable longitudinal study. *Dev. Psychol.,* 30:73–87.

Whalen, C.K., Henker, B., Collins, B.E., McAuliffe, S. & Vaux, A. (1979), Peer interaction in a structured communication task: Comparisons of normal and hyperactive boys and of methylphenidate (Ritalin) and placebo effects. *Child Dev.,* 50:388–401.

Wolf, M. (1991), Naming speed and reading: The contribution of the cognitive neurosciences. *Reading Res. Q.,* 26:123–140.

Wolf, M. (1997), A provisional, integrative account of phonological and naming deficits in dyslexia: Implications for diagnosis and intervention. In: *Cognitive and Linguistic Foundations of Reading Acquisition: Implications for Intervention Research,* ed., B. Blachman. Hillsdale, NY: Erlbaum, pp. 67–92.

Wolraich, M.L., Lindgren, S., Stromquist, A., Milich, R., Davis, C. & Watson, D. (1990), Stimulant medication use by primary care physicians in the treatment of attention deficit hyperactivity disorder. *Pediatrics,* 86:95–101.

Zentall, S.S. (1988), Production deficiencies in elicited language but not in the spontaneous verbalizations of hyperactive children. *J. Abnorm. Child Psychol.,* 16:657–673.

Zentall, S.S., Gohs, D.E. & Culatta, B. (1983), Language and activity of hyperactive and comparison children during listening tasks. *Exceptional Children,* 50:255–266.

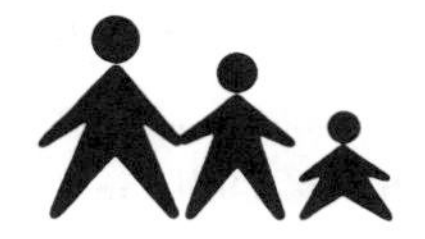

Attention Deficit Hyperactivity Disorder and Ritalin Side Effects: Is Sleep Delayed, Disrupted, or Disturbed?

MARK A. STEIN and MARYLAND PAO

Stimulants such as caffeine, dextroamphetamine, and Ritalin (methylphenidate, MPH) have been known to increase arousal and to interfere with sleep (Rechtschaffen and Maron, 1964). Despite a voluminous literature on the cognitive and behavioral effects of stimulants, as well as the widespread and increasing use of Ritalin to treat symptoms of ADHD (Safer et al., 1996), only a handful of pharmacologic studies have examined sleep in children with ADHD. Nonetheless, it is often assumed by parents of ADHD children as well as clinicians that sleep problems are more prevalent in children with ADHD than in children without ADHD. However, it is unclear whether parent reports of sleep problems are specific to ADHD, because parents of children with a range of psychologic and developmental problems report increased sleep problems relative to normal children (Stein et al., 1994; Obermeyer et al., 1999). This review attempts to answer whether Ritalin contributes or causes delayed (i.e., insomnia), disrupted (i.e., frequent waking), or disturbed (e.g. nightmares, parasomnias) sleep. Before a discussion of the implications of these sleep studies, several issues related to the study of sleep will be highlighted.

First, it should be noted that sleep and sleep disturbances are defined in numerous and sometimes contradictory ways. The task is further complicated by wide intraindividual variability in sleep measures. It is important to distinguish subjective general complaints and perceptions of sleep difficulties from more objective measures of specific types of sleep disturbance. To what extent parents' reports of the child's sleep problems are valid and not primarily the result of inaccurate perception or rater bias, remains an empirical question. Rater bias is a particular concern with ADHD, because maternal depression has been associated with increased perceptions of childhood sleep disturbance (Lozoff et al., 1985; Stoleru et al., 1997) and depressive symptoms are relatively common in the parents of children with ADHD (Roizen et al., 1996).

A second issue that must be considered before medication effects are evaluated is the high base rate of sleep problems in ADHD. Otherwise, base rate differences may be erroneously attributed to treatment. Parent surveys of hyperactive and inattentive children indicate that as many as 56% of hyperactive children are reported by their parents to have difficulties with falling asleep (Ball et al., 1997). Additionally, frequent waking has been reported in as many as 39% of children with ADHD (Kaplan et al., 1987; Trommer et al., 1988). As a result, it is crucial for any study of stimulant side effects to measure sleep problems at baseline and highly desirable to have a second baseline or placebo phase.

A third issue is the variability that appears to characterize individual sensitivity to stimulants. As anyone serving coffee after a late dinner knows, some individuals report severe insomnia following stimulants and need to restrict caffeine, whereas others report no sleep

Center for Neuroscience and Behavioral Medicine, Children's National Medical Center, Washington, D.C.

difficulties whatsoever and order double espressos. In an early study with a more potent stimulant, dextroamphetamine (Dexedrine), administered before bedtime, two of 10 college students were unable to fall asleep after 90 minutes. However, the other subjects had no obvious difficulty falling asleep but displayed less rapid eye movement (REM) sleep (Rechtschaffen and Maron, 1964). The focus of this chapter is whether similar effects occur with a different stimulant, Ritalin, and more specifically in a clinical population of children with ADHD. In an evaluation of the effects of Ritalin on sleep, both grouped data and individual data are helpful, as grouped data may obscure meaningful individual differences.

This review focuses on controlled studies of Ritalin on sleep in children with ADHD. More recent studies using post–*Diagnostic and Statistical Manual of Mental Disorders (DSM), 3rd ed.* diagnostic criteria for ADHD are referenced. Several illustrative case studies are provided, along with recommendations for future research and clinical practice.

RITALIN AND PERCEPTIONS OF SLEEP EFFECTS

One of the most commonly reported side effects of Ritalin is insomnia (Barkley et al., 1990; Ahmann et al., 1993). Insomnia or delayed sleep can be defined in different ways, depending on how the temporal endpoints of going to sleep and falling asleep are measured (Rechtschaffen, 1994). For example, the child's and the parents' perceptions of sleep onset may differ from each other and from polysomnographic evidence of sleep as defined by electroencephalogram, electromyogram, and electro-oculogram activity. The point at which delayed or lengthy sleep onset latency (i.e., the time it takes for sleep to occur) becomes insomnia varies considerably with age, from person to person, and from night to night.

Insomnia in children may be very different from insomnia in adults. In contrast to adult insomnia, insomnia in children may be the result of both temperamental factors and poor limit setting and is often described as the caretaker's complaint rather than the child's (Ferber, 1995; Horne, 1991). Although clinical experience with children with ADHD suggests that many children with ADHD appear tired and frequently report difficulty falling asleep, no studies were found that surveyed sleep from the child's perspective.

Four recent studies of stimulant side effects reported few differences in parental perception of sleep problem between children receiving 0.3 and 0.5 mg/kg/dose of Ritalin twice daily (Barkley et al., 1990), three times daily (Ahmann et al., 1993; Stein et al., 1996; Kent et al., 1995), or between low-dose Ritalin compared with Dexedrine (Efron et al., 1997). These studies all utilized the Stimulant Side Effects Rating Scale (SSRS) (Barkley et al., 1990), a relatively objective parent rating scale developed by Barkley to measure the side effects of stimulant medication. On the SSRS, each item is rated on a 10-point scale from "absent" to "serious." The rates of insomnia and other sleep-related behaviors from these studies are described in Table 1. These studies suggest the following:

1. Using a standardized parent-rating scale of stimulant side effects, parents of children with ADHD report a high prevalence of insomnia or trouble sleeping (range 25% to 54%) at baseline. This does not appear to be an artifact of the SSRS, because similar rates were obtained using other measures. For example, in the study by Ball et al. (1997), sleep problems ranged from 32.9% for the clinic control subjects to 64.2% for the ADHD group being treated with stimulant medication, using the item "problems with sleep" from the Conners Parent Scale to measure sleep problems.
2. There appears to be a negative halo effect with the SSRS in that parents of children with ADHD generally report more behavior problems at baseline than during stimulant treatment.
3. Despite the high prevalence of parental perceptions of insomnia, in >90% of cases, the

TABLE 1. PARENT PERCEPTIONS OF SLEEP PROBLEMS

Reference	*Subjects (n)*	*Baseline (%)*	*Placebo (%)*	*0.3 mg/kg (%)*	*0.5 mg/kg (%)*	*4 P.M. (%)*	*Comment*
Barkley et al., 1990	83						
Drowsiness			18	23	20		
Nightmares			20	20	21		
Insomnia			40	62	68		Severity of side effects mild in most; worse during placebo
Ahmann et al., 1990	234						
Insomnia		38	36.7	58.8	53.2		No difference between low and moderate dose
Stein et al., 1996	25						
Drowsiness		24	17	21		20	
Nightmares		20	17	21		20	
Insomnia		44	50	61		60	No difference between b.i.d. and t.i.d. dosing
Efron et al., 1997							
Drowsiness		25		18			
Nightmares		39		21			
Insomnia	125	54		64			Trouble sleeping increased with stimulants

b.i.d. = twice a day; t.i.d. = three times a day.

insomnia was reported as mild and did not result in termination from the trial. One caveat, however, is that all but one study were short-term studies lasting only several weeks. A second caveat is that the dosage ranges were generally low to moderate (<0.5 mg/kg/dose). Because children are being treated with a wide range of dosages for increasingly long periods of time (e.g., 0.3–1 mg/kg/dose), research is needed that more closely parallels clinical practice.

4. Within the low-to-moderate dosage range examined in the above studies, there do not appear to be significant dose-response relationships. Because of small sample sizes and limited statistical power in studies conducted to date, one cannot rule out mild or more subtle effects that may be dose-related.
5. Nightmares or drowsiness do not appear to be related to, or exacerbated by, short-term, low-to-moderate doses of Ritalin.
6. Contrary to the general perception, taking medication at 4 P.M. does not appear to be associated with more insomnia than taking the medication at noon, based on grouped data. However, there are some individuals who sleep much better when taking a 4 P.M. dose.

RITALIN AND OBJECTIVE MEASURES OF SLEEP

As mentioned previously, parent ratings of sleep problems may not correlate with objective measures of sleep. Several earlier studies with hyperactive children (pre-*DSM-III*) evaluated the effects of MPH on the stages of sleep of hyperactive children using polysomnographic measures. Studies conducted in the sleep laboratory have the advantage of objectively defined sleep stages. In a study of six hyperactive boys, Haig reported that the latency to falling asleep was 18.5 minutes with stimulant medication vs. 8.2 minutes for the nonmedicated, normal control subjects (Haig, 1974). However, the nonmedicated hyperactive group took almost as long to fall asleep: 16.7 minutes. The other significant finding was the latency to first REM period, which was slightly longer with medication (174 minutes) vs. without medication (167 minutes) and still longer relative to the normal control subjects (131 minutes). Dosages and dosing patterns were not controlled, however, as a third of the subjects received only a morning dose. The investigators concluded that "the use of methylphenidate affects the sleep of hyperactive children very little, even with large doses and with administration close to bedtime" (p. 187).

Nahas and Krynicki (1977) came to a similar conclusion after studying the sleep of four child psychiatry inpatients administered 10 mg of Ritalin twice daily. These investigators also found relatively little effect of Ritalin on sleep patterns in the hyperactive group. Interpretation of the above studies should be limited by nonstandardized diagnostic procedures, the small sample sizes, the limited statistical power necessary to detect subtle effects, and the brief time interval studied.

More recent studies of sleep have used *DSM-III-R* or *DSM-IV* criteria for ADHD. In one of the few polysomnographic studies of sleep in children with ADHD, Greenhill et al. (1983) studied nine children with ADHD and 11 control subjects. Few differences were found between 9 ADHD children and 11 control subjects in sleep architecture. Seven children who received MPH twice daily displayed delayed sleep onset, lengthened sleep, and changes in REM sleep variables. This study was noteworthy for using research diagnostic criteria, extensive measurement of sleep architecture, and medication procedures that closely parallel common clinical practices. In this study, prepubertal children were evaluated after 6 months of continuous treatment with moderate dosages that are consistent with clinical practice (mean 0.99 mg/kg/day) administered in the morning and at noon. Mean sleep latency was 39.9 minutes with medication. This was, on average, 10–12 minutes longer than when the same child received no medication or than the sleep latencies reported for the normal control subjects. Of interest, the variability in sleep latency almost doubled during Ritalin administration, increasing from a standard deviation of 0.13 without the drug to 25.5 during Ritalin use. Although the authors conclude that Ritalin does not affect sleep patterns adversely, this conclusion should be tempered by the early, single-dose administration of the drug, which is discrepant from typical clinical practice.

A recent placebo-controlled study found longer sleep duration during baseline and placebo for 10 children with ADHD treated with MPH, as assessed with a wrist actometer, the actigraph (Tirosh et al., 1993). Previously, the actigraph has demonstrated the ability to discriminate between sleep and wake states, has been validated against polysomnography with an agreement rate >90% (Sadeh et al., 1994), and has demonstrated sensitivity to treatment effects in studies of insomnia (Brooks et al., 1993). Although Tirosh, et al. concluded that Ritalin did not affect sleep patterns adversely, this conclusion should again be tempered by the early, single-dose administration of the drug, which is discrepant from typical practice. In addition, for most of the medication period, each child received his or her only dose at 7:30 A.M.

Several studies examine the timing of stimulant dosing and, in particular, the relative benefits of giving a third late-afternoon dose. Kent et al. (1995) examined the effects of a

4 P.M. dose in 12 child psychiatric inpatients and found substantial behavioral improvement in those given the 4 P.M. dose. Average sleep latency determined from a nursing log was 47 minutes for those receiving a placebo, 50 minutes for those who received 10 mg, and 51 minutes for those who received 15 mg. Of interest, the standard deviation for the 15-mg condition was 18.2, relative to 12.6 and 12.1 for the low-dose and placebo conditions, respectively, suggesting increased variability in sleep latency in the high-dose group receiving 15 mg. An additional finding was that the low-dose group was rated as having more adequate sleep than both the group receiving placebo and the group on high dose. Sleep adequacy was defined on the basis of ease of arising and lack of tiredness during the day. The suggestion of a nonlinear dose-response curve for sleep adequacy is intriguing and requires replication.

Using similar dosages, Stein et al. (1996) compared twice-daily administration (8 A.M. and 12 P.M.) with thrice-daily (an additional 4 P.M. dose) dosing in 25 boys with ADHD. On average, children were reported by their parents to sleep 24 minutes less per night on the thrice-daily schedule (M = 9.4 hours) than with placebo (M = 9.8 hours). Trends for shorter sleep duration were found on the thrice-daily dose relative to baseline, and on titration relative to baseline and placebo. Similarly, assessment of sleep estimated from the actigraph revealed a trend toward a dosing schedule effect for total sleep, reflecting a 42-minute difference between placebo (M = 9.4) and thrice-daily dosing (M = 8.7). When given placebo, children fell asleep, on average, 33 minutes faster than with twice-daily dosing and 25 minutes faster than with thrice-daily dosing. Average sleep duration, as assessed with the actigraph, was 18 minutes shorter in the thrice-daily condition than in the twice-daily condition (not significant). Thus, both parent and actigraphic assessment indicated decreased sleep duration associated with Ritalin treatment, but no difference between twice-daily and thrice-daily dosing schedules. Consistent with the findings of Tirosh, et al. (1993), children taking stimulant medication took much longer to fall asleep than those receiving placebo or those at baseline. Parents reported that children in the thrice-daily condition took longer to fall asleep than children receiving placebo, but the more objective actigraphic recording of sleep did not reveal significant group differences. This discrepancy between parent ratings and more objective measures of sleep and behavior is not unique to Ritalin; It has also been observed in studies of theophylline, which is biochemically related to caffeine (Avital et al., 1991).

CASE REPORTS

Reporting percentages of adverse responders and inspection of individual cases can provide additional information on the relationship between stimulant effects and sleep. Moreover, the high standard deviations of medication effects in several studies suggests that there is a great deal of variability in response. Three cases are presented below that highlight individual differences in stimulant response and the value of a multimodal assessment of sleep as a component of a broader medication evaluation.

Case 1: Jeremy

Jeremy was an 8-year-old boy referred to the study by Children and Adults with Attention Deficit Disorders (CHADD), a support group for families of people with ADHD. Jeremy had a long-standing history of problems with inattention, fighting with peers, and oppositional behavior. He also had several motor tics, including eye blinking and shoulder shrugging, which had begun during the previous year. His pediatrician had prescribed Ritalin, 10 mg twice daily for 2 weeks, several weeks before Jeremy entered the study. His parents

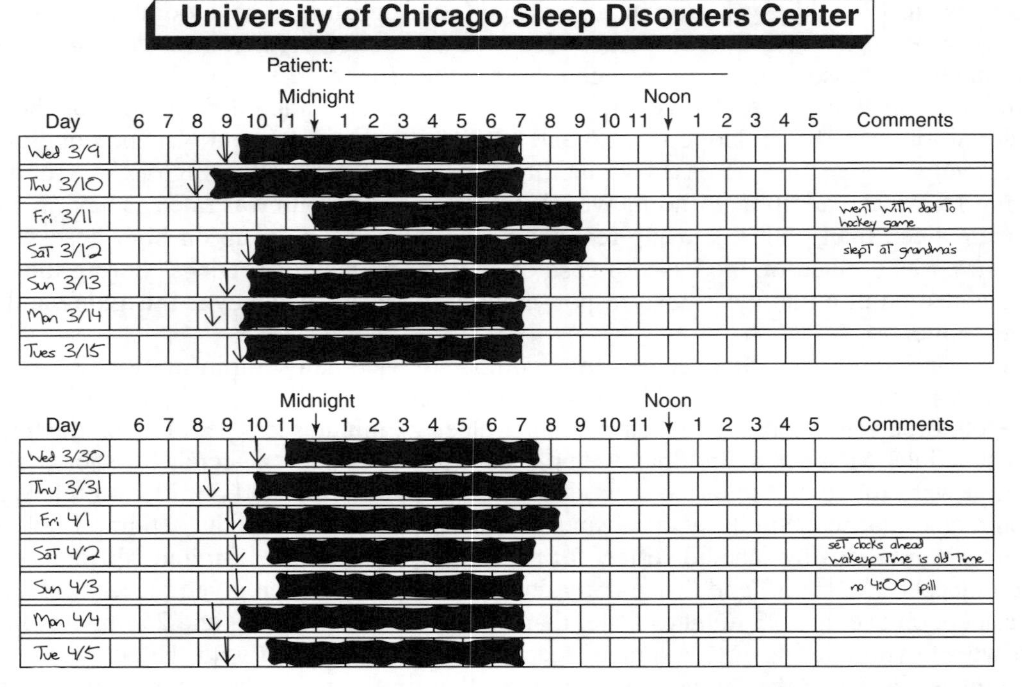

FIG. 1 Jeremy's sleep diaries at baseline and at twice-daily dosing as reported by his mother.

thought the medication "helped" but wanted to know the optimal dose and requested a more thorough medication evaluation.

Jeremy met the criteria for ADHD on the Diagnostic Interview Schedule for Children (DISC) (National Institute of Mental Health, 1992) and had elevations on the Attention Problems (t = 73), Antisocial Problems (t = 70), Thought Problems (t = 70), and Delinquent Behavior (t = 70) factors of the Child Behavior Checklist (CBCL) (Achenbach and Edelbrock, 1983). Similarly, Abbreviated Connors Teacher Rating Scale (ACTRS) teacher ratings indicated significant problems with hyperactivity, attention problems, and oppositional behavior (Ullmann et al., 1984). Dependent measures used to assess sleep included (1) a sleep log completed by the parents; (2) parent ratings on item 42 ("Problems with sleep, can't fall asleep, up too early, up in the night") from the Conners Parent Rating Scale (Conners, 1989); (3) sleep items from the SSRS (Barkley et al., 1990) rated 0 "absent" to 9 "serious and frequent" (insomnia or trouble sleeping, nightmares, and drowsiness); (4) self-report ratings based on items related to sleep from the Child Depression Inventory (Kovacs and Beck 1977) rated 0–2 (e.g. "I have trouble sleeping many nights," "I am tired many days"); and (5) actigraph monitoring (Ambulatory Monitoring, 1990). In addition, actigraphic assessment was conducted on two consecutive 16-hour periods during each week of the protocol. Jeremy wore an actigraph wrist monitor from 4 P.M. until 8 A.M. The actigraph was used to calculate latency to sleep onset (time sent to bed until first minute of sleep), duration of sleep (minutes of quiet sleep time), and number and duration of awakenings.

After baseline, Jeremy received three placebo capsules each day for 1 week. No sleep problems were reported during either baseline or placebo on parent report measures. A sleep log completed by his mother indicated that he went to bed between 8 and 9:30 and was usually asleep before 10 P.M. During week 4, he received twice-daily dosing, with the last dose of Ritalin given at noon and a 4 P.M. placebo. The sleep log completed by his parents

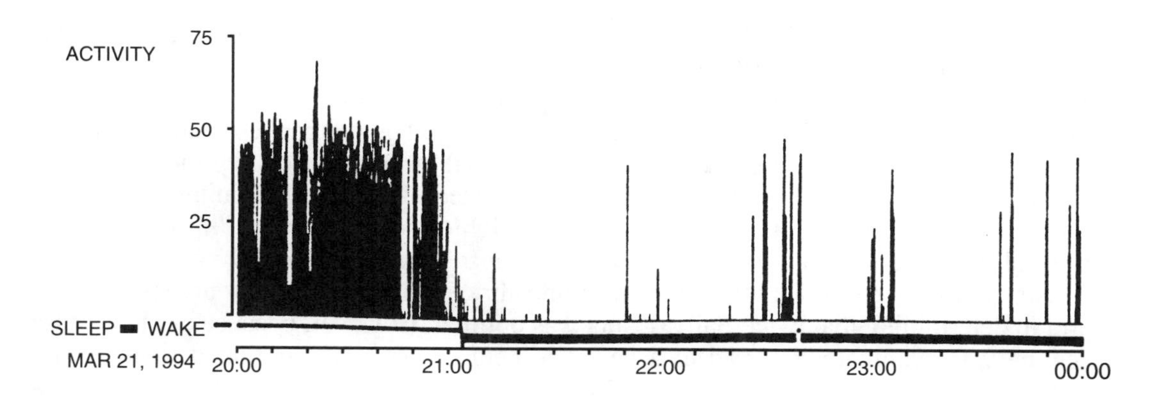

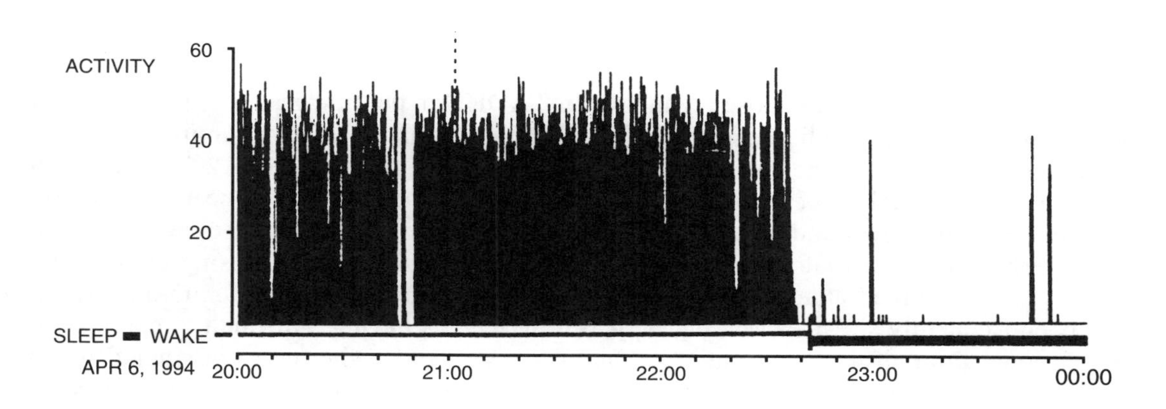

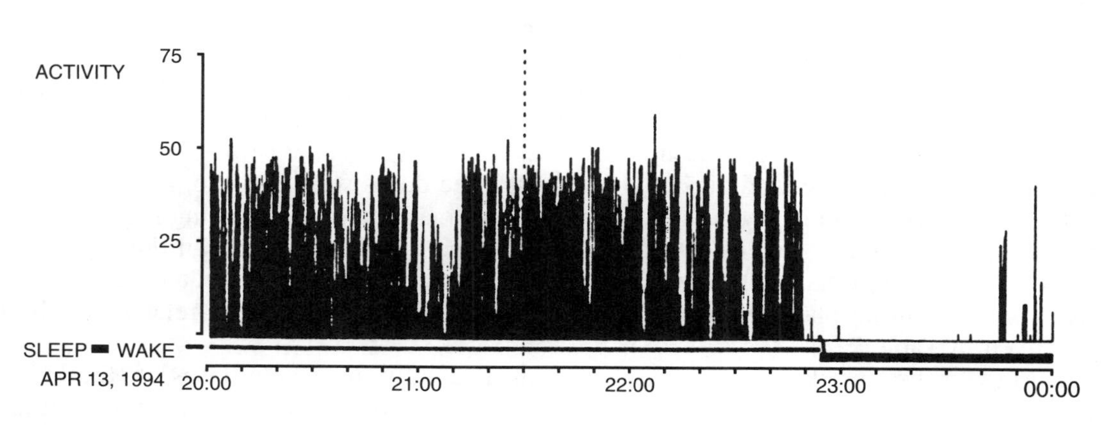

FIG. 2. Jeremy's latency to sleep onset as measured by actigraphic assessment during placebo, twice-daily dosing, and three-times daily dosing with Ritalin.

clearly indicate an increase in sleep latency during twice-daily dosing (Figure 1). This was confirmed by actigraphic assessment (Fig. 2).

During the twice-daily phase, his average sleep latency increased from 78.3 minutes during placebo to 85.1 minutes, as indicated by the actigraph. His mother reported that it took him almost 2 hours to fall asleep during this week. Visual inspection of actigraphic data during the thrice-daily phase indicated a slightly longer sleep latency of 89 minutes when he was given a 4 P.M. dose. In this case, there was a slight objective increase in the length of time to fall asleep associated with a late afternoon dose. Although ADHD symptoms were significantly improved with both twice-daily and thrice-daily dosing, parent reports were helpful in determining that twice-daily dosing was optimal. However, because of an increase in tics, he was eventually referred to a pediatric neurologist, who continued treating him with twice-daily Ritalin, and clonidine before bed. This resulted in a decrease in tics, improved sleep, and continued normalization of ADHD symptoms at home and at school.

According to Kent et al. (1995), "a medium-dose, late-day stimulant can help children settle down more easily and consequently sleep better, whereas higher stimulant doses can induce less-restful sleep than the lower dose" (p. 324). This phenomenon, first reported by Chatoor et al. (1983) in a study of Dexedrine, is illustrated in the following case.

Case 2: Jason

Jason, a 12-year-old boy diagnosed with "severe" ADHD in the first grade, had been treated with several different medications, including Ritalin, Ritalin S-R, Cylert, imipramine, and clonidine. Most recently, he had been prescribed Ritalin: 15 mg at 8 A.M., 12.5 mg at 10:30 A.M., and 10 mg at 1 P.M., with good results at school. However, he appeared to be exhibiting "stimulant rebound," becoming increasingly active and difficult to control in the late afternoons. His pediatrician referred him for a study of stimulant dosing effects. His parents were divorced and he lived with his mother. His birth history was normal. Jason had been frequently sick as an infant; he was described as having a difficult temperament, not sleeping through the night until he was over a year old. Other concerns included decreased appetite and a frequent appearance of being tired. Interpretation of medication effects was complicated by a high degree of family stress and instability.

Jason met the criteria for ADHD and oppositional defiant disorder, based on the DISC (NIMH, 1992). On the CBCL completed by his mother while he was receiving stimulant medication, he had elevations on Aggressive Behavior and Social Problems. In addition, the following items related to sleep were recorded at baseline: nightmares, sleeps less than most children his age, talks in his sleep, and has trouble getting to bed and going to sleep. Sleep-related measures for Jason are given in Table 2.

Following a 1-week washout period, Jason started taking Ritalin again, and his dose was gradually increased over a 7-day period to 10 mg three times daily (8 A.M., 12 P.M., 4 P.M.) by day 6. He remained at this dosage for week 2. During week 3, a placebo was substituted for the 4 P.M. dose, and during week 4, all three doses were placebo. Jason, his parents, his teachers, and his psychologic examiners were all blind to his dosing regimen. Parent and teacher ratings suggested marked improvement and normalization during thrice-daily dosing. Additionally, there were no family conflicts during thrice-daily dosing (vs. five conflicts during placebo and eight during thrice-daily dosing). Sleep-related variables are given in Table 2.

During the first week, when he was receiving gradually increasing doses of Ritalin, on most nights Jason went to bed at 10 P.M. and was asleep by 11 P.M., according to both his mother and actigraphic measures. According to the sleep log completed by his mother, on one night Jason fell asleep on the couch at 10 P.M. and slept until 11 A.M. the next morn-

TABLE 2. SIDE EFFECTS AND SLEEP FOR CASE 2: JASON (AGE 12, 82.5 POUNDS)

	Baseline	*Week 1 (titration)*	*Week 2 (t.i.d.)*	*Week 3 (b.i.d.)*	*Week 4 (placebo)*
Parent ratings					
1. SSRS					
Insomnia	3	0	0	3	2
Nightmares	2	0	0	0	0
Drowsiness	0	0	0	0	0
2. CPRS					
Problems with sleep	3	1	1	1	1
3. Sleep log					
Mean time to fall alseep (hours)	1.2	0.5	0.53	0.70	0.78
Mean hours slept	9.5	10.1	9.5	8.8	9.4
Self ratings					
4. CDI					
Trouble sleeping	0	0	0	0	0
Tiredness	0	0	0	0	0
5. Actigraph					
Latency to sleep onset (minutes)	—	31	47.1	69	126.3
Number of wakes		10	6.5	5	4
Duration of wakes (minutes)		8.5	9.7	1.4	1.3
Total sleep (hours)		11.5	8.5	9.25	9.0

ing. On another night, it was "too hot to sleep," his mother took him grocery shopping at midnight, and he did not get to sleep until 1 A.M.

During the second week, when Jason was taking Ritalin three times a day, his mother reported "a really good week!" with "no problems at all." He had his best week at school, and no sleep problems were reported by his mother or by Jason. Although actigraphic assessment indicated more frequent waking through the night and less total sleep, there were no complaints or concerns. His mother noted that he was falling asleep faster after being sent to bed, generally about half an hour after "lights out" around 10 P.M., which was confirmed by the actigraph.

During week 3, when he received a placebo at 4 P.M., Jason's mother reported that his behavior had deteriorated from the preceeding week. On two days in the afternoon, Jason became so upset he banged his head repetitively on the door and was described as destructive, breaking things, and taking things apart. Questionnaire ratings indicated increased impulsivity and hyperactivity (although significantly better than at baseline). There was a slight increase in sleep latency of 22 minutes from the previous week, and inspection of sleep logs and the actigraphic record indicated that on several nights he went to bed much later.

During the final week, Jason received three placebo capsules. According to his mother, he was "out of control," wound up, and extremely silly. His teacher also noted problems, especially with transitions. His sleep log and actigraphic data indicate that it took him much longer to fall asleep. He went to bed later but did not wake up as much.

In summary, Jason displayed optimal response to thrice-daily dosing using a somewhat lower dosage than he had received previously, but with more frequent dosing. The increased coverage provided by regular stimulant treatment had a dramatic impact on afternoon and evening behavior, with no significant change in sleep. The most significant adverse sleep events occurred at baseline and placebo. Of interest, his history suggests that Jason was always a poor sleeper. In addition to temperamental variables, environmental events and medication wearing off or rebounding may have contributed to his poor sleep habits. Follow-up after a year indicated continued positive responding to thrice-daily dosing.

The final case example suggests that Ritalin can have an adverse effect on sleep latency in some children long after the behavioral effectiveness has worn off.

Case 3: Kevan

Kevan was a 7-year-old boy in a regular second-grade classroom who had been taking 10 mg Ritalin twice daily for several months. He was slow at learning to read but, according to his mother, had displayed some improvement since starting to take Ritalin. His mother referred him to determine whether the medication was helping and because of behavioral concerns and increased "sensitivity" as the medication was wearing off.

Kevan met the criteria for ADHD based on the DISC and was rated in the clinical range on the ACTRS rating scale completed by his teacher. With 5 mg of Ritalin, his behavior was "normalized," as he was not displaying significant behavior problems on any of the "narrow-band" factors from the CBCL. The following sleep-related items from the CBCL were reported to be "very true or often true": trouble sleeping—takes a long time (1–2 hours) to fall asleep, sleeps less than most children, and wets the bed. His mother reported that as an infant, Kevan had slept very little, and beginning at 16 months, he had refused to take naps. Since then, it had always taken Kevan over an hour to fall asleep. Frequently, his mother would lie down with him and rub his back to help him sleep. She noted that he was always moving in his bed. Sleep measures for Kevan are given in Table 3.

Kevan's ADHD symptoms were most improved with thrice-daily dosing. However, Ritalin, even when the last dose was given at noon, exacerbated his insomnia. Given the mild

TABLE 3. SIDE EFFECTS AND SLEEP FOR CASE 3: KEVAN (AGE 7, 61 POUNDS)

	Baseline	*Week 1 (titration)*	*Week 2 (t.i.d.)*	*Week 3 (b.i.d.)*	*Week 4 (placebo)*
Parent ratings					
1. SSRS					
Insomnia	9	2	4	4	2
Nightmares	0	0	0	0	0
Drowsiness	0	0	0	0	0
2. CPRS					
Problems with sleep	3	2	1	2	1
3. Sleep log					
Mean time to fall alseep (hours)	0.82	1.1	1.7	1.3	0.82
Mean hours slept	8.7	9.4	8.7	9.1	8.9
Self ratings					
4. CDI					
Trouble sleeping	2	1	0	0	0
Tiredness	0	0	0	0	0
5. Actigraph					
Latency to sleep onset (minutes)	—	125.2	117	118.4	44
Number of wakes		9	3.5	6	8.5
Duration of wakes (minutes)		1.9	1.4	2.0	2.2
Total sleep (hours)		8.25	8.0	8.0	8.25

severity of his ADHD symptoms, alternative interventions were recommended that had not been tried previously, particularly psychosocial and academic interventions. In terms of sleep side effects, there was little difference between twice-daily and thrice-daily dosing. Both resulted in significant increases in latency to sleep onset compared with when he was taking placebo. However, Kevan's most severe sleep difficulties were reported by his mother to occur at baseline, when he was not taking medication. Inspection of his sleep logs and actigraphic data revealed that although he was put in bed between 8:30 and 9 P.M. on most school nights, he did not fall asleep (or lie still) until after 10 P.M. On weekends, he stayed up significantly longer, often not going to bed till 10:30 or 11 P.M. This extreme variability in his bedtime schedule was a likely contributor to his sleep problems. Behavioral and environmental interventions, including increasing his activity level and exercise in the afternoon, giving him a later bedtime, delaying sending him to bed until he was tired, and keeping him on a more consistent 7-nights-per-week schedule were suggested.

These case reports highlight the wide intraindividual differences in sleep as well as the many confounding factors that can influence the measurement of sleep in addition to stimulant medication. Consistent with Stein et al. (1996) and Kent et al. (1995), neither Kevan nor Jason displayed significant differences between twice-daily and thrice-daily dosing in sleep latency.

CONCLUSION

To summarize, there is little evidence that many or most children with ADHD who do not take medication have *disrupted* sleep. Children with ADHD who take medication do not display more frequent waking or other evidence of disrupted sleep. The question of whether sleep is *disturbed* requires further study over longer time periods. It should be noted, however, that earlier polysomnographic studies were suggestive of delayed and altered REM periods. Previous studies and clinical experience are consistent in suggesting that low to moderate dose of Ritalin often *delay* sleep onset considerably for children with ADHD. On average, however, there are few consistent differences in sleep latency between taking the last dose at noon or 4 P.M.

As with most clinical problems, treatment decisions should be based on treating the symptoms associated with the greatest impairment. For many children with ADHD, increased sleep latency is a tolerable cost relative to greater benefit in terms of reduction in ADHD symptoms. For others, fatigue and other sleep-related behaviors are a major component of their attention difficulties, requiring closer scrutiny to the effects of treatment on sleep. It is particularly important to distinguish sleep deprivation from "true" ADHD before giving stimulant treatment, since the cognitive symptoms of ADHD and sleep deprivation overlap. Otherwise, there is the possibility that Ritalin may be "treating" sleep deprivation. Further research is needed on potential interaction effects between sleep deprivation/satiety and stimulant response.

REFERENCES

Achenbach, T.M. & Edelbrock, C. (1983), *Manual for the Child Behavior Checklist and Revised Child Behavior Profile*. Burlington, VT: University of Vermont.

Ahmann, P., Waltonen, S., Olson, K., Theye, F., Van Erem, A. & LaPlant, R. (1993), Placebo-controlled evaluation of Ritalin side effects. *Pediatrics*, 86:1101–1106.

Ambulatory Monitoring, I. (1990), *Users Guide for the Motionlogger Actigraph Mini, Revision 1.5*. Ardsley, NY: Ambulatory Monitoring, Inc.

Avital, A., Steljes, D.G., Pasterkamp, H., Kryger, M., Sanchez, I. & Chernick, V. (1991), Sleep quality in children with asthma treated with theophylline or cromolyn sodium. *J Pediatr.*, 119:979–984.

Baekeland, F. (1966), The effect of methylphenidate on the sleep cycle in man. *Psychopharmacologia*, 10:179–183.

Ball, J.D., Tiernan, M., Janusz, J. & Furr, A. (1997), Sleep patterns among children with attention-deficit hyperactivity disorder: A reexamination of parent perceptions. *J. Pediatr. Psychol.*, 22:389–398.

Barkley, R.A., McMurray, M.B., Edelbrock, C.S. & Robbins, K. (1990), Side effects of methylphenidate in children with attention deficit hyperactivity disorder: A systematic placebo-controlled evaluation. *Pediatrics*, 86:184–192.

Brooks, J., Friedman, L., Bliwise, D. & Yesavage, J. (1993), Use of the wrist actigraph to study insomnia in older adults. *Sleep*, 16:151–155.

Chatoor, I., Wells, K.C., Conners, C.K., Seidel, W. & Shaw, D. (1983), The effects of nocturnally administered stimulant medication on EEG sleep and behavior in hyperactive children. *J. Am. Acad. Child Adolesc. Psychiatry*, 22:337–342.

Conners, C.K. (1989), *Conners' Rating Scale Manual*. North Tonawanda, NY: Multi-Health Systems.

Efron, D., Jarman, F. & Barker, M. (1997), Side effects of methylphenidate and dextroamphetamine in children with attention deficit hyperactivity disorder: A double blind crossover trial. *Pediatrics,* 100:662–666.

Ferber, R. (1995), Sleeplessness in children. In: *Principles and Practice of Sleep Medicine in the Child*, eds., R. Ferber & M. Kryger. Philadelphia: W.B. Saunders, pp. 79–91.

Greenhill, L.L., Puig-Antich, J., Goetz, R. & Hanlon, C. (1983), Sleep architecture and REM sleep measures in prepubertal children with attention deficit disorder with hyperactivity. *Sleep*, 6:91–101.

Haig, J. (1974), Effects of methylphenidate on hyperactive children's sleep. *Psychopharmacologia*, 37:185–188.

Horne, J. (1991), Sleep and its disorders in children. *J. Child Psychol. Psychiatry*, 33:473–487.

Kaplan, B., McNicol, J., Conte, R. & Moghadan, H. (1987), Sleep disturbance in preschool-aged hyperactive and nonhyperactive children. *Pediatrics*, 80:839–844.

Kent, J.D., Blader, J., Koplewicz, H.S., Abikoff, H. & Foley, C.A. (1995), Effects of late afternoon methylphenidate administration on behavior and sleep in attention-deficit hyperactivity disorder. *Pediatrics*, 96:320–325.

Kovacs, M. & Beck, A.T. (1977), An empirical-clinical approach toward a definition of childhood depression. In: *Depression in Children: Diagnosis, Treatment, and Conceptual Models*, eds., J.G. Shulterbrand & A. Raskin. New York: Raven.

Lozoff, B., Wolf, A.W. & Davis, N.S. (1985), Sleep problems seen in pediatric practice. *Pediatrics*, 75:477–483.

Nahas, A.D. & Krynicki, V. (1977), Effect of methylphenidate on sleep stages and ultradian rhythyms in hyperactive children. *J. Nerv. Ment. Dis.*, 164:66–69.

National Institute of Mental Health (1992), *Diagnostic Interview Schedule for Children (DISC-2.3), Parent Version*. Washington, DC: National Institute of Mental Health.

Obermeyer, W.H., Witkovsky, M. & Benca, R.M. (1999), Sleep and ADHD. In: *Attention Deficits and Hyperactivity in Children and Adults*, eds., P. Accardo, T. Blondis, B. Whitman, & M. Stein. New York: Marcel Dekker.

Rechtschaffen, A. (1994), Sleep onset: Conceptual issues. In: *Sleep Onset*, eds. R. Ogilvie & J. Harsh, Washington, DC: American Psychological Association, pp. 3–17.

Rechtschaffen, A. & Maron, L. (1964), The effect of amphetamine on the sleep cycle. *Electroencephalogr. Clin. Neurophysiol.*, 16:438–445.

Roizen, N.J., Irwin, M., Blondis, T., Rubinoff, A., Kieffer, J. & Stein, M.A. (1996), Incidence of psychiatric and developmental disorders in families of children with ADHD: Utility of parent report. *Arch Pediatr. Adolesc. Med.*, 150:203–208.

Sadeh, A., Sharkey, K. & Carskadon, M. (1994), Activity-based sleep-wake identification: An empirical test of methodological issues. *Sleep*, 17:201–207.

Safer, D.J., Zito, J.M. & Fine, E. (1996), Increased methylphenidate usage for attention deficit disorder in the 1990s. *Pediatrics*, 98:1084–1088.

Stein, M., Blondis, T.A., Schnitzler, E., O'Brien, T., Fishkin, J., Blackwell, B., Szumowski, E. & Roizen, N. (1996), Methylphenidate dosing: Twice daily versus three times daily. *Pediatrics*, 98:748–756.

Stein, M., Mendelsohn, J., Nadelman, D., Schwab, J., Berget, B., Hagerman, L., O'Brien, T., Phillips, W. & Benca, R. (1994), Sleep and behavior problems in elementary school age children. *Soc. Pediatr. Res.*, 35:279.

Stoleru, S., Nottelmann, E.D., Belmont, B. & Ronsaville, D. (1997), Sleep problems in children of affectively ill mothers. *J. Child Psychol. Psychiatry*, 38:831–841.

Stores, G. (1992), Sleep studies in children with a mental handicap. *J. Child Psychol. Psychiatry*, 8:1303–1317.

Tirosh, E., Sadeh, A., Munvez, R. & Lavie, T. (1993), Effects of methylphenidate on sleep in children with attention-deficit hyperactivity disorder. *Am. J. Dis. Child.* 147:1313–1315.

Trommer, B.L., Hoeppner, J.B., Rosenberg, R., Armstrong, K. & Rothstein, J. (1988), Sleep disturbances in children with attention deficit disorder. *Ann. Neurol.*, 24:322–325.

Ullmann, R., Sleator, E.K. & Sprague, R. (1984), A new rating scale for diagnosis and monitoring of ADHD children. *Psychopharmacol. Bull.*, 20:160–164.

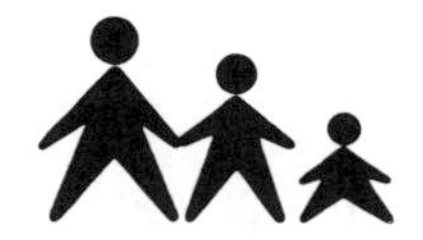

Methylphenidate Treatment for Children with Attention Deficit Hyperactivity Disorder and Tic Disorder: Inadvisable or Indispensable?

JEFFREY SVERD

One of the most controversial issues in pediatric psychopharmacology involves the use of pyschostimulant medication for the treatment of children with attention deficit hyperactivity disorder (ADHD) and comorbid tic disorder or Tourette's disorder (TD) (Cohen and Leckman, 1988; Comings and Comings, 1988; Gadow and Sverd, 1990; Shapiro et al., 1988; Sverd et al., 1989.) The controversy has taken on greater importance as a significant relationship between ADHD and TD becomes apparent, and it is increasingly recognized that TD and tics are far more prevalent in the general population than has been previously recognized (Comings et al., 1990; Kurlan et al., 1994b; McMahon et al., 1996; Spencer et al., 1995). Because practitioners are more frequently called upon to treat children in whom tic disorder coexists with ADHD and behavior problems, better understanding of the controversy is necessary. This chapter reviews the status of the debate through completion of a double-blind placebo-controlled study of the effects of methylphenidate (MPH) in children with comorbid ADHD and tics (Gadow et al., 1995a, 1995b) and preliminary reports of two studies of long-term maintenance MPH treatment (Gadow et al., 1997; Law and Schachar, 1997). In addition, evidence from a survey of children and adolescents referred for clinical evaluation of ADHD symptoms is presented, which suggests that children with ADHD show tic disorder before being treated with stimulant medication. Furthermore, neuropsychiatric disorders (including tics and TD) were present in the families of the children, and the array of disorders was similar to that described in families of patients referred for TD. The combined evidence provides support for the position that (1) a substantial portion of ADHD may be genetically related to TD, (2) tic exacerbation or emergence is relatively uncommon in stimulant-treated children with ADHD, and (3) MPH may be safely used in the treatment of children with ADHD and tic disorder.

TOURETTE'S DISORDER

TD is a common hereditary neurobehavioral spectrum disorder characterized by childhood or adolescent onset of motor and vocal tics (Comings, 1990; Shapiro et al., 1988). The disorder is typified by a fluctuating course and by waxing and waning of tics. The average age at onset of tics is ~7 years, and on average, patients show symptoms of ADHD 2.5–3 years before the onset or recognition of tics. It has been proposed that TD is a result of a genetic defect that causes an imbalance in mesencephalic-mesolimbic dopamine pathways

---

Sagamore Children's Psychiatric Center, State of New York Office of Mental Health, Dix Hills, New York.

Supported in part by a research grant from the National Institute of Mental Health (MH-45358).

and that both hyper- and hypodopaminergic dysfunctions are involved in the pathophysiology of the disorder (Comings, 1987). In addition, evidence exists for a complex interaction between several additional neurotransmitter pathways in the pathogenesis of TD and hyperkinetic movement disorders, including serotonergic, glutamate, and gamma-aminobutyric acid systems (Brito, 1997, Comings, 1990, 1997; Gadow et al., 1995b; Leckman et al., 1997). A model of polygenic inheritance that involves transmission of defective genes from both maternal and paternal sides of the family (bilineal transmission) has also been proposed (Comings, 1997).

Although the diagnosis of TD may be one of the easiest neurobehavioral diagnoses to make, many cases or familial cases of TD may be missed because tics are mild, are suppressible, and may subside and remit in a significant portion of persons by late adolescence or early adulthood (Bruun, 1988; Kerbeshian and Burd, 1992; Kurlan et al., 1987; Comings, 1990; Shapiro et al., 1988). In addition, affected persons and family members may be unaware they have tics or may ignore them (Kurlan et al., 1987, Moldofsky et al., 1974). In some cases, complex tic behaviors that have a semivoluntary quality may be considered to be merely a habit or part of a person's repertoire of habits (Comings, 1990). Finally, some professionals believe that the disorder must be severe or that coprolalia must be present. The latter symptom occurs in as few as 10% to 20% of patients (Cohen et al., 1992; Comings, 1990; Shapiro et al., 1988).

A wide array of neuropsychiatric disturbances is associated with TD and includes ADHD, obsessive compulsive disorder, conduct disorder, temper problems, school difficulties, learning disabilities, mood and anxiety disorders, drug and alcohol abuse, eating disorders, inappropriate sexual behavior, paranoid feelings, hallucinatory experiences, and autistic disorders (Comings, 1990; Comings and Comings, 1984; Kerbeshian and Burd, 1992, 1996; Sverd, 1988, 1989, 1991; Sverd et al., 1988). There is agreement that chronic tic disorder and significant portions of transient tic and obsessive compulsive disorders are genetic expressions of TD (Comings, 1990; Kurlan et al., 1994a; Shapiro et al., 1988), but controversy exists about the relationship between other psychiatric disorders (e.g., affective and anxiety disorders) and TD. Some investigators believe that these associated disorders are variant expressions of TD (Kerbeshian and Burd, 1992, 1996; Comings, 1990, 1994; Sverd, 1989, 1991), whereas others hypothesize that they are coincidental or that the observation of a high frequency of comorbid psychiatric disorders in patients with TD is a result of ascertainment bias (Pauls et al., 1986, 1993, 1994; Shapiro et al., 1988).

SIGNIFICANT RELATIONSHIP BETWEEN ADHD AND TD

A significant relationship between ADHD and TD was suggested by the observation that many patients with TD had preexisting ADHD and received the diagnosis of ADHD before the diagnosis of TD, and 25% to 90% of samples of patients with TD were reported to have comorbid ADHD (Cohen et al., 1992; Comings and Comings, 1988; Sverd et al., 1988). Comings and Comings (1984), at the City of Hope National Medical Center, proposed that TD and many cases of ADHD were genetically related. The hypothesis was based on the observation that of 250 probands, 54% had ADHD, and ADHD was present in siblings who themselves did not have tics (Comings and Comings, 1984, 1988). In a subsequent study, the investigators reported ADHD in 49% of a sample of patients with TD, which included ADHD in 33% of patients whose tics were too mild to treat. In the severe tic disorder subgroup, 83% of the patients had attention deficit disorder (ADD) without hyperactivity, and 71% had ADD with hyperactivity (Comings and Comings, 1987, 1988). Pauls et al. (1986), at Yale, argued that ascertainment bias explained the co-occurrence of the disorders. However, several family studies conducted by Comings and colleagues (Comings, in press; Knell and Comings, 1993) observed significantly higher rates of ADHD in relatives of TS probands compared with relatives of control subjects and results of epidemiologic studies (which eliminated the factor of referral bias) demonstrated the existence of higher rates of ADHD in identified patients with TD and their relatives than in those in the general population (Comings, in press). In a prospective study that eliminated the problem of referral bias, the Yale researchers (Carter et al., 1994) monitored 21 children or siblings of TD probands from age 7 to 10 years before they showed tics and reported that 43% developed tics and 24% had ADHD—rates significantly higher than those in the general population.

Further support for a significant relationship between ADHD and TD was suggested by the finding of high rates of tic disorder in children referred for ADHD. In one study, ≤50% of children with ADHD had chronic motor tics or a family history of tics (Comings and Comings, 1987), and other investigators reported tics in 30% to 35% of children with ADHD whom they evaluated (Conners, 1970; Munir et al., 1987). Sverd et al. (1988) diagnosed TD in nine (11%) of 82 boys referred for evaluation of ADHD. As a result of these findings, the authors proposed that TD constituted a major etiologic subgroup of ADHD (Sverd, 1988). Recent work conducted by Pauls et al. (1993) provided support for the hypothesis of a significant relationship between ADHD and TD, and they agreed that at least a portion of ADHD associated with TD was a result of TD. Additional support for a significant relationship between the disorders comes from the study of comorbid psychiatric disorder in probands with TD and their relatives, and probands with ADHD and their relatives. These studies demonstrated that the spectrum of disorders in families of patients with ADHD and TD is strikingly similar (Biederman et al., 1991; Comings, in press).

THE MPH-TIC CONTROVERSY

Psychostimulants are the medications of choice for the treatment of children with ADHD and are considered to be among the safest psychoactive agents used in child psychiatry (Greenhill, 1995). MPH is the most frequently prescribed stimulant and has proved to be effective in ameliorating the target symptoms of ADHD, including oppositional and aggressive behavior (Greenhill, 1995). The controversy about the use of MPH for the treatment of ADHD in children who have tics or TD or a family history of tics or TD was based on (1) post hoc or retrospective case studies of MPH-associated tic emergence or exacerbation in children with ADHD and (2) questionnaire surveys administered to patients with TD (Shapiro et al., 1988). The latter resulted in reports by some patients that they received psychostimulants before the onset of their tics or experienced tic exacerbation associated with stimulant use. Because TD is believed to be a result of central nervous system hyperdopaminergic dysfunction, and MPH is a dopamine agonist, many researchers and clinicians believed that stimulants were contraindicated for patients with ADHD who had tics or a family history of tics (Cohen and Leckman, 1988; Golden, 1988; Lowe et al., 1982; Shapiro et al., 1988). They urged extreme caution and advised that MPH be stopped if tics emerged or exacerbated (Cohen and Leckman, 1988; Lowe et al., 1982, Golden, 1988). Other investigators believed that the alarm and concern were unwarranted and premature, and they expressed concern that many children would be denied treatment with the safest and most effective pharmacologic agents available (Comings and Comings, 1988; Shapiro et al., 1988; Sverd, 1988).

Inadequate attention has been given to the literature review by Shapiro and Shapiro and colleagues (Shapiro and Shapiro, 1981; Shapiro et al., 1988). This review noted the methodologic limitations and logical inconsistencies in the studies and arguments contributing to the belief that stimulants were contraindicated for children with tic disorder. Regarding case reports, Shapiro et al. (1988) pointed out that people who believed in a causal relationship between stimulant use and tic emergence or exacerbation (Cohen and Leckman, 1988; Golden, 1988; Lowe et al., 1982) failed to account sufficiently for the natural history of TD. ADHD precedes the onset of tics by an average of 2.5–3 years, and many children are first given stimulant medication in the early school years, before the onset or recognition of tics. Therefore, the emergence of tics in some patients would be expected to occur at about the beginning of stimulant treatment. Several studies reported a positive relationship between tic severity and severity of behavioral disorder (Comings and Comings, 1987; Nolan et al., 1996; Singer and Rosenberg, 1989; Sverd et al., 1988). This association might also explain the emergence of tics in some patients, which coincides with the beginning of stimulant treatment. Furthermore, a high percentage of patients experience waxing, waning, and fluctuation of symptoms; temporary remission; and diurnal, seasonal, and stimuli-induced changes in tic status; and some patients unexposed to medication may experience a sudden and explosive onset of tics (Shapiro et al., 1988). Of further interest is the fact that, on average, 36% of patients showed increase in symptoms when treated with placebo (Shapiro et al., 1988).

Regarding questionnaire surveys, Shapiro et al. (1988) noted that ascertainment bias was inherent in the methodology that attempted to establish the percentage of patients with TD who used stimulants before the onset of tics and would result in spuriously high rates of positive response. Patients who had such histories would be more likely to respond to the questionnaire than those who did not have such histories. Moreover, responders to surveys may be more severely afflicted with TD and may have more symptoms in all categories of disturbance, including ADHD. This factor might result in a higher percentage of stimulant use before the onset of TD in responders and would lead to the erroneous conclusion that stimulants cause or invariably exacerbate tics. The findings reported by Shapiro et al. (1988) that 5% of consecutive clinically referred patients had exposure to stimulants before tic onset, compared with 14% of respondents to questionnaire surveys, supported their argument. Additional support for the argument was provided by reports of a positive association between the severity and frequency of psychiatric disorder and ADHD and severity of tic disorder (Comings and Comings, 1987; Nolan et al., 1996; Pierre et al., 1996; Sverd et al., 1988). It must also be acknowledged that the results of surveys of patients' experience while receiving stimulant medication demonstrated that tic response was heterogeneous (Comings and Comings, 1988; Shapiro et al., 1988). Some patients reported amelioration of symptoms. Heterogeneity of response may be more likely a result of the natural waxing, waning, and fluctuating course of TD than a result of the drug. Comings (1990) similarly argued that reporting bias might contribute to the false impression that stimulants cause or exacerbate tics. If 100 children are treated with MPH and five show tic emergence or exacerbation, the five patients who show tics are likely to be reported, and not the 95 children who did not develop tics. If the 95 children are otherwise similar, the argument for a cause-and-effect relationship between stimulants and tics is less than convincing.

Studies conducted of the percentage of children with ADHD who develop tics while receiving MPH are better able to answer the question about the relationship between stimulant use and tic emergence or exacerbation than case reports and questionnaire surveys. Denckla et al. (1976) studied 1520 children with minimal brain dysfunction. Forty-five (3%) of the children had tics before start of medication. Of these children, only 6 (13%) showed worsening of tics, and only 14 (0.9%) of the remaining 1475 patients showed tics while receiving MPH. Of the 20 patients who showed tics, the tics subsided in 13 and, in 4 patients, the tics did not recur when the patients were retreated with the same medication doses. In a retrospective study of 122 children with ADHD treated with stimulants, Lipkin et al. (1994) reported that 11 (9%) children developed tics or dyskinesia while receiving stimulants, nine of whom received MPH. The movement disorder was predominantly transient.

Two additional studies are of interest and do not support the notion that MPH is dangerous for children with tic disorder. Comings and Comings (1984) found that children with TD treated with stimulants before the development of tics had a longer duration from the onset of ADHD symptoms to the onset of tics compared with the same duration for a group of children with TD who did not receive stimulants (5.3 years vs. 3.3 years). These investigators suggested that stimulants might actually delay the onset of tics in some patients. Price et al. (1986) reported on six identical twins in which one twin of each pair received stimulants. Irrespective of stimulant use, both twins in each pair developed TD. The results of this study did not support the authors' prior and subsequent concern about the use of MPH in children with tic disorder (Lowe et al., 1982; Cohen and Leckman, 1988; Riddle et al., 1995).

DOES MPH EXACERBATE TICS? A CONTROLLED STUDY

Given the controversy surrounding the use of MPH in children with tic disorder, we (Sverd et al., 1989) conducted a single-blind, placebo-controlled study of the effects of MPH on four boys with TD and ADHD. We observed worsening of tics in three of the boys taking MPH, followed by tic amelioration when the children received higher doses. In two of the boys, exacerbation was precipitous and dramatic and resembled reports in the literature of tic worsening or emergence in some children with ADHD who were treated with this stimulant (Bremness and Sverd, 1979; Golden, 1974, Lowe et al., 1982; Pollack et al., 1977). The observation of variability of tic status in other experimental conditions of this study suggested that tic change was independent of medication or dose but also the possibility that MPH affected tic status by altering dopamine receptor sensitivity.

To further explore these questions, a double-blind, placebo-controlled study involving a relatively large sample of children with ADHD and diagnosed tic disorder was conducted (Gadow et al., 1995a, 1995b). Participants were assigned at random to various sequences of placebo and three dosages of MPH (0.1 mg/kg, 0.3 mg/kg, and 0.5 mg/kg) twice daily. Each dose was administered for 2 weeks. The investigation consisted of a lengthy battery of tic assessment measures, numerous evaluators, and a variety of settings including the children's natural school setting. The results showed that all 34 children who participated experienced dramatic clinical improvement in inattentive, disruptive, and aggressive behaviors, and on the basis of group data, there was no statistically significant increase in severity of tics as rated by teachers, parents, and physician. Similarly, videotapes of the children performing an academic task 15 minutes long did not reveal any drug-related changes in tic frequency. Regarding school observations, only the classroom setting at the low dose of MPH (0.1 mg/kg) showed a statistically significant increase in tic occurrence, and the magnitude of the effect was small. The physician's 2-minute count of motor tics at the 0.5 mg/kg dose showed a significant increase in tic frequency. Surprisingly, some investigators have interpreted the latter finding as evidence of their position that MPH should be contraindicated in the treatment of children with tics (Riddle et al., 1995). However, as we have previously noted, this observation was of questionable clinical significance because changes in tic frequency were not observed by care providers and trained raters who spent lengthy periods of time with the children at the same dose condition. Moreover, findings from a videotaped 15-minute simulated classroom observation period obtained shortly after the physician interviews were clearly negative. We suggested the possibility that if MPH did produce an adverse effect during the interview, that it might have done so by interacting with somatic (arousal level of child) and environmental variables to produce a transient tic exacerbation. Similarly, although the finding of a slight increase in tic frequency observed in the classroom at the 0.1-mg/kg dose could have been a drug effect, this finding was also of questionable clinical significance. The case reports of MPH-associated tic worsening or onset that generated concern about the safety of stimulants for children with tics more characteristically involved precipitous and dramatic increases in tic frequency and severity. The results of our single-blind and double-blind studies suggested that the precipitous tic worsening observed in the single-blind study was more likely a natural waxing phase of the disorder or, at worst, the result of a transient drug effect of insufficient significance to lead to discontinuation of effective treatment. In support of our conclusion regarding the safety and efficacy of MPH for the treatment of children with ADHD with comorbid tics are the findings of controlled studies conducted by others (Borcherding et al., 1990; Castellanos et al., 1997; Konkol et al.; 1990). Indeed, in one study, the only patient of 12 who had to be dropped from the study was a child who experienced a severe tic exacerbation during the placebo condition, which was the first blinded phase of the study (Castellanos et al., 1997).

Although short-term studies of the effects of MPH support the position that the drug is safe for the majority of children with tic disorder, study of its long-term use is necessary. Riddle and colleagues (Riddle et al., 1995) reported a study of five patients who received MPH for >6 months. The patients' tic status was evaluated by use of an on-medication, off-medication, on-again design, and the investigators reported that tics worsened while patients received MPH. The study suffered from too many limitations to enable any firm conclusions to be drawn. For example, the study did not assess tic disorder periodically over the long term that the drug was used, and the absence of a placebo-controlled, double-blind design could have allowed for parents' and patients' expectations and investigator's bias to influence the patients' tic status. Ironically, the results of this study could be interpreted as providing additional evidence to support the claim that MPH does not lead to permanent tic worsening, because patients were reported to show amelioration of tics when MPH was discontinued. In a 1-year prospective study, which attempted to determine the relationship between MPH use and tic status, Law and Schacher (1997) compared the effects of MPH and placebo in children with ADHD only and in children with ADHD and preexisting tics. They reported that MPH and placebo had similar effects. Fifteen percent of children with ADHD only, treated with MPH, showed emergence of tics compared with 15% of a similar group treated with placebo. In the groups of children with ADHD and preexisting tics, 66% showed improvement and 33% showed worsening. In a 2-year follow-up study of children who participated in a double-blind, placebo-controlled MPH evaluation (Gadow et al., 1997), long-term MPH treatment did not produce changes in the frequency or severity of motor or vocal tics of the children compared with baseline or initial placebo evaluations. Furthermore, behavioral improvements demonstrated during the acute trial were maintained during follow-up.

ARE OTHER DRUGS SAFER?

Another issue frequently overlooked when MPH is considered for children with tics is the safety and efficacy of alternative medications. We have previously addressed this issue and pointed out that all drugs currently in use in child psychiatry are associated with the emergence or exacerbation of tics, including neuroleptics, which have been proved to be effective for the treatment of tic disorder (Gadow and Sverd, 1990). Since the publication of that commentary, additional case reports of psychotropic medication–related tic worsening have been published (Diaz et al., 1992; Dillon, 1990; Scahill et al., 1997). Furthermore, the side effect profiles of other popularly prescribed psychoactive agents are not insignificant. For example, clonidine and desipramine, the two most frequently nominated alternatives to MPH for the treatment of patients with tic disorder, are themselves associated with tic worsening (Gadow and Sverd, 1990) and, more importantly, with serious cardiovascular toxicity (Popper and Zimnitzker, 1995; Varley and McClellan, 1997; Werry, 1995). The reports of sudden death in a few patients who received desipramine led one researcher to suggest that it should not be used in children (Werry, 1995). Regarding clonidine, little controlled evidence exists for its efficacy in the treatment of ADHD or tic disorder, and therefore there is little support for its rapidly increasing use (Cantwell et al., 1997; Popper, 1995). Ironically, one of the staunchest advocates of the use of clonidine over MPH is in agreement with the latter point (see Popper, 1995).

GENERATING A HYPOTHESIS TO RESOLVE THE MPH-TIC CONTROVERSY

Based on evidence for a significant relationship between TD and ADHD, and the finding that a group of boys with behavior disorder only resembled boys with behavior disorder and tics on parent and teacher ratings of behavioral disturbance (Sverd et al., 1988), the author, in agreement with Comings and Comings (1984), hypothesized that many cases of ADHD and TD were genetically related (Sverd, 1988). It was further hypothesized that because tic disorder is underdiagnosed, a significant portion of children with ADHD might have unrecognized tic disorder. If this were the case, the association among stimulant use, ADHD, and tic disorder might be better understood. For example, if most children with ADHD actually have undiagnosed tic disorder, then it would be apparent that the vast majority of children who receive MPH do not experience tic "emergence" or exacerbation. The data of Denckla et al. (1976) indeed suggest that tic emergence occurs infrequently in MPH-treated children with ADHD. If a large portion of Denckla's patients actually had undiagnosed tic disorder, this would support the arguments by Comings, 1990; Shapiro et al., 1988 that reporting and ascertainment bias contributed to the erroneous conclusion that tics are exacerbated or their onset hastened by MPH use. The belief then that stimulants are contraindicated in the presence of tics would be considerably weakened, and the hyperdopaminergic hypothesis of TS as applied by those who urge extreme caution before using MPH in children with tics would require modification. The proposed complex role of central nervous system hypo- and hyperdopaminergic dysfunction and multiple neurotransmitter system involvement in the pathogenesis of TD might explain why clinical doses of MPH do not exacerbate tics, as predicted by the simpler hyperdopaminergic theory (Comings, 1987; Sverd et al., 1989). For example, in regard to the theory of dopaminergic dysfunction, it is hypothesized that hypofunction of mesocortical dopamine pathways results in disinhibition and hypersensitivity of subcortical dopamine pathways and consequent tics and ADHD behaviors (Comings, 1987).

To further investigate the hypothesis that a significant portion of children with ADHD has tics, the author undertook a survey of 102 children and adolescents consecutively referred to a practice of child and adolescent psychiatry for evaluation of ADHD. Because patients were referred to a clinical practice, the experience was considered to approximate that of child and adolescent psychiatrists in private practice and other clinical settings.

CLINICAL SURVEY

Assessment

To be included for study, a patient had to have an IQ >80 and be free of neurologic disorder. The assessment consisted of a clinical interview with the parent or parents, which reviewed the patient's history of ADHD, psychiatric symptoms, medication history, and family history of psychiatric disorder. Because structured interviews were not conducted, no attempt was made to establish *Diagnostic and Statistical Manual of Mental Disorders, (DSM) 4th ed.,* diagnoses other than ADHD. Following a clinical interview with the child, parents were questioned about habit behaviors and tic symptoms in the child and about similar behaviors in themselves and other family members. Children were considered to have ADHD only if the parents did not spontaneously report during the first phase of the interview that the child had tics and the referring professionals sought evaluation for ADHD only.

Subjects

The sample comprised 92 boys and 10 girls; all were Caucasian except two boys who were African-American. The patients ranged in age from 3 to 17 years; the mean age at referral was 10 years. All children met the criteria for *DSM-IV* diagnosis of ADHD. The mean age of onset of ADHD and associated behavioral problems was 3.8 years. Fifty-three (fifty-two percent) of the patients had histories of special education or grade retention and three required resource room help in addition to regular class placement. Four patients were adopted, and information was not available about their natural parents.

Patients' tic status and psychiatric symptoms

Two patients were identified as having tics by the referring school psychologist. In one of those patients (Patient A), a diagnosis of TD had been made previously, but the mother reported that her son no longer had tics. In the second patient, a long-standing history of TD was acknowledged, but a diagnosis had never been made. Three subjects were siblings of patients with TD known to us. The parents of these subjects did not spontaneously report the presence of, or concern about, tics in these individuals. Of the remaining 97 subjects, the parents of eight (8.2%) of the children reported spontaneously that their children had tics. Four of these patients had received stimulants before the referral and after the parents had recognized that the children had tics, and in one patient, mouth tics were observed concurrent with the use of pemoline. In the remaining 89 subjects, none of the parents reported tic disorder, and they were considered to have ADHD only. Nevertheless, on careful questioning in the second phase of the parent interviews and on observation of the patients, tic disorder was present in all 89 children, including the three siblings of patients with TD. Despite the mother's report that patient A no longer had tic behaviors, he was observed to have minor tics. For the entire sample, 75 patients had motor and vocal tics, and 27 had motor tics only. The mean age at onset of tic disorder was estimated to be 5 years. In the patients whose parents could not identify the onset of their children's tics, the onset was estimated as occurring ~2.5–3 years after the onset of the behavior disorder.

Table 1 presents the tics and TD behaviors of 22 randomly selected subjects. The tics and TD behaviors were representative of those in the remaining subjects of the sample. In previous studies, independent verification of tic symptoms was obtained for subjects assessed by the author (Nolan et al., 1996). Many of the TD behaviors observed have been variously termed complex tics, compulsive tics, ritualistic compulsions, repetitive behaviors, or mannerisms by other TD experts (Bruun, 1988; Comings, 1990; Fahn and Erenberg, 1988; Leckman et al., 1997; McMahon et al., 1996; Santangelo et al., 1994). Nevertheless, as can be seen in Table 1, all subjects had multiple behaviors that all would agree were tics. Table 2 lists the frequency of psychiatric symptoms for the entire sample. The array of disorders was similar to that described in other samples of ADHD probands and TD probands (Biederman et al., 1991; Comings, 1990).

TABLE 1. TICS AND TOURETTE'S DISORDER BEHAVIORS OF 22 RANDOMLY SELECTED SURVEY PATIENTS

Patient	*Age at Referral*	*Estimated Age at Onset of Tics*	*Tics and TD Behaviors*
1	9-year-old boy	6.5 years	Lip licking, picks sores, bites nails, bites inside of mouth, holds genitals.
2	17-year-old boy	7 years	Tongue tics, cracks knuckles, picks at scabs, makes sucking movements, taps feet, genital grabbing, twirls hair, makes snorting sounds.
3	8-year-old boy	3 years	Bites lips, picks sores, bites finger- and toe-nails, picks at lips, lip licking, spitting, makes sucking noise, pull at clothing tic, twirls hair, knuckle cracking, mouth tics.
4	12-year-old boy	5 years	Throat clearing, sniffing, biting lip and inside of mouth, cracks knuckles and neck, grooming, picks at shirt, mouth tics, finger tapping, bites nails.
5	13-year-old boy	5 years	Mouth tics, lip licking, neck turning, licks finger tips, cracks neck, back and knuckles, throat clearing, bites nails.
6	13-year-old boy	5 years	Mumbles to self, picks sores, pull at clothing tic, rolls shoulders, bites lip, rocks in chair, constant touching.
7	10-year-old boy	4 years	Pull at clothing tic, tapping, grooming, grinds teeth, sucks thumb, bites nails, picks sores, genital touching.
8	13-year-old boy	8 years	Bites nails, chews on objects, shakes legs, picks at sores, lip licking, eyebrow tics, plays with hair, throat clearing, sniffing, head jerks, eye blinking.
9	6-year-old boy	5 years	Bites lip, head bob tic, cracks knuckles, coughing tic, throat clearing, sniffing.
10	8-year-old boy	6 years	Throat clearing, lip licking, plays with ear, plays with lips.
11	8-year-old boy	3 years	Bites lip, nose tics, chews hair, twirls hair, knuckle cracking, humming, sniffing.
12	17-year-old boy	6 years	Sniffing, coughing, lip licking, tapping, bites nails, twirls hair, head jerks.
13	6-year-old boy	4 years	Bites lip, lip licking, finger tapping, mouth stretch tic, yells out.
14	8-year-old girl	7 years	Bites clothes, bites nails, flaps hands, burping.
15	11-year-old boy	3 years	Forehead tics, eye blinking, eye elevation tics.
16	9-year-old girl	7 years	Burps, finger tapping, sucks on clothing, turns around and taps when leaving a room, picks at sores, cough tic, throat clearing.
17	5-year-old girl	3 years	Mutters to self, throat clearing, sniffing, swings feet, touches face of others, pulls at clothing tic, picks sores, mouth tics.
18	4-year-old boy	2 years	Lip licking, lip biting, sniffing.
19	9-year-old boy	5 years	Mouth tics, eye blinking, shakes leg, grooming, touching, shoulder shrugs, nose tics, cough tic.

(*continued*)

TABLE 1. (*continued*) TICS AND TOURETTE'S DISORDER BEHAVIORS OF 22 RANDOMLY SELECTED SURVEY PATIENTS

Patient	*Age at Referral*	*Estimated Age at Onset of Tics*	*Tics and TD Behaviors*
20	11-year-old boy	6 years	Bites lip, eye widening tics, shakes leg and feet, wipe hand across hair tic, jaw, knuckle and neck cracking, grinds teeth.
21	11-year-old boy	9 years	Eye-rolling tic, throat clearning, sniffing, yells out, bites nails, mouth tics, tongue movement, grooming, nose tics, head and neck writhing.
22	13-year-old	6 years	Lip picking, mouth tics, eye deviation tic, tongue tics, picks lip, bites nail, sniffing, bites lip, twirls hair.

Patients' medication history and tic response

Of the 102 patients, 36 (35%) had received psychoactive medication for ADHD before referral. Of those, 32 patients (88%) had received MPH, and eight of those patients had received another medication. In all, pemoline was used in five patients (13%), dextroamphetamine in three patients (8%), and desipramine in three patients (8%). Of 66 patients who had not received stimulant medications before referral, 37 subsequently received MPH, five pemoline, and one dextroamphetamine.

Of the 36 patients who had received medication before referral, tics were reported spontaneously by parents in four patients (11%). Of the 37 patients who received MPH subsequent to referral, tics were reported in three patients. Thus, for the entire sample of 69 children and adolescents who received MPH, the parents of six children (8.6%) reported that their children showed tics during pharmacotherapy. In all of the cases, the parents indicated that tic behaviors predated the use of MPH. The mean daily dosage of MPH for the sample was 30 mg, and the mean duration of MPH exposure was 1.95 years.

TABLE 2. PATIENTS' COMORBID PSYCHIATRIC SYMPTOMS (N = 102)

Symptom	*No. (%)*
Conduct problem, aggressivity	29 (28)
Depression	8 (7.8)
Major depression	5 (12)
Bipolar disorder	1 (0.9)
Body dysmorphic disorder	1 (0.9)
Obsessive compulsive behavior	9 (8.8)
Suicidal feelings	4 (3.9)
Sexually inappropriate behavior	4 (3.9)
Fireplay	4 (3.9)
History of psychiatric hospitalization	10 (9.8)

TABLE 3. PARENTS' HISTORY OF PSYCHIATRIC SYMPTOMS 98 SETS OF PARENTS

Problem	*Mother: No. (%)*	*Father: No. (%)*
Alcohol	8 (8)	26 (26)
Drugs	8 (8)	5 (5)
Depression	20 (20)	11 (11)
Panic attacks	20 (20)	1 (1)
Obese	5 (5)	2 (2)
"Hyper"	6 (6)	8 (8)
Incarceration	—	3 (3)
Temper problems	—	7 (7)
Sexual or physical abusiveness	—	6 (6)

Parent history of tics and psychiatric symptoms

Because there is evidence that the comorbid psychiatric disorders associated with tic disorder are variant expressions of the same genes that cause TD, the presence or report of a history of tics, obsessive compulsive behaviors, and psychiatric disorders and habits associated with TD were considered evidence that a given parent was a likely carrier of TD genes (Comings, 1990, 1997, in press; Kurlan et al., 1994a; Sverd, 1991). The frequencies of disorders in parents might have been underestimated because not all parents were available to be interviewed and observed. Table 3 shows the parents' psychiatric symptoms. In 25 cases, both parents were reported or observed to have tics. In 46 cases, one parent only had tics, and psychiatric symptoms associated with TD were reported in the other parent in 34 of those 46 cases. In the remaining 27 cases, neither parent had tics, but psychiatric symptoms were reported in both parents in 10 cases and in one parent only in 15 cases. In only two of the latter 27 cases was it considered that both parents had neither tics nor psychiatric symptoms. Thus, bilineal transmission of TD genes might have been present in at least 69 (70%) of 98 cases.

TREATMENT RECOMMENDATIONS

The finding from the survey that tic exacerbation associated with MPH use was uncommon combined with the results of placebo-controlled studies (Borcherding et al., 1990; Castellanos et al., 1997; Gadow et al., 1995a, 1995b; Konkol et al., 1990), and studies of long-term MPH maintenance (Law and Schachar, 1997; Gadow et al., 1997) support the contention that MPH is safe for children with ADHD and tic disorder. Nevertheless, given the longstanding belief that MPH was contraindicated for the treatment of children with tic disorder, it is understandable that clinicians might still be reluctant to prescribe the drug for children with comorbid tic disorder and ADHD. However, if the author's observations are correct, clinicians are already successfully treating with MPH patients who have unrecognized tic disorder. In addition, I believe that the task of treating children with comorbid tics using MPH is a task far less daunting than that associated with the prescription of medications whose side effects include the potential for serious cardiovascular toxicity.

The following is an approach to treating children with ADHD in whom the diagnosis of TD or tic disorder is made. Assuming that tics do not require treatment, MPH is prescribed in much the same manner as for "ADHD only" children. I do encounter children for whom the treatment of tics and ADHD appears indicated but in whom it is first elected to use MPH only. Despite improvement in ADHD, some of the children may require neuroleptic or other psychoactive drug treatment for tics and/or other behavioral problems. This is not uncommon and has been reported by us and others (Castellanos et al., 1997; Comings and Comings, 1988; Shapiro et al., 1988; Sverd et al., 1989). The need for additional medications can be best explained by the fact that many clinically referred children with ADHD and children with tic disorder have complex and comorbid psychiatric disorders (Biederman et al., 1991; Comings, 1990; Nolan et al., 1996; Sverd et al., 1989). The need for additional medications is also consistent with findings that the severity of tic disorder correlates with the severity and complexity of psychopathologic conditions. Data do not exist to support the concern of others that MPH use will result in a need for neuroleptic treatment (Cohen and Leckmen, 1988). When a child shows worsening or emergence of tics while receiving MPH, our approach is to continue the drug and observe the patient's tic status rather than discontinue effective treatment. In many cases, the tic disturbance does not require treatment or may remit. We find very often that when patients show tics requiring treatment, they are patients whose tic disorder and/or psychiatric symptoms were previously considerable (Sverd et al., 1989).

CASE STUDIES

The following are case histories of children with diagnoses of "ADHD only" and represent cases encountered in the clinical practices of physicians and mental health professionals. The histories demonstrated that careful inquiry and observation resulted in the recognition of tics in the patients and some of their parents.

The children in Cases 1 and 2 represented children in whom MPH produced dramatic and long-term improvement in functioning. The histories of these two children also demonstrated that independent confirmation of tics may be obtained during a clinically based assessment (Sprafkin and Gadow, 1993).

Case 1

Philip was 8 years old and attended regular second grade when he was referred for evaluation of his inability to concentrate and remain focused during class lessons. He was academically capable, and his scores on the WISC-R were verbal IQ 117, performance IQ 112, and full-scale IQ 117. He had been a happy child but was beginning to "feel down" because of his struggles at school. His parents did not spontaneously offer information about habits or tics and did not recognize the latter as such. He evidenced tic disorder whose onset was estimated at 5 years and which consisted of lip licking, teeth grinding, throat clearing, and noise making. A school psychologist later reported independently that she believed the latter symptom to be a vocal tic. The family history was positive for TD behaviors and associated psychiatric symptoms. Philip's father had experienced mild depression and had the habit of cracking his knuckles, his sister had an eating disorder, and another sister had an anxiety disorder. Philip's mother had the habit of biting her lip and showed a mild head jerking tic, and her brother had been hospitalized for depression and had eye blinking, tapping his feet, rubbing the area behind his ears, and curling his hair. Philip received MPH $\leq$25 mg daily for 5.5 years without adverse effect on tic behaviors. Indeed, despite discussion about tic disorder at the time of evaluation, the topic of tics was never spontaneously broached by Philip's parents, and Philip's response to medication was excellent.

Case 2

Karl was a 10-year-old fifth-grade boy who was referred because of inattention, failure to complete schoolwork, and poor school achievement despite a full-scale IQ of 110. His mother reported that "from day one he was hyperactive." From kindergarten on he was restless, impulsive, and hard to control in class and caused "grief" at every family outing. His mother reported that at the time of referral the marital relationship was suffering, and she seriously doubted her abilities as a mother. Karl received MPH for 2.5 years and was receiving 20 mg in the morning, 15 mg at noon, and 15 mg at 3:30 P.M. Following the first year of treatment, Karl was reported to be popular, secure, and cooperative with teachers, and his self-esteem had improved greatly. He became better organized and more effective at school, where he had previously done "no work at all." In addition, Karl was able to participate in extracurricular activities. He was playing on his school and town traveling soccer teams. His family history of psychiatric disorder was similar to that seen in subgroups of families with ADHD and TD children. His father had alcohol problems, his mother had experienced depression and panic attacks, his maternal grandmother and aunt had experienced depression and anxiety, and his paternal grandmother had alcohol problems. The patient's brother was diagnosed as having ADHD. Careful questioning of Karl's mother about habits and tic behavior revealed that Karl had the habit of biting his nails, shaking his legs, and wringing his hands. He picked at his mouth and bit his lip and sometimes coughed for no apparent reason. Home movies taken when Karl was 3 years old showed tongue movements and lips that were always chapped, and he presently engaged in occasional lip licking.

Case 3

Brett, a 10-year-old boy, and his parents represented a case of undiagnosed familial TD in which tics were readily observed in the patient and his father during the assessment. His mother also showed evidence that she was a carrier of the TD genes because she had lip biting and throat clearing, played with her fingers and her hair, and had been hyperactive as a child. The parents had previously sought psychiatric intervention because of Brett's long-standing behavioral disturbance. Brett showed lip biting, mouth stretches, knuckle cracking, sniffing, and coughing tics. He had received MPH 10 mg twice daily before the referral, and his behavior was believed to be improved. The patient's tics were not spontaneously reported by parents, were not recognized as such, and were not considered to be influenced by pharmacotherapy. The parents were unable to state with certainty when his tics had begun, but they indicated that they predated the use of medication. Although it might be argued that MPH was responsible for the tics (Lowe et al., 1982), this is highly unlikely because the patient's behavior difficulties had become evident by age 1 year, and both parents showed motor and vocal tics and family histories of neuropsychiatric problems much like those described in families of other TD patients. Brett's father had a history of alcohol and drug abuse and showed eye blinking, mouth and nose tics, and sniffing, and his brother was a substance abuser and had excessive eye blinking.

Case 4

The case of Jim, a 17-year-old boy who showed a dramatic emergence of a head jerking tic while receiving MPH, exemplifies the clinical dilemma that may confront physicians who treat children and adolescents with behavior disorders and captures the many issues involved in the debate over the safety of stimulant use for children with tic disorders. Jim had a long-standing history of hyperactive, impulsive behavior and had required psychiatric hospitalizations. His scores on the WISC-R were verbal IQ 87, performance IQ 85, and full-scale IQ 85. Jim had been placed with a maternal aunt at age 4 because his mother was an alcohol and drug abuser and physically abused him. Little was known about the natural father. MPH in doses ≤60 mg daily was first prescribed when he was 8 years old, but he was not receiving this medication at the time of the current hospitalization. He was questioned about the presence of tics and habits and offered that he had a long history of lip biting, biting the inside of his mouth, sometimes producing sores, knuckle cracking, teeth grinding, leg shaking, and making a "brrring" noise. He showed a clothes pulling tic and had sniffing tics. After receiving MPH 40 mg (SR) and 20 mg SR in the afternoon for 3 months, a precipitous onset of head jerking was reported by staff. It was elected to continue treatment because of the benefits Jim derived from the medication. After 3 days of observation, the tic remitted. Given the belief that MPH can exacerbate or precipitate tics in vulnerable individuals, it is easy to understand why clinicians might discontinue MPH in such a case. In this instance, the belief would have been reinforced because the tic remitted soon after its onset. But Jim's history, taken before MPH treatment was begun, demonstrated that Jim, like other patients who developed tics while receiving MPH, had preexisting tic disorder (Comings, in press; Sprafkin and Gadow, 1993).

Case 5

The case of Darryl, a 10-year-old boy, illustrates comorbid obsessive compulsive behaviors, ADHD, and tic disorder. It is increasingly recognized that obsessive compulsive disorder frequently co-occurs with ADHD (Geller et al., 1996). Because obsessive compulsive disorder is genetically related to TD, it can be expected that many children with ADHD and obsessive compulsive symptoms will also have tic disorder. In Darryl's case, his parents spontaneously reported that he had symptoms of tics and obsessive compulsive disorder. Because of behavioral and learning problems, he was retained in the first grade and required special education placement in third grade. His full-scale IQ was 92. His tics consisted of humming, guttural noises, sniffing, object smelling, mouth tics, nail biting, eye blinking, and foot tics. A diagnosis of TD had never been made. Obsessive compulsive behaviors included concern about germs. For example, he refused to eat a slice of pizza if his mother had touched it. His family history was consistent with the presence of TD on both his mother's and his father's sides of the family. His mother showed throat clearing and mouth and tongue tics, she had episodes of mild depression and anxiety, and her father had alcohol problems. The patient's father abused alcohol and drugs and had been hospitalized for depression. He had the habit of tapping his fingers and picking at sores. Both his parents had alcohol problems, and his brother abused drugs.

DISCUSSION

The clinical experience combined with evidence for a significant relationship between ADHD and TD reviewed above, suggests that tic disorder may be present in the vast majority of children with ADHD. The observation that tic emergence in children treated with MPH is uncommon is in agreement with the results of the Denckla et al. (1976) study. This is particularly striking, given the fact that all patients had tics that predated medication use and had family histories consistent with the presence of familial TD. Most would agree that patients such as these are among the most vulnerable to the development of tics while receiving MPH. These observations should further serve to dispel the notion that MPH causes tics or TD (Golden, 1988; Lowe et al., 1982). When combined with the results of controlled studies, the clinical experience described here supports the contention that MPH does not worsen tic disorder in the vast majority of ADHD patients. The findings from recently reported studies of long-term MPH treatment provide additional support for its safety. The findings of the survey also indicate that the prior belief concerning the relationship between MPH use and tic induction might best be explained by the fact that MPH is the medication most frequently used to treat ADHD. The frequency of its use compared with that of other medications in the children referred to us supports this contention. Although some might suggest that tic disorder was overdiagnosed, it should be noted that others have identified tics in significant subgroups of ADHD children referred to them (Conners, 1970; Munir et al., 1987), and it is well known that tic disorder is easy to miss when it is mild (Comings, 1990; Kurlan et al., 1987; Moldofsky et al., 1974; Sverd, 1988). For example the mother of Patient A, who had observed her son's TD symptoms for 7 years, did not recognize that he still had mild tic disorder at the time of referral and did not recognize that the patient's brother had mild tics. In support of the hypothesis for a highly significant relationship between TD and ADHD is the observation that the spectrum of comorbid psychiatric disorders described in ADHD probands and relatives is the same as that described in TD patients and their relatives (Biederman et al., 1991; Comings, in press). A similar array of disorders was present in our sample of ADHD patients and their parents.

CONCLUSION

In summary, the evidence compiled to date, including the clinical experience described here, may explain the MPH-tic controversy. The author believes that the vast majority of patients with ADHD have unrecognized tic disorder and that some of such patients will eventually evidence recognizable tics, sometimes precipitously. This is consistent with the natural history of TD. It is also believed that the emergence of obvious tics in some patients who receive MPH is best explained as coincidence in the majority of cases. As a result of reporting and ascertainment bias, and acceptance that a simple hyperdopaminergic causation theory of TD had been proved, it was erroneously concluded that a cause-and-effect relationship existed between MPH use and tic worsening. Evidence that complex pathophysiologic mechanisms involving multiple neurotransmitter systems may underlie TD may further explain why evidence does not support the belief that MPH exacerbates or precipitates tics. Indeed, the theory that hypodopaminergic dysfunction contributes to the pathogenesis of TD might explain why some patients may actually experience salutary effects on tic status from MPH use.

ACKNOWLEDGMENTS

The author thanks Kenneth D. Gadow, Ph.D., for his review of the chapter and invaluable comments and Edith E. Nolan, Ph.D., and Joyce Sprafkin, Ph.D., for their collaborative efforts.

REFERENCES

Biederman, J., Newcorn, J. & Sprich, S. (1991), Comorbidity of attention deficit hyperactivity disorder with conduct, depressive, anxiety and other disorders. *Am. J. Psychiatry*, 148:564–577.

Borcherding, B.G., Keysor, C.S., Rapoport, J.L., Elia, J. & Amass, J. (1990), Motor/vocal tics and compulsive behaviors on stimulant drugs: Is there a common vulnerability? *Psychiatry Res.*, 33:84–94.

Bremness, A.B. & Sverd, J. (1979), Methylphenidate-induced Tourette syndrome. *Am. J. Psychiatry*, 136:1334–1335.

Brito, G.N.O. (1997), A neurological model for Tourette syndrome centered on the nucleus accumbens. *Med. Hypotheses*, 49:133–142.

Bruun, R.D. (1988), The natural history of Tourette's syndrome. In: *Tourette's Syndrome and Tic Disorders: Clinical Understanding and Treatment*, eds., D.J. Cohen, R.D. Bruun & J.F. Lechman. New York: John Wiley & Sons, Inc., pp. 21–39.

Cantwell, D.P., Swanson, J. & Connor, D.F. (1997), Case study: Adverse response to clonidine. *J. Am. Acad. Child Adolesc. Psychiatry*, 36:539–544.

Carter, A.S., Pauls, D.L., Leckman, J.F. & Cohen, D.J. (1994), A prospective longitudinal study of Gilles de la Tourette's syndrome. *J. Am. Acad. Child Adolesc. Psychiatry*, 33:377–385.

Castellanos, F.X., Giedd, J.N., Elia, J., Marsh, W.L., Ritcline, G.F., Hamburger, S.P. & Rapoport, J.L. (1997), Controlled stimulant treatment of ADHD and comorbid Tourette's syndrome: Effects of stimulant and dose. *J. Am. Acad. Child Adolesc. Psychiatry*, 36:589–596.

Cohen, D.J. & Leckman, J.F. (1988), Commentary. *J. Am. Acad. Child Adolesc. Psychiatry*, 28:580–582.

Cohen, D.J., Riddle, M.A. & Leckman, J.F. (1992), Pharmacotherapy of Tourette's syndrome and associated disorders. *Psychiatr. Clin. North Am.*, 15:109–129.

Comings, D.E. (1987), A controlled study of Tourette syndrome VII: Summary. A common genetic disorder causing disinhibition of the limbic system. *Am. J. Hum. Genet.*, 41: 839–866.

Comings, D.E. (1990), *Tourette Syndrome and Human Behavior*. Duarte, CA: Hope Press.

Comings, D.E. (1997), Polygenetic inheritance of psychiatric disorders. In: *Handbook of Psychiatric Genetics*, eds., K. Blum, E.P. Noble, R.S. Sparks, J.G. Cull & T. Chen. Boca Raton, FL: CRC Press, pp. 235–260.

Comings, D.E. (1994), Tourette syndrome: A hereditary neuropsychiatric spectrum disorder. *Ann. Clin. Psychiatry*, 6:235–247.

Comings, D.E. (In press), ADHD with Tourette syndrome. In: *Attention Deficit Disorders and Comorbidities in Children*, ed., T. Brown. Washington, DC: American Psychiatric Press.

Comings, D.E. & Comings, B.G. (1984), Tourette's syndrome and attention deficit disorder with hyperactivity: Are they genetically related? *J. Am. Acad. Child Adolesc. Psychiatry*, 23:238–246.

Comings, D.E. & Comings, B.G. (1987), A controlled study of Tourette syndrome: I. Attention deficit disorder, learning disorder and school problems. *Am. J. Hum. Genet.*, 41:701–741.

Comings, D.E. & Comings, B.G. (1988), Tourette's syndrome and attention deficit disorder. In: *Tourette's Syndrome and Tic Disorders: Clinical Understanding and Treatment*, eds., D.J. Cohen, R.P. Bruun & J.F. Leckman. New York: John Wiley & Sons, Inc., pp. 119–135.

Comings, D.E., Himes, J.A. & Comings, B.G. (1990), An epidemologic study of Tourette syndrome in a single school district. *J. Clin. Psychiatry*, 51:463–469.

Conners, C.K. (1970), Symptom patterns in hyperkinetic, neurotic, and normal children. *Child Dev.*, 41:667–682.

Denckla, M.B., Bemporad, J.R. & MacKay, M.C. (1976), Tics following methylphenidate administration. *JAMA*, 235:1349–1351.

Diaz, J.M., Smith, K.G. & Maccario, M. (1992), Exacerbation of motor tic and induction of new tic by haloperidol use. *West. J. Med.*, 156:198–199.

Dillon, J.E. (1990), Self-injurious behavior associated with clonidine withdrawal in a child with Tourette's disorder. *J. Child Neurol.*, 5:308–310.

Fahn, S. & Erenberg, G. (1988), Differential diagnosis of tic phenomena: A neurologic perspective. In: *Tourette's Syndrome and Tic Disorders: Clinical Understanding and Treatment*, eds., D.J. Cohen, R.D. Bruun & J.F. Leckman. New York: John Wiley & Sons, Inc., pp. 41–54.

Gadow, K.D., Nolan, E., Sprafkin, J. & Sverd, J. (1995a), School observations of children with attention deficit hyperactivity disorder and comorbid tic disorder: Effects of methylphenidate treatment. *Dev. Behav. Pediatr.*, 16:167–176.

Gadow, K.D. & Sverd, J. (1990), Stimulants for ADHD in child patients with Tourette's syndrome: The issue of relative risk. *Dev. Behav. Pediatr.*, 11:269–271.

Gadow, K.D., Sverd, J., Sprafkin, J., Nolan, E.E. & Ezor, S.N. (1995b), Efficacy of methylphenidate for attention-deficit hyperactivity disorder in children with tic disorder. *Arch. Gen. Psychiatry*, 52:444–455.

Gadow, K.D., Sverd, J., Sprafkin, J., Nolan, E.E. & Ezor, S. (1997), Follow-up study of methylphenidate treatment in children with Tourette's disorder. Presented at the Annual Meeting of the American Academy of Child and Adolescent Psychiatry, Toronto.

Geller, P.A., Biederman, J., Griffin, S., Jones, J. & Lefkowitz, J.D. (1996), Comorbidity of juvenile onset obsessive-compulsive disorder with disruptive behavior disorders. *J. Am. Acad. Child Adolesc. Psychiatry*, 35:1637–1646.

Golden, G.S. (1974), Gilles de la Tourette's syndrome following methylphenidate administration. *Dev. Med. Child. Neurol.*, 16:76–78.

Golden, G.S. (1988), The use of stimulants in the treatment of Tourette's syndrome. In: *Tourette's Syndrome and Tic Disorders: Clinical Understanding and Treatment*, eds., D.J. Cohen, R.D. Bruun & J.F. Leckman. New York: John Wiley & Sons, Inc., pp. 317–325.

Greenhill, L.L. (1995), Attention-deficit hyperactivity disorder: The stimulants. *Child. Adolesc. Psychiatr. Clin. North Am.*, 4:123–168.

Kerbeshian, J. & Burd L. (1992), Epidemiology and comorbidity: The North Dakota prevalence studies of Tourette syndrome and other developmental disorders. In: *Advances in Neurology, vol. 58: Tourette Syndrome: Genetics Neurobiology, and Treatment*, eds., T.N. Chase, A.J. Friedhoff & D.J. Cohen. New York: Raven Press, pp. 271–281.

Kerbeshian, J. & Burd, L. (1996), Case study: Comorbidity among Tourette's syndrome, autistic disorder and bipolar disorder. *J. Am. Acad. Child Adolesc. Psychiatry*, 35: 681–685.

Konkol, R.J., Fischer, M. & Newley, R.F. (1990), Double-blind placebo-controlled stimulant trial in children with Tourette's syndrome and attention-deficit hyperactivity disorder (abstract). *Ann. Neurol.*, 28:424.

Knell, E. & Comings, D.E. (1993), Tourette syndrome and attention deficit hyperactivity disorder: Evidence for a genetic relationship. *J. Clin. Psychiatry*, 54:331–337.

Kurlan, R., Behr, J., Medved, L., Shoulson, I., Pauls, D. & Kidd, K.K. (1987), Severity of Tourette's syndrome in one large kindred. *Arch. Neurol.*, 44:268–269.

Kurlan, R., Eapen, V., Stern, J., McDermott, M.P. & Robertson, M.D. (1994a), Bilineal transmission in Tourette's syndrome families. *Neurology*, 44:2336–2342.

Kurlan, R., Whitmore, D., Irvine, C., McDermott, M.P. & Como, P.G. (1994b), Tourette's syndrome in a special education population: A pilot study involving a single school district. *Neurology*, 44:669–702.

Law, S. & Schachar, R. (1997), Does methylphenidate cause tics? Presented at the Annual Meeting of the American Academy of Child and Adolescent Psychiatry, Toronto.

Leckman, J.F., Peterson, B.S., Anderson, G.M., Arnstein, A.F.T., Pauls, D.L. & Cohen, D.J. (1997), Pathogenesis of Tourette's syndrome. *J. Child Psychol. Psychiatry*, 38:119–142.

Lipkin, P.H., Goldstein, I.J. & Adesman, A.R. (1994), Tics and dyskinesias associated with stimulant treatment in attention-deficit hyperactivity disorder. *Arch. Pediatr. Adolesc. Med.*, 148:859–861.

Lowe, T.L., Cohen, D.J., Detlor, J., Kremmitzer, M.W. & Shaywitz, B.A. (1982), Stimulant medications precipitate Tourette's syndrome. *JAMA*, 247:1729–1731.

McMahon, W.M., van de Wetering, B.J., Filloux, F., Betit, K., Coon, H. & Leppert, M. (1996), Bilineal transmission and phenotypic variation of Tourette's disorder in a large pedigree. *J. Am. Acad. Child Adolesc. Psychiatry*, 35:672–680.

Moldofsky, H., Tullis, C. & Lamon, R. (1974), Multiple tic syndrome (Gilles de la Tourette's syndrome): Clinical, biological and psychosocial variables and their influence with haloperidol. *J. Nerv. Ment. Dis.*, 151:282–292.

Munir, K. Biederman, J. & Knere, D. (1987), Psychiatric comorbidity in patients with attention deficit disorder: A controlled study. *J. Am. Acad. Child Adolesc. Psychiatry*, 26:844–848.

Nolan, E.E., Sverd, J., Gadow, K.D., Sprafkin, J. & Ezor, S.N. (1996), Associated psychopathology in children with both ADHD and chronic tic disorder. *J. Am. Acad. Child Adolesc. Psychiatry*, 35:1622–1630.

Pauls, D.L., Hurst, C.R., Kruger, S.D., Leckman, J.F., Kidd, K.K. & Cohen, D.J. (1986), Gilles de la Tourette's syndrome and attention deficit disorder with hyperactivity: Evidence against a genetic relationship. *Arch. Gen. Psychiatry*, 43:1177–1179.

Pauls, D.L., Leckman, J.F. & Cohen, D.J. (1993), Familial relationship between Gilles de la Tourette's syndrome, attention deficit disorder, learning disabilities, speech disorders, and stuttering. *J. Am. Acad. Child Adolesc. Psychiatry*, 32:1044–1050.

Pauls, D.L., Leckman, J.F. & Cohen, D.J. (1994), Evidence against a genetic relationship between Tourette's syndrome and anxiety, depression, panic and phobic disorders. *Br. J. Psychiatry*, 164:215–221.

Pierre, C.B., Nolan, E.E., Gadow, K.D., Sverd, J. & Sprafkin, J. (1996), Comparison of internalizing and externalizing symptoms in ADHD children with and without comorbid tic disorder. Presented at the Annual Meeting of the American Academy of Child and Adolescent Psychiatry, Philadelphia.

Pollack, M.A., Cohen, N.L. & Friedhoff, A.J. (1977), Gilles de la Tourette's syndrome: Familial occurrence and precipitation by methylphenidate therapy. *Arch. Neurol.*, 34: 630–632.

Popper, C.W. (1995), Combining methylphenidate and clonidine: Pharmacologic questions and news reports about sudden death. *J. Child Adolesc. Psychopharmacol.*, 5:157–166.

Popper, C.W. & Zimnitzker, B. (1995), Sudden death putatively related to desipramine treatment in youth: A fifth case and a review of speculative mechanisms. *J. Child Adolesc. Psychopharmacol.*, 5:283–300.

Price, R.A., Leckman, J.F., Pauls, D.L., Cohen, D.J. & Kidd, K.K. (1986), Tics and central nervous system stimulants in twins and non-twins. *Neurology*, 36:232–237.

Riddle, M.A., Lynch, K.A., Scahill, L., DeVries, A., Cohen, D.J. & Leckman, J.F. (1995), Methylphenidate discontinuation and reinitiation during long-term treatment of children with Tourette's disorder and attention-deficit hyperactivity disorder: A pilot study. *J. Child. Adolesc. Psychopharmacol.*, 5:205–214.

Santangelo, S.L., Pauls, D.L., Goldstein, J.M., Faroone, S.V., Tsuang, M.D. & Leckman, J.F. (1994), Tourette's syndrome: What are the influences of gender and comorbid obsessive-compulsive disorder? *J. Am. Acad. Child Adolesc. Psychiatry*, 33:795–804.

Scahill, L., Riddle, M.A., King, R.A., Hardin, M.T., Rasmussen, A., Makuch, R.W. & Leckman, J.F. (1997), Fluoxetine has no marked effect on tic symptoms in patients with Tourette's syndrome: A double-blind placebo-controlled study. *J. Child Adolesc. Psych. Pharmacol.*, 7:75–85.

Shapiro, A.K. & Shapiro, E. (1981), Do stimulants provoke cause or exacerbate tics and Tourette syndrome? *Comp. Psychiatry*, 22:265–273.

Shapiro, A.K., Shapiro, E.S., Young, J.G. & Feinberg, T.E. (1988), *Gilles de la Tourette Syndrome*. New York: Raven Press.

Singer, H.S. & Rosenberg, L.A. (1989), Development of behavioral and emotional problems in Tourette syndrome. *Pediatr. Neurol.*, 5:41–44.

Sprafkin, J. & Gadow, K.D. (1993), Four purported cases of methylphenidate-induced tic exacerbation: Methodological and clinical doubts. *J. Child. Adolesc. Psychopharmacol.*, 3:231–244.

Spencer, T., Biederman, J., Harding, M., Wilens, T. & Farraone, S. (1995), The relationship between tic disorders and Tourette's syndrome revisited. *J. Am. Acad. Child Adolesc. Psychiatry*, 34:1133–1139.

Sverd, J. (1988), Tourette syndrome and attention deficit disorder: Relationship and treatment with methylphenidate. Presented at the Annual Meeting of the American Academy of Child and Adolescent Psychiatry, Seattle.

Sverd, J. (1989), Clinical presentations of the Tourette syndrome diathesis. *J. Multihandicapped Person*, 2:311–326.

Sverd, J. (1991), Tourette syndrome and autistic disorder: A significant relationship. *Am. J. Med. Genet.*, 39:173–179.

Sverd, J., Curley, A.D., Jandorf, L. & Volkersz, L. (1988), Behavior disorder and attention deficits in boys with Tourette syndrome. *J. Am. Acad. Child Adolesc. Psychiatry*, 27:413–417.

Sverd, J., Gadow, K.D. & Paolicelli, L.M. (1989), Methylphenidate treatment of attention-deficit hyperactivity disorder in boys with Tourette's syndrome. *J. Am. Acad. Child. Adolesc. Psychiatry*, 28:574–579.

Varley, C.K. & McClellan, J. (1997), Case study: Two additional sudden deaths with tricyclic antidepressants. *J. Am. Acad. Child Adolesc. Psychiatry*, 36:390–394.

Werry, J.S. (1995), Resolved: Cardiac arrhythmias make desipramine an unacceptable choice in children. *J. Am. Acad. Child Adolesc. Psychiatry*, 34:1239–1241.

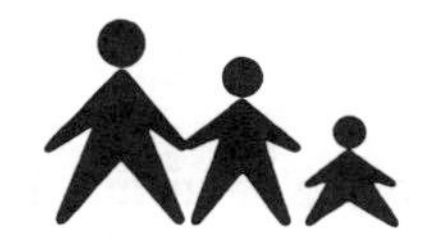

Ritalin: An Energetic Factor?

JOSEPH SERGEANT[1] and JAAP J. VAN DER MEERE[2]

In the previous edition of this chapter, we expressed the hope that the locus and effect of methylphenidate (MPH) (Ritalin) would be placed in a strict cognitive model. Our review of the literature leads us to the sober conclusion that we are unable to explain definitively the effect of Ritalin in terms of our cognitive model, a point noted by others using other cognitive models (Rapport and Kelly, 1991). Similarly, attempts at integrating both animal and human research with MPH have led to proposals, but no definitive conclusions on the neuropsychopharmacologic mechanisms of methylphenidate (Solanto, 1998), its neuronal imaging (Matochik et al., 1994), or its biochemistry (Patrick and Markowitz, 1997) can yet be drawn. That having been said, the reader is encouraged to go a step further and review the reasons why we have come to this conclusion.

Without doubt, Ritalin has been demonstrated under controlled conditions to have a positive effect on the ratings of both teachers and parents of children with attention deficit hyperactivity disorder (ADHD). One may conclude that Ritalin is an ecologically valid therapy, considered to improve inattention rather than motor activity (Taylor et al., 1987; Buitelaar et al., 1995). However, it is well established that halo effects play a role in ratings and that the long-term benefits of MPH are modest (Mannuzza et al., 1988; Gillberg et al., 1997). Thus, while parent and teacher ratings are useful, they will not provide insight into which process(es) are remedied by Ritalin. To reach this goal, the Continuous Performance task (CPT) and the Go No-Go tasks (among others) have been used as objective measures of the effect of Ritalin. We first present these tasks as a measure of effect and evaluate their contribution to understanding the locus of Ritalin.

MEASURING DRUG EFFECTS WITH THE CPT AND GO NO-GO

It has been consistently reported that hyperactive children commit more errors than do control children in a CPT (Anderson et al., 1973; Horn et al., 1989; Klee and Garfinkel, 1983; Klorman et al., 1979; Levy and Hobbes, 1981; Loiselle et al., 1980; Michael et al., 1981; Nuechterlein, 1983; O'Dougherty et al., 1984; Schachar et al., 1988; Sostek et al., 1980; Sykes et al., 1973; Zentall and Meyer, 1987) or variants thereof (Firestone and Douglas, 1975; Hoy et al., 1978; Prior et al., 1985). Poor performance in the CPT by ADHD children is highly dependent on the supervision or absence of the experimenter (Gomez and Sanson, 1994; van der Meere et al., 1995b). Two studies have reported, unexpectedly, that reward does not have an explanatory role in CPT performance (Corkum et al., 1996; van der Meere et al., 1995a) and that knowledge of results does not explain ADHD performance deficits.

Reports of studies using Ritalin and the CPT in hyperactive children suggest that the attentional defects of such children could be successfully overcome with this treatment.

[1]Department of Clinical Neuropsychology, Vrije Universiteit; and [2]Laboratory of Experimental Clinical Psychology, University of Amsterdam, Amsterdam, The Netherlands.

Rapoport et al. (1980) compared the effect of d-amphetamine on hyperactive children, control children, and college students using the CPT. They found a comparable time decrement effect and improvement in performance when this drug was used in hyperactive and control children. The same type of finding has been reported in ADHD children with and without epilepsy (van der Meere et al., 1996; Gross-Tsur et al., 1997).

Solanto et al. (1997) using a CPT, reported a tendency for the combination of reward for correct responses and response cost for errors to improve d′ but to have no effect on deterioration of performance over time. β decreased over time-on-task irrespective of contingencies or MPH. In contrast, MPH improved performance over time. However, van der Meere et al. (1995a) used a CPT with both reward and nonreward conditions and reported that ADHD children not comorbid for conduct disorder (CD) did not differ from control children in the effect of reward. However, ADHD+CD children differed both from controls and ADHD children in being more sensitive to the effect of reward (improvement in performance) with time-on-task, in contrast to the report by Solanto et al. (1997).

Klorman et al. (1979), using the CPT, showed that methylphenidate significantly reduced false positive results and speeded reaction times in the X only version of the CPT. Klorman et al. (1988) found that in both a CPT-X and a double CPT, MPH improved the accuracy and the speed of performance to an equal degree in hyperactive children with and without aggressive features. Losier et al. (1996) conducted a meta-analysis of 15 published CPT studies investigating the effect of MPH in ADHD children. On average, it was calculated, ADHD children commit 39% fewer errors while taking MPH compared with placebo and have 29% fewer commissions when given MPH compared with placebo. More recently, O'Toole et al. (1997) reported that commission errors were significantly reduced with low-dose MPH, whereas omission errors were not medication sensitive. Given the high number of commissions compared with omissions in this study, this effect is probably due to an uncontrolled strategy (β) effect. Interestingly, Losier, et al. (1996) noted that the effect on omissions was greatest in reports with short target exposures, fewer trials, and higher target probabilities.

Using convergent measures, such as event-related potentials, MPH increased the amplitude of the electrocortical potential P300, which was smaller in the ADDH children than in control children (Klorman et al., 1983; Holcomb et al., 1985; Loiselle et al., 1980; Taylor et al., 1993). Strandburg, et al. (1996) replicated this finding in a single-target CPT but found in a double-target CPT that the P300 amplitude did not differ between their ADHD group and the control group. This is of interest, because if *increases* in attentional demands (single vs. double target conditions) do not lead to differences between ADHD and control children, two points may be drawn. First, this finding replicates the attentional findings using the additive factor method (see for review Sergeant & van der Meere, 1990b) and thus provides confirmation that an *attentional* factor is not the crucial factor in ADHD. Second, if increases in processing load are equated with effort allocation in ADHD, this study argues against the effort pool as being responsible for the ADHD deficit. This finding is consistent with an early study showing that *both* ADHD and control children made equally more errors of omission in an A-X vs. an X-only CPT (Sykes et al., 1971).

Coons, et al. (1981) used both the X and double CPT (A-X) with normal young adults. In their first study, there was no effect of MPH on CPT performance or P300. Their second study replicated this finding for the simple X version. The double version was prolonged, and MPH decreased omissions and increased P300 amplitude. A later study of adolescents diagnosed with attention deficit disorder with hyperactivity (ADDH) as children replicated the effect of MPH on improving perceptual sensitivity and found that the P300 amplitude increased with MPH administration (Coons et al., 1987). When Strauss et al. (1984) used the CPT double with an uninterrupted vigil of 45 minutes, a time decrement was observed for omissions as well as d′ in the placebo condition. An interaction between drug and placebo with time-on-task was significant and indicated that MPH reduced the time decrement effect. In accordance with the habituation hypothesis, P300 amplitude interacted with drug and time-on-task. Amplitude did not decline in the MPH condition but did so in the placebo condition. In this long, double CPT, MPH had the additional effect that the latency of P300 remained relatively constant, whereas in the placebo condition, latency increased. Verbaten, et al. (1994) reported a significant enhancing effect of MPH on the parietal P300 but no effect upon reaction times to targets. Verbaten, et al. also found that the frontal N2 component in the same CPT was under the influence of MPH, which was restricted to target stimuli. Consequently, there is evidence that MPH influences both early and late ERPs.

The results reviewed above are encouraging but hardly specific. It should be observed that differences in CPT performance are not specific to hyperactive children. For instance, children at risk for schizophrenia have also been differentiated from control children with the CPT (Freidman et al., 1978). Some research suggests that ADHD and ADHD+CD groups have more omissions on the CPT than do pure CD children. More important for the present discussion is that one cannot define where and on which cognitive process Ritalin is operating from these CPT studies. This is because the task variables that need to be manipulated in order to determine process specificity have not been used in standard CPT research in ADHD.

A similar remark can be made of Go No-Go studies, in which ADHD children are instructed to respond on Go signal trials and to refrain from responding on No-Go trials. ADHD children commit more No-Go responses, or errors of commission (Iaboni et al. 1995; Milich et al., 1994; Shue and Douglas, 1992; Trommer et al., 1991). Higher proportions of No-Go responses have also been reported in children with "attentional" problems (Grünewald-Züberbier et al., 1978). Thus, several studies show that this task can distinguish ADHD children from normal children. This task also differentiates children with early and continuously treated phenylketonuria from normal children (Stemerdink et al., 1995). However, less successful has been the demonstration with this task for the effect of MPH (van der Meere et al., 1999). In the context of this chapter, the critical issue is that the mechanism involved in committing more No-Go responses is unclear from this task and makes the Go No-Go task unhelpful in determining the locus of MPH action. In order to be more specific on the locus of MPH, we introduce the cognitive-energetic model as a means of establishing greater specificity than by using the CPT and Go No-Go tasks.

THE COGNITIVE-ENERGETIC MODEL AND ATTENTION

Cognitive-energetic model

The cognitive-energetic model (Sanders, 1983, 1998) has its origins in the stage model of Sternberg (1969), known more generally as the additive factor method (AFM). This model has been reviewed by us with respect to clinical research in general (Sergeant and van der Meere, 1990a). With respect to the diagnostic issue of hyperactivity (Sergeant and van der Meere, 1990b; van der Meere, 1996) the model has been discussed in terms of ecologic validity (Sergeant and van der Meere, 1994) and its relation to response disinhibition (Sergeant et al., 1999). We shall outline the logic here only briefly.

The cognitive-energetic model contains three levels: (1) a management or executive function level; (2) a middle level containing three energetic pools (effort, arousal, and activation); and (3) a bottom layer, which contains three general stages of information processing (encoding, central processing [memory search and decision], and response organization). The hallmark of the model is that each level is associated with task variables and specific physiologic activity. Management is associated with knowledge of results, error detection, correction, and monitoring. Effort is measured by dilation of the pupils (Kahneman, 1973) and deceleration of the heart rate (Jennings et al., 1992; van der Molen et al., 1991). Arousal and activation are defined, according to Pribram and McGuiness (1975), as, respectively, phasic and tonic activity to task stimuli. Encoding is manipulated by varying the quality of stimulus input or levels of processing (Posner, 1978). Central processing contains memory search (number of items in short-term memory) and a decision: A target is present or absent. Motor organization is manipulated by variables affecting motor preparation, motor initiation, motor selection, and response execution. This general model follows a logic known as the AFM (Sternberg, 1969).

Sternberg (1969) proposed that when two task variables are found to have independent effects on the dependent variable, reaction time, the two task variables can be said to be localized in *independent* stages in the information chain. However, when two task variables, besides being main effects, are also found to interact significantly, they can be said to operate on a *common* stage.

Attention

The theoretical link between the AFM and the definition of attention was made when it was shown that the central stages of search and decision of Sternberg's model were crucial to selective attention (Schneider and Shiffrin, 1977; Shiffrin and Schneider, 1977). Shiffrin and Schneider defined attention as a limitation in the rate at which information could be processed within working memory. They noted that there are two general modes of information processing: controlled and automatic. Controlled information processing requires that a task be performed slowly, serially, and usually with some effort. Hence, attention demands are characterized by slowing down the rate at which the system can meet such demands. Automatic processing is characterized by fast, parallel, effortless processing.

This operationalization of attention as controlled processing led Schneider and Shiffrin to identify two general deficits of attention. The first is the divided attention deficit. When cognitive load increases, the number of elements that require processing of attention can be met only by dividing the attention pool over the elements. This can occur only through slowing down the processing, because, in the controlled mode, information must be processed in series. The second deficit of selective attention is the focused attention deficit. The subject, by directing attention to a particular point or object, is hindered in processing when the target is present at an invalid location. By limiting the veridical processing to specific input locations, stimuli that are the usual targets and appear on invalid positions make it difficult for subjects to ignore the invalid input. This is called a focused attention deficit.

The third type of attention deficit that concerns research in ADDH is the sustained attention deficit. This refers to maintaining attention over time. This definition is empirical, not theoretic. Fisk and Schneider (1981) argued and demonstrated that sustained attention means the maintenance of controlled processing over time.

Cognitive-energetic model and methylphenidate

The basic logic of using drugs with cognitive tasks is to show the specificity of the drug effect. Obviously, models that have discrete cognitive processes and predict how to interpret effects are to be preferred over models that lack specificity and have little predictive power. The cognitive-energetic model has the advantage that task variables are well defined and the locus of their effects reasonably robust. Hence, the use of a drug with such task variables follows the basic logic of the AFM, namely, that when a drug and a task variable have acted as two main effects without interaction, it is said that the drug acts on a stage other than the task variable. When the drug and the task variable are significant main effects and have a significant interaction, then it is said that the drug and the task variable act on the same stage. This will enable the locus of the drug in the information processing chain to be located.

Strategy

It should be noted that performance decrements in speed of processing can be compensated for by trading accuracy for speed. This is referred to as a strategy effect and not a process effect of attention (Sergeant and Scholten, 1985b). In the CPT research noted above, the measure used for response strategy is β. When β is large, many commissions have been committed; when β is low, few commissions have been committed. Most studies fail to report this measure and consequently make it difficult to know whether the effect of methylphenidate is *solely* on d′ or also on β.

Attempts to disentangle CPT measures adjuvanated by reaction times have been conducted by Halperin et al. (1988). We have discussed the construct validity *impulsive*, *inattention* errors elsewhere (Sergeant et al., 1999). Suffice it to say that the operationalization of impulsivity according to Halperin et al. (1988) is partly based on the assumption that *both* fast and inaccurate responding (A not X errors) and slow and inaccurate responding (slow A-only errors) are valid indices of the inability to suppress responding to inappropriate stimuli. We argue that the claim that fast commission errors reflect *only* impulsivity depends on showing that fast commission errors reflect an impulsive strategy and are not a failure in one of the information processing stages. The use of these refined measures of the CPT show that MPH positively influences all measures of impulsivity and dyscontrol in ADHD children (Nigg et al., 1996). Hence, MPH does not have a specific locus, in terms of these CPT measures.

We now apply the cognitive-energetic model to the available data and attempt to determine the locus of MPH.

MODEL AND FINDINGS

Encoding

Using undrugged subjects, Sergeant and Scholten (1985a) found that encoding did not differentiate hyperactive from control children, although there was some evidence that attention deficit children without hyperactivity did have an encoding defect. It was suggested that this group might have shown a strategy difference from the control group, rather than a true processing deficit. Weingartner et al. (1980) used free recall from word lists and suggested that a possible higher-order encoding deficit was ameliorated by the administration of amphetamine. However, the same group recently reported that neither MPH nor d-amphetamine at either a high or a low dose interacted with encoding (Borcherding et al., 1988). Using a Posner physical and name identity task in a double-blind crossover design with MPH, Ballinger et al. (1984) found an effect for the drug that failed to interact with level of encoding.

Four studies of hyperactive and normal children have further confirmed that encoding is unlikely to be the locus of the ADHD deficit or of the remedial effect of MPH/amphetamine. Using a depth-of-processing task, Reid and Borkowski (1984) found no interaction between depth of processing and drug-placebo condition. Benezra and Douglas (1988) have reported that hyperactive subjects are comparable with control subjects in their encoding speed and patterns of spontaneous decay of verbal traces. A second study (Peeke et al., 1984) using the depth-of-processing model (Posner and Boies, 1971) has shown that MPH has independent effects on depth of processing. This has been replicated by another study (Malone et al., 1988). Also, de Sonneville et al. (1991) investigated encoding by using the classic stimulus intact-degraded and employing a double-blind crossover design with MPH. No interaction was found between MPH and stimulus intact-degraded. Thus, using various encoding task variables, and on grounds of interactions with d-amphetamine and MPH, the available evidence seems to rule out encoding as either the site of the ADHD deficit or the locus of the remedial effects of these drugs.

This conclusion has been questioned by Losier et al. (1996) on the basis of a meta-analysis of the CPT. They argued that since d′ was lower in ADHD children and that MPH had its beneficial effects on d′, this implicated a deficit in encoding. However, since encoding variables were not manipulated in the studies reviewed in that meta-analysis, our conclusion remains correct until a study shows an interaction between ADHD and encoding variables.

Central processing

There is strong evidence that hyperactive children do not have a central processing deficit during automatic processing (Van der Meere and Sergeant, 1988b) or during controlled processing with focused attention (Van der Meere and Sergeant, 1988a; Tannock et al., 1993) or with divided attention demands (Sergeant and Scholten, 1983, 1985b; van der Meere and Sergeant, 1987; van der Meere et al., 1989). Adolescents previously diagnosed in childhood as being hyperactive (Coons et al., 1987) cannot be differentiated from ADDH children, ADDH+CD children, and control children when using these central stages (Werry et al., 1975). Coons et al. (1987) reported that MPH did not influence the rate of search and decision in their sample of adolescents. Confirmation that MPH does not operate on search and decision was provided by early studies with hyperactive subjects (Sprague et al., 1970; Werry and Aman, 1975) and by Callaway (1983) using normal subjects and by Klorman et al. (1988). It should be noted, however, that in the latter study the effect of MPH on reaction time was confined to normal young adults. These studies suggest that the effect of MPH is located at a stage subsequent to the central stages of search and decision.

An important effect of memory scanning is to prolong P300 latency. This effect is independent of the effects of amphetamines and MPH (Brumaghim et al., 1987; Callaway, 1983, 1984; Coons et al., 1987; Klorman et al., 1988; Peloquin and Klorman, 1986). This effect has been found in a variety of samples: adults, adolescents previously diagnosed as being hyperactive, and normal children (Klorman et al., 1992). In view of the additive effects of these stimulants on stimulus evaluation and a reduction in reaction time, it was concluded that stimulants affected postevaluation processes. This picture became less clear following two reports from Klorman's laboratory. The first, by Brumaghim et al. (1987), found that MPH interacted with search and decision in such a manner that the negative slope became slower and the positive slope became faster. In terms of Shiffrin and Schneider's model of controlled processing, MPH produced greater controlled processing (negative slope greater than positive slope). The second report, by Fitzpatrick et al. (1988) found that with larger levels of load than had been used previously, thus requiring more controlled processing, load increased the latency of P300 to targets and speeded-up nontargets. However, MPH had no effect upon latency of P300. This fails to replicate the effect of methylphenidate upon latency P300 reported by Brumaghim et al. (1987). In the study by

Fitzpatrick et al. (1988), stimulus-response compatibility factor interacted with load (incompatibility increased P300 latency in low levels of load). There was no interaction with MPH. Taylor et al. (1993) reported that P3a and P3b latencies were significantly longer in ADHD children and that with the administration of MPH there was no difference in latency compared with a control group. Using a single and double-target CPT, Strandburg et al. (1996) reported that the latency of the P300 for ADHD children was longer than that of control subjects in the nontarget condition, indicating an interaction with response type. Processing of a nontarget suggests that a decision-response selection is involved in the ADHD deficit, consistent with earlier suggestions of a dysfunction in late stages of processing (van der Meere et al., 1989).

Thus, P300 latency research suggests that the hyperactivity deficit occurs beyond the central stages. Further, the evidence available suggests that the locus of the effect of MPH is also at some stage beyond the central stages. This evidence converges with that reported by van der Meere et al. (1989) that the response choice stage (which follows the central stages) interacts with hyperactivity.

Motor organization

The stage subsequent to the central stages is motor organization. A task variable used to determine the functioning of this stage is stimulus-response compatibility. Stimulus-response compatibility-incompatibility requires that the subject first map stimulus location symmetrically to response side (target right-response right hand) and then reverse the pattern. During the reversal phase, the previous dominant response requires suppression. It was reported by van der Meere et al. (1989) that ADHD children, compared with control subjects and learning-disabled non-ADHD children were slower in the incompatible condition. This finding implicated a deficiency in motor selection for the ADHD group. Brandeis et al. (1998) reported a partial replication of the stimulus-response compatibility interaction with ADHD (inattentive subtype). A second study, using separate groups of pure ADHD without reading disability, a reading disability group without ADHD, and a control group, reported a full replication of the original differential ADHD interaction with stimulus-response compatibility (Hall et al., 1997). Further, Nigg et al. (1998) have used a composite score of standardized Porteus maze, Rey-Osterreith, and motor-leg test scores and found that ADHD children perform significantly poorer on these tests than control subjects, even after controlling for IQ and age. These results are consistent with the above studies in that they suggest a motor planning deficiency in ADHD. In contrast, Zahn et al. (1991) did not find a stimulus response incompatibility interaction in boys with disruptive behavior disorders. Oosterlaan and Sergeant (1995) also failed to replicate the interaction of stimulus-response incompatibility in ADHD children. They argued that this was due to the event rate used, since van der Meere et al. (1992) demonstrated that event rate interacted with ADHD, with ADHD children becoming *slower* in this task in the slow event rate. Because event rate influences the activation pool (Sanders, 1983), this finding suggests that task performance of ADHD children reflects a dysfunction in activation.

The role of amphetamines in motor organization was first studied by Frowein (1981) using normal adult subjects. Frowein demonstrated that a stimulant (phentermine HCl) did not interact with stimulus degradation; hence, encoding was not influenced by this d-amphetamine. It did interact with stimulus-response compatibility and in particular with movement time. It was concluded that this drug had its locus on the output side of the system. A further interaction with time uncertainty suggested that d-amphetamine affects the motor decision and output of the system. Thus, these results suggested that the locus of the effect of phentermine was not at the input but at the output. Using load and stimulus-response compatibility and five response mappings, Fitzpatrick et al. (1988) found that load and compatibility interacted. In their study, the assumption of stage independence was broken slightly. Nevertheless, using reaction time, Fitzpatrick et al. (1988) were able to replicate that MPH administered to students did not influence search but did speed up decision and response selection. These studies suggest that the locus of the MPH effect is at the output side of the information processing chain.

It should be noted that the output side of the information processing chain has been subdivided into four separate stages: response selection, motor programming, motor loading, and motor adjustment (see Sanders, 1990). Recent research, despite clear task effects, has shown that stimulus-response frequency did not differentiate ADHD children from control children (van der Meere et al., 1996) and that MPH did not affect this task variable or stimulus sequence (Smithee et al., 1998). Smithee, et al. also showed that MPH decreased commissions and premature responding, primarily in young children, as well as a general speeding of reaction time. These two studies suggest that this aspect of motor processing is not deficient in ADHD and is not influenced by MPH. Further, the results are suggestive of an overall improvement in energetic performance. This argument is supported by the finding in the study by Smithee, et al. that the late P300 (P471) was sensitive to stimulus probability and sequence but, contrary to prediction, MPH had no clear-cut effect on the amplitude of this component.

Some suggestive evidence of the effect of motor preparation as a crucial variable has been provided by a study that examined the effect of cueing on sitmuli presented to the left and right visual half fields (Nigg et al., 1997). These authors reported that responses to *cued* targets revealed a visual field interaction with dose. This was interpreted as indicating that both the right and left hemispheres reach optimal levels of performance in response to cueing, which affects motor preparation. This finding requires replication, but it is consistent with the hypothesis that MPH has its locus on motor-energetic output factors.

Motor processes and activation

Since motor output processes are dependent on the energetic pools (Sanders, 1983, 1998), the output dysfunction in the ADHD child may be caused by an activation/effort dysfunction. Activation may be manipulated by differences in event rate (Sanders, 1983). Therefore, evidence concerning the energetic part of the system will be restricted to event rate studies.

It has been known for some time that the speed at which stimuli are presented in a task generally improves performance, whereas slow presentations lead to poorer performance (Broadbent, 1971). Dalby and colleagues (1977) reported that in a paired-associate learning task, the faster the event rate the better the hyperactive child learns per unit time. The importance of pacing a task has been noted by van der Meere, et al. (1992). In that study, a fast event rate led to a similar performance level in hyperactive, learning-disabled, and control children, but a slow event rate clearly differentiated these three groups, with ADHD having poorer performance. Using a CPT with fast and slow event rates, van der Meere et al. (1995c) demonstrated that ADHD subjects with and without tics were differentiated from control subjects, especially in the slow event rate. The same study showed that there was a tendency for ADHD children without tics to be more inaccurate in the slow event rate than those with tics. These results suggest that ADHD children have a deficiency in activation, but it is not entirely clear whether this is confined to the group without tics. Further, van der Meere et al. (1995b) showed that event rate and MPH interact, thus suggesting that MPH is an energetic variable.

Recently, time production, a motor variable, has been used with ADHD children, whereby the subjects are required to reproduce time intervals between 12 and 60 seconds (Barkley et al., 1997). Normal children were reported as being significantly more accurate than ADHD children in temporal reproductions, especially at the longer intervals. MPH did not improve temporal reproduction in a small sample of ADHD children (Barkley et al., 1997). One possible reason is that MPH appears to improve EF (executive functioning) measures only in the medium range of event rates and not in extremely slow event rates (see Management, below).

Another method by which motor processing and MPH have been studied is the Stop-Signal Task (Logan and Cowan, 1984; Logan et al., 1984). Oosterlaan et al. (1998) reported a meta-analysis of the Stop-Signal task in groups of children with psychopathologic conditions. The main conclusion from that study was that ADHD children could be significantly differentiated from control children by this task. However, the meta-analysis also indicated that CD children were also significantly impaired in this task compared with control children. Further, ADHD and CD children could not be distinguished from one another in the Stop-Signal task.

An important finding was that MPH has a significant positive effect on the inhibition slope and, importantly, the primary inhibition Stop signal reaction time (Tannock et al., 1989). In a related paradigm, the change paradigm, in which both a Stop response and a Go response are required, it was found that MPH significantly improved both response execution and inhibitory processes (Tannock et al., 1995b). Both high and low doses enhanced response inhibition as measured by Stop-Signal reaction time, whereas probability of inhibition was not differentially affected by dosage. Similarly, the change response showed a drug effect but no dosage effect. Not all these effects are easily explained, but they suggest that MPH operates on output-related motor inhibition but may also in addition have a nonspecific energetic effect. This point is further discussed in Effort, below.

Effort

At various points in this chapter, the term *effort* has been used. We noted the definition of this concept used by Kahneman (1973) and its place in the cognitive-energetic model. It should be noted that increases in processing load are not the equivalent of measuring effort. To illustrate: effort is best measured by pupil dilation; the greater the dilation, the more effort was being applied to the task. Pupil dilation occurs when processing load is below 7 to-be-recalled digits, but constriction occurs when load is increased beyond this point (Granholm et al., 1996). Thus, not all increases in processing load reflect effort allocation. There is some evidence that heart rate deceleration and respiratory sinus arrhythmia (Jennings et al., 1992; van der Molen et al., 1991) may reflect the operation of effort. Using a version of the Stop-Signal task, accompanied with indices of heart rate change, Jennings et al. (1997) reported that ADHD and control children had similar changes in interbeat interval while performing Go responses in this task. It was expected that Stop signals would induce less heart rate deceleration in ADHD if these children were less able to inhibit their repsonses compared with control children. No evidence was found for smaller changes in ADHD children's interbeat interval. Indeed, ADHD children were found to have greater cardiac deceleration than control children to both Go and Stop signals. This argues against a deficiency in effort in ADHD children as an explanation of their disinhibitory behavior.

A well-established information processing paradigm is the Eriksen precue paradigm (Eriksen and Schultz, 1979). This paradigm was used by Tannock, et al. (1993) with four levels of precueing (one or four locations on display precued) in a study of ADHD children at two levels of dosage (0.3 mg/kg and 1.0 mg/kg) with MPH. Tannock, et al. also reported the data from 1 and 2.5 hours after testing. The paradigm requires that subjects either focus attention at a particular location or divide their attention over the four locations. Transition from focused to divided attention is measured by a dog-leg function. If MPH has a nonspecific effect, placebo and MPH will appear as two parallel dog-leg functions (two ascending but broken levels of improvement). If MPH is specific, there will appear an interaction between drug and placebo and the number of precue locations. Tannock, et al. displayed their data separately for the 1- and 2.5-hour periods. Time-on-task clearly interacted with both dose and number of target locations that were precued. At the shorter time-on-task, MPH had no dose effect, and on reaction time for the number of precues, MPH speeded overall performance compared with placebo. After 2.5 hours, ADHD children performed more poorly than at 1 hour, noticeably at the lower-load (focused) one and two precue locations. ADHD children in the placebo condition were approximately 70 milliseconds slower in these two processing levels. In contrast, precue at three and four locations led to virtually no difference or were even faster after 2.5 hours than 1 hour. MPH speeded up processing more for one and two precue locations than for four. These results suggest that the energetic demands of a task clearly interact with drug-nondrug conditions. Second, the beneficial effects of MPH do not correspond with *increases* in processing load in this task, but facilitate energetic allocation, particularly at low processing levels of load. These data strongly suggest that MPH has an energetic rather than a process-specific effect.

Further support stems from a study using the change task, during which heart rate was measured in ADHD children receiving three levels of MPH (Tannock et al., 1995). Heart rate was linearly related to dose: The rate increased with dose. This finding suggests that MPH has a nonspecific energetic effect, which positively influences the inhibitory performance of ADHD children.

Obviously, alternative energetic explanations are possible and require study. For example, Ornitz, et al. (1997) reported in a startle habituation task that ADHD children failed to maintain tonic heart rate (activation) in the same way as control subjects, suggesting a possible activation deficiency in ADHD. Iaboni et al. (1997) observed that control children increased heart rate when rewarded and increased skin conductance when reward was absent. In contrast, ADHD children displayed faster heart rate habituation to reward and increased skin conductance level during extinction. Using a variant of the Go No-Go task, Iaboni et al. (1995) used reward and response costs in ADHD children. It was reported that ADHD children made significantly more commission errors than control children in all four conditions of reward and response cost. In contrast, omission errors were significantly absent in both the response cost and reward only conditions. This suggests that strategy may interact with energetic variables such as reward and response cost in ADHD children. No significant main effect was found by Iaboni, et al. for response speed, again consistent with the hypothesis that effort is intact in ADHD children.

Management

Interest in the frontal functioning of hyperactive subjects was stimulated by Mattes (1980), who reviewed research using the contingent negative variation and suggested that hyperactive children had a dysfunction associated with motor and frontal processing (Grünewald-Zuberbier et al., 1975, 1978). However, using the bereitschafts potential (also an electrophysiologic measure of motor functioning), Rothenberger (1984) found that frontal differences between hyperactive and control subjects were not specific, since children with tics also showed such differences. Using BEAM (brain electrical analysis method) methodology and an event-related potential: processing negativity (for review, see Naatanen and Picton, 1987), Satterfield, et al. (1988) reported that the processing negativity measured at the frontal lobe differs between hyperactive and control boys. Tannock (1998) reviewed 14 studies of structural neuroimaging in ADHD and concluded that "Given the diverse methodologies and subject characteristics of the available studies to date, most cannot be directly compared" (p. 77). Swanson et al. (1998) reported the standardized effect size for many of the same neuroimaging studies. The authors noted that not only the frontal lobes but also the basal ganglia and corpus callosum had an 8% to 10% decrease in size in ADHD children compared with control children. Tannock noted in her review that other electrophysiologic evidence, particularly from event-related potentials such as the P300, suggested an energetic deficit in ADHD children. The effect of stimulants on brain metabolism at present is unclear, because of conflicting findings (Matochik et al., 1993, 1994). Thus, currently, there appears to be evidence that morphologic and metabolic differences in ADHD and the locus of MPH are not solely confined to the frontal lobes but involve both basal ganglia and other subcortical structures (Brandeis et al., 1998).

A major current hypothesis concerning the cause of ADHD is that it is an executive function deficit (Pennington and Ozonoff, 1996). Executive functioning has been defined in 33 different ways, and it has been conceived as primarily a psychologic construct (Eslinger, 1996). In line with this admonition, the cognitive-energetic model portrays executive functioning to be part of the management system. A critical control mechanism of executive functioning is the detection and correction of errors and the effect of such detection-correction on subsequent behavior. ADHD children can detect and correct errors like normal children (Sergeant and van der Meere, 1988). The same study reported, however, that the effect of such executive functioning for subsequent speed of processing was markedly different between ADHD and control children. Control children adjusted subsequent processing to ensure correct processing by becoming slower. ADHD children failed to adjust their processing after making errors. Krusch et al. (1996) demonstrated that the effect of MPH in ADHD subjects was to ensure that these subjects slowed down their processing after making errors. This demonstrates that MPH operates on this management, or executive functioning, of ADHD subjects.

Another executive function studied in ADHD children with MPH is working memory (Tannock et al., 1995a). These authors showed that working memory performance deteriorated with event rate. Second, the magnitude of the improvement of MPH on working memory performance was dependent on both dosage and event rate. High dosages of MPH (0.9 mg/kg) were more effective than low dosages (0.3 mg/kg), especially in the fast event rate condition. These data suggest two things. First, apparent executive functioning such as working memory may be dependent on the energetic demands of the task, slow event rates producing poorer performance in the ADHD group. Second, when a fast event rate is used, energetic supply improves interactively with high-dosage MPH. This indicates that at least in this executive functioning task, MPH interacts with the critical energetic variable, suggesting that MPH may be considered as having a general energetic effect. The study by Tannock et al. used event rates that were at least four times faster than the fastest event rate in the study by Barkley et al. (1997) timing study. This suggests that negative findings of MPH in long event rates may reflect an inherent limitation in currently available preparations.

This finding has further significance, namely, that there is evidence that MPH is not located specifically at motor processes but also has effects in the energetics and higher management system. Of interest is the fact that when MPH is given to ADHD children, the right hemisphere dysfunction found in these children with a cancellation task is no longer evident (Malone et al., 1994). Given the proposed holistic function of the right compared with the left hemisphere (Tucker and Williamson, 1984), alleviation of right hemisphere dysfunction is consistent with executive functioning difficulties in ADHD. The degree to which this is associated with learning disabilities, as in the report by Malone et al., is unclear, since others have been able to partial out reading disorder and maintain differentiation of ADHD children from comorbid oppositional defiant disorder/CD children and control subjects on a neuropsychologic test battery. How higher management may be influenced by the combination of MPH and reinforcement is not currently clear (Pelham et al., 1986) and is a point in need of urgent research. Consequently, the current evidence suggests that MPH is a diffuse central and output-related substance.

DISCUSSION

Taylor (1984) critically examined the relation between drug response and diagnostic validation. Of Taylor's several points of criticism concerning the evaluation of medication, three issues are discussed here: (1) the poor measurement of attention/impulsivity, (2) the use of responders only, and (3) the short-term/long-term drug responder distinction. To these issues may be added the issue of fatigue and the process strategy distinction.

It is clear from a review of the literature that many investigators use a task such as the CPT with little theoretic knowledge of what the task measures (Sergeant and van der Meere, 1990b). Alternatively, a wide variety of "cognitive tasks" is often used to measure the effect of MPH, usually with the clear finding that all tasks improve under MPH compared with placebo (Rapport et al., 1993). In order for pediatric psychopharmacology research to advance, it is necessary to use tasks that have a well-defined theoretic framework in order to identify the locus of the effect of medication.

In terms of the cognitive-energetic model, MPH does not seem to influence encoding and has its effect relatively on the output side of the information processing system, but it also involves the two energetic systems: activation and effort (the latter probably to a lesser extent than the former). Within the cognitive-energetic model, the evidence seems to indicate that some executive functions are improved by MPH (see, for example, Krusch et al., 1996). Thus, from management through effort, into the activation-motor output axis, there is evidence of a generalized energetic effect of MPH. The role of effort as a primary deficiency in ADHD seems to be less than previously claimed (Douglas, 1988), because ADHD children perform tasks that increase in cognitive load with the same degree of efficiency as control children (Sergeant and Scholten, 1983, 1985a, 1985b; van der Meere and Sergeant, 1987). In addition, in a more difficult CPT, P300 amplitude did not differ between ADHD and control children (Strandburg et al., 1996). In contrast, in an effortless task, activation declined in ADHD children (Ornitz et al., 1997) or there was greater cardiac deceleration in ADHD children than in control children to Stop and Go signals (Jennings et al., 1997). These data argue against an effort explanation of the ADHD deficit. Further, the finding that heart rate increases linearly with dose (Tannock et al., 1995) suggests that activation, not effort, is crucial in localizing the MPH effect. Nevertheless, we consider this conclusion preliminary, since alternative explanations can be offered.

Taylor's criticism of using and reporting responders is still relevant to current research. A taxonomy of the sensitivity and specificity of levels of MPH to tasks has not yet been constructed. This endangers attempts such as we have made here to localize the effects. It is a fair argument that because the effects appear to be stronger in the responder group, this does not take into account the proportion of nonresponders, which could be as large as or larger than the number of responders. Little research has examined the clinical (group) specificity of MPH (Klorman et al., 1994; Tannock et al., 1995). This too is needed in greater detail for adequate evaluation and theoretical definition of the action of MPH.

Tasks are performed over time, at various rates, and with different instruction sets. Both these factors and fatigue, event rate, and speed-accuracy instructions are seldom taken into proper account when attentional studies and the effect of MPH are reported. We urge that more detailed study of these factors be made to clarify the role of the two energetic pools, effort and activation, in ADHD. Such research can determine the locus of MPH, enhance our understanding of its therapeutic effects and limitations, and lay the cornerstone for empiric determination of drug administration to ADHD children. This is particularly evident in view of the epidemic character of current clinical decision making on the administration of MPH.

REFERENCES

Anderson, R.P., Halcombe, C.G. & Doyle, R.B. (1973), The measurement of attentional deficits. *Exceptional Children,* 39:539–543.

Ballinger, C.T., Varley, C.K. & Nolen, P.A. (1984), Effects of methylphenidate on reading in children with attention deficit disorder. *Am. J. Psychiatry*, 141:1590–1593.

Barkley, R.A., Koplowitz, S., Anderson, T. & McMurray, M.B. (1997), Sense of time in children with ADHD: Effects of duration, distraction and stimulant medication. *J. Int. Neuropsychol. Soc.*, 3:359–369.

Benezra, E. & Douglas, V.I. (1988), Short-term serial recall in ADDH, normal, and reading disabled boys. *J. Abnorm. Child Psychol.*, 16:511–526.

Borcherding, B., Thompson, K., Kruesi, M., Bartko, J., Rapoport, J.L. & Weingartner, H. (1988), Automatic and effortful processing in attention deficit hyperactivity disorder. *J. Abnorm. Child Psychol.*, 16:333–346.

Brandeis, D., van Leeuwen, Th., Rubia, K., Vitacco, D., Steger, J., Pascual-Marqui, R.D. & Steinhausen, H-Ch. (1998), Neuroelectric mapping reveals precursor of stop failures in children with attention deficits. *Behav. Brain Res.,* 94:111–125.

Broadbent, D.E. (1971), *Decision and Stress*. New York: Academic Press.

Brumaghim, J.T., Klorman, R., Strauss, J., Lewine, J.D. & Goldstein, M.G. (1987), Does methylphenidate affect information processing? Findings from two studies on performance and P3b latency. *Psychophysiology*, 24:361–373.

Buitelaar, J.K., van der Gaag, R.J., Swaab-Barneveld, H. & Kuiper, M. (1995), Prediction of clinical response to methylphenidate in children with attention-deficit hyperactivity disorder. *J. Am. Acad. Child Adolesc. Psychiatry*, 34:1025–1032.

Callaway, E. (1983), The pharmacology of human information processing. *Psychophysiology*, 20:359–370.

Callaway, E. (1984), Human information processing: Some effects of methylphenidate, age and dopamine. *Biol. Psychiatry*, 19:649–662.

Coons, H.W., Klorman, R. & Borgstedt, A.D. (1987), Effects of methylphenidate on adolescents with a childhood history of attention deficit disorder: 2. *J. Am. Acad. Child Psychiatry*, 26:368–374.

Coons, H.W., Peloquin, L.J., Klorman, R., Bauer, L.O., Ryan, R.M., Perlmutter, R.A. & Salzman, L.F. (1981), Effect of methylphenidate on young adults vigilance and event-related potentials. *Electroencephalogr. Clin. Neurophysiol.*, 51:373–387.

Corkum, P.V., Schachar, R.J. & Siegel, L.S. (1996), Performance on the continuous performance task and the impact of reward. *J. Attention Disorders*, 1:114–121.

Dalby, J.I., Kinsbourne, M., Swanson, J.M. & Sobel, M.P. (1977), Hyperactive children's underuse of learning time: Correction by stimulant treatment. *Child Dev.*, 48:1448–1453.

de Sonneville, L.M.J., Njiokiktjien, C. & Hilhorst, R.C. (1991), Methylphenidate induced changes in ADDH information processors. *J. Child Psychol. Psychiatry*, 32:285–296.

Douglas, V.I. (1988), Cognitive deficits in children with attention Deficit Disorder with hyperactivity. In: *Attention Deficit Disorder: Criteria, Cognition, Intervention,* eds., L.M. Bloomingdale & J.A. Sergeant, Oxford: Pergamon Press, pp. 65–82.

Eriksen, C.W. & Schultz, D.W. (1979), Information processing in visual search: A continuous flow conception and experimental results. *Perception Psychophysics*, 25:249–263.

Eslinger, P.J. (1996), Conceptualizing, describing, and measuring components of executive function: A summary. In: *Attention, Memory, and Executive Function*, eds., G.R. Lyon & N.A. Krasnegor. Baltimore: Paul H. Brookes, pp. 367–395.

Firestone, P. & Douglas, V.I. (1975), The effects of reward and punishment on reaction times and autonomic activity in hyperactive and normal children. *J. Abnorm. Child Psychol.*, 3:201–215.

Fisk, A.D. & Schneider, W. (1981), Control and automatic processing during tasks requiring sustained attention: A new approach to vigilance. *Hum. Factors*, 23:737–750.

Fitzpatrick, P., Klorman, R., Brumaghim, J.T. & Keefover, R.W. (1988), Effects of methylphenidate on stimulus evaluation and response processes: Evidence from performance and event-related potentials. *Psychophysiology*, 25:292–304.

Freidman, D., Vaughan, H. & Erlenmeyer-Kimling, L. (1978), Task-related cortical potentials in children in two kinds of vigilance tasks. In: *Multidisciplinary Perspectives in Event-Related Brain Potential Research*, ed., D.A. Otto. Washington, DC: U.S. Government Printing Office, pp. 309–313.

Frowein, H.W. (1981), *Selective Drug Effects on Information Processing*. Thesis, University of Tilburg.

Gomez, R. & Sanson, A.V. (1994), Effects of experimenter and mother presence on attentional performance and activity of hyperactive boys. *J. Abnorm. Child Psychol.*, 22: 517–529.

Granholm, E., Asarnow, R.F., Sarkin, A.J. & Dykes, K.L. (1996), Pupillary responses index cognitive resource limitations. *Psychophysiology*, 33:457–461.

Gross-Tsur, V. Manor, O., van der Meere, J.J., Joseph, A. & Shalev, R.S. (1997), Epilepsy and attention deficit hyperactivity disorder: Is methylphenidate safe and effective? *J. Pediatr.*, 130:40–44.

Grünewald, G., Grünewald-Züberbier, E. & Netz, J. (1978), Late components of average evoked potentials in children with different abilities to concentrate. *Electroencephalogr. Clin. Neurophysiol.*, 44:617–625.

Grünewald-Züberbier, E., Grünewald, G. & Rasche, A. (1975), Hyperactive behavior and EEG arousal reactions in children. *Electroencephalogr. Clin. Neurophysiol.*, 38:149–159.

Grünwald-Züberbier, E., Grünewald, G., Rasche, A. & Netz, J. (1978), Contingent negative variation and alpha attenuation responses in children with different abilities to concentrate. *Electroencephalogr. Clin. Neurophysiol.*, 44:37–47.

Hall, S.J., Halperin, J.M., Schwartz, S.T. & Newcorn, J.H. (1997), Behavioral and executive functions in children with attention-deficit hyperactivity disorder. *J. Attention Disorders*, 1:235–244.

Halperin, J.M., Wolf, L.E., Pascualvaca, D.M., Newcorn, J.H., Healey, J.M., O'Brien, J.D., Morganstein, A. & Young, J.G. (1988), Differential assessment of attention and impulsivity in children. *J. Am. Acad. Child Adolesc. Psychiatry*, 27:326–329.

Holcomb, P.J., Ackerman, P. & Dykman, R. (1985), Cognitive event-related potentials in children with attention and reading deficits. *Psychophysiology,* 31:656–667.

Horn, W.F., Wagner, A.E. & Ialongo, N. (1989), Sex differences in school-aged children with pervasive attention deficit hyperactivity disorder. *J. Abnorm. Child Psychol.*, 17:109–125.

Hoy, E., Weiss, G., Minde, K. & Cohen, N. (1978), The hyperactive child at adolescence: Cognitive, emotional, and social functioning. *J. Abnormal Child Psychol.*, 67:311–324.

Iaboni, F., Douglas, V.I. & Baker, A.G. (1995), Effects of reward and response costs on inhibition in ADHD children. *J. Abnorm. Psychol.*, 104:232–240.

Iaboni, F., Douglas, V.I. & Ditto, B. (1997), Psychophysiological response of ADHD children to reward and extinction. *Psychophysiology*, 34:116–123.

Jennings, J.R., van der Molen, M.W., Brock, K. & Somsen, R.J.M. (1992), On the synchrony of stopping motor responses and delaying heartbeats. *J. Exp. Psychol.*, 18:422–436.

Jennings, J.R., van der Molen, M.W., Pelham, W., Brock-Debski, K. & Hoza, B. (1997), Psychophysiology of inhibition in boys with attention deficit disorder. *Dev. Psychol.*, 33:308–318.

Kahneman, D. (1973), *Attention and Effort*. Englewood Cliffs, NJ: Prentice Hall.

Klee, S.H. & Garfinkel, B.D. (1983), The computized CPT: A new measure for inattention. *J. Abnorm. Child Psychol.*, 11:487–493.

Klorman, R., Brumaghim, J.L., Coons, H.W., Peloquin, L.-J., Strauss, J., Lewine, J.D., Borgstedt, A.D. & Goldstein, M. (1988), The contributions of event-related potentials to understanding the effects of stimulants on information processing in attention deficit disorder. In: *Attention Deficit Disorder, vol. 5*, eds., L.F. Bloomingdale & J.A. Sergeant. Oxford: Pergamon Press, pp. 199–218.

Klorman, R., Brumaghim, J.L., Fitzpatrick, P.A., Borgstedt, A.D. & Strauss, J. (1994), Clinical and cognitive effects of methylphenidate on attention deficit disorders as a function of aggression/oppositionality and age. *J. Abnorm. Psychol.*, 103:206–221.

Klorman, R., Salzman, L.F., Bauer, L.O., Coons, H.W., Borgstedt, A.D. & Halpern, W.I. (1983), Effects of two doses of methylphenidate on cross-situationals and borderline hyperactive children's evoked potentials. *Electroencephalogr. Clin. Neuropsychol.*, 56:169–185.

Klorman, R., Salzman, L.F., Pass, H.L., Borgstedt, A.D. & Dainer, K.B. (1979), Effects of methylphenidate on hyperactive children's evoked response during passive and active attention. *Psychophysiology*, 16:23–29.

Krusch, D.A., Klorman, R., Brumaghim, J.T., Fitzpatrick, P.A., Borgstedt, A.D. & Strauss, J. (1996), Slowing during and after errors in ADD: Methylphenidate slows reactions of children with attention deficit disorder during and after an error. *J. Abnorm. Child Psychol.*, 24:633–650.

Levy, F. & Hobbes, G. (1981), The diagnosis of attention deficit disorder (hyperkinesis) in children. *J. Am. Acad. Child Psychiatry*, 20:376–384.

Logan, G.D. & Cowan, W.B. (1984), On the ability to inhibit thought and action: A theory of an act of control. *Psychol. Rev.*, 91:295–327.

Logan, G.D., Cowan, W.B. & Davis, K.A. (1984), On the ability to inhibit thought and action: A model and a method. *J. Exp. Psychol.*, 10:276–291.

Loiselle, D.L., Stamn, J.S., Matinsky, S. & Whipple, S. (1980), Evoked potential and behavioral signs of attentive dysfunctions in hyperactive boys. *Psychophysiology*, 17:193–201.

Losier, B.J., McGrath, P.J. & Klein, R.M. (1996), Error patterns on the continuous performance test in non-medicated and medicated samples of children with and without ADHD: A meta-analytic review. *J. Child Psychol., Psychiatry*, 37:971–988.

Malone, M., Couitis, J., Kershner, J.R. & Logan, W.J. (1994), Right hemisphere dysfunction and methylphenidate effects in children with attention-deficit/hyperactivity disorder. *J. Child Adolesc. Psychopharmacol.*, 4:245–253.

Malone, M., Kershner, J.R. & Siegal, L. (1988), The effects of methylphenidate on levels of processing and laterality in children with attention deficit disorder. *J. Abnorm. Child Psychol.*, 16:379–395.

Mannuzza, S., Gittelman Klein, R., Bonagura, N., Horowitz Konig, P. & Shenker, R. (1988), Hyperactive boys almost grown up. *Arch. Gen. Psychiatry*, 45:13–18.

Matochik, J.A., Liebenauer, L.L., King, C., Szymanski, H.V., Cohen, R.M. & Zematkin, A.J. (1994), Cerebral glucose metabolism in adults with attention deficit hyperactivity disorder after chronic stimulant treatment. *Am. J. Psychiatry*, 151:658–664.

Matochik, J.A., Nordal, T.E., Gross, M., Semple, W.E., King, A.C., Cohen, R.M. & Zematkin, A.J. (1993), Effects of acute stimulant medication in cerebral metabolism in adults with hyperactivity. *Neuropsychopharmacology*, 8:377–386.

Mattes, J.A. (1980), The role of frontal lobe dysfunction in childhood hyperkinesis. *Comprehen. Psychol.*, 21:358–368.

Michael, R.L., Klorman, R., Salzman, L.F., Borgstedt, A.D. & Dainer, K.B. (1981), Normalizing effects of methylphenidate on hyperactive children's vigilance performance and evoked potentials. *Psychophysiology*, 18:665–677.

Milich, R., Hartung, C.M., Martin, C.M. & Haigler, E.D. (1994), Behavioral disinhibition and underlying processes in adolescents with disruptive behavior disorders. In: *Disruptive Behavior Disorders in Childhood: Essays Honoring Herbert C. Quay*, ed., D.K. Routh. New York: Plenum Press, pp. 109–138.

Naatanen, R. & Picton, T.W. (1987), The NI wave of the human electric and magnetic response to sound: A review and an analysis of the component structure. *Psychophysiology*, 24:375–425.

Nigg, J.T., Hinshaw, S.P., Carte, E.T. & Treuting, J.F. (1998), Neuropsychological correlates of childhood attention-deficit hyperactivity disorder: Explainable by comorbid disruptive behavior or reading problems. *J. Abnorm. Psychol.*, 107:468–480.

Nigg, J.T., Hinshaw, S.P. & Halperin, J.M. (1996), Continuous performance test in boys with attention deficit hyperactivity disorder: Methylphenidate dose response and relations with observed behaviors. *J. Clin. Child Psychol.*, 25:330–340.

Nigg, J.T., Swanson, J.M. & Hinshaw, S.P. (1997), Covert visual spatial attention in boys with attention deficit hyperactivity disorder: Lateral effects, methylphenidate response and results for parents. *Neuropsychologia*, 35:165–176.

Nuechterlein, K. (1983), Signal detection in vigilance tasks and behavioral attributes among offspring of schizophrenic mothers and among hyperactive children. *J. Abnorm. Psychol.* 92:4–28.

O'Dougherty, M., Nuechterlein, K.H. & Drew, B. (1984), Hyperactive and hypoxic children: Signal detection, sustained attention, and behavior. *J. Abnorm. Psychol.*, 93: 178–191.

Oosterlaan, J., Logan, G.D. & Sergeant, J.A. (1998), Response inhibition in ADHD, CD, comorbid ADHD+CD, anxious and normal children: A meta-analysis of studies with the stop task. *J. Child Psychol. Psychiatry*, 39:411–426.

Oosterlaan, J. & Sergeant, J.A. (1995), Response choice and inhibition in ADHD, anxious and aggressive children: The relationship between S-R compatibility and stop signal task. In: *European Approaches to Hyperkinetic Disorder: Eunethydis*, ed., J.A. Sergeant. Zurich, Switzerland: Fotorotar, pp. 225–240.

Ornitz, E.M., Gabikian, P., Russell, A.T., Guthrie, D., Hirano, C. & Gehricke, J.G. (1997), Affective valence and arousal in ADHD and normal boys during a startle habituation experiment. *J. Am. Acad. Child Adolesc. Psychiatry*, 36:1698–1705.

O'Toole, K., Abramowitz, A., Morris, R. & Dulcan, M. (1997), Effects of methylphenidate on attention and non-verbal learning in children with attention-deficit hyperactivity disorder. *J. Am. Acad. Child Adolesc. Psychiatry*, 36:531–538.

Patrick, K.S. & Markowitz, J.S. (1997), Pharmacology of methylphenidate, amphetamine enantiomers and pemoline in attention-deficit hyperactivity disorder. *Hum. Psychopharmacol.*, 12:527–546.

Peeke, S., Halliday, R., Callaway, E., Prael, R. & Reks, V. (1984), Effects of two doses of methylphenidate on verbal information processing in hyperactive children. *J. Clin. Psychopharmacol.*, 4:82–88.

Pelham, W.E., Milich, R. & Walker, J.L. (1986), Effects of continuous and partial reinforcement and methylphenidate on learning in children with attention deficit disorder. *J. Abnorm. Psychol.*, 95:319–325.

Peloquin, L.J. & Klorman, R. (1986), Effects of methylphenidate on normal children's mood, event-related potentials, and performance in memory scanning and vigilance. *J. Abnorm. Psychol.*, 95:88–98.

Pennington, B.F. & Ozonoff, S. (1996), Executive functions and developmental psychopathology. *J. Child Psychol. Psychiatry*, 37:51–87.

Posner, M.I. & Boies, S.J. (1971), Components of attention. *Psychol. Rev.*, 78:391–408.

Posner, M.I. (1978), *Chronometric Explorations of Mind*. Hillsdale, NJ: Erlbaum.

Pribram, K.H. & McGuiness, D. (1975), Arousal, activation and effort in the control of attention. *Psychol. Rev.*, 82:116–149.

Prior, A., Sanson, A., Freethy, L. & Geffen, G. (1985), Auditory attentional abilities in hyperactive children. *J. Child Psychol. Psychiatry*, 26:289–304.

Rapoport, J.L., Buchsbaum M.S., Weingartner H., Zahn T.P. & Ludlow C. (1980), Dextroamphetamine: Cognitive and behavioral effects in normal and hyperactive boys and normal men. *Arch. Gen. Psychiatry,* 37:933–943.

Rapport, M.D., Carlson, G.A., Kelly, K.I. & Pataki, C. (1993), Methylphenidate and desipramine in hospitalized children: I. Separate and combined effects on cognitive function. *J. Am. Acad. Child Adolesc. Psychiatry*, 32:333–342.

Rapport, M.D. & Kelly, K. (1991), Psychostimulant effects on learning and cognitive function: Findings and implications for children with attention deficit hyperactivity disorder. *Clin. Psychol. Rev.,* 11:61–92.

Reid, M.K. & Borkowski, J.G. (1984), Effects of methylphenidate (Ritalin) on information processing in hyperactive children. *J. Abnorm. Child Psychol.*, 12:169–186.

Rothenberger, A. (1984), Bewegungsbezogene Veranderungen der elektrischen Hirnaktivitat bei Kinder mit multiplen Tics and Gilles de la Tourette-syndrom. Thesis, University of HE.

Sanders, A.F. (1983), Towards a model of stress and performance. *Acta Psychol.*, 53:61–97.

Sanders, A.F. (1990), *Elements of Human Performance*. Mahwah, NJ: Erlbaum.

Sanders, A.F. (1998), *Elements of Human Performance: Reaction Processes and Attention in Human Skill*. Mahwah, NJ: Erlbaum.

Satterfield, J.H., Schell, A.M., Backs, R.W. & Hidaka, K.C. (1988), A cross-sectional and longitudinal study of age effects of electrophysiological measures in hyperactive and normal children. *Biol. Psychiatry*, 19:973–990.

Schachar, R., Logan, G., Wachsmuth, R. & Chajzyk, D. (1988), Attaining and maintaining preparation: A comparison of attention in hyperactive, normal, and disturbed control children. *J. Abnorm. Child Psychol.*, 16:361–370.

Schneider, W. & Shiffrin, R.M. (1977), Controlled and automatic human information processing: 1. Detection, search and attention. *Psychol. Rev.*, 84:1–66.

Sergeant, J.A., Oosterlaan, J. & van der Meere, J. (1999), Information processing and energetical factors in attention deficit hyperactivity disorder. In: *Handbook of Disruptive Behavior Disorders*, eds., Herbert C. Quay & Ann E. Hogan. New York: Plenum Press, pp. 75–104.

Sergeant, J.A. & Scholten, C.A. (1983), A stages-of-information processing approach to hyperactivity. *J. Child Psychol. Psychiatry*, 22:49–60.

Sergeant, J.A. & Scholten, C.A. (1985a), On data limitations in hyperactivity. *J. Child Psychol. Psychiatry*, 26:111–124.

Sergeant, J.A. & Scholten, C.A. (1985b), On resource strategy limitations in hyperactivity: Cognitive impulsivity reconsidered. *J. Child Psychol. Psychiatry*, 26:97–109.

Sergeant, J.A. & van der Meere, J.J. (1988), What happens after a hyperactive commits an error? *Psychiatry Res.*, 28:157–164.

Sergeant, J.A. & van der Meere, J.J. (1990a), Convergence of approaches in localizing the hyperactivity deficit. In: *Advancements in Clinical Child Psychology, vol. 13*, eds., B.B. Lahey & A.E. Kazdin. New York: Plenum Press, pp. 207–245.

Sergeant, J.A. & van der Meere, J.J. (1990b), Additive factor methodology applied to psychopathology with special reference to hyperactivity. *Acta Psychol.*, 74:277–295.

Sergeant, J.A. & van der Meere, J.J. (1994), Towards an empirical child psychopathology. In: *Disruptive Behavior Disorders in Childhood: Essays Honoring Herbert C. Quay*, ed., D.K. Routh. New York: Plenum Press, pp. 59–85.

Shiffrin, R.M. & Schneider, W. (1977), Controlled and automatic human information processing: 1. Detection, search and attention. *Psychol. Rev.*, 84:979–987.

Shue, K.L. & Douglas, V.I. (1992), Attention deficit hyperactivity disorder and the frontal lobe syndrome. *Brain Cognition*, 20:104–124.

Smithee, J.A., Klorman, R., Brumaghim, J.T. & Borgstedt, A.D. (1998), Methylphenidate does not modify the impact of response frequency or stimulus sequence on performance and event-related potentials of children with attention deficit hyperactivity disorder. *J. Abnorm. Child Psychol.*, 26:233–245.

Solanto, M.V. (1998), Neuropsychopharmacological mechanisms of stimulant drug action in attention-deficit hyperactivity disorder: A review and integration. *Behav. Brain Res.*, 94:127–152.

Solanto, M.V., Wender, E.H. & Bartell, S.S. (1997), Effects of methylphenidate and behavioral contingencies on vigilance in AD/HD: A test of the reward dysfunction hypothesis. *J. Child Adolesc. Psychopharmacol.*, 7:123–136.

Sostek, A.J., Buchsbaum, M.S. & Rapoport, J.L. (1980), Effects of amphetamine on vigilance performance in normal and hyperactive children. *J. Abnorm. Child Psychol.*, 8:491–500.

Sprague, R.L., Barnes, K.R. & Werry, J.S. (1970), Methylphenidate and thioridazine: Learning, reaction time, and classroom behavior in disturbed children. *Am. J. Orthopsychiatry*, 40:615–628.

Stemerdink, B.A., van der Meere, J.J., van der Molen, M.W., Kalverboer, A.F., Hendrikx, M.M.H., Huisman, J., van der Schot, L.W.A., Slijper, F.M.E., van Spronsen, F.J., & Verkerk, P.H. (1995), Information processing in patients with early and continuously treated phenylketonuria. *Pediatrics,* 154:739–746.

Sternberg, S. (1969), Discovery of processing stages: Extensions of Donders' method. In: *Attention and Performance, vol. II*, ed., W.G. Koster. Amsterdam: North Holland, pp. 276–315.

Strandburg, R.J., Marsh, J.T., Brown, W.S., Asarnow, R.F., Higa, J., Harper, R., & Guthrie, D. (1996), Continuous-processing related ERPs in children with Attention Deficit Disorder. *Biological Psychiatry,* 40:964–980.

Strauss, J., Lewis, J.L., Klorman, R., Peloquin, L.J., Perlmutter, R.A. & Salzman, L.F. (1984), Effects of methylphenidate on young adults' performance and event-related potentials in a vigilance and a paired-associates learning test. *Psychophysiology*, 21:609–621.

Swanson, J.M., Sergeant, J.A., Taylor, E., Sonuga-Barke, E.J.S., Jensen, P.S. & Cantwell, D.P. (1998), Attention-deficit disorder and hyperkinetic disorder. *Lancet*, 351:429–433.

Sykes, D.H., Douglas, V.I. & Morgenstern, G. (1973), Sustained attention in hyperactive children. *J. Child Psychol. Psychiatry*, 14:213–220.

Sykes, D.H., Douglas, V.I., Weiss, G. & Minde, K.K. (1971), Attention in hyperactive children and the effect of methylphenidate (Ritalin). *J. Child Psychol. Psychiatry*, 12:129–139.

Tannock, R. (1998), Attention deficit hyperactivity disorder: Advances in cognitive, neurobiological, and genetic research. *J. Child Psychol. Psychiatry*, 39:65–99.

Tannock, R., Ickowicz, A. & Schachar, R. (1995a), Differential effects of methylphenidate on working memory in ADHD children with and without comorbid anxiety. *J. Am. Acad. Child Adolesc. Psychiatry*, 34:886–896.

Tannock, R., Schachar, R. & Logan, G. (1993), Does methylphenidate induce overfocusing in hyperactive children? *J. Clin. Child Psychol.*, 22:28–41.

Tannock, R., Schachar, R. & Logan, G. (1995b), Methylphenidate and cognitive flexibility: Dissociated dose effects in hyperactive children. *J. Abnorm. Child Psychol.*, 23:235–266.

Tannock, R., Schachar, R.J., Carr, R.P., Chajczyk, D. & Logan, G.D. (1989), Effects of methylphenidate on inhibitory control in hyperactive children. *J. Abnorm. Child Psychology*, 17:473–491.

Taylor, E. (1984), Drug response and diagnostic validation. In: *Developmental Psychiatry*, ed. M. Rutter. New York: Guilford Press, pp. 280–329.

Taylor, E., Schachar, R., Thorley, G., Wisselberg, M., Everitt, B. & Rutter, M. (1987), Which boys respond to stimulant medication? A controlled trial of methylphenidate in boys with disruptive behaviour. *Psychol. Med.*, 17:121–143.

Taylor, M.J., Voros, J.G., Logan, W.J. & Malone, M.A. (1993). Changes in event-related potentials with stimulant medication in children with attention deficit hyperactivity disorder. *Biol. Psychology*, 36:139–156.

Trommer, B.L., Hoeppner, J.B. & Zecker, S.G. (1991), The Go-No-Go test in attention deficit disorder is sensitive to methlyphenidate. *J. Child Neurol.*, 6(supp):126–129.

Tucker, D.M. & Williamson, P.A. (1984), Asymmetric neural control systems in human self-regulation. *Psychol. Rev.*, 91:185–215.

van der Meere, J.J. (1996), The role of attention. In: *Monographs in Child and Adolescent Psychiatry. Hyperactivity Disorders of Childhood*, ed. S.T. Sandberg. Cambridge: Cambridge University Press, pp. 109–146.

van der Meere, J.J., Gunning, B. & Stemerdink, N. (1999), The effect of methylphenidate and clonidine on response inhibition and state regulation in children with ADHD. *J. Child Psychol. Psychiatry*, 40:291–298.

van der Meere, J.J., Gunning, W.B. & Stemerdink, N. (1996), Changing a response set in normal development and in ADHD children with and without tics. *J. Abnorm. Child Psychol.*, 24:767–786.

van der Meere, J.J., Hughes, K.A., Börger, N. & Sallee, F.R. (1995a), The effect of reward on sustained attention in ADHD children with and without CD. In: *European Approaches to Hyperkinetic Disorder: Eunethydis*, ed., J. Sergeant. Zürich: Fotorator, pp. 241–253.

van der Meere, J.J. & Sergeant, J.A. (1987), A divided attention experiment in pervasively hyperactive children. *J. Abnorm. Child Psychol.*, 16:379–391.

van der Meere, J.J. & Sergeant, J.A. (1988a), A focused attention experiment in pervasively hyperactive children. *J. Abnorm. Child Psychol.*, 16:627–639.

van der Meere, J.J. & Sergeant, J.A. (1988b), Acquisition of attentional skill in pervasively hyperactive children. *J. Child Psychol. Psychiatry*, 29:301–310.

van der Meere, J.J., Shalev, R., Börger, N. & Gross-Tsur, V. (1995b), Sustained attention, activation and MPH in ADHD. *J. Child Psychol. Psychiatry*, 36:697–703.

van der Meere, J.J., Stemerdink, N. & Gunning, B. (1995c), Effects of presentation rate of stimuli on response inhibition in ADHD children with and without tics. *Perceptual Motor Skills*, 81:259–262.

van der Meere, J.J., van Baal, M. & Sergeant, J.A. (1989), The additive factor method: A differential diagnostic tool in hyperactivity and learning disablement. *J. Abnorm. Child Psychol.*, 17:409–422.

van der Meere, J.J., Vreeling, H.J. & Sergeant, J.A. (1992), A motor presetting study in hyperactives, learning disabled and control children. *J. Child Psychol. Psychiatry*, 34:1347–1354.

van der Molen, M.W., Bashore, T.R., Halliday, R. & Callaway, E. (1991), Chronophysiology: Mental chronometry augmented by physiological time markers. In: *Handbook of Cognitive Psychophysiology: Central and Autonomic Nervous System Approaches*, eds., J.R. Jennings & M.G.H. Coles. Chichester, UK: John Wiley & Sons, Inc., pp. 9–178.

Verbaten, M.N., Overtoom, C.C.E., Koelega, H.S., Swaab-Barneveld, H., van der Gaag, R.J. & van Engeland, H. (1994), Methylphenidate influences on both early and late ERP waves of ADHD children in a continuous performance test. *J. Abnorm. Child Psychol.*, 22:561–578.

Weingartner, H., Rapoport, J.L., Buchsbaum, M.S., Bunney, W.E., Ebert, M.H., Mikkelsen, E.J. & Caine, E.D. (1980), Cognitive processes in normal and hyperactive children and their response to amphetamine treatment. *J. Abnorm. Child Psychol.*, 89:25–37.

Werry, J.S. & Aman, M.G. (1975), Methylphenidate and haloperidol in children: Effects on attention, memory and activity. *Arch. Gen. Psychiatry*, 32:790–795.

Zahn, T., Kruesi, M.J.P. & Rapoport, J.L. (1991), Reaction time indices of attention deficits in boys with disruptive behavior disorders. *J. Abnorm. Child Psychol.*, 19:233–252.

Zentall, S.S. & Meyer, M.J. (1987), Self-regulation of stimulation for ADD-H children during reading and vigilance task performance. *J. Abnorm. Child Psychol.*, 15:519–536.

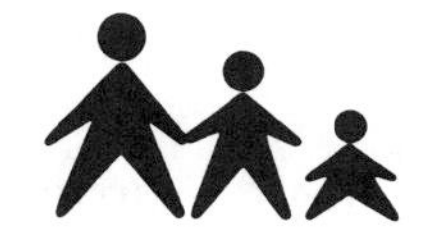

Diagnostic Comorbidity, Attentional Measures, and Neurochemistry in Children with Attention Deficit Hyperactivity Disorder

VANSHDEEP SHARMA,[1] JEFFREY H. NEWCORN,[1] and JEFFREY M. HALPERIN[1,2]

DIAGNOSTIC CO-MORBIDITY: ADHD, DISORDERS OF CONDUCT AND COGNITIVE PROBLEMS

In past decades, children with behavior disorders and/or poor academic achievement were described by a variety of nonspecific diagnostic terms such as minimal brain dysfunction, hyperkinetic disorder, and learning disabilities. In *Diagnostic and Statistical Manual of Mental Disorders* (*DSM*) *3rd ed.,* (American Psychiatric Association, 1980), specific, operationally defined symptom clusters were introduced in an attempt to define more discrete diagnostic entities. The use of multiple diagnoses within the same individual was encouraged when these symptom clusters overlapped. Diagnostic criteria for these disorders have evolved over the various iterations of *DSM*, although the core features have not changed substantially. The current categories for these syndromes are attention deficit hyperactivity disorder (ADHD), oppositional defiant disorder (ODD), conduct disorder (CD), and several Axis II specific developmental disorders (SDDs) (APA, 1994).

In *DSM-IV*, ADHD is identified by a persistent, severe pattern of inattention and/or hyperactivity-impulsivity symptoms, compared with other children of the same gender and at a comparable developmental level. The age at onset of some of the symptoms must be younger than 7 years. Furthermore, some symptoms causing impairment in either social or academic/occupational functioning must be evident in more than one setting. The ADHD category is further divided into three subtypes: combined, in which threshold criteria for both inattention and hyperactivity/impulsivity are present; primarily inattentive, in which threshold symptomatology for inattention is reached, with five or fewer hyperactivity/impulsivity symptoms present (six are required for diagnosis); and primarily hyperactive/impulsive, in which the threshold for hyperactive/impulsive symptoms is reached, but there are five or fewer inattention symptoms (again, with six required for diagnosis).

The essential feature of CD is a persistent pattern of behavior in which the basic rights of others or major age-appropriate societal norms or rules are violated. Three symptoms (one in the past 6 months) are required from a rather lengthy and heterogeneous list of behaviors. As is the case for ADHD, CD symptoms are seen in more than one setting and cause significant impairment in functioning. Subtypes of CD are determined on the basis of age at onset. Childhood-onset CD is diagnosed in children who show at least one of the behaviors before 10 years of age, while the adolescent-onset subtype is characterized by

[1]Department of Psychiatry, Division of Child and Adolescent Psychiatry, The Mount Sinai School of Medicine, New York, New York.

[2]Neuropsychology Graduate Program, Queens College, City University of New York, Flushing, New York

the absence of any CD behaviors before 10 years of age. The essential feature of ODD is a recurrent pattern of negativistic, defiant, and hostile behavior toward authority figures. Often there is a mixture of CD and ODD symptoms. Children with SDD are characterized by poor academic, linguistic, speech, or motor skills that are not due to demonstrable neurologic disorders, pervasive developmental disorders, mental retardation, or lack of educational opportunities.

The rationale for placing ADHD, CD, and ODD together in the attention deficit disruptive behavior disorders (AD-DBDs) group is that similar types of problems are present in children with these disorders. Also, among the three disorders that constitute the AD-DBD group, there is a high rate of comorbidity. Data from several epidemiologic studies (Szatmari et al., 1989; Esser et al., 1990; Kashani et al., 1987; Anderson et al., 1987; Bird et al., 1988) indicate that ODD and/or CD are present in 40% to 70% of children with ADHD. Conversely, among children with ODD and/or CD in these same studies, 40% to 60% are estimated to also have ADHD. Overlap of ODD and CD symptomatology is so frequent that these two diagnoses are not made together. Children who meet the criteria for CD and ODD are diagnosed with CD only.

Comorbidity between the AD-DBD group and other diagnostic categories is also quite common (Jensen et al., 1988; Kovacs et al., 1988, Livingston et al., 1990; Woolston et al., 1989). It has been estimated that 15% to 20% of children with ADHD have comorbid mood disorders (Barkley et al., 1991; Biederman et al., 1991a, 1991b, 1992), 20% to 25% have anxiety disorders (Biederman et al., 1991b, 1991c, 1992; Pliszka, 1992) and 6% to 20% have learning disabilities (Forness et al., 1992). However, when a broader definition of academic underachievement is used, the rates show a wide variability to ≤90% (Cantwell & Baker, 1991; Hinshaw, 1992; McGee & Share, 1988; Semrud-Clikeman et al., 1992). Other conditions that may occur comorbidly with the AD-DBDs include Tourette's disorder (TD) (Pauls et al., 1986; Comings and Comings, 1984, 1987), drug and alcohol abuse syndromes (Wood et al., 1983; Eyre et al., 1982; Alterman et al., 1984) and mental retardation (Hunt and Cohen, 1988; Koller et al., 1983). Thus, in our current diagnostic nomenclature, the majority of children who are diagnosed with ADHD have at least one other comorbid diagnosis. Also, the clinical presentation of ADHD children may differ considerably as a function of this comorbidity.

Perhaps owing to this high degree of comorbidity, attempts to establish the discriminant validity of ADHD with respect to other psychiatric disorders have been fraught with difficulties. Whereas several measures significantly distinguish between ADHD children and normal control subjects, few measures consistently distinguish between ADHD children and those with other psychiatric disorders (Koriath et al., 1985; Werry et al., 1987). Furthermore, despite the high degree of reliability and overall consistency of the ADHD syndrome, there is considerable variability in presenting symptoms (APA, 1994), response to treatment (Barkley, 1977; Halperin et al., 1986), and long-term outcome (Gittelman et al., 1985; Weiss et al., 1985). This has caused some people to question the validity of ADHD as a discrete syndrome (Prior and Sanson, 1986). Others maintain that these differences are accounted for by associated features (Biederman et al., 1991b; August and Garfinkel, 1989).

One approach to unraveling this heterogeneity and attempting to identify more homogeneous subgroups of ADHD children has been to study the impact of different patterns of comorbidity on the overall syndrome. Comorbidity is defined by the presence of more than one diagnosis in a single patient, and suggests that the child has symptom patterns characteristic of all of his/her comorbid diagnoses. Children in whom two syndromes occur comorbidly should have the defining symptoms of both syndromes and should resemble both diagnostic groups in terms of correlates of the disorder. However, a variety of other possibilities exists. For example, children with certain patterns of comorbidity may have symptoms that are specific to the comorbid group rather than any of the individual diagnoses.

This latter possibility suggests that children in the comorbid group may represent a distinct subgroup with a slightly different disorder. Alternatively, it is possible that what we call "comorbidity" of two disorders is a reflection of the fact that these disorders are actually related and not truly independent. For example, the nature and/or defining characteristics of the two disorders may overlap sufficiently that comorbidity is virtually guaranteed. In this case, comorbidity would not truly describe two separate disorders but rather would represent an artifact of a poorly constructed diagnostic system. A variation on this theme is that two distinct disorders might appear to overlap because of problems in measurement, either because of difficulties in obtaining accurate and specific information or because information that might distinguish different disorders might not have been included in the diagnostic algorithm (Achenbach et al., 1991). Another possibility is that one disorder could serve as a predisposing factor in the development of a second disorder, making the two disorders interrelated and therefore more likely to co-occur, even if their defining characteristics are fundamentally different (Caron and Rutter, 1991).

To clarify the nature of comorbidity in children with AD-DBDs, and to determine which of the above possibilities exists, it is necessary to closely examine the specific symptoms that constitute the various syndromes. A comprehensive review (Hinshaw, 1987) of the relationship between inattention/hyperactivity and aggression in children indicates that, while these symptom dimensions often overlap in the same child, they have distinct correlates, suggesting their validity as independent and clinically meaningful symptom dimensions. Inattention/hyperactivity is associated with greater learning and cognitive problems, whereas aggressive behavior is associated with social disadvantage, family conflict, parental sociopathy, and poorer long-term outcome. Yet, if these dimensions are truly independent, why do they coexist with such great frequency?

CLINICAL ASSESSMENT OF DISRUPTIVE DISORDERS

One important methodological problem related to the task of disentangling ADHD, ODD, and CD is that establishing diagnoses often requires the collection of data from several sources. Symptoms of these disorders are frequently not visible in the clinician's office, and may occur differently in different settings. The most commonly used assessment tools have been behavior rating scales and clinical interviews.

Behavior rating scales permit the systematic acquisition of information from parents and teachers and have been a mainstay in the clinical assessment of ADHD children for >20 years. Yet, because of halo effects, children with behavior disorders may be erroneously rated as impaired across multiple symptom domains. For example, children who are disruptive and defiant are frequently rated by teachers as inattentive and overactive even if they are not (Schacher et al., 1986, Abikoff et al., 1993). Thus, information derived from rating scales may indicate that children with behavioral problems have symptoms of multiple *DSM* diagnoses, whether or not they actually do. In particular, teacher ratings are likely to overestimate the presence of ADHD in children with ODD and CD.

Comorbidity has also been evaluated by use of structured diagnostic interviews; in the case of AD-DBDs, this generally involves interviewing the parents. However, excessive reliance on structured interviews can also be problematic. For one thing, parents may not understand the subtle differences among symptoms, and they may not have adequate information about behavior in other settings (e.g., school) to respond accurately (Mitsis et al., 1997). Certainly, there is no reason to believe that parents' subjective impressions are better than teachers' for discriminating among inattentive and disruptive behaviors. Yet, for practical purposes, parents are generally the source of this information. While there are no studies documenting the presence of halo effects in clinical interviews, parent reports in the assessment of ADHD have poor reliability (Rapoport et al., 1986). Consequently, the possibility that selective symptom identification in clinical interview data is inaccurate must be considered. If this were true, it might contribute to an artificially inflated rate of comorbid diagnoses within the disruptive behavior disorder domain.

NEUROPSYCHOLOGICAL ASSESSMENT

Neuropsychological assessment can provide assistance in evaluating symptoms in children with attention deficits and/or disruptive behavior. This approach provides a more objective assessment of attention, inhibitory control, and learning abilities, and it is far less likely to be susceptible to rater bias and halo effects. Neuropsychological assessments generally include tests of intelligence (e.g., WISC-III), academic achievement, and more specific aspects of linguistic, perceptual/motor, and attentional functioning. Many clinicians and investigators have turned to neuropsychological tests to elicit data that can be helpful in diagnosing ADHD. However, while neuropsychological test data are frequently useful for planning treatment, and should not be overlooked as an important source of information, these tests rarely yield data that clearly distinguish ADHD from other related disorders. In this regard, it is important to note that no single neuropsychological test is pathognomonic for ADHD.

The WISC-III is a test of overall intellectual functioning. Factor analytic studies have found that the WISC-III subtests generate orthogonal Verbal Comprehension, Perceptual Organization, Freedom from Distractibility (FDI), and Processing Speed (PSI) indices. Poor performance on the FDI, which is composed of the Arithmetic and Digit Span subtests, and the PSI, composed of the Coding and Symbol Search subtests, may be indicative of ADHD. However, this interpretation must be made with extreme caution because children with learning disabilities also perform worse than control subjects on both of these indices. No consistent pattern of subtest scores on the WISC-III has been found to uniquely distinguish ADHD children from non-ADHD children (Wechsler, 1991).

Paper-and-pencil target cancellation tests are also frequently used in the assessment of attention. These tests, which come in a variety of forms, typically require the child to scan a page with letters, numbers, or geometric figures, and cross off as many of the designated targets as possible. Thus, these tests require vigilance, perceptual-motor speed, visual search, and selection. Dependent measures include speed, accuracy, or both. Some data suggest that cancellation test performance may distinguish ADHD children from control subjects (Aman and Turbott, 1986). Yet, these tests have more consistently been found to distinguish children with learning problems (Rudel et al., 1978). One study (Matier et al., 1994) designed to assess the psychometric properties and clinical utility of a cancellation test, the Target Detection Test (TDT), found performance to be age-related between 6 and 11 years, with no gender effects. Furthermore, factor analysis of the six TDT subtests yielded two factors that differentially correlated with inattention, impulsivity, and academic achievement deficits. Thus, as with most measures of cognitive processing, cancellation tests are multidimensional, and performance on them may be affected by a variety of cognitive (perceptual speed, ability to organize a search, and visual-motor speed) and behavioral (activity level, impulse control) factors, in addition to attention.

The Matching Familiar Figures Test (MFF) has also been used to distinguish ADHD children from control subjects. This test of Impulsivity-Reflectivity requires children to perform a matching-to-sample task in which latency to respond and number of errors are measured. Presumably, impulsive children respond quickly, with a high number of errors, whereas reflective children respond slowly with few errors. The MFF has been shown to distinguish ADHD children from control subjects, but data have been inconsistent with regard to which measure appears deviant (Douglas, 1983). Some studies have found ADHD children to have a shorter response latency, and other studies have found a greater number of errors. Relatively few studies have found ADHD children to differ on both measures, which would be required to clearly define impulsivity. Furthermore, differences between ADHD children and control subjects are not specific. A variety of other patient groups, including those with learning problems and CD, have been shown to differ from normal control subjects on the MFF.

For nearly 20 years, investigators have hypothesized that deficits in executive function are involved in the pathophysiology of ADHD and that this dysfunction is mediated by circuits involving the prefrontal cortex (PFC). These hypotheses have been supported by more recent MRI data (Castellanos et al., 1996; Castellanos, 1997; Giedd et al., 1994; Hynd et al., 1993) indicating that the right PFC in children with ADHD may be smaller than in control subjects, and positron emission tomography data (Zametkin et al., 1993) indicating diminished glucose metabolism in the PFC of adults with ADHD. As a consequence, a burgeoning literature examining the performance of ADHD children on neuropsychological measures of PFC function has emerged in the last several years. Although a recent review (Barkley, 1997) concluded that considerable data provide evidence for the presence of inhibitory control and executive function deficits in children with ADHD relative to control subjects, it is notable that this literature is replete with inconsistent findings. Some investigators have attempted to reconcile these inconsistencies by examining the task demands of different neuropsychological tests. However, different studies report discrepant results from the same test, suggesting that some of the inconsistent findings may be due to sample, rather than test, characteristics.

Variability of findings in studies of executive function across different samples is consistent with the hypothesis that ADHD is diagnosed in a heterogeneous group of children, and that executive function deficits are present only in one or more subgroups of ADHD children. Several studies have therefore examined neuropsychological functioning in ADHD children with and without specific cognitive impairment. Some investigators have suggested that ADHD children with and without reading disabilities (RDs) constitute distinct subgroups that differ on measures of cognitive/neuropsychological and behavioral functioning (Purvis and Tannock, 1997; Pisecco et al., 1996; Hynd et al., 1995). Recently, Pennington, et al. (1993) reported a dissociation such that RD children with or without ADHD performed poorly on measures of phonological processing but not on measures of executive functioning. ADHD children without RD showed the opposite pattern: deficits on tests of executive function but not phonological processing. Recent data from our laboratory are consistent with the hypothesis that ADHD children without RD have PFC-related executive function deficits. Using a computerized version of Luria's Competing Motor Program task, we found that ADHD children without RD, unlike children in the RD group or the comorbid ADHD+RD groups, were selectively impaired in their ability to generate a response that was incompatible with stimulus characteristics (Hall et al., 1997). Additionally, the comorbid group was found to be different from the RD group, a finding not reported by others (McGee et al., 1989; Pennington et al., 1993). Overall, these data suggest that some, but not all, children with ADHD may have executive function deficits and that these children may represent an etiologically distinct subgroup.

ASSESSMENT OF CORE ADHD SYMPTOMS

Activity level has long been considered a central component of children's behavior disorders. Yet, the relative importance of overactivity, in comparison with inattention, in ADHD children has been the topic of considerable debate. Much of the research on children's activity level is derived from behavior ratings of motor activity (with questionable validity). There are many objective measures of activity level in children, but they have significant drawbacks as well. Examples include limitations on setting for stabilimeter chairs (Kendall and Brophy, 1981) and the requirement that highly trained observers be available to use direct observational methods (Abikoff et al., 1980). Actigraphs also have a long and checkered history. However, newer technology has provided a more accurate and versatile method of assessing activity, using acceleration-sensitive actigraphs with solid-state memory. These devices have facilitated the objective measurement of motor activity in a variety of settings over long periods of time. Research using actigraphs has demonstrated that ADHD boys are more active than control subjects (Porrino et al., 1983a) and that activity level is reduced following the administration of stimulant medication (Porrino et al., 1983b).

Although the use of actigraphs in a naturalistic setting may not be practical for clinical neuropsychological evaluations, reliable and valid measures of activity level obtained during a structured test session could be useful in both clinical and research efforts. To determine whether attention and activity level are distinct, it is advantageous to study them in a nonreferred sample because these children are more likely to have a wider range of attentional capacities and activity levels. Accordingly, we (Reichenbach et al., 1992) studied a group of nonreferred 6- to 13-year-old children using actigraph measures of activity and continuous performance test (CPT) measures of inattention (see below). Test-retest reliability of the actigraph during structured test sessions ($r = 0.85$, $p < 0.001$) was excellent. Furthermore, objective measures of activity level and attention were both correlated with age ($r = -0.57$, $p < 0.001$; $r = -0.46$, $p < 0.001$) but unrelated to each other after controlling for age ($r = -0.01, p > 0.10$). Finally, activity level, as measured by the actigraph, was significantly correlated with both parent and teacher ratings of hyperactivity but not with measures of cognitive function.

As briefly noted above, CPTs have been widely used as an objective measure of sustained attention. These tests require the subject to monitor a lengthy series of stimuli and to respond manually whenever a designated target stimulus appears. Despite its extensive use and considerable intuitive appeal, the neuropsychological processes assessed by the CPT remain unclear. Most investigators agree that CPT omission errors reflect deficits in attention, while commission errors reflect impulsive responding.

Like other purported measures of attention, the CPT discriminates several patient populations from normal control subjects (Werry et al., 1987). However, its ability to distinguish among distinct patient groups has not been conclusively demonstrated. Our laboratory has done extensive work with the CPT in an attempt to (1) refine the measures generated by the CPT and provide evidence of construct validity for these measures, and (2) determine the utility of the CPT for defining discrete symptom dimensions that may be used to identify more homogeneous subgroups of ADHD children.

Our experience using the *A-X* CPT, patterned after Rosvold et al. (Rosvold et al., 1956), suggested that, whereas many commission errors do indicate impulsive behavior, other psychologic processes may be operative. Unlike omission errors, which all occur under similar conditions, commission errors can occur in several different contexts. Specifically, there are four different situations under which a commission error can occur within the *A-X* paradigm: a child may erroneously respond to (1) letters other than *X* following an *A* (A-not-X error), (2) the letter *A* prior to the onset of the next letter (A-only error), (3) *X* not preceded by *A* (X-only error), or (4) letter sequences containing neither *A* nor *X* (Random error). We hypothesized that CPT commission errors do not constitute a unitary measure that is indicative of a single deficit (e.g., impulsivity) but rather that different subtypes of commission errors reflect deficits in different psychologic processes. Furthermore, we predicted that these differences in underlying psychologic processes would be reflected by different reaction times (RTs) for the distinct error subtypes.

CPT commission error subtypes were initially studied in a heterogeneous sample of child psychiatric patients. The number of omission errors, each of four hypothesized types of commission errors, and RTs were computed. All the hypothesized subtypes of commission errors occurred and were characterized by significantly different RTs as predicted (Halperin et al., 1991a).

Subsequently (Halperin et al., 1988; Halperin et al., 1991b), in a larger sample of nonreferred school children, these CPT subtypes were replicated and found to be differentially associated with teacher ratings of inattention and impulsivity. Misses and X-only commission errors were selectively correlated with ratings of inattention, whereas A-not-X commission errors were correlated with ratings of impulsivity, hyperactivity, and conduct problems. A-only and Random errors were unrelated to teacher ratings of behavior. Thus, the dimensions of inattention and impulsivity could be distinctly assessed with this objective measure.

We next attempted to explore the distinctions between behaviorally disturbed subgroups of children based on patterns of comorbidity using these newly developed CPT measures of inattention and impulsivity, as well as measures of academic achievement (Halperin et al., 1990a). A sample of 85 nonreferred school children was divided into four groups using the Inattention/Overactivity (I/O) and Aggression (A) scales of the IOWA Conners Teaching Rating Scale (Loney and Milich, 1982). The Pure ADHD group consisted of children with high I/O and low A ratings; the Pure Aggressive group consisted of children with high A and low I/O ratings; the Mixed ADHD/Aggressive group consisted of children with high scores on both scales; and control subjects had low ratings on both scales. The Pure ADHD group was found to be significantly more inattentive than all other groups, and the ADHD/Aggressive group was found to be significantly more impulsive than the Pure Aggressive and control groups. The Pure Aggressive group did not differ from the control group on any CPT measure. Although there were no significant group differences on either measure of academic achievement, there was a trend for the ADHD group to have lower reading scores.

These data indicate that many children who receive high scores on teacher rating scales, consistent with ADHD, are not inattentive as measured by the CPT. Furthermore, they suggest a dissociation between inattention and aggressive (or disruptive) behavior in children and raise the possibility that children can receive ratings consistent with ADHD by being *either* inattentive *or* disruptive, while relatively fewer children are *both* inattentive *and* impulsive as measured by the CPT.

To further explore the relationship of objectively assessed inattention to ADHD, a new sample of 72 nonreferred children was divided into two groups on the basis of teachers' ratings of *DSM-III-R* symptoms for ADHD (Halperin et al., 1990b). Children with at least eight of the 14 ADHD symptoms were entered into the ADHD group. Those with four or fewer symptoms were placed in the control group. Children rated as having five to seven ADHD symptoms were eliminated from the study in order to achieve separation of ADHD and control groups. Children were further divided into objectively assessed inattentive and noninattentive groups on the basis of their CPT performance. In addition, each child was rated by the Conners Teacher (CTQ) and Parent (CPQ) Questionnaires (Goyette et al., 1978) and tested with the WISC-R. Among the ADHD group, 47.4% were inattentive according to the CPT, compared with 13.6% of the control subjects (Chi-square = 6.57, $p = 0.01$). Thus, significantly more ADHD children than control subjects were objectively assessed as inattentive, but about half of the ADHD children were not found to be inattentive.

Two-way (ADHD × CPT-Inattention) analyses of variance were conducted examining the relationships of ADHD and objectively assessed inattention to behavioral and cognitive functioning. As expected, the ADHD children were rated significantly higher than control subjects on all factors of the CTQ, and on the Conduct Problems, Impulsivity/Hyperactivity, and Learning Problems factors of the CPQ. However, in addition to these main effects, significant ADHD × Inattention interactions were found selectively for the Conduct Problems factors of both the CTQ and the CPQ. On the CTQ, the noninattentive ADHD group was rated significantly higher than the inattentive ADHD group, and on the CPQ, only noninattentive ADHD children were rated as having more conduct problems than control subjects. With regard to cognitive functioning, there was a trend ($p < 0.10$) for an ADHD × Inattention interaction such that the inattentive ADHD group had a lower WISC-R FSIQ than the other three groups.

These data suggested that ADHD children do not constitute a homogeneous group with regard to attentional dysfunction and raised the question whether children with comorbid ADHD + conduct problems may not have the same presenting features as children with "pure" ADHD (i.e., the comorbid group may not be inattentive). Thus, within the larger category of ADHD, there appeared to be subgroups of Inattentive/Cognitively Impaired and Impulsive/Aggressive (but noninattentive) ADHD children. Objectively determined inattentive ADHD children were found to have low IQ scores, and noninattentive ADHD children were rated as aggressive. These findings were specific for the role of objectively assessed inattention among ADHD children; inattentive and noninattentive control children did not differ on measures of cognitive or behavioral functioning.

ASSESSMENT OF ATTENTION, IMPULSIVITY, AND ACTIVITY LEVEL IN REFERRED ADHD CHILDREN

Overall, our research with a nonreferred sample of children with ADHD suggested that (1) the dimensions of inattention, impulsivity, and hyperactivity could be distinctly assessed, and (2) these symptom domains may be differentially present in subgroups of children with ADHD. This latter conclusion is consistent with the *DSM-IV* approach of having a bidimensional symptom list for ADHD rather than the unidimensional, polythetic approach of *DSM-III-R*. However, for a clearer understanding of the variability of ADHD symptoms in different subgroups of children who were diagnosed with ADHD, it was necessary to study clinical populations. Therefore, a series of studies was conducted, using the objective measures described above, in a consecutive sample of children referred to an urban child psychiatry outpatient clinic. The objectives of this study were to determine (1) to what extent the symptoms of inattention, impulsivity, and overactivity are *uniquely characteristic* of children with ADHD and (2) whether the presentation of these ADHD core symptoms vary as a function of comorbidity and/or other associated features.

Two approaches were used to address the first question. Initially, 102 children (84 patients referred to a child psychiatry clinic and 18 normal control subjects) were studied (Halperin et al., 1992). Each child was administered a 1-hour psychometric test battery along with a CPT. Activity level was measured throughout the test session. The patients were divided into two groups according to the presence or absence of ADHD and, by use of the three objective measures, were compared with a sample of normal control subjects recruited from a local school. Both patient groups were found to be inattentive relative to control subjects but indistinguishable from each other. However, the ADHD group was more active than both non-ADHD patients and normal subjects, who did not differ from each other. Finally, the ADHD patients were significantly more impulsive than the control subjects, while the non-ADHD patient group did not differ from the other two groups.

These data suggested that children with ADHD were uniquely hyperactive but also raised questions regarding the extent to which both inattention and impulsivity were unique characteristics of ADHD patients. The fact that non-ADHD patients were inattentive on the CPT relative to control subjects and indistinguishable from those with ADHD suggested that inattention may be a nonspecific symptom of a psychopathologic condition in children. Further, the data indicated that children with ADHD were impulsive relative to control subjects but raised the possibility that at least some non-ADHD patients might also be impulsive, because these patients fell midway between the ADHD and control groups.

However, the possibility that these results were confounded by high rates of comorbidity in both the ADHD and non-ADHD patient groups remained. To eliminate this important confound, we reexamined the symptoms of inattention and impulsivity, as measured by the CPT, as a function of comorbidity. Three groups of patients were identified and were compared along with our existing sample of nonreferred control subjects. The three patient groups were composed of (1) ADHD children without any other comorbid disruptive, anxiety, or mood disorder; (2) ODD or CD children, without ADHD, mood disorders, or anxiety disorders; and (3) children with an anxiety disorder but no comorbidity with any of the AD-DBDs or mood disorders. Consecutive admissions (n = 244) to our clinic were screened for this purpose (Halperin et al., 1993a). The majority of children had comorbidity across conditions and could not be included in this study. However, a subgroup of 50 children was identified and divided into discrete ADHD-only, CD+ODD-only, and anxiety-only groups. These children were compared with those in a nonreferred control group. All three patient groups were found to have cognitive and academic achievement difficulties relative to the control group. In this relatively restricted, "pure" groups of patients, children with ADHD were found to be selectively inattentive and impulsive compared with those with other psychiatric disorders and controls. That is, the ADHD children made significantly more CPT inattention and impulsivity errors relative to the other patient groups and the nonreferred control subjects. These data supported the discriminant validity of a small subgroup of "pure" ADHD children (without any comorbidity) and demonstrated that as a group, these children could be distinguished from patients with anxiety as well as other disruptive disorders on objective measures. The fact that the larger group of children with ADHD (i.e., those including comorbidity) could not be distinguished from non-ADHD patients suggested that comorbid conditions might affect the symptoms in children with ADHD.

Consequently, we examined the extent to which comorbidity with other disruptive and anxiety disorders affected the symptoms of children with ADHD. Similarly to Pliszka (1992), we found that ADHD children with comorbid anxiety disorders were highly inattentive and hyperactive but were not impulsive as measured by the CPT. In contrast, children with ADHD+ODD/CD were both impulsive and inattentive and not appreciably different on CPT from ADHD children without comorbid disruptive disorders (suggesting that this group was truly comorbid). However, when these same children were redivided according to the presence or absence of aggressive behavior in the form of physical fighting, rather than by the presence or absence of the ODD/CD diagnoses, a different picture emerged. Two-way (ADHD × Fighting) analyses of variance indicated a significant main effect for ADHD for the objective measures of inattention, impulsivity, and activity level. In addition, there was a significant main effect for Fighting for the CPT-impulsivity measure such that children who fought were impulsive whether or not they had ADHD. Finally, there was a significant ADHD × Fighting interaction for CPT-inattention such that nonaggressive ADHD children were inattentive, but ADHD children who engaged in frequent fights were not. These data suggested that hyperactivity is unique and relatively consistent among children with ADHD. However, inattention is primarily present in ADHD who are not physically aggressive. Finally, while impulsivity is an independent characteristic of children with ADHD and children who fight, ADHD children who fight were clearly the most impulsive (Halperin et al., 1995).

Taken together, these data suggest that children with ADHD have characteristic core symptoms of inattention, impulsivity, and hyperactivity, as ascertained by objective measures, and that this pattern of symptoms is less clearly present in children with other psychiatric disorders but not ADHD. However, these symptom dimensions are not uniformly high across all children with ADHD. Rather, there appear to be distinct subgroups of children with ADHD, some of whom are primarily inattentive and others who are primarily impulsive. Whereas impulsivity appears to be differentially associated with aggressive behavior among ADHD children, the data (principally from our nonreferred samples) suggest that inattention is more closely associated with cognitive impairment. This differentiation of inattentive/cognitively impaired and impulsive/aggressive children with ADHD closely parallels the distinction between primarily "behavioral" and "cognitive" subtypes described by other investigators (August and Garfinkel, 1989; Shaywitz and Shaywitz, 1991). We subsequently hypothesized that these two groups of ADHD children were distinct not only with regard to symptom presentation but also with regard to their underlying pathophysiologic states (Halperin et al., 1991c).

One possible limitation of this research must be appreciated. The studies described above were conducted using the *DSM-III*-R definition of ADHD, which required a fixed number of ADHD symptoms to be present but did not stipulate that inattention, impulsivity, and hyperactivity symptoms all had to be present in equal proportions. That type of definition would seem to accentuate any problem with heterogeneity. This is not the case in *DSM-IV*, in which requisite numbers of inattention and hyperactivity/impulsivity symptoms are required to meet the criteria for the combined subtype of ADHD. Therefore, one might expect similar studies using the *DSM-IV* for ADHD, combined subtype, rather than *DSM-III-R* critieria, to result in decreased variability in symptomatic presentation. However, we believe that the new structure of the ADHD diagnosis would not greatly alter these findings because of the many problems described earlier in assessing specific symptoms reliably, halo effects from ratings, etc. Indeed, our initial investigations using the *DSM-IV* criteria for ADHD have continued to indicate heterogeneity among ADHD children on objective measures of core symptom domains (Marks et al., 1997).

NEUROBIOLOGIC MECHANISMS IN INATTENTIVE/COGNITIVELY IMPAIRED AND IMPULSIVE/AGGRESSIVE SUBGROUPS OF CHILDREN WITH ADHD

We (Halperin et al., 1991c) previously hypothesized that inattentive/cognitively impaired (IN/CI) and impulsive/aggressive (IMP/AGG) subgroups of children with ADHD would differ with regard to noradrenergic (NA) and serotonergic (5-HT) function such that the IN/CI group would be impaired on measures of NA function whereas the IMP/AGG group would be deficient in central 5-HT function. These hypotheses were based on an extensive literature in animals (Soubrie, 1986; Higley et al., 1992; Mehlman et al., 1994) and adults (Linnoila et al., 1993; Coccaro et al., 1989; Brown and Linnoila, 1990; Virkkunen et al., 1995) indicating an association between diminished 5-HT function and impulsive aggression, and studies in animals (Aston-Jones, 1985; Berridge et al., 1993) and adults (Posner and Petersen, 1990; Clark et al., 1987) indicating a central role for the NA-rich locus coeruleus (LC) in the regulation of attention.

To test these hypotheses, central 5-HT function was assessed in children with ADHD by the prolactin response to a challenge dose of the 5-HT releaser/reuptake inhibitor fenfluramine (Halperin et al., 1994), and NA function was assessed by plasma levels of the NA metabolite methoxyhydroxyphenylglycol (MHPG) (Halperin et al., 1993b). The data provided partial support for the hypothesized distinctions but suggested that the heterogeneity among children with ADHD cannot be accounted for fully by this simple bivariate dissociation.

Importantly, in this new sample, completely distinct IN/CI and IMP/AGG subgroups could not be formed. When the sample was divided according to the presence or absence of cognitive disabilities, as ascertained by measures of academic achievement, the cognitively impaired group tended to be less aggressive. Yet, when divided according to the presence or absence of aggressive behavior, the subgroups did not differ significantly on measures of cognitive function. Therefore, parallel analyses were conducted, examining separately the relationship of aggression and cognitive dysfunction to neurochemistry in these children with ADHD.

With regard to NA function, the data were highly consistent. Among children with ADHD, those with cognitive dysfunction, as determined by the presence of a learning disability, had higher levels of the NA metabolite MHPG than children without learning problems (Halperin et al., 1993b). This finding, which has been replicated in an independent sample (Halperin et al., 1997b), is consistent with data from other investigators who have found that children with ADHD tend to fall into distinct "high" and "low" subgroups with regard to urinary MHPG (Shekim et al., 1979; Khan and Dekirmenjian, 1981). We hypothesized that this distinction may be related to the nature of the NA dysfunction in the different subgroups of children with ADHD. Specifically, ADHD children characterized primarily by attentional problems and cognitive dysfunction may have dysregulation of the NA-rich LC, primarily via disruption to presynaptic alpha-2 receptors. This in turn results in dysfunction of the "posterior attentional system" (Posner et al., 1987). Some investigators have embraced this mechanism as the core dysfunction in all children with ADHD (Mefford and Potter, 1989; Pliszka et al., 1996). In contrast, our hypothesis—that children with ADHD who have primarily behavioral, but not cognitive, dysfunction have a different NA deficit—was more consistent with the findings of Arnsten and colleagues (Arnsten et al., 1996). Lesion studies in animals indicate that diminished function of the LC results in a deafferentation of alpha-2 receptors in the prefrontal cortex, with supersensitive postsynaptic receptors. This, in turn, results in the impulsive/disorganized behavior characteristic of children with ADHD.

Although distinct NA mechanisms are hypothesized for the different subgroups of children with ADHD, both should be improved by treatment with stimulant medications, such as methylphenidate and amphetamine, which have powerful effects on central NA transmission. Furthermore, postjunctional alpha-2 receptors, which are stimulated via NA projections emanating from the LC, are located on non-NA fibers in the PFC and may particularly affect dopamine (DA)-rich neurons (Arnsten and Goldman-Rakic, 1985; Gresch et al., 1995). Several recent genetic studies of ADHD also highlight the importance of DA mechanisms in the pathophysiology of ADHD (Swanson et al., 1998) The fact that stimulant medications have robust effects on both NA and DA systems, and are particularly well suited to regulating NA/DA homeostasis, may explain their powerful effect in treating ADHD. The multiple neurotransmitter model also serves to explain why stimulant medications appear to be more effective than most purer NA medications such as the tricyclic antidepressants (Rapoport et al., 1974) and the alpha-2 adrenergic agonists, clonidine and guanfacine (Hunt, 1987).

The role of 5-HT in the pathophysiology of ADHD is less clear. The data suggest that although central 5-HT function is intimately involved in aggression, this is, to a large extent, independent of ADHD. We initially reported that central 5-HT responsivity was elevated in aggressive compared with nonaggressive ADHD children (Halperin et al., 1994). This finding is in the opposite direction of that typically reported in animals and adults, where aggression has been found to be associated with reduced 5-HT function. Nonetheless, the finding of increased 5-HT function associated with aggression in youths was replicated in two other studies. One of these studies (Castellanos et al., 1994) was also conducted in a sample of children with ADHD; it assessed central 5-HT function via cerebrospinal fluid levels of the 5-HT metabolite 5-HIAA. The other study (Pine et al., 1997), which measured the prolactin response to fenfluramine challenge, examined a nonreferred sample of siblings of adjudicated adolescents. Contrary to these results, we did not replicate the finding of increased 5-HT responsivity in a second sample of ADHD children (Halperin et al., 1997b), and others have reported reduced rather than enhanced 5-HT function in aggressive youths (Kruesi et al., 1990, 1993).

While the precise nature of the association between ADHD, aggression, and 5-HT function in youth is not clear at this point, a systematic examination of data across studies suggests that ADHD does not appear to account for the inconsistency of findings (Schulz et al., 1998). We (Halperin et al., 1997b) and others (Pine et al., 1997) have speculated that developmental factors may account in part for the directional difference in findings between children and adults (i.e., elevated rather than blunted serotonergic function). It is possible that the 5-HT system, which may initially be overactive in aggressive youth, may downregulate more rapidly as these aggressive children grow older. However, examination of our data and that of others indicates that aggressive children (with or without ADHD) are highly variable with regard to 5-HT function and casts some doubt as to whether a simple downregulation model can explain the findings. Certainly, in our data set, and to some extent across studies, aggressive children may have either relatively low or high 5-HT responsivity. Furthermore, there is no characteristic pattern of 5-HT responsivity in nonaggressive children, who also may demonstrate relatively high or low function.

While this pattern of results might seem to indicate that there is not a consistent or meaningful relationship between 5-HT and aggression in children, subgroup analyses in our data as well as others suggest that 5-HT function may be an important moderator of outcome in aggression, rather than a state marker for this behavior. It may be that among aggressive children, those with low 5-HT function (which is characteristic of aggressive adults) are more likely to develop more severe aggression over time, whereas children with high 5-HT responsivity are less likely to become aggressive adults. This hypothesis is supported by data indicating that, among aggressive children, low 5-HT function is associated with several risk factors for the persistence of this maladaptive behavior. When samples across studies are compared, those in whom aggression was associated with low 5-HT function (Kruesi et al., 1990, 1993) were far more aggressive than the samples in any of the studies finding a positive association between 5-HT and aggression (Halperin et al., 1994; Castellanos et al., 1994; Pine et al., 1997). In addition, we found that aggressive children with relatively low 5-HT function, compared with aggressive children with relatively high 5-HT function, (1) were rated as more aggressive and are more likely to have CD (Halperin et al., 1997a), (2) were more likely to have aggressive parents (Halperin et al., 1997a), (3) were more likely to be aggressive in multiple settings (i.e., home and school) (McKay et al., 1996), (4) were more affectively labile and impulsive (Newcorn et al., 1996), and (5) had a threefold increase in the incidence of aggressive/antisocial behavior in their first- and second-degree relatives (McKay et al., 1995). Thus, among aggressive children, low 5-HT function is associated with several known risk factors for the persistence of this maladaptive behavior. The fact that only about half of aggressive children progress to increased aggressive behavior and antisocial personality disorder as adolescents and adults, while the remainder desist in their aggression (Loeber et al., 1993; Fergusson et al., 1996), raises the possibility that differences in 5-HT function in childhood may have differential predictive value with regard to long-term outcome.

CONCLUSIONS: IMPLICATIONS OF HETEROGENEITY AMONG ADHD CHILDREN FOR DIAGNOSIS AND TREATMENT

We have described an initial group of studies that used the CPT to further our understanding of the relationship of objectively measured symptoms of inattention and impulsivity to the diagnostic entity of ADHD. The results of these studies challenged the notion that ADHD children constitute a unitary group and led to the hypothesis that ADHD children may constitute distinct inattentive/cognitively impaired and impulsive/aggressive subgroups. We subsequently conducted research that has attempted to elucidate the neurobiologic underpinnings of these different ADHD subgroups. Although not all our *a priori* hypotheses regarding the neurochemical substrates of these different ADHD symptom domains were fully confirmed, several important directions emerged. The findings indicate that ADHD children with and without cognitive impairment differ with regard to noradrenergic function (a finding that has held in several different studies conducted by our group, using different measures of NA function), and that at least some impulsive/aggressive children have a dysfunction mediated by serotonergic mechanisms.

These data clearly indicate that ADHD children are heterogeneous with regard to behavioral, cognitive, and neurochemical function. Furthermore, although the full pattern of interrelationships is not yet apparent, variability across these three domains is not orthogonal (i.e., variability in these domains is not independent). As such, it is unlikely that future studies comparing normal control subjects with the large, diverse group of children labeled as having ADHD will substantially further our understanding of the neural basis of this disorder. Rather, future research should focus either on more homogeneous subgroups of children currently labeled as having ADHD, or on the distinct symptom dimensions believed to be impaired in these children. Such research could potentially provide data that would allow us to move away from the current atheoretical approach to diagnosis and lead to a more hypothesis-driven approach to treatment of this condition, using selective pharmacologic interventions that are individually tailored to a child's constellation of presenting symptoms and/or neurobiologic status.

REFERENCES

Abikoff, H., Courtney, M., Pelham, W.E. & Koplewicz, H.S. (1993), Teachers' ratings of disruptive behaviors: The influence of halo effects. *J. Abnorm. Child Psychol.* 21:519–533.

Abikoff, H., Gittelman, R. & Klein, D.F. (1980), Classroom observation code for hyperactive children: A replication of validity. *J. Consult. Clin. Psychol.*, 48:555–565.

Achenbach, T.M., Howell, C.T., Quay, H.C. & Conners, C.K. (1991), National survey of problems and competencies among four- to sixteen-year-olds: Parents' reports for normative and clinical samples. *Monogr. Soc. Res. Child Dev.*, 56:1–131.

Alterman A.I., Tarter, R.E., Baughman, T.G., Bober, B.A. & Fabian, S.A. (1984), Differentiation of alcoholics high and low in childhood hyperactivity. *Drug Alcohol Dependence*, 15:111.

Aman, M.G. & Turbott, S.H. (1986), Incidental learning, distraction, and sustained attention in hyperactive and control subjects. *J. Abnorm. Child Psychol.,* 14:441–455.

American Psychiatric Association (1980), *Diagnostic and Statistical Manual of Mental Disorders, 3rd ed.* Washington, DC: American Psychiatric Association.

American Psychiatric Association (1994), *Diagnostic and Statistical Manual of Mental Disorders, 4th ed.* Washington, DC: American Psychiatric Association.

Anderson, J.C., Williams, S.M., McGee, R. & Silva, P.A. (1987), *DSM-III* disorders in preadolescent children: Prevalence in a large sample from the general population. *Arch. Gen. Psychiatry*, 44:69–76.

Arnsten, A.F.T. & Goldman-Rakic, P.S. (1985), Alpha-2 adrenergic mechanisms in prefrontal cortex associated with cognitive decline in aged nonhuman primates. *Science*, 230:1273–1276.

Arnsten, A.F.T., Steere, J.C. & Hunt, R.D. (1996), The contribution of α-2-noradrenergic mechanisms to prefrontal cortical cognitive function: Potential significance for attention-deficit hyperactivity disorder. *Arch. Gen. Psychiatry*, 53:448–455.

Aston-Jones, G. (1985), Behavioral functions of locus coeruleus derived from cellular attributes. *Physiol. Psychol.,* 13:118–126.

August, G.J. & Garfinkel, B.D. (1989), Behavioral and cognitive subtypes of ADHD. *J. Am. Acad. Child Adolesc. Psychiatry*, 28:739–748.

Barkley, R.A. (1977), A review of stimulant drug research with hyperactive children. *J. Child Psychol. Psychiatry*, 18:137–165.

Barkley, R.A. (1997), Attention-deficit/hyperactivity disorder, self-regulation, and time: Toward a more comprehensive theory. *J. Dev. Behav. Pediatr.,* 18:271–279.

Barkley, R.A., Fischer, M., Edelbrock, C. & Smallish, L. (1991), The adolescent outcome of hyperactive children diagnosed by research criteria: III. Mother–child interactions, family conflicts and maternal psychopathology. *J. Child Psychol. Psychiatry*, 32:233–255.

Berridge, C.W., Arnsten, A.F. & Foote, S.L. (1993), Noradrenergic modulation of cognitive function: Clinical implications of anatomical, electrophysiological and behavioural studies in animal models. *Psychol. Med.,* 23:557–564.

Biederman, J., Faraone, S.V., Keenan, K. & Steingard, R. (1991c), Familial association between attention deficit disorder and anxiety disorders. *Am. J. Psychiatry*, 148:251–256.

Biederman, J., Faraone, S.V., Keenan, K. & Tsuang, M.T. (1991a), Evidence of familial association between attention deficit disorder and major affective disorders. *Arch. Gen. Psychiatry*, 48:633–642.

Biederman, J., Faraone, S.V. & Lapey, K. (1992), Comorbidity of diagnosis in attention-deficit hyperactivity disorder. In: *Attention-Deficit Hyperactivity Disorder,* ed., G. Weiss. Philadelphia: W.B. Saunders, pp. 335–360.

Biederman, J., Newcorn, J. & Sprich, S. (1991b), Comorbidity of attention deficit hyperactivity disorder with conduct, depressive, anxiety, and other disorders. *Am. J. Psychiatry*, 148:564–577.

Bird, H.R., Canino, G., Rubio-Stipec, M. & Gould, M.S. (1988), Estimates of the prevalence of childhood maladjustment in a community survey in Puerto Rico: The use of combined measures. *Arch. Gen. Psychiatry*, 45:1120–1126.

Brown, G.L., Ebert, M.H., Goyer, P., Jimerson, D., Klein, W., Bunney WE & Goodwin, F. (1982), Aggression, suicide, and serotonin: Relationships to CSF amine metabolites. *Am. J. Psychiatry*, 139:741–746.

Brown, G.L. & Linnoila, M.I. (1990), CSF serotonin metabolite (5-HIAA) studies in depression, impulsivity, and violence: Symposium. Serotonin and its effects on human behavior (1989, Atlanta, Georgia). *J. Clin. Psychiatry*, 51(Suppl):31–41.

Cantwell, D.P. & Baker, L. (1991), Association between attention deficit-hyperactivity disorder and learning disorders. *J. Learn. Disabil.*, 24:88–95.

Caron, C. & Rutter, M. (1991), Comorbidity in child psychopathology: Concepts, issues and research strategies. *J. Child Psychol. Psychiatry*, 32:1063–1080.

Castellanos, F.X. (1997), Neuroimaging of attention-deficit hyperactivity disorder. *Child Adolesc. Psychiatr. Clin. North Am.,* 6:383–411.

Castellanos, F.X., Elia, J., Kruesi, M.J., Gulotta, C.S., Mefford, I., Potter, W., Ritchie, G. & Rapoport, J.L. (1994), Cerebrospinal fluid monoamine metabolites in boys with attention-deficit hyperactivity disorder. *Psychiatr. Res.,* 52:305–316.

Castellanos, F.X., Giedd, J.N., Marsh, W.L. & Hamburger, S.D. (1996), Quantitative brain magnetic resonance imaging in attention-deficit hyperactivity disorder. *Arch. Gen. Psychiatry*, 53:607–616.

Clark, C.R., Geffen, G.M. & Geffen, L.B. (1987), Catecholamines and attention: I. Animal and clinical studies. *Neurosci. Biobehavior. Rev.*, 11:341–352.

Coccaro, E.F., Siever, L.J., Klar, H.M., Maurer, G., Cochrane, K., Cooper, T.B., Mohs, R.C. & Davis, K.L. (1989), Serotonergic studies in patients with affective and personality disorders: Correlates with suicidal and impulsive aggressive behavior. *Arch. Gen. Psychiatry*, 46:587–599.

Comings, D.E. & Comings, B.G. (1984), Tourette's syndrome and attention deficit disorder with hyperactivity: Are they genetically related? *J. Am. Acad. Child Adolesc. Psychiatry*, 23:138–146.

Comings, D.E. & Comings, B.G. (1987), A controlled study of Tourette syndrome: I. attention deficit disorder, learning disorders, and school problems. *Am. J. Hum. Genet.,* 41:701–741.

Donnelly, M., Rapoport, J.L., Potter, W.Z. & Oliver, J. (1989), Fenfluramine and dextroamphetamine treatment of childhood hyperactivity: Clinical and biochemical findings. *Arch. Gen. Psychiatry*, 46:205–212.

Douglas, V.I. (1983), Attentional and cognitive problems. In: *Developmental Neuropsychiatry*, ed., M. Rutter. New York: Guilford Press, pp. 280–329.

Esser, G., Schmidt, M.H. & Woerner, W. (1990), Epidemiology and course of psychiatric disorders in school-age children: Results of a longitudinal study. *J. Child Psychol. Psychiatry*, 31:243–263.

Eyre, S.L., Rounsaville, B.J. & Kleber, H.D. (1982), History of childhood hyperactivity in a clinic population of opiate addicts. *J. Nerv. Ment. Dis.*, 170:522–529.

Fergusson, D.M., Lynskey, M.T. & Horwood, L.J. (1996), Factors associated with continuity and changes in disruptive behavior patterns between childhood and adolescence. *J. Abnorm. Child Psychol.*, 25:533–553.

Forness, S.R., Swanson, J.M., Cantwell, D.P. & Youpa, D. (1992), Stimulant medication and reading performance: Follow-up on sustained dose in ADHD boys with and without conduct disorders. *J. Learn. Disabil.*. 25:115–123.

Giedd, J.N., Castellanos, F.X., Casey, B.J. & Kozuch, P. (1994), Quantitative morphology of the corpus callosum in attention deficit hyperactivity disorder. *Am. J. Psychiatry*, 151:665–669.

Gittelman, R., Mannuzza, S., Shenker, R. & Bonagura, N. (1985), Hyperactive boys almost grown up: I. Psychiatric status. *Arch. Gen. Psychiatry*, 42:937–947.

Goyette, C.H., Conners, C.K., & Ulrich, R.F. (1978). Normative data on revised Conners Parent and Teacher Rating Scales. *J. Abnorm. Child Psychol.,* 6:221–236.

Gresch, P.J., Sved, A.F., Zigmond, M.J. & Finlay, J.M. (1995), Local influence of endogenous norepinephrine on extracellular dopamine in rat medial prefrontal cortex. *J. Neurochem.*, 65:111–116.

Hall, S.J., Halperin, J.M., Schwartz, S.T. & Newcorn, J.H. (1997), Behavioral and executive functions in children with attention-deficit hyperactivity disorder and reading disability. *J. Attention Disorders*, 1:235–247.

Halperin, J.M., Gittelman, R., Katz, S. & Struve, F.A. (1986), Relationship between stimulant effect, electroencephalogram, and clinical neurological findings in hyperactive children. *J. Am. Acad. Child Adolesc. Psychiatry*, 25:820–825.

Halperin, J.M., Matier, K., Bedi, G. & Sharma, V. (1992), Specificity of inattention, impulsivity, and hyperactivity to the diagnosis of attention-deficit hyperactivity disorder. *J. Am. Acad. Child Adolesc. Psychiatry*, 31:190–196.

Halperin, J.M., Newcorn, J.H., Kopstein, I., McKay, K.E., Schwartz, S.T., Siever, L.J. & Sharma, V. (1997a), Serotonin, aggression, and parental psychopathology in children with attention-deficit hyperactivity disorder. *J. Am. Acad. Child Adolesc. Psychiatry*, 36:1391–1398.

Halperin, J.M., Newcorn, J.H., Matier, K. & Bedi, G. (1995), Impulsivity and the initiation of fights in children with disruptive behavior disorders. *J. Child Psychol. Psychiatry*, 36:1199–1211.

Halperin, J.M., Newcorn, J.H., Matier, K. & Sharma, V. (1993a), Discriminant validity of attention-deficit hyperactivity disorder. *J. Am. Acad. Child Adolesc. Psychiatry*, 32:1038–1043.

Halperin, J.M., Newcorn, J.H., Schwartz, S.T. & McKay, K.E. (1993b), Plasma catecholamine metabolite levels in ADHD boys with and without reading disabilities. *J. Clin. Child Psychol.*, (Special Issue: *The Neuropsychologicalal Basis of Disorders Affecting Children and Adolescents*) 22:219–225.

Halperin, J.M., Newcorn, J.H., Schwartz, S.T., Sharma, V., Siever, L.J., Koda, V. & Gabriel, S. (1997b), Age-related changes in the association between serotonergic function and aggression in boys with ADHD. *Biol. Psychiatry*, 41:682–689.

Halperin, J.M., Newcorn, J.H. & Sharma, V. (1991c), Ritalin: Diagnostic comorbidity and attentional measures. In: *Ritalin: Theory and Patient Management*, eds. L.L., Greenhill & B.B. Osman. Larchmont, NY: Mary Ann Liebert, pp. 15–24.

Halperin, J.M., Newcorn, J.H., Sharma, V. & Healey, J.M. (1990b), Inattentive and noninattentive ADHD children: Do they constitute a unitary group? *J. Abnorm. Child Psychol.,* 18:437–449.

Halperin, J.M., O'Brien, J.D., Newcorn, J.H. & Healey, J.M. (1990a), Validation of hyperactive, aggressive, and mixed hyperactive/aggressive childhood disorders: A research note. *J. Child Psychol. Psychiatry*, 31:455–459.

Halperin, J.M., Sharma, V., Greenblatt, E. & Schwartz, S.T. (1991b), Assessment of the Continuous Performance Test: Reliability and validity in a nonreferred sample. *Psychol. Assess.*, 3:603–608.

Halperin, J.M., Sharma, V., Siever, L.J. & Schwartz, S.T. (1994), Serotonergic function in aggressive and nonaggressive boys with attention deficit hyperactivity disorder. *Am. J. Psychiatry*, 151:243–248.

Halperin, J.M., Wolf, L.E., Greenblatt, E.R. & Young, G. (1991a), Subtype analysis of commission errors on the continuous performance test in children. *Dev. Neuropsychol.*, 7:207–217.

Halperin, J.M., Wolf, L.E., Pascualvaca, D.M. & Newcorn, J.H. (1988), Differential assessment of attention and impulsivity in children. *J. Am. Acad. Child Adolesc. Psychiatry*, 27:326–329.

Higley, J.D., Mehlman, P.T., Taub, D.M. & Higley, S.B. (1992), Cerebrospinal fluid monoamine and adrenal correlates of aggression in free-range rhesus monkeys. *Arch. Gen. Psychiatry*, 49:436–441.

Hinshaw, S.P. (1987), On the distinction between attentional deficits/hyperactivity and conduct problems/aggression in child psychopathology. *Psychol. Bull.*, 101:443–463.

Hinshaw, S.P. (1992), Academic underachievement, attention deficits, and aggression: Comorbidity and implications for intervention. (Special Section: Comorbidity and Treatment Implications.) *J. Consult. Clin. Psychol.,* 60:893–903.

Hunt, R.D. (1987), Treatment effects of oral and transdermal clonidine in relation to methylphenidate: An open pilot study in ADD-H. *Psychopharmacol. Bull.*, 23:111–114.

Hunt, R.D. & Cohen, D.J. (1988), Attentional and neurochemical components of mental retardation: New methods for an old problem. In: *Mental Retardation and Mental Health: Classification, Diagnosis, Treatment Services*, eds., J.A. Stark, F.J. Menolascino, M.H. Albaralli, et al. New York: Springer-Verlag.

Hynd, G.W., Hern, K.L., Novey, E.S. & Eliopulos, D. (1993), Attention deficit-hyperactivity disorder and asymmetry of the caudate nucleus. *J. Child Neurol.*, 8:339–347.

Hynd, G.W., Morgan, A.E., Edmonds, J.E. & Black, K. (1995), Reading disabilities, comorbid psychopathology, and the specificity of neurolinguistic deficits. *Dev. Neuropsychol.*, 11:311–322.

Jensen, J.B., Burke, N. & Garfinkel, B.D. (1988), Depression and symptoms of attention deficit disorder with hyperactivity. *J. Am. Acad. Child Adolesc. Psychiatry*, 27:742–747.

Kashani, J.H., Beck, N.C., Hoeper, E.W. & Fallahi, C. (1987), Psychiatric disorders in a community sample of adolescents. *Am. J. Psychiatry*, 144:584–589.

Kendall, P.C. & Brophy, C. (1981), Activity and attentional correlates of teacher ratings of hyperactivity. *J. Pediatr. Psychol.*, 6:451–458.

Khan, A.U. & Dekirmenjian, H. (1981), Urinary excretion of catecholamine metabolites in hyperkinetic child syndrome. *Am. J. Psychiatry,* 138:108–110.

Koller, H., Richardson, S.A., Katz, M. & McLaren, J. (1983), Behavior disturbance since childhood among a 5-year birth cohort of all mentally retarded young adults in a city. *Am. J. Ment. Deficiency*, 87:386–395.

Koriath, U., Gualtieri, C.-T. & Van-Bourgondien, M.-E. (1985), Construct validity of clinical diagnosis in pediatric psychiatry: Relationship among measures. *J. Am. Acad. Child Adolesc. Psychiatry*, 24:429–436.

Kovacs, M., Paulauskas, S., Gatsonis, C. & Richards, C. (1988), Depressive disorders in childhood: III. A longitudinal study of comorbidity with and risk for conduct disorders. *J. Affect. Disorders* (Special Issue: *Childhood Affective Disorders*), 15:205–217.

Kruesi, M.J., Hibbs, E.D., Zahn, T.P. & Keysor, C.S. (1993), A 2-year prospective follow-up study of children and adolescents with disruptive behavior disorders: Prediction by cerebrospinal fluid 5-hydroxyindoleacetic acid, homovanillic acid, and autonomic measures. *Ann. Prog. Child Psychiatr. Child Dev.*, 1993: 284–300.

Kruesi, M.J., Rapoport, J.L., Hamburger, S. & Hibbs, E.D. (1990), Cerebrospinal fluid monoamine metabolites, aggression, and impulsivity in disruptive behavior disorders of children and adolescents. *Arch. Gen. Psychiatry*, 47:419–426.

Linnoila, M., Virkkunen, M., George, T. & Higley, D. (1993), Impulse control disorders:. International Scientific Symposium. Depression, OCD, Anxiety (1993, Mainz, Germany). *Int. Clin. Psychopharmacol.*, 8(suppl 1):S1–S56.

Livingston, R.L., Dykman, R.A. & Ackerman, P.T. (1990), The frequency and significance of additional self-reported psychiatric diagnoses in children with attention deficit disorder. *J Abnorm. Child Psychol.*, 18:465–478.

Loeber, R., Wung, P., Keenan, K. & Giroux, B. (1993), Developmental pathways in disruptive child behavior.X *Dev. Psychopathol.* (Special Issue: *Toward a Developmental Perspective on Conduct Disorder*), 51:103–133.

Loney, J. & Milich, R. (1982), Hyperactivity, inattention, and aggression in clinical practice. *Adv. Dev. Behav. Pediatr.*, 3:113–147.

Marks, D.J., Himelstein, J., Newcorn, J.H. & Halperin, J.M. (1997), Identification of AD/HD subtypes using laboratory symptom measures: A cluster analysis. *J. Abnorm. Child Psychol.*

Matier, K., Wolf, L.E. & Halperin, J.M. (1994), The psychometric properties and clinical utility of a cancellation test in children. *Dev. Neuropsychol.*, 10:165–177.

McGee, R. & Share, D.L. (1988), Attention deficit disorder-hyperactivity and academic failure: Which comes first and what should be treated? *J. Am. Acad. Child Adolesc. Psychiatry*. 27:318–325.

McGee, R., Williams, S., Moffitt, T. & Anderson, J. (1989), A comparison of 13-year-old boys with attention deficit and/or reading disorder on neuropsychological measures. *J. Abnorm. Child Psychol.,* 17:37–53.

McKay, K.E., Newcorn, J. & Halperin, J.M. (1996), Situationally vs. pervasively aggressive boys: Behavioral, cognitive, and neurochemical differences. *Scientific Proceedings of the Annual Meeting of the American Academy of Child & Adolescent Psychiatry*, 12:102.

McKay, K.E., Newcorn, J., Schulz, K., Kopstein, I., Schwartz, S.T. & Halperin, J.M. (1995), Serotonin, aggression, and family psychopathology in ADHD boys. *Scientific Proceedings of the Annual Meeting of the American Academy of Child & Adolescent Psychiatry*, 11:111.

Mefford, I.N. & Potter, W.Z. (1989), A neuroanatomical and biochemical basis for attention deficit disorder with hyperactivity in children: A defect in tonic adrenaline mediated inhibition of locus coeruleus stimulation. *Med. Hypotheses*, 29:33–42.

Mehlman, P.T., Higley, J.D., Faucher, I. & Lilly, A.A. (1994), Low CSF 5-HIAA concentrations and severe aggression and impaired impulse control in nonhuman primates. *Am. J. Psychiatry*, 151:1485–1491.

Mitsis, E.M., McKay, K.E., Schulz, K.P., Newcorn, J.H. & Halperin, J.M. (1997), Parent–teacher concordance on structured interview for disruptive behavior disorders. *Scientific Proceedings of the Annual Meeting of the American Academy of Child & Adolescent Psychiatry*, 13:142.

Newcorn, J., McKay, K.E., Loeber, R., Bonafina, M., Sharma, V. & Halperin, J.M. (1996), Emotionality and serotonergic function in aggressive and non-aggressive ADHD children. *Scientific Proceedings of the Annual Meeting of the American Academy of Child & Adolescent Psychiatry*, 12:94.

Pauls, D.L., Hurst, C.R., Kruger, S.D. & Leckman, J.F. (1986), Gilles de la Tourette's syndrome and attention deficit disorder with hyperactivity: Evidence against a genetic relationship. *Arch. Gen. Psychiatry*, 43:1177–1179.

Pennington, B.F., Groisser, D. & Welsh, M.C. (1993), Contrasting cognitive deficits in attention deficit hyperactivity disorder versus reading disability. *Dev. Psychol.*, 29:511–523.

Pine, D.S., Coplan, J.D., Wasserman, G.A., Miller, L.S., Fried, J.E., Davies, M., Cooper, T.B., Greenhill, L., Shaffer, D. & Parsons, B. (1997), Neuroendocrine response to fenfluramine challenge in boys: Associations with aggressive behavior and adverse rearing. *Arch. Gen. Psychiatry*, 54:839–846.

Pisecco, S., Baker, D.B., Silva, P.A. & Brooke, M. (1996), Behavioral distinctions in children with reading disabilities and/or ADHD. *J. Am. Acad. Child Adolesc. Psychiatry,* 35:1477–1484.

Pliszka, S.R. (1992), Comorbidity of attention-deficit hyperactivity disorder and overanxious disorder. *J. Am. Acad. Child Adolesc. Psychiatry*, 31:197–203.

Pliszka, S.R., McCracken, J.T. & Maas, J.W. (1996), Catecholamines in attention-deficit hyperactivity disorder: Current perspectives. *J. Am. Acad. Child Adolesc. Psychiatry,* 35:264–272.

Porrino, L.J., Rapoport, J.L., Behar, D., Ismond, D.R. & Bunney, W.E. Jr. (1983b), A naturalistic assessment of the motor activity of hyperactive boys: II. Stimulant drug effects. *Arch. Gen. Psychiatry*, 40:688–693.

Porrino, L.J., Rapoport, J.L., Behar, D., Sceery, W., Ismond, D.R. & Bunney, W.E. Jr. (1983a), A naturalistic assessment of the motor activity of hyperactive boys: I. Comparison with normal controls. *Arch. Gen. Psychiatry*, 40:681–687.

Posner, M.I., Inhoff, A.W., Friedrich, F.J. & Cohen, A. (1987), Isolating attentional systems: A cognitive-anatomical analysis. *Psychobiology*, 15:107–121.

Posner, M.I. & Petersen, S.E. (1990), The attention system of the human brain. *Ann. Rev. Neurosci.*, 13:25–42.

Prior, M. & Sanson, A. (1986), Attention deficit disorder with hyperactivity: A critique. *J. Child Psychol. Psychiatry*, 27:307–319.

Purvis, K.L. & Tannock, R. (1997), Language abilities in children with attention deficit hyperactivity disorder, reading disabilities, and normal controls. *J. Abnorm. Child Psychol.*, 25:133–144.

Rapoport, J.L., Donnelly, M., Zametkin, A. & Carrougher, J. (1986), "Situational hyperactivity" in a U.S. clinical setting. *J. Child Psychol. Psychiatry*, 27:639–646.

Rapoport, J.L., Quinn, P.O., Bradbard, G., Riddle, K.D. & Brooks, E. (1974), Imipramine and methylphenidate treatments of hyperactive boys: A double-blind comparison. *Arch. Gen. Psychiatry*, 30:789–93.

Reichenbach, L.C., Halperin, J.M., Sharma, V. & Newcorn, J.H. (1992), Children's motor activity: Reliability and relationship to attention and behavior. *Dev. Neuropsychol.*, 8:87–97.

Rosvold, H.E., Mirsky, A.F. & Sarason, I., et al. (1956), A continuous performance test of brain damage. *J. Consult. Psychol.*, 20:343–350.

Rudel, R.G., Denckla, M.B. & Broman, M. (1978), Rapid silent response to repeated target symbols by dyslexic and nondyslexic children. *Brain Language*, 6:52–62.

Schachar, R.J., Sandberg, S. & Rutter, M. (1986), Agreement between teachers' ratings and observations of hyperactivity, inattentiveness, and defiance. *J. Abnorm. Child Psychol.*, 14(2), 331–345.

Schulz, K.P., Newcorn, J.H., McKay, K.E., Koda, V., Himelstein, J., Sharma, V., Siever, L. & Halperin, J.M. (1998), Central serotonergic function and aggression in boys: Effect of ADHD. *Scientific Proceedings of the Annual Meeting of the American Academy of Child & Adolescent Psychiatry*, 14:91.

Semrud-Clikeman, M., Biederman, J., Sprich-Buckminster, S. & Lehman, B.K. (1992), Comorbidity between ADDH and learning disability: A review and report in a clinically referred sample. *J. Am. Acad. Child Adolesc. Psychiatry*, 31:439–448.

Shaywitz, B.A. & Shaywitz, S.E. (1991), Comorbidity: A critical issue in attention deficit disorder. *J. Child Neurol.*, 6 Suppl:S13–22.

Shekim, W.O., Dekirmenjian, H., & Chapel, J.L. (1979), Urinary MHPG excretion in minimal brain dysfunction and its modification by d-amphetamine. *Am. J. Psychiatry*, 136:667–671.

Soubrie, P. (1986), Reconciling the role of central serotonin neurons in human and animal behavior. *Behav. Brain Sci.*, 9:319–335.

Swanson, J.M., Sunohara, G.A., Kennedy, J.L., Reino, R., Fineberg, E., Wigal, T., Lerner, M., Williams, L., LaHoste, G.J. & Wigal, S. (1998), Association of the dopamine receptor D4 (DRD4) gene with a refined phenotype of attention deficit hyperactivity disorder (ADHD): A family-based approach. *Mol. Psychiatry*, 3:38–41.

Szatmari, P., Offord, D.R. & Boyle, M.H. (1989), Ontario Child Health Study: Prevalence of attention deficit disorder with hyperactivity. *J. Child Psychol. Psychiatry*, 30:219–230.

Virkkunen, M., Goldman, D., Nielsen, D.A. & Linnoila, M. (1995), Low brain serotonin turnover rate (low CSF 5-HIAA) and impulsive violence. *J. Psychiatry Neurosci.*, 20:271–275.

Wechsler, D. (1991), *The Wechsler Intelligence Scale for Children, 3rd ed.*, New York: The Psychological Corporation.

Weiss, G., Hechtman, L., Milroy, T. & Perlman, T. (1985), Psychiatric status of hyperactives as adults: A controlled prospective 15-year follow-up of 63 hyperactive children. *J. Am. Acad. Child Adolesc. Psychiatry*, 24:211–220.

Werry, J.S., Reeves, J.C. & Elkind, G.S. (1987), Attention deficit, conduct, oppositional, and anxiety disorders in children: I. A review of research on differentiating characteristics. *J. Am. Acad. Child Adolesc. Psychiatry*, 26:133–143.

Wood, D., Wender, P.H. & Reimherr, F.W. (1983), The prevalence of attention deficit disorder, residual type, or minimal brain dysfunction, in a population of male alcoholic patients. *Am. J. Psychiatry*, 140:95–98.

Woolston, J.L., Rosenthal, S.L., Riddle, M.A. & Sparrow, S.S. (1989), Childhood comorbidity of anxiety/affective disorders and behavior disorders. *J. Am. Acad. Child Adolesc. Psychiatry*, 28:707–713.

Zametkin, A.J., Liebenauer, L.L., Fitzgerald, G.A. & King, A.C. (1993), Brain metabolism in teenagers with attention-deficit hyperactivity disorder. *Arch. Gen. Psychiatry*, 50:333–340.

Section 6

The Pharmacology of Ritalin and Future Research

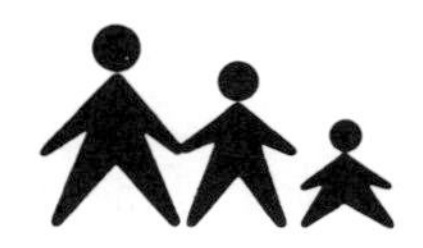

Generic Methylphenidate Versus Brand Ritalin: Which Should Be Used?

BENEDETTO VITIELLO[1] and LAURIE B. BURKE[2]

METHYLPHENIDATE PRODUCTS ON THE MARKET

Methylphenidate (MPH) is currently available as brand Ritalin (by Novartis, formerly Ciba-Geigy) and generic MPH (by MD Pharmaceuticals, Danbury Pharma, and Mallinckroot). Immediate-release tablets (5 mg, 10 mg, and 20 mg) and a slow-release formulation (20 mg) are available as both generic and brand-name preparations (Food and Drug Administration [FDA], 1998).

According to the National Prescription Audit of IMS America (IMS, 1996), out of a total projected 10.9 million prescriptions for MPH dispensed in 1996, 30% were for brand Ritalin and 70% for the generic product. The National Prescription Audit surveys retail pharmacies across the United States. Out of the universe of approximately 50,000 pharmacies, a sample of 40% was actually sampled.

PHARMACEUTICAL AND THERAPEUTIC EQUIVALENTS

According to the FDA standards, brand Ritalin and generic MPH are pharmaceutically and therapeutically equivalent. This equivalency implies that they can be substituted with the full expectation that each product will produce the same clinical effect and safety profile as the other.

Drug products are *pharmaceutically equivalent* if they contain the same active ingredient(s) in the same amount, meet all the applicable standards of quality and purity, and are meant to be used at the same dosage and through the same route of administration (FDA, 1998). Pharmaceutically equivalent products can differ in certain other features, such as excipients, shape, packaging, and expiration time. If pharmaceutical equivalents can be expected to produce the same clinical effects when given to patients for the therapeutic indications specified in the labeling, they are considered to be also *therapeutically equivalent.* Therapeutic equivalents must be *bioequivalent*; that is, they must possess the same rate and extent of absorption. The FDA considers two or more compounds to be bioequivalent if (1) they do not present any known or potential bioequivalent problems (and because of this,

[1]Child and Adolescent Treatment and Preventive Intervention Research Branch, National Institute of Mental Health, Bethesda, Maryland.

[2]Center for Drug Evaluation and Research, Food and Drug Administration, Washington, D.C.

The opinions and assertions contained herein are the private views of the authors and are not to be construed as official or reflecting the views of the National Institute of Mental Health or of the Food and Drug Administration.

an *in vivo* bioequivalency test has not been done, as it has been considered unnecessary) or (2) they have presented potential bioequivalency problems and have been subjected to a test of *in vivo* bioequivalence that has demonstrated comparable rate and extent of absorption. Generic medications that qualify according to the former criterion are placed by the FDA into Category A, whereas medications that qualify on the basis of a successful bioequivalency test are in Category B. Drugs are in Category AB if they were first thought not to present potential bioequivalence problems and were classified in Category A, but were later suspected to have possible bioequivalence problems, were consequently subjected to a bioequivalence test, and finally were found to meet all the bioequivalence criteria. As we will see, this is the case for MPH, which is currently classified in bioequivalence Category AB.

A test of bioequivalence is usually done by conducting a plasma pharmacokinetics study in healthy adult male volunteers. Similar doses of the compounds to be tested are administered, and standard pharmacokinetics parameters, such as area under the curve (AUC_{inf}, or AUC throughout the text), peak concentration (C_{max}), time at which peak concentration occurs (T_{max}), elimination half-life (T_{half}), and rate of absorption (K_a) and elimination (K_e), are computed. The AUC is the most important parameter in the determination of drug bioequivalency. According to FDA standards, for two drug products to be considered bioequivalent, their AUCs must not differ >20% from one another. In fact, most drugs submitted to the FDA for bioequivalency determination differ <5% in their AUC. The C_{max} is also important in bioequivalency determinations, but no *a priori* maximum allowable difference has been set. In order for a generic drug product to be approved as bioequivalent, it must meet the regulatory 80% to 125% bioequivalence acceptance criteria in both C_{max} and AUC.

When generic MPH was first introduced in 1976, it was considered bioequivalent under Category A. An in vitro dissolution test done at that time evidenced no potential absorption problems of clinical relevance, and an *in vivo* bioequivalency test was therefore deemed to be unnecessary. After the product had been marketed, however, several anecdotal reports were filed by physicians and families of children who were given generic MPH that raised the possibility that the product might be more rapidly absorbed and eliminated. Many of these reports mentioned that the generic preparation was wearing off too soon, with an earlier than expected reemergence of inattention and hyperactivity. Following these reports, the FDA commissioned a bioequivalence study that was conducted by M. Meyer and his colleagues at the University of Tennessee in Memphis (FDA, 1989).

BIOEQUIVALENCE STUDY OF GENERIC METHYLPHENIDATE IMMEDIATE RELEASE

Twenty healthy male volunteers (ages 20–33 years) were given, on separate occasions, two single doses of both Ritalin 20 mg and generic MPH 20-mg immediate-release tablets (FDA, 1989). The sample size provided adequate power to detect a ≥20% difference in AUC and C_{max} between products. Blood samples were drawn at close intervals until 10 hours after drug administration. Methylphenidate was assayed by a specific gas chromatography—mass spectrometry method with a lower level of sensitivity of 1.0 ng/ml. AUC_{inf} was calculated using the usual method: AUC (0–10 hours) + $C10/K_e$. Elimination half-life was calculated using the formula $T_{half} = 0.693/K_e$. As shown in Figure 1 and summarized in Table 1, generic MPH, compared with brand Ritalin, was found to have a faster absorption with consequent earlier plasma peak (on average, half an hour earlier). The extent of absorption (i.e., same AUC) and elimination (T_{half}) were the same. There was, however, more inter-

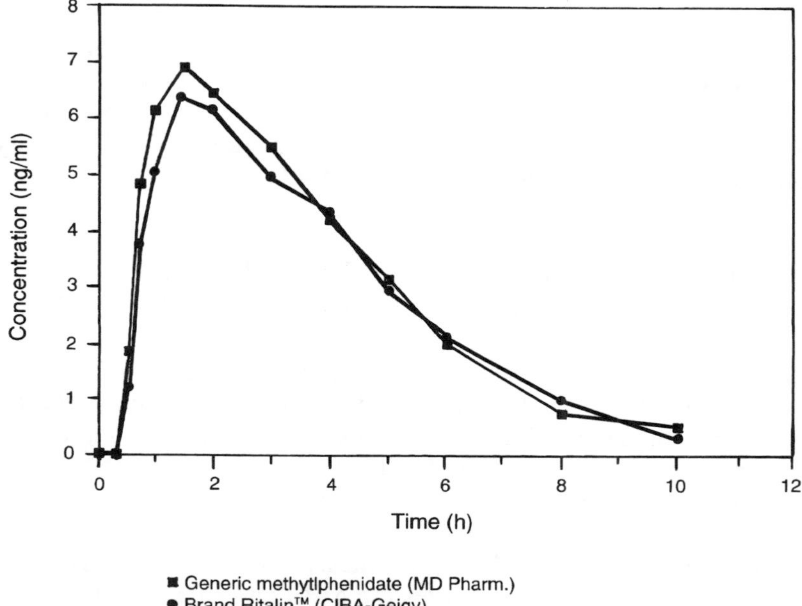

FIG. 1. Plasma pharmacokinetics of immediate-release generic methylphenidate (20 mg orally; n = 20; mean drug levels).

subject variation in C_{max} and AUC after generic MPH (1.5–2 times greater than brand Ritalin).

The finding of a more rapid absorption rate of generic MPH is consistent with the result of a dissolution test that was conducted also in 1989 (FDA, 1989). This *in vitro* test was conducted in three different media: water, simulated gastric fluid without enzymes, and simulated intestinal fluid without enzymes. It was found that generic MPH dissolved more rapidly than brand Ritalin, although both products met the specifications set by the United States Pharmacopeia.

TABLE 1. BIOEQUIVALENCE TEST OF GENERIC METHYLPHENIDATE VS. BRAND RITALIN 20-MG TABLETS: PLASMA PHARMACOKINETICS PARAMETERS (n = 40, 20 SUBJECTS RECEIVING EACH DRUG ON 2 OCCASIONS, MEAN ± SD) (FDA 1989)

	Generic (MD Pharm.)	*Brand (Ciba-Geigy)*	*Ratio Generic/Brand*	
				90% C.I.
C_{max}*	7.08	6.46	1.10	99.4–119.4
AUC_{inf}*	33.22	30.73	1.08	99.3–116.1
				p (t test)
T_{max}, hr	1.55 ± 0.59	1.97 ± 0.76	0.80	<0.05
T_{half}, hr	2.56 ± 0.75	2.47 ± 0.72	1.04	NS
K_a	3.94 ± 4.36	2.54 ± 1.80	1.55	<0.05
K_e	0.29 ± 0.08	0.30 ± 0.09	0.96	NS

*Geometric mean; C_{max} = peak concentration; T_{max} = time to peak; K_a = constant of absorption; AUC_{inf} = area under the curve; T_{half} = elimination half-life; K_e = constant of elimination.

In conclusion, the results of the study indicate that generic MPH meets all the criteria to be considered bioequivalent to brand Ritalin, because both the extent of absorption and the peak concentration of the two products do not differ >20%. Generic MPH, however, is more rapidly absorbed, and plasma peak concentration is achieved about half an hour earlier than with brand Ritalin. In addition, there is greater intersubject variability in pharmacokinetics following the administration of generic MPH.

BIOEQUIVALENCE STUDY OF GENERIC METHYLPHENIDATE SUSTAINED-RELEASE

A bioequivalence study was also conducted on the generic sustained-release formulation of MPH (Patrick et al., 1989). Each of the 18 healthy male volunteers who participated in the study was given, on three separate occasions, (1) a generic sustained-release 20-mg tablet (MP Pharmaceuticals), (2) a brand Ritalin sustained-release 20-mg tablet (Ciba-Geigy), and one brand Ritalin immediate-release 10-mg tablet (Ciba-Geigy), followed by another similar 10-mg tablet 5 hours after the first dose. Blood samples were obtained until 16 hours after dosing, and plasma MPH was measured using a chromatographic method.

As shown in Figure 2, generic sustained-release MPH and Ritalin sustained-release formulations have superimposable plasma pharmacokinetics curves and are, in every respect, bioequivalent. In the same experiment, the administration of immediate-release Ritalin shows that higher plasma levels are achieved following the second dosing. The terminal half-life was 3.1 hours for the slow-release preparations and 2.6 hours for the immediate-release Ritalin. The extent of absorption of the three products (i.e., AUC_{inf}) did not differ >5% of each other.

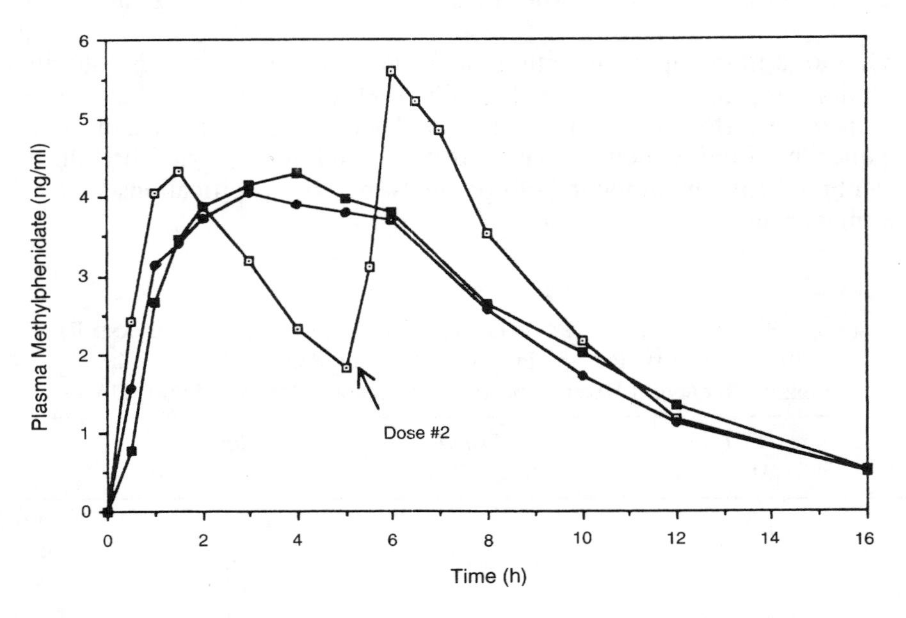

FIG. 2. Plasma pharmacokinetics of sustained-release generic methylphendidate (MPH) (n = 18; mean drug levels). 20-mg sustained-release generic MPH (black squares); 20-mg sustained-release brand Ritalin (circles); 10-mg immediate-release brand Ritalin given twice daily (open squares). From Patrick, K.S. et al. (1989), The absorption of sustained-release MPH formulations compared to an immediate-release formulation. In: *Biopharmaceutics & Drug Disposition, Vol. 10*, p. 170. Copyright © John Wiley & Sons, Limited. Reproduced with permission.

This study indicates that the sustained-release tablets of generic MPH and brand Ritalin are bioequivalent without significant differences in pharmacokinetics.

COST OF GENERIC VS. BRAND RITALIN

As is usually the case with generic products, generic MPH is usually less expensive than the brand name. Medication costs charged to the patient vary according to several factors, such as wholesale distributor, pharmacy, amount of drug bought, and insurance prescription plan. The wholesale price charged by distributors for 100 tablets of generic MPH is about $30 for 5-mg tablets (vs. $34.21 for Ritalin), $40 for 10 mg tablets (vs. $48.81 for Ritalin), $60 for 20-mg tablets (vs. $70.21 for Ritalin), and $95 for 20-mg extended-release (vs. $107.46 for Ritalin). These numbers indicate that the generic product is 11% to 18% cheaper, at least based on the wholesale price.

WHICH ONE TO USE?

According to all the currently accepted standards, generic and brand-name MPH are comparable. The more rapid absorption of the generic immediate-release formulation is not considered to be of clinical significance, in general. The bioequivalence studies on which these conclusions are based were conducted in young adults, but it is considered unlikely that a similar study in children would lead to significantly different results. No pharmacodynamics study comparing the duration of action of generic MPH with that of brand Ritalin has been reported. Anecdotal reports of shorter duration of action of generic MPH exist, but they are relatively few, given the extent this product is used.

If the value and limitation of the available data are considered, it can be concluded that there is no *a priori* pharmacologic or therapeutic reason to choose one product over the other. In treating individual patients, however, it cannot be excluded that for some individual patients, the faster absorption of the generic immediate-release formulation can translate into a shorter duration of action of the pharmacologic activity with a negative impact on the patient's functioning. This situation is more likely to emerge when patients are switched from brand Ritalin to generic MPH. In these cases, attention to the drug's duration of action after dosing is recommended. Some patients may do better with one formulation than the other, although no predicting factors have been identified. It is up to the treating physician to recognize such cases based on information provided by patient, family, and school, and to treat them accordingly.

REFERENCES

Food and Drug Administration, Center for Drug Evaluation and Research (1998), *Approved Drug Products with Therapeutic Equivalence Evaluations, 18th ed.* Washington, DC: U.S. Department of Health and Human Services.

Food and Drug Administration, Division of Bioequivalence (1989), *Review of a Bioequivalence Study*. FDA Contract No. 223-87-1802 (report on file at the FDA).

IMS (1996), National Prescription Audit, IMS America, Ltd., Plymouth Meeting, PA.

Patrick, K.S., Straughn, A.B., Jarvi, E.J., Breese, G.R. & Meyer, M.C. (1989), The absorption of sustained-release methylphenidate formulations compared to an immediate-release formulation. *Biopharm. Drug Dispos.*, 10:165–171.

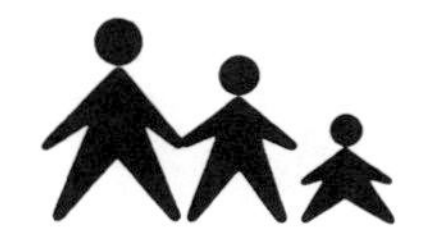

Methylphenidate: The Role of the d-Isomer

DECLAN M.P. QUINN

Few people are aware that methylphenidate (MPH) (Ritalin), a stimulant medication in the treatment of attention deficit hyperactivity disorder (ADHD), is a complex racemic drug with two different isomers. Recent research has allowed for the isolation of these isomers, determination of their pharmacologic properties, and establishment of the role of the isomers in children with ADHD. It has become apparent that there is a selective uptake of one isomer in the brain, which may, over time, allow a better understanding of the neurochemical basis for ADHD. This chapter highlights research over the last decade in our understanding of the role of the different isomers.

MPH (dl-threo-methyl-2-phenyl-2-[2-piperidyl]) acetate is a potent central nervous stimulant in the treatment of ADHD in children. Until recently, the role of the individual isomers of MPH was poorly understood and hardly recognized. Meier et al. (1954) first described the pharmacology of MPH. However, only in the last few years have we begun to understand the pharmacokinetics of the individual isomers and the relevance they may have to the understanding of and treatment interventions with ADHD.

CHEMISTRY

MPH has two chiral carbon centers, giving rise to four different optical isomers: d-threo, l-threo, d-erythro, and l-erythro forms. When synthesized, it yields a ratio of 80% dl-erythro and 20% dl-threo MPH. The dl-erythro MPH is not active and was believed to have undesirable side effects on blood pressure. Consequently, in the early 1960s, this form was eliminated. The commercially available MPH (Ritalin) contains only the dl-threo preparation (Patrick et al., 1987) (Figure 1). It is extensively metabolized by de-esterification, primarily to ritalinic acid. These esterases are stereospecific. The metabolic product is not believed to be clinically active. Several practical and technical problems made the isolation of the different isomers difficult, and an assay to measure the plasma levels of the isomers was developed only in 1986 (Lim et al., 1986). However, substantial evidence was accumulating from laboratory studies that these isomers had different properties. It was believed that the therapeutic effect of dl-threo MPH resided with the d-isomer from earlier work, even though this was not demonstrated in clinical studies (Pan et al., 1994; Ritz et al., 1987; Schweri et al., 1985; Patrick et al., 1987). In 1985, Schweri et al. (1985) described a specific d-methylphenidate receptor site.

Department of Psychiatry, College of Medicine, University of Saskatchewan, Saskatoon, Saskatchewan, Canada.

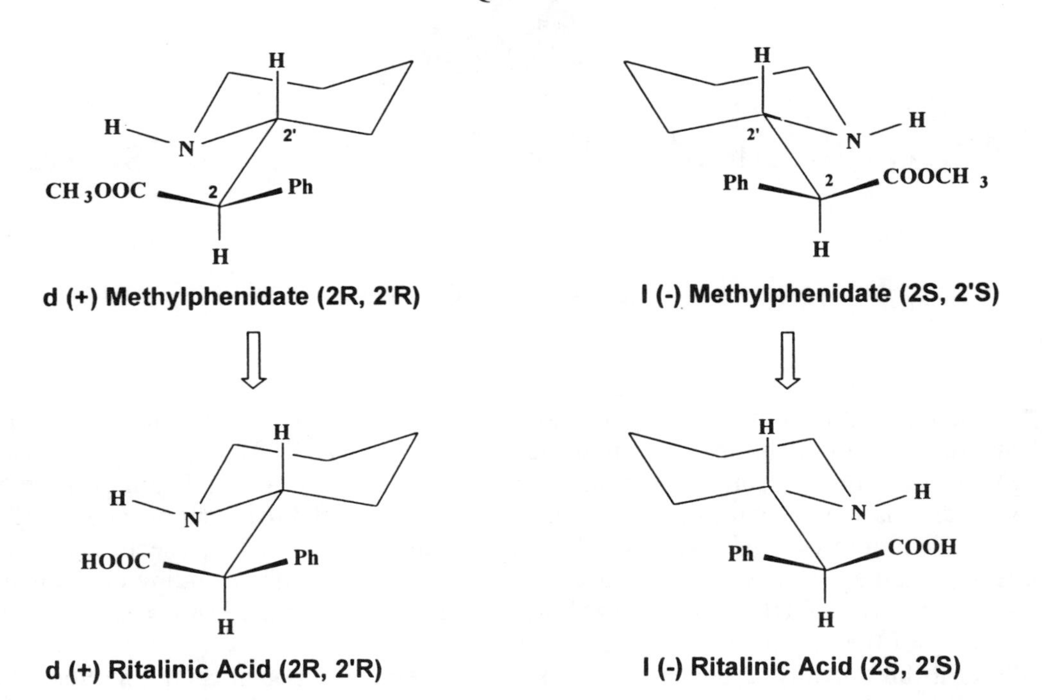

FIG. 1. Stereochemistry of d-methylphenidate and 1-methylphenidate and their primary metabolic products.

PLASMA STUDIES OF THE ISOMERS OF THREO-METHYLPHENIDATE

Plasma measurements of the d and l-isomers of methylphenidate in human subjects and children with ADHD

In 1986, at the University of Saskatchewan, Lim et al. (1986) developed the first assay to measure the individual isomers of MPH in plasma after the oral administration of the racemic mixture. A pilot study showed profound distortion in the plasma levels of the ratio of the isomers in plasma: The d-isomer plasma level was many times higher than the l-isomer.

After the initial pilot study, a more definitive study was undertaken in six children receiving regular immediate-release MPH (MPH-IR) for ADHD (Srinivas et al., 1987). These children had all been taking MPH for ADHD and were considered to be positive responders. The results of analysis of the plasma levels of the isomers supported the initial pilot study: the levels were at least five times greater for the d-isomer than for the l-isomer in all six children (Figure 2).

In a subsequent study with six other children with ADHD, we investigated the plasma levels of the isomers again, but after a racemic mixture of the sustained release preparation of MPH (MPH-SR) (Hubbard et al., 1989). These children had been taking MPH-SR, were considered positive responders and had a clinical diagnosis of ADHD. Analysis of the data again demonstrated the same pronounced distortion in the plasma levels of the isomers: the d-isomer was 8- to 10-fold higher than the l-isomer.

To clarify the metabolism of MPH in non-ADHD individuals, a study of the plasma levels of the isomers in healthy humans was undertaken. Eleven adult subjects were given MPH intravenously, or orally as immediate-release preparation or sustained-release prepa-

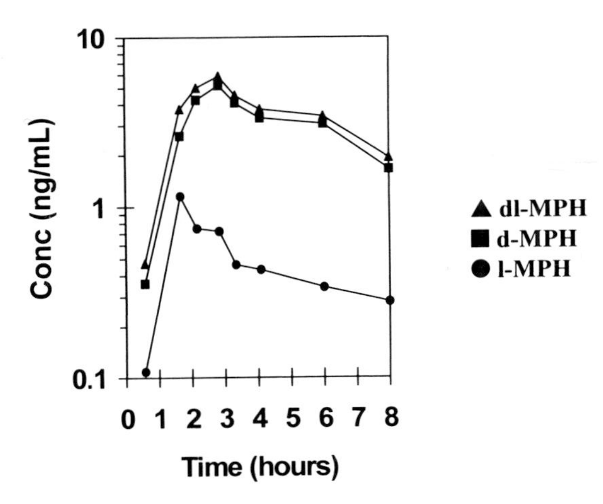

FIG. 2. Differences in plasma levels of d- and l-methylphenidate over time.

ration, either swallowed or chewed. Plasma levels of the d-isomer were substantially higher in all individuals, compared with the l-isomer (Srinivas et al., 1993).

A more definitive study was then undertaken to examine the effect of the different isomers in children with ADHD. Nine boys with a diagnosis of ADHD were given d-

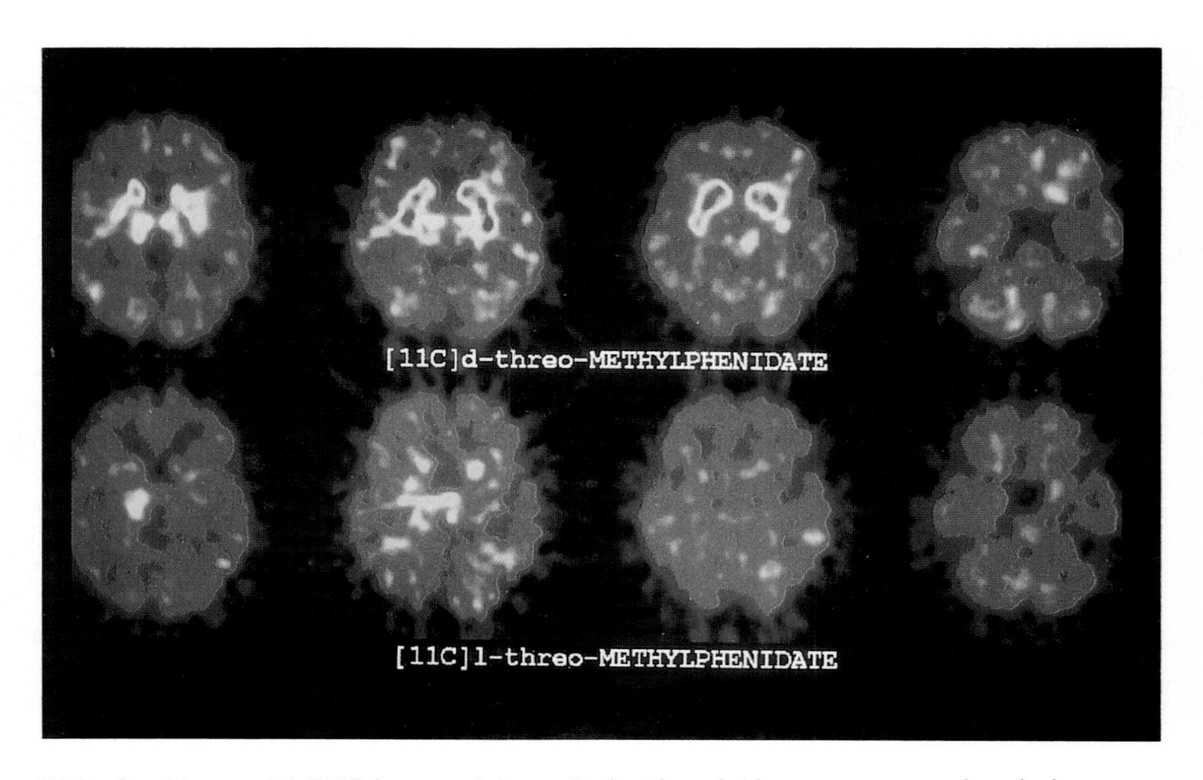

FIG. 3. Transaxial PET images (planes 8, 9, 10 and 12 on an averaged emission scan representing the activity from 10 to 90 min) of the human brain after the injection of ^{11}C-d-threo-methylphenidate (top panel) and ^{11}C-l-threo-methylphenidate (bottom panel). Images are from top of the brain to the base of the skull (left to right). Notice the high accumulation of radioactivity in the basal ganglia for the d-isomer compared with the l-isomer. (Courtesy of Dr. Y.-S. Ding, Brookhaven National Laboratory.)

methylphenidate, l-methylphenidate, dl-methylphenidate, or placebo in a double-blind, four-way, randomized, crossover design (Srinivas et al., 1992). A drug effect for children using a sustained task of attention was seen with the dl-methylphenidate and the d-methylphenidate, and none was seen with the l-isomer of MPH, which was comparable to placebo, suggesting that the effectiveness of racemic MPH rests exclusively with the d-isomer. In that study, there was no evidence of interconversion between the isomers. A study by Ayomi et al. (1994) also suggests that intraconversion between the different isomers does not occur. Whether the l-isomer would have had a clinical effect if plasma levels had been higher was not answered. The pharmacokinetic values for the isomers of MPH are reported elsewhere (Srinivas et al., 1993; Hubbard et al., 1989; Srinivas et al., 1987).

MECHANISM OF ACTION

MPH works at the dopamine transporter and blocks the reuptake of dopamine from the synaptic vesicle (Ding et al., 1997). It differs from d-amphetamine, which not only blocks dopamine reuptake but also stimulates dopamine release. There appears to be a specific d-methylphenidate receptor site on the dopamine transporter. The role of d-methylphenidate appears to be different from that of the l-isomer, which has a different profile. From the work of Ding and colleagues (1997), the primary site of action appears focused and localized to the basal ganglia. The d-methylphenidate isomer is selectively taken up in the basal ganglia, in comparison to the l-isomer, which has nonspecific binding in the brain (Figure 3).

DISCUSSION

From these studies, the following conclusions may be tentatively reached. The clinical effectiveness of racemic MPH in ADHD seems to reside exclusively in the d-isomer of MPH. There is extensive presystemic metabolism, particularly of the l-isomer. The plasma levels of the d- to l-isomers show profound distortion, with d-methylphenidate substantially higher than l-methylphenidate. It is possible that the l-isomer is effective at higher plasma levels, but that would require substantially higher oral doses to achieve such plasma levels. Ding et al. (1997) contend that it would be preferable to use only one isomer in the treatment of ADHD. Reasons given include the unknown side effects of the inactive isomer, such as the granulocytopenia seen with racemic dopa but not with levo-dopa, the use of R(-) methadone in heroin addicts with liver disease, and the phocomelia associated with the use of the d-isomer of thalidomide when it is given to pregnant women (the l-isomer has a sedative therapeutic effect). Other advantages include smaller doses and a superior pharmacologic profile of the active isomer.

The role of the l-isomer in racemic MPH is unclear. It could account for a different side effect profile. It could have an antagonistic effect on the role of the d-isomer. The anecdotal information from individuals who have abused racemic MPH suggests a "high" only when it is used intravenously or "snorted" through the nasal membranes, but not when it is taken orally.When taken this way, it bypasses first-stage metabolism, and plasma levels of the isomers are similar. These individuals have reported side effects of headache, tachycardia, and nausea when large doses are taken orally but not when the drug is used intravenously or snorted. Elimination of the abuse potential needs to be examined by elimination of the l-isomer.

The role of the d-isomer in the treatment and management of ADHD warrants further study in subjects with ADHD. Whether the reported abuse occurs with the different isomers is unclear and needs further studies. At this time, the role of the l-isomer suggests it has no therapeutic effect. Since the introduction of MPH in the 1950s, it has taken almost 40 years to appreciate and understand the role of the different isomers. Future studies need to look at the exclusive use of the d-isomer, the issue of side effects, the abuse potential, the role of inhibition of the d-methylphenidate isomer in the basal ganglia, and the role of dopamine in ADHD.

REFERENCES

Aoyami, T., Hajime, K., Sawada, Y. & Iga, T. (1994), Stereospecific distribution of methylphenidate enantiomers in rat brain: Specific binding to dopamine reuptake sites. *Pharmacol. Res.*, 11:407–411.

Ding, Y.S., Fowler, J.S., Volkow, N.D., Dewey, S.L., Wang, G.J., Logan, J., Gatley, S.J. & Pappas, N. (1997), Chiral drugs: Comparison of the pharmacokinetics of [11C]d-threo and l-threo-methylphenidate in the human and baboon brain. *Psychopharmacol. Berl.*, 131:71–78.

Hubbard, J.W., Srinivas, N.R., Quinn, D. & Midha, K.K. (1989), Enantioselective aspects of the disposition of dl-threo-methylphenidate after the administration of a sustained-release formulation to children with attention deficit-hyperactivity disorder. *J. Pharm. Sci.*, 78:944–947.

Lim, H.K., Hubbard, J.W. & Midha, K.K. (1986), Development of an enantioselective gas chromatographic quantitation assay dl-threo-methylphenidate in biological fluids. *J. Chromatogr.*, 378:109–123.

Meier, R., Gross, F. & Tripod, J. (1954), Ritalin, eine neuartige synthetische Verbinding mit spezifischer zentralerregender Wirkungskomponente. *Klin. Wochenschr.*, 32:445–450.

Pan, D., Gatley, S.J., Dewey, S.L., Chen, R., Alexoff, D.A., Ding, Y.S. & Fowler, J.S. (1994), Binding of bromine substituted analogs of methylphenidate to monoamine transporters. *Eur. J. Pharmacol.*, 264:177–182.

Patrick, K.S., Caldwell, R.W., Ferris, R.M. & Bresse, G.R. (1987), Pharmacology of the enantiomers of threo-methylphenidate. *J. Pharmacol. Exp. Ther.*, 241:152–158.

Ritz, M.C., Lamb, R.J., Goldberg, S.R. & Kuhar, M.J. (1987), Cocaine receptors on dopamine transporters are related to self-administration of cocaine. *Science*, 237:1219–1223.

Schweri, M.M., Skolnick, P., Rafferty, M.F., Rice, K.C., Janowsky, A.J. & Paul, S. (1985), [H]Threo-(+/−)-methylphenidate binding to 3,4-dihydroxyphenyethylamine uptake site in corpus striatum: Correlation with stimulant properties of ritalinic acid esters. *J. Neurochem.*, 45:1062–1070.

Srinivas, N.R., Hubbard, J.W., Korchinski, E.D. & Midha, K.K. (1993), Enantioselective pharmacokinetics of dl-threo-methylphenidate in humans. *Pharmaceutical Res.*, 10:14–21.

Srinivas, N.R., Hubbard, J.W., Wuinn, D. & Midha, K.K. (1992), Enantioselective pharmacokinetics and pharmacodynamics of dl-threo-methylphenidate in children with attention deficit hyperactivity disorder. *Clin. Pharmacol. Ther.*, 52:561–568.

Srinivas, N.R., Quinn, D., Hubbard, J.W. & Midha, K.K. (1987), Stereoselective disposition of methylphenidate in children with attention-deficit disorder. *J. Pharmacol. Exp. Ther.*, 241:300–306.

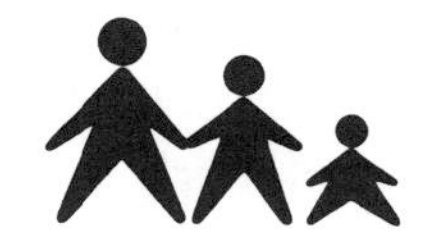

Brain Imaging Studies of the Action of Methylphenidate and Cocaine in the Human Brain

MONIQUE ERNST,[1] ALYSSA EARLE,[2]
and ALAN ZAMETKIN[2]

In June 1995, a research article appeared in the *Archives of General Psychiatry* (Volkow et al., 1995) and asked the provocative question "Is methylphenidate like cocaine?" This question was addressed by examining the cerebral location and time course of the effects of these drugs by use of functional neuroimaging. The answer is not simple. Although in many ways, both drugs have similar mechanisms of action, it is the more subtle differences that make methylphenidate (MPH) a safe and effective medication for the treatment of attention deficit hyperactivity disorder (ADHD) and cocaine an addictive and dangerous agent.

To help appreciate the brain imaging literature, we will briefly review the pharmacology of cocaine and MPH, the basic principles of brain imaging techniques, and the strategies used to map and quantify the effects of pharmacologic agents in the living human brain. The reader will be introduced to the dopamine system, which is the main neural target of cocaine and MPH.

PHARMACOLOGY

Routes of administration

A fundamental concept in psychopharmacology is the importance of the route of administration (e.g., intravenous, oral, intranasal) for an agent's psychologic effect (Koob and Bloom, 1988). For example, MPH administered orally can almost be considered to be a different medication from MPH administered intravenously or intranasally (used only when the medication is abused). However, oral use of MPH can lead to abuse and dependence when the dosage is escalated and only after long periods of sustained use with large doses. Throughout this chapter, the reader must be critically aware that much of the research involved in the study and comparison of both MPH and cocaine used methods in which the drugs were given intravenously. Although these studies clarify the mechanism and site of action of these drugs, the translation of the findings to the clinical domain with respect to ADHD treatment (stable regimen of orally administered MPH at low doses) is not straightforward. The generalization of the information based on intravenous administration may be misleading. Intravenous MPH was shown to induce restlessness in adult control subjects

[1]NIDA Brain Imaging Center, National Institute on Drug Abuse, Baltimore, Maryland.
[2]Office of Clinical Director, National Institutes of Health, Bethesda, Maryland.

(Volkow et al., 1997b), to have reinforcing effects (Bergman et al., 1989), and to produce a "high" (Wang et al., 1997), whereas oral MPH reduces hyperactivity in both control subjects and ADHD individuals, is devoid of addictive properties, and does not produce a "high." Similarly, the oral ingestion of cocaine is essentially devoid of psychotropic effects (save the chewing of coca leaves) and has little relevance to the epidemic of intranasal cocaine abuse.

Pharmacokinetics (what the body does to the drug: peak effects, half-life, metabolism, excretion)

After a single oral dose of MPH, the MPH blood level peaks at 60–120 minutes, and the half-life ranges from 2.3 to 4.2 hours (mean 3.4 hours) (Gualtieri and Hicks, 1985). Changes in MPH blood levels over time closely parallel the clinical activity of the drug (Swanson et al., 1978) but vary greatly from one individual to the other. In contrast, after intravenous administration of MPH, MPH blood level peaks at 4–10 minutes for 15–20 minutes. Intravenous cocaine has a blood level peak uptake at 2–8 minutes for 2–4 minutes. Cocaine has a half-life in brain tissue of only 20 minutes compared with 90 minutes for MPH (Table 1). This difference has critical implications for the abuse liability of these drugs.

Pharmacodynamics (what the drug does to the body: target and mechanism of action)

The common and biologically most salient target of action of cocaine and MPH is the dopamine transporter (DAT).

To help understand the mechanism of action of these drugs, some basic aspects of brain function are reviewed. The brain is the most complex organ of the body. It is composed of support cells (glia) and nerve cells (neurons). All brain functions are mediated by neurons, the number of which is estimated to reach ~100 billion. Neurons connect with each other at synapses (specialized gaps between cells), which are the primary units of brain function. The carriers of information between neurons are neurotransmitters. A neurotransmitter is a chemical that is synthesized in a neuronal cell and is released by that neuron at synapses in response to electrical impulses (depolarization of the presynaptic nerve membrane). There, it diffuses across the synapse and acts on other neurons by binding to specialized receptor proteins located on cell membranes. The action of neurotransmitters in the synapse is terminated either by enzymatic degradation or by transport back into the presynaptic nerve cell (reuptake by a transporter, e.g., dopamine transporter) (Figure 1) (Kuhar et al., 1991). Up to 100 different molecules may function as neurotransmitters. In this chapter,

TABLE 1. PHARMACOKINETICS OF METHYLPHENIDATE AND COCAINE INTRAVENOUSLY

Drug (0.375 mg/kg iv)	*Peak Uptake (min)*	*Peak Duration*[a] *(min)*	*Ki*[b] *(nM)*	*DAT Occupancy (%)*	*Striatal Half-Life (min)*
Cocaine	2–8	2–4	640	65	20
Methylphenidate	4–10	15–20	390	84	90

[a]Peak duration = Length of time during which the peak concentration is maintained.
[b]Ki = Affinity constant; concentration at which the drug occupies 50% of the dopamine transporters (DAT).

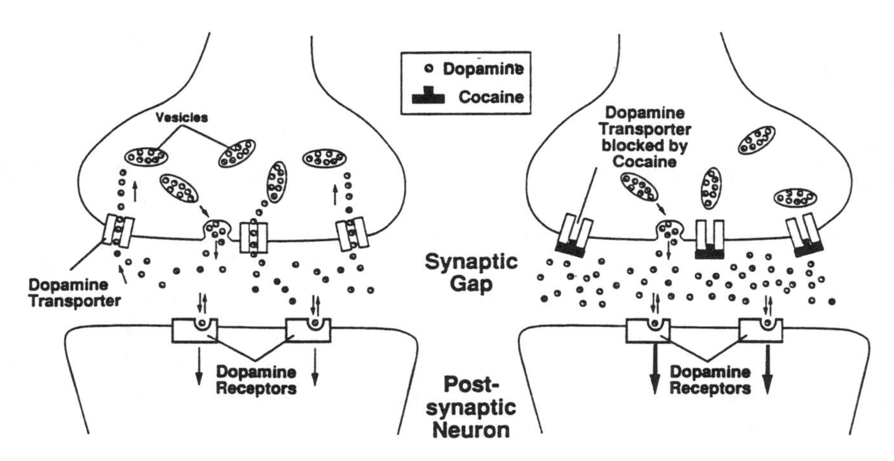

FIG. 1. The dopamine hypothesis of drug reinforcement. Cocaine binds to the transporter and blocks the reuptake of dopamine in the mesolimbocortical pathways. This potentiates dopaminergic neurotransmission and begins the sequence of events that ultimately causes the rewarding effects of the drug. (Reprinted with permission from Kuhar, M.J. et al. (1991), The dopamine hypothesis of the reinforcing properties of cocaine. *Trends Neurosci.*, 14:299–302.

we focus on the neurotransmitter dopamine because of its major role in MPH and cocaine actions. Dopamine transmission is inactivated mainly by its reuptake in the presynaptic cell, which is mediated by a molecule located on the membrane of the presynaptic cell, the DAT. Because of its critical importance in dopamine transmission, this molecule has been the object of intensive investigation. Its molecular structure, subcellular localization, and physiology have been well characterized (Kuhar et al., 1990; Shimada et al., 1991).

Cocaine and MPH bind to the DAT and inhibit the reuptake of dopamine into the cell. Furthermore, the affinity for the DAT is similar in both drugs (Ritz et al., 1987; Bergman et al., 1989). This blockade of the DAT results in the accumulation of dopamine in the synaptic cleft and has been linked to the psychostimulant properties of MPH (Solanto, 1997) and the abuse liability of cocaine (Koob and Bloom, 1988; DiChiara and Imperato, 1988; Kuhar et al., 1990; Shimada et al., 1991). The therapeutic efficacy of MPH in the treatment of ADHD has been proposed to be mediated by the increased levels of extracellular dopamine. However, the exact mechanism, i.e., the cascade of events engendered by this increase, as well as the contribution of other neurotransmitter systems, is unclear. In fact, opposite theories of deficit and excess of dopaminergic transmission have been proposed for the pathophysiology of ADHD. Whereas it is easy to understand how MPH would correct a dopaminergic deficit, the normalization of dopaminergic excess requires a more complex model. This model hypothetizes the activation of inhibitory dopamine receptors by low-dose stimulants (Solanto, 1986; Grace, 1995; Castellanos, 1997). This theory is based on the identification of two types of dopaminergic receptors: (1) excitatory and located on the postsynaptic cell membrane, and (2) inhibitory, also called autoreceptors, located mainly on the presynaptic cell membrane. Presynaptic receptors exert an inhibitory feedback on dopaminergic transmission by inhibiting the synthesis and release of dopamine; postsynaptic receptors mediate dopaminergic transmission. Presynaptic receptors are significantly more sensitive to dopamine (higher affinity) than postsynaptic receptors. Thus, low doses of MPH, within the therapeutic range, would activate preferentially (indirectly) these inhibitory presynaptic receptors, and higher nontherapeutic doses would enhance dopaminergic transmission through postsynaptic receptor stimulation. This last proposition may also account for the reinforcing properties of cocaine. Hence, the quandary addressed in this chapter is the differential addictive liability of cocaine and MPH in the face of similar pharmacologic actions.

BASIC PRINCIPLES OF POSITRON EMISSION TOMOGRAPHY

Positron emission tomography (PET) is a functional brain imaging technique, like single photon emission computed tomography (SPECT) or functional magnetic resonance imaging (fMRI). The development of PET was made possible by the discoveries of Sokoloff (1978) and Kety (1960) that related glucose metabolism and blood flow to synaptic activity and permitted the quantitative measurement of cerebral metabolic rate of glucose (CMRglc) and cerebral blood flow (CBF). At present, PET permits the mapping and quantification of a large number of neurochemical processes in addition to those of CMRglc and CBF.

PET is a nuclear medicine technique that uses molecules tagged with radionuclides (e.g., ^{11}C, ^{15}O, ^{18}F). These molecules can mimic the behavior of biologic chemicals (tracers, e.g., [^{18}F]fluorodeoxyglucose for glucose, [^{18}F]fluoroDOPA for DOPA) or mark molecular processes such as the binding to neurotransmitter receptors or transporters (ligands, e.g., [^{11}C]raclopride for D2/D3 dopamine receptors; [^{11}C]β-CIT or [^{11}C]MPH for DAT). The radioactivity emitted by these tracers or ligands is detected by the PET scanner and reconstructed by high-power computers in the three-dimensional (3D) space of a brain. The radioactivity's distribution in this 3D space reflects the behavior of the molecule under study and is quantified by complex mathematical models. For example, [^{11}C]MPH (Ding et al., 1994) and [^{11}C]cocaine (Fowler et al., 1989) bind to DATs and are localized in the brain regions that are rich in dopaminergic innervation, such as the striatum. The quantification of the radioactivity will reflect the number of transporters available to be bound by [^{11}C]MPH or [^{11}C]cocaine. Thus, it is possible to compare the behavior of MPH with that of cocaine in the brain. This example is one of the most sophisticated and ingenious uses of PET at the present time. More common are the studies of regional CBF (rCBF) and CMRglc (rCMRglc). As mentioned above, these measures of rCBF and rCMRglc reflect synaptic activity, indiscriminately of the underlying biochemical processes. Therefore, these measures inform researchers the integrated functional activity of the brain, whether at rest, during the performance of a task (motor or cognitive), or in response to pharmacologic challenges. This last experimental paradigm has been used for the study of the cerebral effects of cocaine and MPH and will be reviewed below.

EFFECTS OF MPH AND COCAINE ON THE INTEGRATED ACTIVITY OF THE BRAIN (rCMRglc AND rCBF)

Comparison of the effects of cocaine and MPH on rCMRglc and rCBF needs to account for the difference in the populations studied. For obvious reasons of ethics and safety, cocaine is not administered to cocaine-naive subjects; thus, studies of acute cocaine administration are few and have been conducted almost exclusively in substance abusers. In contrast, studies of MPH have been performed in control subjects and ADHD individuals, for the most part.

Reduction of global CMRglc was reported after the intravenous administration of cocaine (40 mg intravenously) to polydrug abusers (London et al., 1990). Similarly, decreased global CBF occurred after the intravenous administration of MPH (0.5 mg/kg) to healthy adult control subjects (Wang et al., 1994). Although it is difficult to assess the relative contribution of neural activity vs. direct drug-related vasoactive effect in blood flow measures, this overall decrement of neural activity has been postulated to mediate, in part, the euphorigenic effect of these drugs. Indeed, reduction of overall brain-glucose metabolism has also been reported after the short-term intramuscular administration of a euphorigenic dose of opiate (morphine 30 mg) to polydrug abusers (London et al., 1990), suggesting that if a relationship exists between global cerebral activity and subjective "high," it is not drug specific. In contrast to the intravenous injection of MPH, the oral administration of MPH at therapeutic doses failed to alter global CMRglc and produced only few rCMRglc changes (Matochik et al., 1993; Matochik et al., 1994). This lack of global effects is likely to reflect the route of administration of MPH, which does not elicit euphoria at therapeutic doses, as well as the nature of the parameter studied (CMRglc vs. CBF). In an attempt to identify neurochemical contributors to MPH-related changes in rCMRglc, Volkow et al. (1997b) assayed in the same subjects regional D2 dopamine receptor availability as well as rCMRglc effects of intravenous MPH. The influence of intravenous MPH for a sustained period of time (scan performed after two sequential injections of MPH, 90 minutes apart, to image the effects of sustained dopaminergic disruption rather than the effects of acute changes) on global CMRglc varied among subjects. However, a relationship was found between D2 dopamine receptor availability and the influence of MPH on rCMRglc in the frontal, temporal, and cerebellar regions: in individuals with *high* D2 dopamine receptor availability, MPH *increased* rCMRglc; whereas in individuals with *low* D2 dopamine receptor availability, MPH *decreased* rCMRglc. These findings suggested that MPH-induced changes in rCMRglc depended, in part, on dopaminergic function. The next set of experiments focused more specifically on the quantitative assessment of the dopaminergic effects of MPH and cocaine.

EFFECTS OF MPH AND COCAINE ON THE DOPAMINERGIC NEUROTRANSMITTER SYSTEM

Dopaminergic presynaptic function, particularly the DAT system, has been the target of these studies.

As mentioned above, cocaine and MPH can be tagged with a radionuclide (^{11}C) to serve as ligands and to provide measures of their binding to DAT (Ding et al., 1994; Fowler et al., 1989). Cocaine binding results in DAT blockade and subsequent accumulation of dopamine in the synaptic cleft. These physiologic measures can be directly related to the behavioral effects (feelings of being "high," experiencing a "rush") induced by the administration of the ligands. The relationship between transporter binding and subjective feelings represents the invaluable bridge between basic and clinical neuroscience now made possible by the advent of neuroimaging techniques.

Regional distribution and kinetics of DAT binding

The regional distribution of ^{11}C-MPH in the human brain is almost identical with that of ^{11}C-cocaine, highest in the striatum and relatively low in the cortex and cerebellum (Fowler et al., 1989; Volkow et al., 1995; Volkow et al., 1996a) (see Table 1). The time to reach peak uptake in the brain was 8–10 minutes for MPH and 4–6 minutes for cocaine. The peak concentration in the brain plateaued 15–20 minutes for ^{11}C-MPH and only 2–4 minutes for cocaine. In the striatum, the half-peak clearance was 90 minutes for MPH and 20 minutes for cocaine.

Although cocaine and MPH have similar affinities for DAT (Shimada et al., 1991; Bergman et al., 1989), a common a binding site on DAT for cocaine and MPH remains in question. Two observations tend to support the hypothesis of a common binding site. First, cocaine and MPH substitute for each other on discriminative experiments; second, they compete for binding at the DAT level: pretreatment with MPH decreases binding of ^{11}C-cocaine in the striatum, and conversely pretreatment with cocaine decreases striatal binding of ^{11}C-MPH (Volkow et al., 1995).

However, there is some evidence that the extent and the mode of competition between cocaine and dopamine, and between MPH and dopamine at the DAT level, are different. Dopamine depletion was found to increase striatal binding of ^{11}C-cocaine (Gatley et al., 1995b) but not of ^{11}C-MPH (Gatley et al., 1995a) in similar experiments with baboons.

The translation of DAT blockade to behavior has been studied primarily in the context of the subjective "high" secondary to intravenous cocaine or intravenous MPH.

DAT binding and subjective experience ("high")

Volkow et al. (1995) described a tight coupling of the time course of DAT occupancy, particularly during the uptake process, and the subjective "high" following intravenous cocaine and intravenous MPH. Despite the significant difference in the rates of clearance between cocaine and MPH (20 vs. 90 minutes), the duration of the subjective "high" after intravenous injection was similar for both drugs, i.e., the "high" paralleled the fast uptake of both drugs but declined rapidly despite the continuous binding of ^{11}C-MPH in the brain (Volkow et al., 1995). It is possible that the difference in rates of clearance contributes to the greater abuse liability of cocaine relative to MPH. The higher rate of clearance would stimulate the repeated and frequent self-administration of cocaine. A dissociation between subjective "high" and rate of clearance, such as that seen after intravenous MPH, was also documented for cocaine when its concentration in the brain was maintained constant (Ambre, 1989; Chow et al., 1985), suggesting the development of a phenomenon of tolerance or indirect adaptive mechanisms nonspecific to MPH.

The level of occupancy necessary to produce a subjective feeling of "high" was assessed in a subsequent PET study of intravenous cocaine (Volkow et al., 1997a). By 30 minutes after intravenous cocaine injection, DAT occupancy was still close to 50%, but the subjective "high" was reduced to $<20\%$ of its optimum. Below this level, subjects could not experience a "high" any more. This finding suggested that a minimum of 50% of DAT occupancy (blockade) was needed for a "high" to be perceived.

Given this initial threshold of DAT binding for initiating a "high", it becomes important to assess the level of DAT binding at which the system becomes refractory, i.e., the inability to elicit a "high" from a second injection of MPH or cocaine after the blockade of a substantial number of DAT by a first injection. This question has great relevance for the substance abuse field, as it would encourage the development of substitute medication for cocaine. MPH was chosen to address this question because of its longer-lasting binding to DAT and lesser problematic use than cocaine. Volunteers received two MPH injections 60 minutes apart. The second injection produced a "high" identical with that of the first injection despite a residual DAT occupancy of 75% (Volkow et al., 1996b). Furthermore, a greater DAT occupancy did not predict a more intense "high" and the subjective experience differed qualitatively (aversive vs. pleasurable) among subjects. Possible explanations include the stimulation of receptors that mediate aversive subjective effects at high levels of DAT occupancy (e.g., dynorphin), the development of adaptive responses of DAT upon preexposure to stimulants, or the contribution of other factors than DAT blockade, such as activation of different modulatory systems as a function of levels of synaptic or extracellular dopamine. The influence of the amount of synaptic dopamine concentration on the clinical expression of MPH or cocaine administration has stimulated the development of a very ingenious paradigm to assess the amount of dopamine synaptic release (Volkow et al., 1997b).

Measures of changes of dopamine concentration in the synaptic cleft

The excess of dopamine in the synapse following MPH-related blockade of DAT was assessed by monitoring changes in postsynaptic receptor binding. The basic principle consists in comparing the degree of receptor binding of a ligand (e.g., ^{11}C-raclopride, which binds to D2 and D3 dopamine receptors) before and after stimulant-induced changes of dopamine concentration in the synaptic cleft. The basic concept is that of competition for receptor binding between endogenous dopamine and ligand: the higher the concentration of endogenous dopamine, the smaller the number of receptors available for ligand binding, providing that the affinity of the ligand for the dopamine receptor is lower than that of endogenous dopamine (i.e., endogenous dopamine will displace the ligand from the receptor). Such experimentation showed that the magnitude of changes in ^{11}C-raclopride binding associated with the administration of MPH (0.5 mg/kg intravenous) was quite variable between subjects, ranging from 10% to 47% (Volkow et al., 1994; Volkow et al., 1997b). This wide interindividual variability was postulated to reflect the baseline dopaminergic state, which determines the sensitivity of the system of MPH challenge. Indeed, correlation analyses showed that high anxiety and restlessness at baseline, possibly linked to a dopaminergic supersensitivity state, predicted large changes in ^{11}C-raclopride binding after intravenous MPH challenge. However, they did not predict the nature of the subjective experience associated with MPH administration.

CONCLUSION

Several points emerge from the comparison of brain imaging studies of cocaine and MPH:

1. The route of administration (intravenous vs. oral) is critical to consider for the interpretation of findings and the generalization to the clinical domain. Most studies used intravenous MPH that does not apply to the therapeutic regimen of MPH.
2. Cocaine and MPH are likely to bind to a common site at the DAT, because there is evidence for direct competition between both drugs at the DAT. However, dopamine depletion increases striatal binding of cocaine but not of MPH, suggesting a different extent and mode of competition between cocaine and dopamine, and between MPH and dopamine at the DAT level.
3. Like cocaine, intravenous MPH decreases global cerebral activity, although this finding may be confounded by the direct vasoactive effect of MPH. A global decrease in cerebral activity has been associated with the experience of euphoria induced by drugs of abuse, independently of the type of drug.
4. The pharmacokinetics of intravenous cocaine and intravenous MPH are very similar. Both drugs bind and block the DAT with similar affinities and with similar uptake rate. The main difference between these drugs is the rapid clearance of cocaine (20 minutes) compared with the slow off-rate of MPH (90 minutes). This difference in drug clearance may contribute to the repeated self-administration of cocaine in substance abusers, and less so in intravenous MPH users.
5. In both MPH and cocaine, >50% of the DAT needs to be blocked for a subjective "high" to be experienced. Furthermore, the residual blockade of 50% of DAT does not prevent a subsequent injection of iv MPH to elicit a second "high."

6. The increase of dopamine release in the synaptic cleft secondary to DAT blockade by MPH was quite variable from one individual to the other but was predicted by baseline levels of anxiety and restlessness. Levels of anxiety and restlessness may reflect dopaminergic state, which would determine the sensitivity of the dopaminergic system to MPH challenge.

There is a scarcity of neuroimaging studies of MPH administered orally, because the most frequent use of MPH in this research field has been dedicated to substance abuse, particularly with respect to cocaine. The intravenous administration of MPH produces effects similar to those of cocaine through similar mechanisms of action. However, MPH is rarely a drug of abuse, and it is possible that the few differences in its pharmacokinetics relative to cocaine can explain, in part, the rarity of the compulsive repeated self-administration of this drug.

REFERENCES

Ambre, J.J. (1989), Cocaine kinetics in humans. *Cocaine, Marijuana, Designer Drugs, Chemistry, Pharmacology and Behavior*, eds., K.K. Redda, C.A. Walker & G. Barrett. Boca Raton, FL: CRC Press, pp. 53–69.

Bergman, J., Madras, B.K., Johnson, S.E. & Spealman, R.D. (1989), Effects of cocaine and related drugs in nonhuman primates: III. Self-administration by squirrel monkeys. *J. Pharmacol. Exp. Ther.*, 251:150–155.

Castellanos, F.X. (1997), Towards a pathophysiology of attention-deficit hyperactivity disorder. *Clin. Pediatr.*, 36:381–393.

Chow, M.J., Ambre, J.J., Ruo, T.I., Atkinson, A.J., Jr., Bowsher, D.J. & Fischman, M.W. (1985), Kinetics of cocaine distribution, elimination, and chronotropic effects. *Clin. Pharmacol. Ther.*, 38:318–324.

DiChiara, G. & Imperato, A. (1988), Drugs abused by humans preferentially increase synaptic dopamine concentrations in the mesolimbic system of freely moving rats. *Proc. Nat. Acad. Sci. USA*, 85:5274–5278.

Ding, Y.S., Fowler, J.S., Volkow, N.D., Gatley, S.J., Logan, J., Dewey, S.L., Alexoff, D., Fazzini, E. & Wolf, A.P. (1994), Pharmacokinetics and in vivo specificity of [^{11}C]dl-threo-methylphenidate for the presynaptic dopaminergic neuron. *Synapse*, 18:152–160.

Fowler, J.S., Volkow, N.D., Wolf, A.P., Dewey, S.L., Schlyer, D.J., MacGregor, R.R., Hitzemann, R., Logan, J., Bendriem, B., Gatley, S.J. & Christman, D. (1989), Mapping cocaine binding sites in human and baboon brain *in vivo*. *Synapse*, 4:371–377.

Gatley, S.J., Ding, Y.S., Volkow, N.D., Chen, R., Sugano, Y. & Fowler, J.S. (1995a), Binding of d-threo-[^{11}C]methylphenidate to the dopamine transporter *in vivo*: Insensitivity to synaptic dopamine. *Eur. J. Pharmacol.*, 281:141–149.

Gatley, S.J., Volkow, N.D., Fowler, J.S., & Dewey, S.L. (1995b), Sensitivity of striatal [^{11}C] cocaine binding to decreases in synaptic dopamine. *Synapse*, 20:137–144.

Grace, A.A. (1995), The tonic/phasic model of dopamine system regulation: Its relevance for understanding how stimulant abuse can alter basal ganglia function. *Drug Alcohol Depend.*, 37:111–129.

Gualtieri, C.T. & Hicks, R.E. (1985), Neuropharmacology of methylphenidate and a neural substrate for childhood hyperactivity. *Psychiatr. Clin. North Am.*, 8:875–892.

Kety, S.S. (1960), The cerebral circulation. In: *Handbook of Physiology: Neurophysiology, vol. III*, eds., J. Field, H.W. Magoun & V.E. Hall. Washington, DC: American Physiological Society, pp. 1751–1760.

Koob, G.F. & Bloom, F.E. (1988), Cellular and molecular mechanisms of drug dependence. *Science*, 242:715–723.

Kuhar, M.J., Ritz, M.C. & Boja, J.W. (1991), The dopamine hypothesis of the reinforcing properties of cocaine. *Trends Neurosci.*, 14:299–302.

Kuhar, M.J., Sanchez-Roa, P.M., Wong, D.F., Dannals, R.F., Grigoriadis, D.E., Lew, R. & Milberger, M. (1990), Dopamine transporter: biochemistry, pharmacology and imaging. *Eur. Neurol.*, 30(suppl 1):S15–S20.

London, E.D., Cascella, N.G., Wong, D.F., Phillips, R.L., Dannals, R.F., Links, J.M., Herning, R., Grayson, R., Jaffe, J.H. & Wagner, H.N., Jr. (1990), Cocaine-induced reduction of glucose utilization in human brain. A study using positron emission tomography and [fluorine 18]fluorodeoxyglucose. *Arch. Gen. Psychiatry*, 47:567–574.

Matochik, J.A., Liebenauer, L.L. & King, A.C. (1994), Cerebral glucose metabolism in adults with attention deficit hyperactivity disorder after chronic stimulant treatment. *Am. J. Psychiatry*, 151:658–664.

Matochik, J.A., Nordahl, T.E., Gross, M., Semple, W.E., King, A.C., Cohen, R.M. & Zametkin, A.J. (1993), Effects of acute stimulant medication on cerebral metabolism in adults with hyperactivity. *Neuropsychopharmacology*, 8:377–386.

Ritz, M.C., Lamb, R.J., Goldberg, S.R. & Kuhar, M.J. (1987), Cocaine receptors on dopamine transporters are related to self-administration of cocaine. *Science*, 237:1219–1223.

Shimada, S., Kitayama, S., Lin, C.-L., Patel, A., Nanthakumar, E., Gregor, P., Kuhar, M. & Uhl, G. (1991), Cloning and expression of a cocaine-sensitive dopamine transporter complementary DNA. *Science*, 254:576–578.

Sokoloff, L. (1978), Mapping cerebral functional activity with radioactive deoxyglucose. *Trends Neurosci.*, 1:75–79.

Solanto, M.V. (1986), Behavioral effects of low-dose methylphenidate in childhood attention deficit disorder: Implications for a mechanism of stimulant drug action. *J. Am. Acad. Child Adolesc. Psychiatry*, 25:96–101.

Solanto, M. (1997), Neuropsychopharmacological mechanisms of stimulant drug action in attention deficit/hyperactivity disorder: A review and integration. *Behav. Brain Res.*, 94:127–152.

Swanson, J., Insbourne, M. & Roberts, W. (1978), Time-response analysis of the effect of stimulant medication on the learning ability of children referred for hyperactivity. *Pediatrics*, 61:21–29.

Volkow, N.D., Ding, Y.-S., Fowler, J.S. & Wang, G.-J. (1996a), Cocaine addiction: Hypothesis derived from imaging studies with PET. *J. Addict. Dis.* 15:55–71.

Volkow, N.D., Ding, Y.-S., Fowler, J.S., Wang, G.-J., Logan, J., Gatley, J.S., Dewey, S., Ashby, C., Liebermann, J., Hitzemann, R. & Wolf, A.P. (1995), Is methylphenidate like cocaine? Studies on their pharmacokinetics and distribution in the human brain. *Arch. Gen. Psychiatry*, 52:456–463.

Volkow, N.D., Wang, G.J., Fischman, M.W., Foltin, R.W., Fowler, J.S., Abumrad, N.N., Vitkun, S., Logan, J., Gatley, S.J., Pappas, N., Hitzemann, R. & Shea, C.E. (1997a), Relationship between subjective effects of cocaine and dopamine transporter occupancy. *Nature*, 386:827–830.

Volkow, N.D., Wang, G.-J., Fowler, J.S., Gatley, S.J., Ding, Y.-S., Logan, J., Dewey, S.L., Hitzemann, R. & Lieberman, J. (1996b), Relationship between psychostimulant-induced high and dopamine transporter occupancy. *Proc. Natl. Acad. Sci. USA*, 93:10388–10398.

Volkow, N.D., Wang, G.J., Fowler, J.S., Logan, J., Gatley, S.J., Hitzemann, R., Chen, A.D.,

Dewey, S.L. & Pappas, N. (1997b), Decreased striatal dopaminergic responsiveness in detoxified cocaine-dependent subjects. *Nature* 386:830–833.

Volkow, N.D., Wang, G.J., Fowler, J.S., Logan, J., Schlyer, D., Hitzemann, R., Lieberman, J., Angrist, B., Pappas, N. & MacGregor, R. (1994), Imaging endogenous dopamine competition with [^{11}C]raclopride in the human brain. *Synapse*, 16:255–262.

Wang, G.J., Volkow, N.D., Fowler, J.S., Ferrieri, R., Schyler, D.J., Alexoff, D., Pappas, N., Lieberman, J., King, P., Warner, D., Wong, C., Hitzemann, R.J. & Wolf, A.P. (1994), Methylphenidate decreases regional cerebral blood flow in normal human subjects. *Life Sci.*, 54:143–146.

Wang, G.J., Volkow, N.D., Hitzemann, R., Wong, C., Angrist, B., Burr, G., Pascani, K., Pappas, N., Lu, A., Cooper, T. & Lieberman, J. (1997), Behavioral and cardiovascular effects of intravenous methylphenidate in normal subjects and cocaine abusers. *Eur. J. Addict. Res.* 3:49–54.

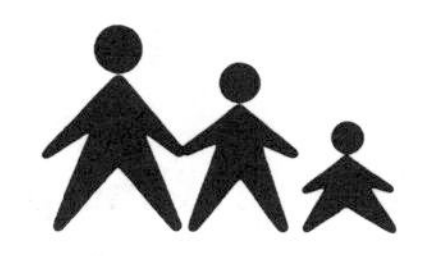

Randomized Clinical Trials of Long-Duration Stimulant Medications: Design Considerations

LAURENCE L. GREENHILL,[1] JEFFREY M. HALPERIN,[2] and HOWARD ABIKOFF[3]

Four Immediate-release (IR) stimulant medications—methylphenidate (MPH), dextroamphetamine (DEX), Adderall, and pemoline (PEM)—are available to clinicians with a package insert indication for the treatment of attention deficit hyperactivity disorder (ADHD) in children. These four medications were approved by the Food and Drug Administration (FDA) for use in children with ADHD more than 20 years ago, even though a brief duration of action produces time-response problems and forces in-school administration for the shorter-duration stimulants (Richters et al., 1995). Existing long-duration stimulants (LDS)—MPH-SR and Dexedrine Spansules—have not solved the late day dosing or time-action problems (Spencer et al., 1996b). Not until 1996 was a new drug application (NDA) for a different longer-duration stimulant filed with the FDA (Laughren, 1997).

One recent review reported robust short-term stimulant-related improvements in ADHD symptoms in 161 randomized controlled trials (RCTs) encompassing five preschool, 140 school-age, seven adolescent, and nine adult trials (Spencer et al., 1996b). Although early articles suggested that stimulant medications uniquely and paradoxically calmed school-age children with ADHD, these drugs have proved effective for diverse age groups. Improvement has been noted in 65% to 75% of the 5,899 patients assigned to stimulant treatment, vs. only 4% to 30% of those assigned to placebo for MPH (n = 133 trials), DEX (n = 22 trials), and PEM (n = 6 trials).

However, the generalizability of these studies has been limited by their failure to use the design and analytic strategies that have become the standard for state-of-the-art clinical trials, such as manualized therapies, large numbers, multiple sites, and parallel designs. A methodological review using standards of randomized clinical trials used by the FDA identified 75 RCT ADHD child stimulant trials but found numerous deficiencies that limited their "validity, relevance, precision and therefore, their clinical application" (McMaster University Evidence-Based Practice Center). Most stimulant studies in ADHD children have a very short duration (often weeks to a few months), small numbers, within-group comparisons, and single-site populations; involve mainly Caucasian male subjects; and fail to include ADHD children with the full range of impairment and other disorders often encoun-

[1]Department of Psychiatry, Division of Child and Adolescent Psychiatry, New York State Psychiatric Institute; and Disruptive Behavior Disorders Clinic, Columbia-Presbyterian Medical Center, New York, New York.

[2]Department of Psychiatry, Division of Child and Adolescent Psychiatry, The Mount Sinai School of Medicine, New York, New York; and Neuropsychology Graduate Program, Queens College, City University of New York, Flushing, New York.

[3]New York University Child Study Center; and Division of Child and Adolescent Psychiatry, New York University Medical Center, New York, New York.

Supported in part by Grant No. 5 UO1-MH50454-02 (Dr. Greenhill) from the National Institute of Mental Health.

tered in clinic-based samples. There is a growing public focus on the increasing numbers of children being treated with stimulants (Safer et al., 1996), so that bringing new stimulant preparations onto the market requires more reliable trial methodology.

METHODS

To further determine what elements of trial design would be needed for trials of new LDS, a Medline search was conducted for randomized clinical stimulant medication trials of children, adolescents, and adults with ADHD. Search terms included methylphenidate, Ritalin, Dexedrine, dextroamphetamine, pemoline, Cylert, and Adderall, each coupled with attention deficit hyperactivity disorder and clinical trial. The dates ranged from 1985 to September 1998. When studies that included comparisons with nonstimulant drugs or other therapies were excluded, and multiple publications of the same study were considered, the search yielded 23 articles that met minimal criteria for RCTs: they compared stimulants with placebo and used double-blind ratings. Four additional RCTs (Abikoff and Hechtman, unpublished; Gillberg et al., 1997; MTA Cooperative Group, in press; Schachar, et al., 1997) were identified from other sources.

THERAPEUTIC EFFECTS OF APPROVED STIMULANTS

Stimulant drugs affect behavior cross situationally (classroom, lunchroom, playground, and home) when they are repeatedly administered throughout the day. In the classroom, stimulants decrease interrupting, fidgetiness, and finger tapping and increase on-task behavior (Abikoff and Hechtman, unpublished). At home, stimulants improve parent–child interactions, on-task behaviors, and compliance. In social settings, stimulants ameliorate peer nomination rankings of social standing and increase attention during baseball (Richters et al., 1995). Stimulants decrease response variability and impulsive responding on cognitive tasks (Tannock et al., 1995a); increase the accuracy of performance; and improve short-term memory, reaction time, seatwork computation, problem-solving games with peers (Whalen et al., 1989), and sustained attention. Studies of time-action stimulant effects show different patterns of improvement for behavioral and attentional symptoms, with behavior affected more than attention. For example, a controlled, analog classroom trial (n = 30) of Adderall (Swanson et al., 1998) showed rapid improvements on teacher ratings and math performance 1.5 hours after administration, with time of peak effects and duration of action dependent on dose. While stimulant drugs show a large 0.8–1.0 effect size for behavioral measures, smaller 0.6–0.8 effect sizes are reported on cognitive measures (Spencer et al., 1996b).

Children with ADHD demonstrate low placebo response rates during clinical drug trials, ranging between 3% (Spencer et al., 1996b) and 30% (Gillberg et al., 1997), with a mode of 10%. This leads to large placebo-active drug differences, enabling small number, single-site, controlled trial designs to identify significant drug effects. The drugs' very short elimination half-lives make stimulants highly eligible for crossover designs (Swanson et al., 1998), because pharmacokinetic carryover of active drug into placebo periods is unlikely.

Stimulant adverse events

Stimulants show a 4% adverse event rate in controlled studies of children with ADHD. Prominently cited are delay of sleep onset, reduced appetite, stomachache, headache, and dizziness (Barkley et al., 1990). No additional delay in sleep onset was seen after the addition of a third, midafternoon dose of MPH to standard twice-daily dosing regimens (Kent et al., 1995). Staring, daydreaming, irritability, anxiety, or nailbiting may decrease with increasing stimulant dose, suggesting that these symptoms may be part of the ADHD disorder rather than stimulant-related adverse events. No consistent reports of behavioral rebound, motor tics, compulsive picking of nose or skin, dose-related emotional or cognitive constriction, or dose-related growth delays have been found in controlled studies (Spencer et al., 1996a). However, this low rate of stimulant side effects emerges from short-term trials that do not account for the cases with poor compliance or with treatment failure (Mayes et al., 1994).

Stimulant-related growth delays have been reported in ADHD children receiving long-term stimulant treatment. Small weight decrements are reported during short-term trials (Gillberg et al., 1997), but prospective follow-up into adult life (Manuzza et al., 1991) has revealed no significant impairment of height attained. Furthermore, the growth rate delays attributed to medication may be a developmental artifact associated with the disorder. ADHD children, either stimulant treated or not, have demonstrated slower growth rate advances than in normal children (Spencer et al., 1996a).

Hepatic tumors in rodents occur when the animals are treated with high oral doses of 4–47 mg/kg of MPH (Dunnick and Hailey, 1995), but are not in stimulant-treated preschool or school age children. However, altered liver function tests have been reported in 44 children treated with PEM (Berkovitch et al., 1995), with 11 experiencing liver failure. As a result, PEM is no longer advised as a first-line treatment for ADHD.

Additional concerns exist about the abuse potential for the psychostimulants. Laboratory evidence suggests that MPH has moderate addiction potential for laboratory animals, which may be species dependent. National surveys indicate that high school seniors may experiment by snorting ground-up MPH tablets, but far less frequently than they experiment with marijuana or cocaine. The actual abuse potential of MPH for adolescents with ADHD has not been evaluated in any controlled, prospective manner. The addiction potential for DEX in adults, on the other hand, has been documented (Sannerud and Feussner, this volume, pp. 27–42).

Stimulant effects on comorbid conditions

Two thirds of ADHD children have one or more comorbid Axis I psychiatric disorders—primarily oppositional defiant disorder, conduct disorder, or anxiety disorder—whereas published stimulant RCTs often enroll children with "pure" ADHD (Richters et al., 1995). Comorbid symptoms may alter the response to IR stimulants. ADHD children with comorbid anxiety disorders have been reported to show increased placebo response rates (DuPaul et al., 1994; Pliszka, 1992), a greater incidence of side effects, or poorer improvements on cognitive tests (Tannock et al., 1995b) during RCTs MPH trials. Controlled studies in ADHD children with Tourette's syndrome have shown either worsening (Schachar et al., 1997) or improving tic frequency patterns (Gadow et al., 1995). Ratings of antisocial behavior specific to conduct disorder were significantly reduced by MPH treatment even when baseline ADHD symptoms were covaried in a controlled study of 84 boys with ADHD and conduct disorder (Klein et al., 1997). Thus, new RCTs, to be ecologically valid, must include children with comorbidities. With large samples now being required by the FDA for efficacy studies, it will be possible to determine moderator effects of comorbid conditions on treatment response to LDS medications.

LIMITATIONS OF STIMULANTS NOW AVAILABLE

There are important limitations in the current stimulant pharmaceopeia. First, IR MPH tablets have a 4-hour duration of action, requiring multiple dosing during school (Swanson et al., 1998). This creates a risk of being ridiculed by peers and irregular supervision by busy school personnel. Time-action effects can produce drug wear-off during the late morning, midafternoon, or evening, with return of the ADHD symptoms. Given too late in the day, stimulants suppress appetite at dinner and delay sleep onset. As a result, parents are reluctant to use them late in the day to help with evening homework inattention and noncompliance. Longer-acting PEM treatment is hampered by concerns about hepatotoxicity appearing late during long-term treatment. The efficacy of combination IR and sustained-release stimulant preparations, though very popular in practice, has been tested in only one controlled study and found to be no different than monotherapy (Fitzpatrick et al., 1992).

Second, the most troublesome stimulant side effects, including anorexia, weight loss, headaches, insomnia, and tics, affect many children and do not improve over time (Schachar, et al., 1997). Third, MPH and DEX are classified as Schedule II medications with "high abuse potential with severe psychic or physical dependence liability." Fourth, these drugs show differential responses across settings and domains in the same child (Pelham et al., 1991), made all the more problematic because reliability predictors of drug response are not available (Jacobvitz et al., 1990).

Trial methodology: limitations

When the four marketed stimulants were developed more than 20 years ago, most phase 1 (safety) and phase II (dosing and early efficacy) data were collected in animals and adults. As a result, modern NDA phase I studies (e.g., effect of fatty diet on absorption and basic pharmacokinetics in children), phase II studies (e.g., combined pharmacokinetic/pharmacodynamic), or phase III studies (e.g., population pharmacokinetics) were not carried out for those stimulants now in use for children with ADHD.

Without the demands of the NDA approval process, the stimulant trials published in the last decade did not consistently use the design features or analytic approaches used in multisite RCTs submitted to the FDA for drug approval. For example, the ethnicity of the samples was not mentioned, nor were representative child patient samples included that would allow the findings to be generalizable. Most studies lasted less than 12 weeks and therefore could not inform maintenance treatment of children with ADHD. Many studies did not report comorbid disorders, which can alter the response to medication. Others did not report the fidelity with which the treatments were administered by staff, nor did they always list results of the compliance measures used. Parallel-design methodology, optimal titration of stimulant doses for each patient, and intent-to-treat designs were not used (Richters et al., 1995). Other details were not listed by most studies, such as the exact method of randomization (including a central randomization group apart from the site) and details of dropouts. The methodological strengths and limitations of the 24 most recent stimulant RCTs are detailed in Table 1.

Methodology: improvements

The design of randomized controlled trials of LDS medications can be improved by the ten practices that follow.

Table 1. Design Features of Randomized Controlled Trials of Stimulants in Children

Study	*Design*	*New?*	*Duration*	*Dosing*	*Representative Sample?*	*Comorbid?*	*Impairment?*	*Multiple Domains*	*Compliance?*	*ITT*	*History?*	*Setting*
Abikoff (1995) School	xver	No	8 weeks	Opt/BID	N/A	N/A	N/A	School only	N/A	N/A	N/A	
Abikoff (1998)	parallel	Yes	104 weeks	Opt/TID	Yes	Yes	Yes, C-GAS	Yes	Saliva levels	Yes	Respon	Clinic
Barkley (1989)	xver	No	4 weeks	Fix/OD	N/A	N/A	N/A	Yes	Pill counts	No	No	Clinic
Barkley (1991)	xver	No	6 weeks	Fix/BID	N/A	N/A	N/A	Yes	Pill counts	N/A	N/A	Clinic
Castellanos (1997)	xver	Yes	9 weeks	Fix/BID	Boys	Yes; TS	Yes, C-GAS	Yes	Staff adm	N/A	Yes	Lab
Douglas (1988)	xver	No	2 weeks	Fix/OD	N/A	Yes	N/A	Yes	Staff adm	N/A	Respon	Lab
Douglas (1995)	xver	No	4 weeks	Fix/OD	N/A	N/A	N/A	Yes	Staff adm	N/A	N/A	Clinic
DuPaul (1993)	xver	No	6 weeks	Fix/BID	N/A	N/A	N/A	No, school	Staff adm	N/A	N/A	Clinic
DuPaul (1994)	xver	No	6 weeks	Fix/OD	N/A	N/A	N/A	No, school	Parent report	N/A	N/A	Clinic
Elia (1991)	xver	No	9 weeks	Fix/BID	Boys; N/A	Yes	CGAS	Yes	Staff adm	N/A	Yes	Lab
Gadow (1995)	xver	No	8 weeks	Fix/BID	Yes	Yes	N/A	ADHD	Pill counts	N/A	Yes	Clinic
Gillberg (1997)	parallel	Yes	60 weeks	Opt/OD	Yes	Yes	N/A	Yes	Pill counts	Yes	Yes	Clinic
Klein (1997)	parallel	Yes	5 weeks	Opt/BID	N/A	Yes	N/A	Yes	N/A	No	N/A	Clinic
Klorman (1990)	xver	No	3 weeks	Fix/TID	Yes	Yes	N/A	Yes	Staff adm	N/A	Yes	Clinic
MTA (1995)	parallel	Yes	56 weeks	Opt/TID*	Yes	Yes	Yes	Yes	Saliva levels	Yes	Yes	Clinic
Musten (1997)	xver	No	3 weeks	Fix/BID	No	Yes	N/A	Yes	pill counts	N/A	N/A	Clinic
Pelham (1990)	xver	No	4 weeks	Fix/OD	N/A	Yes	N/A	Yes	Staff adm	N/A	Yes	STP
Pelham (1995)	xver	No	7 weeks	Fix/OD	N/A	N/A	N/A	Yes	Staff adm	N/A	N/A	Lab
Rapport (1988)	xver	No	5 weeks	Fix/OD	N/A	N/A	N/A	School, lab	Staff adm	N/A	Respon	Lab
Rapport (1994)	xver	No	6 weeks	Fix/OD	Yes	N/A	N/A	School	Envelope counts	N/A	Yes	Clinic
Schachar (1998)	parallel	Yes	52 weeks	Opt	N/A	N/A	N/A	School/ home	Pill counts	N/A	Yes	Clinic
Spencer (1995)	xver	No	7 weeks	Fix/TID	N/A	N/A	N/A	ADHD, dep, anx	Serum samples	N/A	N/A	Clinic
Swanson (1988)	xver	Yes	7 weeks	Fix/OD	N/A	N/A	N/A	N/A	Staff adm	N/A	Yes	Lab
Tannock (1995)	xver	No	4 days	Fix/OD	N/A	Yes	N/A	Cognitive	Staff adm	N/A	Yes	Lab

(*continued*)

TABLE 1. (*continued*) DESIGN FEATURES OF RANDOMIZED CONTROLLED TRIALS OF STIMULANTS IN CHILDREN

Study	*Design*	*New?*	*Duration*	*Dosing*	*Representative Sample?*	*Comorbid?*	*Impairment?*	*Multiple Domains*	*Compliance?*	*ITT*	*History?*	*Setting*
Taylor (1987)	xver	No	6 weeks	Opt/Flex	Boys; N/A	No	N/A	Yes	N/A	N/A	N/A	Clinic
Whalen (1989)	xver	No	5 weeks	Fix/BID	Boys; N/A	Yes	N/A	Peer judgment	Staff adm	N/A	N/A	STP

Scale Legend: Design = type of design (i.e., parallel); New? = did study include a new method for handling placebo?; Duration = length of study, e.g. did study exceed 3 months?; Dosing = type of dosing (fixed, did study optimize child's dose?); Representative Sample? = did study use representative samples?; Comorbid? = did study evaluate comorbidity?; Impairment? = did study use measure of impairment?; Multiple domains = did study use multi-informant, multidomain outcome measures?; Compliance? = did study measure fidelity or compliance?; ITT = did study use intent-to-treat measures; History? = does study include a measure of previous stimulant treatment history?; Setting = study in clinic, laboratory, or summer treatment program (STP); N/A = not addressed in the journal article or not applicable. * = daily switching of stimulant dose; ABBREVIATIONS: xver = crossover design; fix = fixed dose; Opt = each child on his/her optimal dose; OD = once a day; BID = twice daily; TID = thrice daily; CGAS = Children's Global Assessment Scale; Anx = children had a comorbid diagnosis of anxiety.

Replacing crossover design trials with parallel designs

A crossover design enables a small study (n = 20–30) to have adequate power to test a single hypothesis because subjects act as their own controls. This is particularly suitable for a rare disorder—which ADHD is not—because it tests the response to drug in a smaller sample than is required for other controlled designs. In addition, very short-acting drugs, such as DEX and MPH, are optimal for crossover trials because their powerful effects do not last long or carry over into the placebo period (Greenhill et al., 1996). Also, the crossover design addresses parental concerns about placebo assignment because all children who enter the trial will be given the active drug (Fava, 1996). Although all subjects are assigned to placebo in a crossover trial, assignment is brief: typically 2–3 weeks vs. the 8 weeks necessary in a parallel design.

However, crossover designs are vulnerable to carryover effects even for stimulants. Brain catecholamine receptor densities take days to weeks to revert after prolonged stimulant treatment (Pliszka et al., 1996). Also, rater effects lag in crossover trials. A given ADHD symptom behavior—e.g., a moderate level of disruptiveness—may be perceived and rated quite differently following placebo (when it may receive mildly negative ratings) than when it follows successful stimulant treatment (when ratings may be strongly negative). Crossover designs do not always control for this by determining whether the child returns to baseline at the onset of each new treatment condition. For these reasons, the FDA reviews data from drug trials for treatment by period effects. If these are found, then only the data collected before the crossover point are accepted (Laughren, 1997).

Newer stimulants will have a much longer duration of action, making them even more prone to carryover effects. For these reasons, pivotal efficacy trials of new LDS medications will have to use parallel-design methodologies.

Using new designs for control arm of study

Controlled double-blind, parallel-design trials require random assignment of a subgroup to a control condition (placebo, active drug, or a waiting list). Children with ADHD in RCTs show placebo responses from 3% to 40%, so the phase III pivotal efficacy trials for new long-duration stimulants will need to be placebo-controlled to be interpretable. Furthermore, placebo control is the optimal comparison for phase III pivotal trials, for it permits the assessment of the stability of symptoms in the absence of treatment (Laughren, 1997), which is particularly important when comorbid conditions may intermittently contribute to impairment.

However, placebo treatments in pediatric drug trials make it harder to recruit cases (Fava, 1996). The longer duration of action of LDSs, coupled with a need to study the drug in a much longer clinical trial, will require much longer assignment to a placebo control condition than did the traditional 6-week crossover design found in the stimulant literature. Parents may reject a study in which their children may be assigned to treatment with an ineffective agent. The ethical concern of withholding an effective treatment for 6–8 weeks is another important issue.

Alternatives in trial design that favor strong patient recruitment—e.g., using IR MPH for an "active" control or running a discontinuation design—may not solve this problem. Discontinuation trials have not been accepted as a proof of drug efficacy by the FDA. Using another stimulant as an active control may not be an adequate test of the efficacy of the new LDS. No study to date has been able to demonstrate significant differences between different stimulants or between IR and sustained-release stimulants (Greenhill et al., 1997). While a new LDS may provide much better coverage late in the day, the conventional IR stimulant control is likely to produce almost identical global ratings from parents and teachers, making it difficult to show greater benefits for the new LDS.

What will be needed are innovative designs that utilize alternative control conditions, such as that used by the National Institute of Mental Health (NIMH) multimodal treatment study of attention deficit hyperactivity disorder (MTA Cooperative Group, in press). The subgroup of MTA children with ADHD (n = 146) randomly assigned to the control condition were referred out for care by community providers, rather than to placebo, which would have delayed effective treatment for 14 months (Arnold et al., 1997). For other studies, recruitment into a parallel-design study involving placebo can be made more attractive to families by providing each family with incentives that will make the wait for effective interventions worthwhile. Such innovative designs might include a thorough, written, free evaluation of the child with ADHD at the end of the study, parent training for the control group, or weekly supportive visits for the parents with the study physician.

Increasing the duration of the trial

Although the majority of published controlled stimulant trials show robust benefits and only a 4% rate of adverse events, 96% of these lasted less than 4 months (Schachar et al., 1993). longer trials have reported more mixed results. These include retrospective open studies, carried out before 1983, reporting that children receiving stimulants showed no advantage over unmedicated ADHD children in emotional adjustment, delinquency, academic failure, ratings of hyperactivity, and family ratings at the follow-up assessments. However, these used open designs, failed to randomly assign children to drug and no-drug conditions, showed high (30% to 50%) rates of subject attrition, had low compliance rates (12% to 28%) for continuing to take medication, failed to track academic and peer impairment, failed to include relevant control groups, and failed to use standardized, published outcome measures (Jacobvitz et al., 1990).

The four recent prospective multisite studies that used periods between 12 and 24 months show that stimulants continue to exert their effects as long as they are taken (Abikoff and Hechtman, unpublished; Gillberg et al., 1997; MTA Cooperative Group, in press; Schachar, unpublished). Attrition rates in these trials ranged from 7% (MTA Cooperative Group, unpublished) to 30% (Schachar, 1997). They addressed previous methodological limitations by using multiinformant measures across several domains of functioning, randomly assigning children to treatment conditions, including relevant control groups, and prospectively monitoring children with ADHD who receive stimulant treatment.

One of these trials tested the long-term efficacy of racemic amphetamine using a 15-month, prospective, randomized, double-blind, placebo-controlled, discontinuation design (Gillberg et al., 1997). Sixty-two children with ADHD were openly titrated to racemic amphetamine over 3 months. In a randomized, double-blind protocol, 30 were assigned to placebo while 32 continued to receive amphetamine for 12 months of treatment. Study endpoint—need to be removed from the protocol and given open treatment—occurred for 71% of those assigned to placebo vs. 29% assigned to AMP ($p < 0.05$). This trial lacked *a priori* criteria for discontinuation, included children comorbid for pervasive developmental disorder, and did not explain lack of deterioration for AMP responders switched to placebo after 12 months.

The other three RCTs used a prospective, parallel design. One of them used IR MPH in a two-year, parallel, 3-arm, dual-site, multimodal design involving 103 patients (Abikoff and Hechtman, unpublished), and revealed that medication effects lasted as long as children took MPH. Another used IR MPH in a single-site, 12 month, four-arm multimodal design involving 92 patients, and found that the side effects of MPH continue as long as the drug is taken and are a major reason for patient noncompliance (Schachar, 1997). The fourth and largest prospective clinical drug RCT, the NIMH MTA Study, used a six-site, 14 month, four-arm, multimodal parallel design involving 579 patients. The medication strategy provided an algorithm for selecting MPH, DEX, PEM or imipramine (MTA Cooperative Group, in press). These three trials most closely approach the de facto standards used by the FDA for evaluating randomized controlled trials for the approval of new medications.

Just as these four RCTs showed maintenance of both beneficial and adverse drug effects, so too the drug development programs for LDS will need a minimum of 12 months to evaluate their safety, establish the stability of improvements, detect late-appearing side effects, and to determine its long-term acceptability of the LDS drug.

Optimizing each child's drug dose

Many single-site stimulant trials began by giving all treated ADHD children the same dose, titrated using identical dose steps and identical dosing administration times. Modification of dose or timing was allowed to manage side effects. Dosing decisions depended on the protocol, not on the patient's response. Practitioners, on the other hand, individually optimize medication doses for each child. Because of their standardization methods, clinical research offers little advice about selecting starting doses for titration, picking the best times for stimulant administration, or specifying the doses to be given at different times.

Like the published controlled studies of stimulants, protocols submitted to the FDA need to use standardized dosing methods to ensure good internal validity (Laughren, 1997). However, individual optimization can greatly benefit each child in a study and this prevents dropouts while resembling what is done in a clinician's office. Several long-term stimulant RCTs maintained internal validity while individually optimizing each child's dose (Abikoff and Hechtman, unpublished; Gillberg et al., 1997; MTA Cooperative Group, unpublished). Algorithms were used in the NIMH MTA study to standardize the dose and drug optimization process (Greenhill et al., 1996). Similar algorithms can be used for assigning each child his or her "best dose" in a large-number, multisite, placebo-controlled, parallel-design, randomized efficacy study of a new LDS-medication.

Recruiting more representative samples of patients

Treatment studies of children with psychiatric disorders have depended on samples of convenience and suffer because sampling methods are biased or unknown. Patient demographics, socioeconomic status (SES), parent education, family composition, or ethnicity of ADHD children are described in only a few stimulant studies (Gadow et al., 1995; Gillberg et al., 1997) but not in most (Pliszka, 1992). Although IQ and SES do not predict adult outcome in untreated ADHD children, these factors may directly affect compliance with treatment, which then could affect outcome. Ethnicity may influence access to stimulant treatment. Maryland Medicaid prescription records reveal that African-American children receive about one third the number of MPH prescriptions as do Caucasian children (Zito et al., 1997). Parental education, living situation, or single-parent status may be related to attitudes toward treatment and affect patient compliance with treatment instructions.

New LDS drug RCTs will benefit from the inclusion of broad representative samples for clinical and public health relevance. Both treatment-naive patients and those exposed to stimulant treatment in the past should be included. In addition, the sample should be heterogeneous with respect to gender, social class, ethnicity, and comorbidity. This means active recruitment of girls, minority children, and ADHD patients with comorbid internalizing, aggressive, and learning disorders. This will allow investigators to determine how culturally based attitudes toward stimulant medications can be related to outcomes. It will be necessary to translate study instruments for significant minorities such as families whose primary language is Spanish. Exclusion criteria should be limited to factors that interfere with treatment or assessment, such as absence from school (unable to gather teacher's ratings), current participation in another study (confounding of assessments), or parental stimulant abuse.

Including comorbid patients

Comorbid Axis I disorders affect response during stimulant treatment, as suggested by controlled studies that have stratified ADHD children by comorbid diagnosis (DuPaul and Barkley, 1990; Klorman et al., 1990; Tannock et al., 1995a). However, it is not clear whether the reduced effect size for stimulants in ADHD children with comorbid anxiety disorder is the result of increased placebo response (Pliszka, 1992) or an increase in side effects (Tannock et al., 1995b). Only large studies have the power to evaluate the interactions of combined medication/psychosocial treatment and comorbidity in ADHD (Richters et al., 1995).

Multisite trials provide the sample size necessary for assessing the effects of patient comorbid disorders on the response to a new stimulant preparation. Phase III efficacy trials for new drugs for ADHD provide an opportunity to mount multisite patient samples with diverse diagnoses. The study sample can be stratified for Axis I comorbid diagnoses, such as anxiety disorders, or Axis II comorbid disorders, such as learning disabilities, which may have a different pattern of drug response (Laughren, 1997). This approach enhances ecologic validity by including children with comorbid disorders while protecting against type 2 error by prior stratification.

Including a measure of impairment

A common approach for establishing eligibility in treatment studies of ADHD has been to set a cut score on a continuous measure of ADHD symptoms coupled with a categorical measure to determine conformity to *Diagnostical and Statistical Manual of Mental Disorders* (*DSM*) criteria for ADHD. Symptoms listed in *DSM-IV* must produce impairment in two different situations for the child to meet the criteria for ADHD. However, the development of criterion-based diagnostic instruments such as the DISC-2.3 (Shaffer et al., 1996) now makes it possible to ensure that the overall criteria for ADHD are satisfied in a standardized fashion.

It is also possible to consider alternative approaches to ascertaining severity. Impairment can be measured and, by extension, clinical improvement. Symptom count may relate to severity of disorder, but the relationship may be quite weak. An earlier study demonstrated that attention-deficit disorder children who were being treated with MPH showed a significant reduction in symptom severity with no concomitant reduction in measures of global impairment (C-GAS) (Shaffer et al., 1983). There could be a lag between changes in ADHD symptoms and reduction in impairment, because the impairment may be determined by other causes—for example, poverty or learning disability—not related to the ADHD.

Future clinical stimulant trials would benefit by adding measures of impairment as a secondary outcome measure. Studies of new stimulants can determine whether symptomatic improvement is matched by reductions in social and academic impairment. Instruments that inquire about impairments in specific domains, such as the Columbia Impairment Scale, may prove to be more treatment sensitive.

Including primary outcome measures that tap multiple informants and domains

In planning clinical trials, investigators may choose baseline assessment batteries that address several domains, use multiple informants, and combine global behavioral and impairment ratings from parents, teachers, and clinicians (Richters et al., 1995). The NIMH MTA study, for example, carefully characterized the sample by assessing school achievement and educational performance, parent and family processes, peer relations, social functioning, externalizing symptoms, internalizing symptoms, cognitive and attentional processes, impairment, and service utilization patterns for each family.

Additional measures collected at baseline may include academic performance ratings; an "objective" measure (continuous performance task or a direct academic performance rating, such as a test of speed and accuracy at a simple math task); ratings of internalizing comorbid disorders (anxiety or depression); vital signs; side effects; and a measure of impairment, e.g., the Columbia Impairment Scale (Bird et al., 1995). Interim ratings should include abbreviated parent and teacher ratings of externalizing behaviors, vital signs, and side effects.

At the end of the study, the investigator repeats a subset of these measures to determine the effects of the treatment. Ideally, one or two of these baseline measures are chosen, before the study starts, to also serve as the primary outcome measures. One of these outcome measures should tap multiple informants and multiple domains. Primary measures most often used in large, pivotal NDA trials for FDA review—and likely to be the ones recommended for RCTs of new LDS medications—include a global clinician-based measure of improvement synthesized from multiple informants (teachers, parents) over several domains. Sometimes the clinical global improvement (CGI) is used for this purpose, plus an ADHD disorder-specific clinician rating scale that is *DSM-IV* based, such as the SNAP-IV (Laughren, 1997).

Including measures of fidelity and compliance

The new LDS study must include descriptions of the research staff's fidelity in delivering the theraply plus a measure of the child's and family's compliance in adhering to the treatment arm. These factors account for much variance in pediatric psychopharmacologic RCTs. Although sophisticated monitoring techniques are available that use electronic recording of pill bottle openings for tracking the time of pill administration, there is no agreement on a single "gold standard" method for monitoring compliance. For the published studies in Table 1, methods for monitoring exposure of patients to the medication treatment varied from having study staff give all pills (Elia et al., 1991; Tannock et al., 1995a and b; Whalen et al., 1989) to counting pills in the returned bottles of medication at each visit when parents administered the pills (Barkley et al., 1991; Barkley et al., 1989; Klorman et al., 1990; Rapport et al., 1994; Spencer et al., 1995; Taylor et al., 1987). While staff delivery assures high compliance rates, this method is less ecologically valid than clinic-based studies where parents administer the medication. Other studies (Abikoff and Gittelman, 1985; Douglas et al., 1988; Pelham et al., 1990; Pelham et al., 1995; Rapport et al., 1988) list no specific compliance measure.

The NIMH MTA study used three methods of compliance, including parent reports of pill taking, pill counts using returned blister packages during the titration phase (Greenhill et al., 1996), and random MPH saliva assays (Greenhill and Cooper, 1987) collected during the long-term maintenance phase. In addition, fidelity to the protocol was ensured by use of the treatment manuals; audiotaped monitoring of all pharmacotherapy visits by on-site supervisors; and weekly, national, cross-site teleconferences to develop and maintain a common treatment culture.

For pivotal efficacy studies of new LDS medications, both fidelity to the protocol and the patient's adherence to protocol will need to be documented. It is more ecologically valid for the parents to administer the medications. Compliance can be tracked by pill counts of bottles at each weekly visit during the RCT.

Using an intent-to-treat design

Completer analyses, wherein only those who finish the study are included in the analyses, were used in the majority of the small-number, single-site, crossover designs in Table 1. This is because only cases that complete all phases of study in a crossover design trial can be included in the analysis. Modern clinical trials using parallel design methods use analyses that include all children randomized into the study, regardless of their level of participation. To facilitate this, the last recorded data point—sometimes called the "last observation carried forward,"—may be used as the end-of-study measure. Thus, the trend in modern multisite RCTs is to use "intent-to-treat" analyses that include all randomized subjects, rather than use a completer analysis.

Families may stop their participation for a variety of reasons that may affect the overall acceptibility of the drug: severe side effects, inability of the child to swallow the study capsule, or the expectation of major improvements within too short a time and subsequent disappointment. If these families drop out because of an early prohibitive side effect, while the completing patients have minimal side effects, a research report that includes only the completers will suggest a falsely low side effect rate. As a secondary analysis, patients who receive a "sufficient exposure" to the new stimulant treatment can be analyzed separately. The constraints of an "intent-to-treat" approach means that investigators will have to redouble their efforts to keep all subjects in the study until the end of the new LDS drug trial. This is good clinical practice.

CONCLUSIONS

The field of stimulant medication treatment of children with ADHD is "mature," with multiple controlled studies of marketed stimulants—already approved more than 20 years ago—showing good efficacy and safety across the lifespan (Spencer et al., 1996b). However, the many studies that were conducted in an era when drug approval was not the goal used methods and designs that fall short of the standards of modern clinical trials. The limitation of IR stimulants—their brief duration—will mean that new longer-acting stimulant preparations need to be developed, tested, and approved that have a full-day benefit from a single administration. For purposes of FDA review of new LDS medication clinical trials, the traditional stimulant trial methods—small-number, crossover, single-site designs—will not be satisfactory. Instead, pivotal efficacy clinical trials for drug approval will need parallel designs with longer-term assignments to placebo and the inclusion of subjects in the analysis who are not classified as dropouts. More representative samples, including girls, minorities, and children with comorbid disorders need to be recruited. The drugs' effects on impairment need to be measured for key domains, including academics, peer relationships, and family life. Outcome measures should involve multiple informants and domains, and pivotal studies should be run in a school or clinic, not only in a laboratory. This modern clinical trial method will bring pediatric psychopharmacology into a new era, better suited to determine the efficacy of LDS medications for the treatment of children with ADHD.

REFERENCES

Abikoff, H. & Gittelman, R. (1985), Hyperactive children treated with stimulants: Is cognitive training a useful adjunct? *Arch. Gen. Psychiatry*, 42:953–961.

Abikoff, H. & Hechtman, L. (unpublished), *Multimodal Treatment for Children with ADHD: Effects on ADHD and Social Behavior and Diagnostic Status.*

Arnold, L., Jensen, P., Richters, J., Abikoff, H., Conners, K., Greenhill, L.L., Hechtman, L., Hinshaw, S., Pelham, W. & Swanson, J. (1997), The National Institute of Mental Health collaborative multisite multimodal treatment study of children with attention deficit hyperactivity disorder (MTA): II. methods. *Arch. Gen. Psychiatry*, 54:865–870.

Barkley, R., DuPaul, G. & McMurray, M. (1991), Attention deficit disorder with and without hyperactivity: Clinical response to three dose levels of methylphenidate. *Pediatrics*, 87:519–531.

Barkley, R., McMurray, M., Edelbroch, C. & Robbins, K. (1989), The response of aggressive and non-aggressive children to two doses of methylphenidate. *J. Am. Acad. Child Adolesc. Psychiatry*, 28:873–881.

Barkley, R., McMurray, M., Edelbroch, C. & Robbins, K. (1990), Side effects of MPH in children with attention deficit hyperactivity disorder: A systematic placebo-controlled evaluation. *Pediatrics*, 86:184–192.

Berkovitch, M., Pope, E., Phillips, J. & Koren, G. (1995), Pemoline-associated fulminant liver failure: Testing the evidence for causation. *Clin. Pharmacol. Ther.*, 57:696–698.

Bird, H. & Gould, M. (1995), The use of diagnostic instruments and global measures of functioning in child psychiatry epidemiologic studies. In: *The Epidemiology of Child and Adolescent Psychopathology*, eds., F.C. Verhulst and H.M. Koot. Oxford: Oxford University Press, pp. 86–103.

Castellanos, X., Giedd, J., Elia, J., Marsh, W., Ritchie, G., Hamburger, S. & Rapoport, J. (1997), Controlled stimulant treatment of ADHD and comorbid Tourette's syndrome: Effects of stimulant and dose. *J. Am. Acad. Child Adolesc. Psychiatry*, 36:589–596.

Douglas, V.I., Barr, R.G., Amin, K., O'Neill, M.E. & Britton, B.G. (1988), Dose effects and individual responsivity to methylphenidate in attention deficit disorder. *J. Child Psychol. Psychiatry*, 29:453–475.

Douglas, V., Barr, R.G., Desilets, J. & Sherman, E. (1995), Do high doses of stimulants impair flexible thinking in ADHD? *J. Am. Acad. Child Adolesc. Psychiatry*, 34:877–885.

Dunnick, J. & Hailey, J. (1995), Experimental studies on the long-term effects of methylphenidate hydrochloride. *Toxicology*, 103:77–84.

DuPaul, G.J. & Barkley, R.A. (1990), Medication therapy. In: *Attention Deficit Hyperactivity Disorder: A Handbook for Diagnosis and Treatment*, ed., R.A. Barkley. New York: Guilford Press, pp. 573–612.

DuPaul, G., Barkley, R. & McMurray, M. (1994), Response of children with ADHD to methylphenidate: Interaction with internalizing symptoms. *J. Am. Acad. Child Adolesc. Psychiatry*, 33:894–903.

DuPaul, G. & Rapport, M. (1993), Does MPH normalize the classroom performance of children with attention deficit disorder? *J. Am. Acad. Child Adolesc. Psychiatry*, 32:190–198.

Elia, J., Borcherding, B., Rapoport, J. & Keysor, C. (1991), Methylphenidate and dextroamphetamine treatments of hyperactivity: Are there true non-responders? *Psychiatry Res.*, 36:141–155.

Fava, M. (1996), Traditional and alternative research designs and methods in clinical pediatric psychopharmacology. *J. Am. Acad. Child Adolesc. Psychiatry*, 35: 1292–1303.

Fitzpatrick, P., Klorman, R., Brumaghim, J. & Borgstedt, A. (1992), Effects of sustained-release and standard preparations of methylphenidate on attention deficit disorder. *American Academy of Child and Adolescent Psychiatry, Scientific Proceedings of the Annual Meeting*, 31:226–234.

Gadow, K., Sverd, J., Sprafkin, J., Nolan, E. & Ezor, S. (1995), Efficacy of methylphenidate for attention deficit hyperactivity in children with tic disorder. *Arch. Gen. Psychiatry*, 52:444–455.

Gillberg, C., Melander, H., von Knorring, A., Janols, L., Thernlund, G., Heggel, B., Edievall-Walin, L., Gustafsson, P. & Kopp, S. (1997), Long-term central stimulant treatment of children with attention-deficit hyperactivity disorder: A randomized double-blind placebo-controlled trial. *Arch. Gen. Psychiatry*, 54:857–864.

Greenhill, L.L., Abikoff, H., Conners, C.K., Elliott, G., Hechtman, L., Hinshaw, S., Hoza, B., Jensen, P., Kraemer, H., March, J., Newcorn, J., Pelham, W., Richters, J., Schiller, E., Severe, J., Swanson, J., Vereen, D. & Wells, K. (1996), Medication treatment strategies in the MTA: Relevance to clinicians and researchers. *J. Am. Acad. Child Adolesc. Psychiatry*, 35:444–454.

Greenhill, L.L., & Cooper. (1987), Methylphenidate salivary levels in children. *Psychopharmacol. Bull.*, 23:115–119.

Greenhill, L.L., Halperin, J. & March, J. (1997), Psychostimulants. In: *Psychiatry*, eds., A. Tasman, J. Kay and J. Lieberman. Philadelphia: W.B. Saunders, pp. 1659–1682.

Jacobvitz, D., Srouge, L.A., Stewart, M. & Leffert, N. (1990), Treatment of attentional and hyperactivity problems in children with sympathomimetic drugs: A comprehensive review. *J. Am. Acad. Child Adolesc. Psychiatry*, 29:677–688.

Kent, J., Blader, J., Koplewicz, H., Abikoff, H. & Foley, C. (1995), Effects of late-afternoon methylphenidate administration on behavior and sleep in attention-deficit hyperactivity disorder. *Pediatrics*, 96:320–325.

Klein, R., Abikoff, H., Klass, E., Ganales, D., Seese, L. & Pollack, S. (1997), Clinical efficacy of methylphenidate in conduct disorder with and without attention deficit hyperactivity disorder. *Arch. Gen. Psychiatry*, 54:1073–1080.

Klorman, R., Brumagham, J., Fitzpatrick, P. & Burgstedt, A. (1990), Clinical effects of a controlled trial of methylphenidate on adolescents with attention deficit disorder. *J. Am. Acad. Child Adolesc. Psychiatry*, 29:702–709.

Laughren, T. (1997), Design and conduct of ADHD drug treatment trials: Regulatory considerations [abstr.]. *Scientific Proceedings of the Annual Meeting of the American Academy of Child and Adolescent Psychiatry*, 13:70.

Manuzza, S., Klein, R., Bonagura, N., Malloy, P., Giampino, T. & Addlii, K. (1991), Hyperactive boys almost grown up: V. Replication of psychiatric status. *Arch. Gen. Psychiatry*, 48:77–83.

Mayes, S., Crites, D., Bixler, E., Humphrey, B. & Mattison, R. (1994), Methylphenidate and ADHD: influence of age, IQ and neurodevelopmental status. *Dev. Med. Child Neurol.*, 36:1099–1107.

McMaster University Evidence-Based Practice Center. *The Treatment of Attention-Deficit/Hyperactivity Disorder: An Evidence Report* (contract 290-97-0017). Washington, D.C.: U.S. Agency for Health Care Policy and Research, unpublished.

MTA Cooperative Group (1999), 14-Month randomized clinical trial of treatment strategies for attention deficit hyperactivity disorder. *J. Am. Acad. Child Adolesc. Psychiatry*, in press.

Musten, L., Firestone, P., Pisterman, S., Bennett, S. & Mercer, J. (1997), Effects of methylphenidate on preschool children with ADHD: Cognitive and behavioral functions. *J. Am. Acad. Child Adolesc. Psychiatry*, 36:1407–1415.

Pelham, W.E., Greenslade, K.E., Vodde-Hamilton, M.A., Murphy, D.A., Greenstein, J.J., Gnagy, E.M. & Dahl, R.E. (1990), Relative efficacy of long-acting stimulants on ADHD children: A comparison of standard methylphenidate, Ritalin-SR, Dexedrine spansule, and pemoline. *Pediatrics*, 86:226–237.

Pelham, W.E. & Milich, R. (1991), Individual differences in response to Ritalin in classwork and social behavior. In: *Ritalin: Theory and Patient Management*, eds. L.L. Greenhill & B.B. Osman. Larchmont, NY: Mary Ann Liebert, Inc., pp. 203–222.

Pelham, W., Swanson, J., Furman, M. & Schwint, H. (1995), Pemoline effects on children with ADHD: A time response by dose-response analysis on classroom measures. *J. Am. Acad. Child Adolesc. Psychiatry*, 34:1504–1514.

Pliszka, S.R. (1992), Comorbidity of attention-deficit hyperactivity disorder and overanxious disorder. *J. Am. Acad. Child Adolesc. Psychiatry*, 31:197–203.

Pliszka, S., McCracken, J. & Maas, J. (1996), Catecholamines in attention-deficit hyperactivity disorder: Current perspectives. *J. Am. Acad. Child Adolesc. Psychiatry*, 35:264–272.

Rapport, M., Denney, C., DuPaul, G. & Gardner, M. (1994), Attention deficit disorder and methylphenidate: Normalization rates, clinical effectiveness and response prediction in 76 children. *J. Am. Acad. Child Adolesc. Psychiatry*, 33:882–893.

Rapport, M., Stoner, G., DuPaul, G., Kelly, K., Tucker, S. & Schoder, T. (1988), Attention deficit disorder and methylphenidate: A multi-step analysis of dose-response effects on children's impulsivity across settings. *J. Am. Acad. Child Adolesc. Psychiatry*, 27: 60–69.

Richters, J., Arnold, L., Abikoff, H., Conners, C., Greenhill, L., Hechtman, L., Hinshaw, S., Pelham, W. & Swanson, J. (1995), The National Institute of Mental Health Collaborative Multisite Multimodal Treatment Study of Children with Attention-Deficit Hyperactivity Disorder (MTA): I. Background and rationale. *J. Am. Acad. Child Adolesc. Psychiatry*, 34:987–1000.

Safer, D., Zito, J. & Fine, E. (1996), Increased methylphenidate usage for attention deficit hyperactivity disorder in the 1990s. *Pediatrics*, 98:1084–1088.

Schachar, R., *Treatment of ADHD with Methylphenidate and Parent Programs* (unpublished).

Schachar, R. & Tannock, R. (1993), Childhood hyperactivity and psychostimulants: A review of extended treatment studies. *J. Child Adolesc. Psychpharmacol.*, 3:81–97.

Schachar, R., Tannock, R., Cunningham, C. & Corkum, P.V. (1997), Behavioral, situational, and temporal effects of treatment of ADHD with methylphenidate. *J. Am. Acad. Child Adolesc. Psychiatry,* 36:754–763.

Schachar, R.J., Ickowicz, A. & Tannock, R. (1997), Pharmacotherapy of ADHD. In: *Handbook of Disruptive Behavior Disorders*, eds., H. Quay and A. Hogan. New York: Plenum Press, pp. 555–565.

Shaffer, D., Fisher, P., Dulcan, M., Davies, M., Piacentini, J., Schwab-Stone, M., Lahey, B., Bourdon, K., Jensen, P., Bird, H., Canino, G. & Regier, D. (1996), The NIMH diagnostic interview schedule for children version 2.3 (DISC-2.3): Description, acceptibility, prevalence rates, and performance in the MECA Study. *J. Am. Acad. Child Adolesc. Psychiatry*, 35:865–877.

Shaffer, D., Gould, M.S., Brasic, J., Ambrosini, P., Fisher, P., Bird, H. & Aluwahlia, S. (1983), A children's global assessment scale (CGAS). *Arch. Gen. Psychiatry*, 40:1228–1231.

Spencer, T., Biederman, J., Harding, M., Faraone, S. & Wilens, T. (1996a), Growth deficits in ADHD children revisited: Evidence for disorder related growth delays. *J. Am. Acad. Child Adolesc. Psychiatry*, 35:1460–1467.

Spencer, T., Biederman, J., Wilens, T., Harding, M., O'Donnell, D. & Griffin, S. (1996b),

Pharmacotherapy of attention-deficit hyperactivity disorder across the life cycle. *J. Am. Acad. Child Adolesc. Psychiatry*, 35:409–432.

Spencer, T., Wilens, T., Biederman, J., Farone, S., Ablen, S. & Lapey, K. (1995), A double-blind, crossover comparison of methylphenidate and placebo in adults with childhood onset ADHD. *Arch. Gen. Psychiatry*, 52:434–443.

Swanson, J., Wigal, S., Greenhill, L., Browne, R., Waslik, B., Lerner, M., Williams, L., Flynn, D., Agler, D., Crowley, K., Feinberg, B., Baren, M. & Cantwell, D. (1998), Analog classroom assessment of Adderall in children with ADHD. *J. Am. Acad. Child Adolesc. Psychiatry*, 37:1–8.

Tannock, R., Ickowicz, A. & Schachar, R. (1995a), Differential effects of MPH on working memory in ADHD children with and without comorbid anxiety. *J. Am. Acad. Child Adolesc. Psychiatry*. 34:886–896.

Tannock, R., Schachar, R. & Logan, G.D. (1995b), Methylphenidate and cognitive flexibility: Dissociated dose effects in hyperactive children. *J. Abnorm. Child Psychol.*, 23:235–267.

Taylor, E., Schachar, R., Thorley, G., Wieselberg, H.M., Everitt, B. & Rutter, M. (1987), Which boys respond to stimulant medication? A controlled trial of methyphenidate in boys with disruptive behavior. *Psychol. Med.*, 17:121–143.

Whalen, C., Henker, B., Buhrmester, D., Hinshaw, S., Huber, A. & Laski, K. (1989), Does stimulant medication improve the peer status of hyperactive children? *J. Consult. Clin. Psychol.*, 57:545–549.

Zito, J.M., Safer, D., Riddle, M. & dosReis, S. (1997), Methylphenidate patterns among Medicaid youths. *Psychopharmacol. Bull.*, 33:143–147.

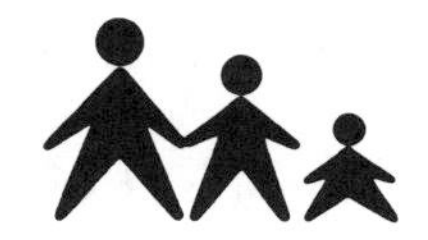

Patterns of Use of Clonidine Alone and in Combination with Methylphenidate

ROLAND REGINO,[1] MARTIN BAREN,[2] DANIEL F. CONNOR,[3]
and JAMES M. SWANSON[1]

The initial report on the effectiveness of clonidine to treat children with ADHD (Hunt et al., 1985) suggested that this pharmacologic treatment was about equal to the standard treatment with methylphenidate (MPH) for reducing symptoms of ADHD. The initial reports of the use of clonidine in combination with MPH also suggested that the addition of clonidine may be effective to treat specifically the nonattentional (hyperactive/impulsive) symptoms of ADHD, the highly associated features of aggression and defiance (Hunt et al., 1985), the treatment-emergent side effects of MPH such as tics (Steingard et al., 1993), and insomnia (Rubinstein et al., 1994; Wilens et al., 1994). However, evidence from controlled trials for the efficacy of clonidine used alone or in combination with MPH is meager. Although some positive study results have been reported, a meta-analysis showed that the sizes of the reported effects decline with the control and rigor of the study methods (Connor et al., submitted).

We have noted elsewhere that by 1995, the prescription of clonidine to treat ADHD in children had increased to over 150,000 per year, and the prescriptions of clonidine in combination with MPH also increased to over 60,000 per year. At the end of 1995, questions about the safety of the combination of MPH and clonidine had arisen (Swanson et al., 1995; Cantwell et al., 1997; Hunt et al., 1985). In this chapter, we review our concern about the use of clonidine and present some data about the pattern of use reflected in the Scott-Levin surveys of physicians, in a large pediatric specialty practice, and in a survey of our clinical trials sample at the University of California, Irvine Child Development Center (see chapter by Swanson et al., this volume, 405–427).

First, we shall review our concern about the combination of clonidine and MPH. Methylphenidate and clonidine have opposite effects on noradrenergic action (increased versus decreased), on the sympathetic nervous system (increased versus decreased alertness, wakefulness, and heart rate), on side effects of anorexia and insomnia, and on blood pressure. Thus, when each medication exerts its direct effect surrounding the peak effect, some opposing effects may operate to cancel the side effects of either medication used alone. Our concern about the safety of combining MPH with clonidine is based on the side effects of these two medications as they wear off, not when their therapeutic effects are at the maximum. Clonidine may have "bounce back" effects, which result in increased heart rate and blood pressure as the initial effects dissipate. If this occurs when the effects of MPH are at a maximum, the side effects of the two medications may combine rather than cancel. This may produce "adrenergic overdrive" (see Cantwell et al., 1997).

[1]University of California, Irvine, Child Development Center, Centerpointe; and [2]Department of Pediatrics, University of California Medical Center, Irvine, California.
[3]Department of Psychology, University of Massachusetts Medical Center, Worcester, Massachusetts.

We have reviewed the spontaneous reports of sudden deaths in patients treated with the combination (Swanson et al., 1995; Cantwell et al., 1997). From mid-1994 to mid-1995, four sudden unexplained deaths were reported to the MedWatch program of the U.S. Food and Drug Administration: on 8/29/94, an 8-year-old girl receiving an unspecified dose of MPH and 0.2 mg/day of clonidine; on 1/30/95, a 7-year-old boy receiving 15 mg MPH three times a day and 0.1 mg/day of clonidine; on 2/25/95, a 9-year-old girl receiving 20 mg of MPH and 0.9 mg/day of clonidine; on 7/30/95, a 10-year-old boy receiving 10 mg MPH three times a day and 0.2 therapeutic transdermal system of clonidine. All had some complicating factor: recent anesthesia, heart murmur and fibrosis, concurrent treatment with high doses of multiple medications, and history of syncope and cardiac malformation. These preexisting conditions and concurrent treatments may "explain" these sudden deaths, but we are not convinced that these complicating factors were necessarily the cause of death. Our reviews of published reports in multiple areas suggested plausible mechanisms associated with the combination.

The pros and cons of the use of the combination have been discussed elsewhere (Wilens et al., 1999; Swanson et al., 1999), so this debate not repeated here. Instead, we describe the patterns of use, on which we have accumulated data from three sources:

1. A specialty pediatric practice in 1996
2. A clinical trials sample
3. Scott-Levin Report, showing in 1998 about 4.9% of the methylphenidate prescriptions were for the combination with clonidine

In 1996, we surveyed a specialty pediatric practice (M.B.). We located the charts of 1167 subjects who had prescriptions for MPH, clonidine, or the combination. Of those, 65 (5.6%) had a prescription for clonidine alone, 74 (6.3%) had a prescription for the combination of

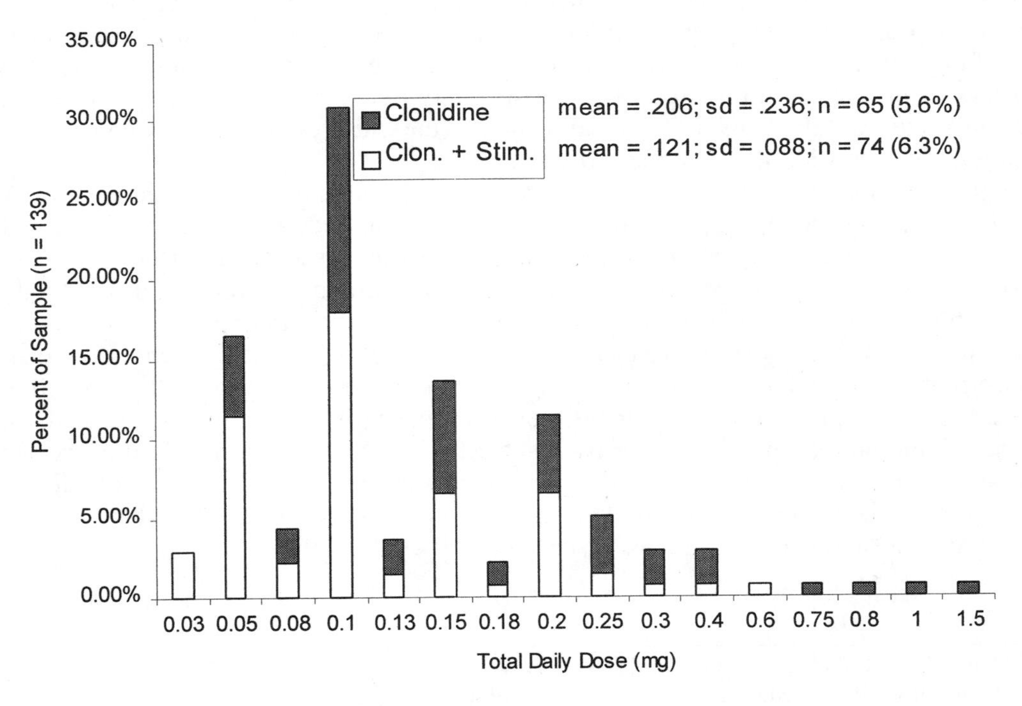

FIG. 1. Clonidine use in a large clinical practice sample.

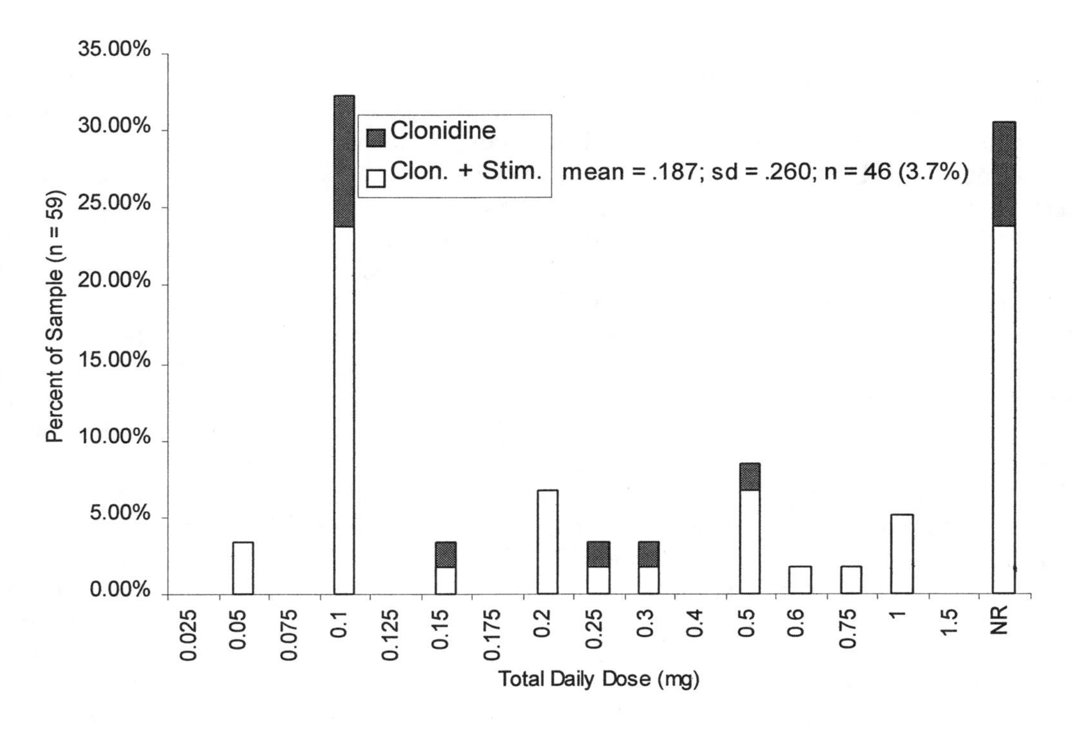

FIG. 2. Clonidine use in a large clinical research sample (n = 1228).

clonidine and MPH, and most (1167 − 139 = 1028 = 88.1%) had a prescription for MPH and not for clonidine. As shown in Figure 1, the modal dose of clonidine was 0.1 mg in this sample, for clonidine alone as well as in combination with stimulants. The mean dose for the combination was lower (0.12 mg) than for clonidine alone (0.21 mg).

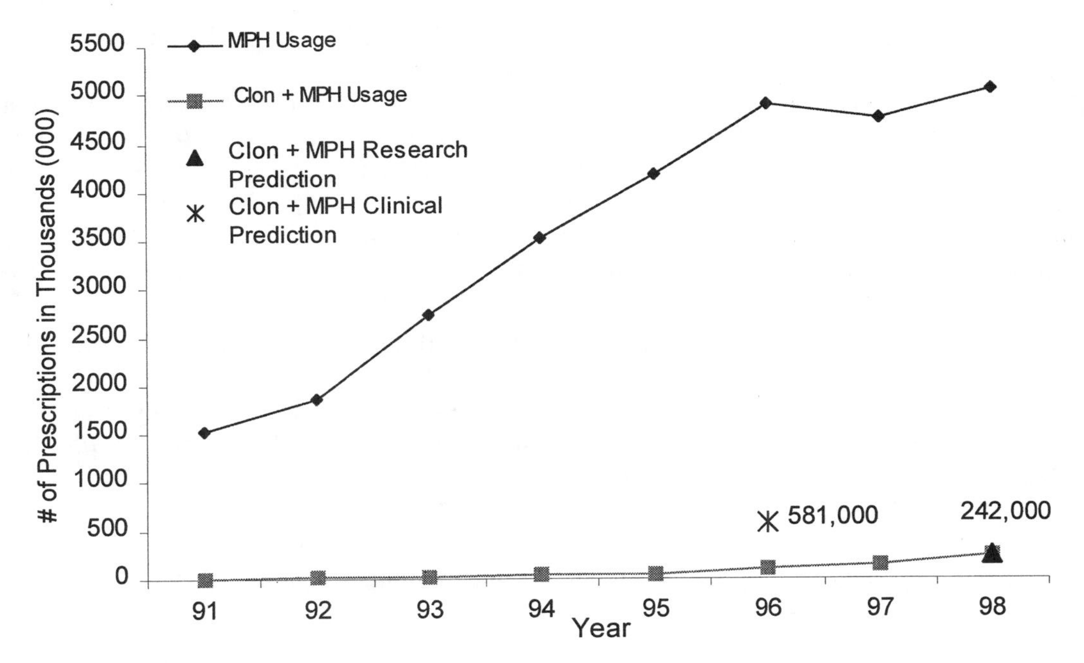

FIG. 3. Scott-Levin report on methylphenidate and clonidine use.

In 1998, we screened a large number of patients for entry into clinical trials being conducted as part of a clinical trials program at University of California, Irvine. We had information on 1228 children. Of those, 13 (1.1%) reported the use of clonidine alone, 46 (3.7%) reported the use of clonidine in combination with MPH, and most (1228 − 59 = 1169 = 95.2%) reported a prescription for MPH but not for clonidine. The modal dose for clonidine was 0.1 mg, whether taken alone or in combination with MPH. As shown in Figure 2, the mean was higher when clonidine was taken in combination with stimulants (0.187) than when taken alone (0.130 mg).

The Scott-Levin Report surveyed a group of physicians who reported on the patients seen and evaluated in an entire day. This representative sample is used to estimate the number of cases in the population. As shown in Figure 3, by 1996 about 5 million prescriptions were being issued per year. After a dramatic increase (see Swanson et al., 1994) that lasted approximately 5 years (see Figure 3), the use of MPH has remained constant. Over this time, the use of clonidine in combination with MPH has increased, so that in 1998 about 4.8% of the prescriptions for MPH were each accompanied by a prescription for clonidine. This figure is almost identical to the figure obtained from the clinical trials sample.

These data indicate that the use of the combination is still relatively rare. However, the small percentage (4.8%) of a large total (5 million) generates large absolute numbers of prescriptions for the combination (0.048 × 5,000,000 = 240,000). Despite this rapid increase, there has not been a reported sudden death. This may be due to precautions set in place by our recommendations (see Cantwell et al., 1997), or it may reflect that our speculations were incorrect.

In the absence of clear demonstration of efficacy from controlled studies, we still question the use of clonidine alone or in combination with MPH. Two studies are now being conducted to evaluate their efficacy and safety, and until the results of these controlled studies are available to guide clinical practice, we consider the use of the combination of MPH and clonidine to be ill advised.

REFERENCES

Cantwell, D.P., Swanson, J.S. & Connor, D.P. (1997), Case study: Adverse response to clonidine. *J. Am. Acad. Child Adolesc. Psychiatry*, 36:1–6.

Hunt, R.D., Minderaa, R.B. & Cohen, D. (1985), Clonidine benefits children with attention deficit hyperactivity disorder. *J. Am. Acad. Child Adolesc. Psychiatry*, 24:617–629.

Rubinstein, S., Silver, L.B. & Locamele, W.L. (1994), Clonidine for stimulant-related sleep problems. *J. Am. Acad. Child Adolesc. Psychiatry*, 33:281–282.

Steingard, R., Biederman, J., Spencer, T., Wilens, T., & Gonzales, A. (1993), Comparison of clonidine response in the treatment of ADHD with and without comorbid tic disorders. *J. Am. Acad. Child Adolesc. Psychiatry*, 32:350–353.

Swanson, J.M., Connor, D.F., Cantwell, D. (1999). Ill-advised. *J. Am. Acad. Child Adolesc. Psychiatry,* 38:5.

Swanson, J.M., Flockhart, D., Udrea, D., Cantwell, D.P., Connor, D. & Williams, L. (1995), Clonidine in the treatment of ADHD: Questions about safety and efficacy. *J. Child Adolesc. Psychopharmacology*, 5:301–304.

Wilens, T.E., Biederman, J. & Spencer, T. (1994), Clonidine for sleep disturbances associated with ADHD. *J. Am. Acad. Child Adolesc. Psychiatry*, 33:424–426.

Wilens, T.E., Spencer, T.J. (1999). A clinically sound medication option. *J. Am. Acad. Child Adolesc. Psychiatry,* 38:5.

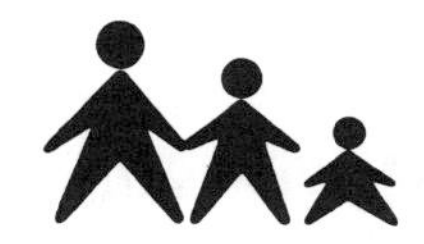

University of California, Irvine, Laboratory School Protocol for Pharmacokinetic and Pharmacodynamic Studies

JAMES M. SWANSON, DAVE AGLER, ERICK FINEBERG, SHARON WIGAL, DAN FLYNN, KATRINA FINEBERG, YVONNE QUINTANA, and HANI TALEBI

The University of California, Irvine, (UCI) Laboratory School Protocol (LSP) was developed for investigations of stimulant medications in the treatment of children with attention deficit hyperactivity disorder (ADHD). Highly controlled studies are necessary to define the pharmacokinetic (PK) and pharmacodynamic (PD) properties of medications, and the LSP provides control by maintaining a consistent setting in an analog classroom, in which surrogate measures of response can be obtained at precise times after administration of medication. In this chapter, we outline the background and the current status of the LSP. Descriptions are provided of the facility, the schedule of activities, and the cognitive and behavioral measurement instruments used. Some examples of highly controlled studies of methylphenidate (MPH) and amphetamine will be presented to show how the LSP has been utilized for several clinical trials for pharmaceutical companies in programs to develop new medications for children with ADHD.

BACKGROUND

Our use of a laboratory school setting to study children with ADHD was initiated in 1977 at the Hospital for Sick Children in Canada, where there was a fleeting interest in the PK and PD properties of stimulant medications (see Swanson, 1985). Our publications on the investigations of MPH (Soldin et al., 1979a,b; Chan et al., 1980 and 1983) and pemoline (Tompkins et al., 1979; Collier et al., 1985) emphasized the PK aspects of this research. Only limited information on the PD aspects of this work has been published (see Swanson, 1985; Swanson, 1988; Pelham et al., 1995).

After a hiatus of almost two decades, there was a revival of interest in PK/PD studies of stimulant medications, because of two converging events: Food and Drug Administration (FDA) encouragement of the evaluation of medications in samples of children (see Jensen, Vietello, Leonard, and Laughren, 1994), and the increase in recognition and treatment of ADHD in the United States (see Swanson et al., 1995; Safer et al., 1996). In response to this, in 1994, we initiated a program of clinical trials at the UCI, Child Development Center (UCI-CDC). For this research, we developed and refined the LSP, which from 1994 to 1998, was used in 11 clinical trials with more than 350 children with ADHD participating as subjects. These recent clinical trials were supported by pharmaceutical companies, and the results of the initial two studies have been published. The first application of the LSP

University of California, Irvine, Child Development Center, Centerpointe, Irvine, California.

was supported by ALZA Corporation and investigated drug delivery patterns of MPH (see Swanson et al., 1998a; Wigal et al., 1998; Swanson et al., 1999). The second application was supported by Richwood Pharmaceutical Company and investigated the time-response and dose-response effects of amphetamine (see Swanson et al., 1998b; Swanson et al., 1999; Wigal et al., 1999).

In this chapter, we will describe the procedures we use to implement the LSP. Three of our recent clinical trials involve multiple sites (UCI, Northwestern University, and the University of Saskatchewan; UCI and Harvard University; UCI and Columbia University), and the transfer of the procedures from UCI to other sites led to the development of a generic LSP manual. This chapter is based on that manual.

The LSP is used for efficacy studies in a highly controlled setting, rather than for effectiveness studies in the natural environment (Hoagwood, et al., 1995). In most LSP studies of short-acting stimulant drugs, a crossover design is used in which subjects experience multiple conditions, which are evaluated in daylong sessions on successive Saturdays (i.e., once every 7 days). A typical schedule is shown in Table 1. After screening and consent, homogeneous age groups (e.g., 6 to 8 years and 9 to 12 years) of children are identified and assigned to classrooms. On each evaluation day, multiple probes are scheduled to capture the time-course effects after dosing, and across days, the different conditions are scheduled in a counterbalanced fashion to evaluate other factors, such as dose-related effects or effects of different drug delivery patterns of a particular daily dose. We describe the LSP procedures for this type of schedule for implementing an efficacy study of pharmacologic treatments of ADHD children.

PROCEDURES FOR IMPLEMENTING THE LSP

Subjects

For our program of clinical trials, we use a general but broad recruitment strategy to identify potential subjects with a diagnosis of ADHD and a history of clinical response to stimulant medication (see Swanson et al., 1998a,b,c, Swanson et al., 1999). Our strategy generates referrals from multiple sources (clinic referrals, newspaper advertisements, etc.). For each referral meeting the screening criteria (age, medication status, etc.), we obtain consent for a diagnostic assessment to identify children who qualify as potential subjects based on general inclusion criteria. Included in these are a current diagnosis of ADHD confirmed by structured psychiatric interview using the Diagnostic Interview Schedule for Children (DISC) (See Shaffer et al., 1989), an IQ of at least 80 according to the Wechsler Intelligence Scale for Children (WISC), and a history of clinical response to stimulant medication. We also set exclusion criteria (e.g., specific comorbid disorders; history of clinical failure on stimulant medication). A second consent process is used to present a specific clinical trial to each qualified subject. Some characteristics of our recruitment and initial assessment procedures are shown in Table 2 (see Swanson et al., 1998c).

TABLE 1. THE GENERAL SCHEMATIC FOR A PK/PD STUDY USING THE LSP

Protocol development	*Practice day (7:00 A.M. to 3:00 P.M.)*	*Experimental days (1 to 7) (6:30 A.M. to 6:00 P.M.)*
IRB approval	Familiarize children	Conditions randomized
Subject recruitment	Staff training	Probes at hourly intervals
Staff selection		

IRB = Institution Review Board.

TABLE 2. GENERAL RECRUITMENT FOR CLINICAL TRIALS OVER A 12-MONTH PERIOD

Number screened	792			
Number meeting general criteria	157			
Number assessed	136			
Male:female ratio	107:29 (3.7:1)			
Average no. of ADHD symptoms	7.8 Inattentive			
	7.5 Hyperactive/impulsive			
Subtypes of ADHD	82% Combined			
	16% Inattentive			
	2% Hyperactive/impulsive			
Comorbid ODD	47%			
Age distribution	*Age (yr)*	n	*Percent*	*M:F*
	6–7	7	5.0	6:1
	7–8	12	8.8	10:2
	8–9	26	19.1	20:6
	9–10	20	14.7	15:5
	10–11	34	25.0	29:5
	11–12	24	17.6	18:6
	12–13	13	9.6	9:4
Dose of methylphenidate	Average initial dose = 14.5 mg			
	Average daily dose = 28.9 mg			
	Average frequency of dosing = 2.3/day			

ODD = oppositional defiant disorder.

For a typical clinical trial study (see Table 1), up to 16 children are identified to form a cohort of subjects. All subjects in a cohort attend a practice day at the laboratory school at the UCI-CDC, to become acquainted with each other, with the staff, and with the procedures of the LSP. For some trials, 2 cohorts are established based on age. Young (6 to 8 years) and old (9 to 11 years) groups are formed, so that up to 32 subjects can be evaluated on the same Saturday test days.

Staff and facility

The staff for the LSP is divided into four areas by function: administrative, school, recess, and medical. Before the LSP is implemented, a full-time administrative staff designs the study with the pharmaceutical company, helps to develop the case report forms (CRFs), adapts the generic LSP for the specific clinical trial, submits applications to the Institutional Review Boards (IRBs), negotiates budgets with contracts and grants office, and recruits subjects. During the implementation of a particular clinical trial, the administrative staff also schedules families to attend the Saturday test days, trains the part-time staff, conducts the practice day, and checks the CRFs for accuracy and completion.

TABLE 3. RECOMMENDED STAFF FOR THE UCI-LSP

Administrative: Investigator, coordinators for each of the 3 areas
School: 1 teacher and 2 raters per cohort
Recess: 1 lead counselor and up to 8 counselors (1 for every 2 subjects), food technician
Medical: 1 physician, 1 pharmacist, 2 nurses, 2 phlebotomists, 1 technician

To implement the LSP on the Saturday test days, a large staff is necessary to establish the tight control for an efficacy study. In contrast to the administrative staff, the other staff members are part time and work just on the Saturdays when a clinical trial is being conducted. For a cohort of 16 subjects, the recommended Saturday staff members are shown in Table 3. The roles of these staff members are discussed in the following three sections.

School staff

Each member of the school staff has specific roles and responsibilities. The school coordinator is responsible for the standardization and implementation of the classroom activities, which includes training the classroom staff, working to establish reliability measures during the study, assisting with the removal of disruptive and aggressive students from the classroom, and serving as a substitute for classroom staff members in the event of an absence. The teacher prepares materials for each class session, sets up the classroom for each study day, and conducts the class sessions (e.g., instructs the students when to start and stop written tests and leads the academic group games). The observers/raters prepare materials for each study day, observe, record frequency counts and anecdotal notes regarding student behavior in the classroom, and complete the Swanson, Kotkin, Agler, M-Flynn, and Pelham (SKAMP) rating scale for each subject, immediately following each classroom session.

Each clinical trial has a training day for staff to learn about the specific duties in the LSP and a practice day for subjects and staff to become acquainted. At the beginning of the practice day, students are given the general rules of the classroom (be quiet and listen when a quiet symbol is given; no talking while teacher is talking; stay seated unless given permission to get up; raise hand and wait to be acknowledged to say something in class discussion).

In addition to the written individual seatwork provided by a 10 minute Math test (see Swanson 1998a), each classroom session has a group academic activity presented. A transition game is also played at the beginning and end of each session. On each study day, the same series of group academic activities may be presented across the day (to hold constant any difference in materials that may be present), or a counterbalanced or random order of these group academic activities may be used (to average across any differences). For example, in a clinical trial with ten classroom sessions scheduled across the day, a fixed or random order set of academic games can be used (see Table 4): Sound Baskets, Math Bingo, Hangman, Word Scramble, Phonics Jeopardy, Zoom In, Story Comprehension Game, Phonics Bingo, Concentration and Family Feud. In contrast with the Math test, which is a static, silent, individualized activity, the academic games are somewhat dynamic, interactive, and group oriented. This contrast serves to represent a range of classroom activities and allows for a variety of displayed behaviors. In Table 4, we outline the content and materials needed for these academic games. Transition games such as I Spy and Question, Guess, or Clue are played during the first and last 5 minutes of the classroom session and are not included in the rating period. These games provide a "buffer" at the beginning and end of the period, so that the Math test can be administered at a precise time, even when some children arrive a little late (i.e., because of a longer than expected physical exam) or must leave a little early (i.e., for a time-critical blood sample to capture peak serum concentrations).

Recess staff

The recess staff (counselors) monitor children during their activities outside of the classroom. Their primary responsibility is to entertain the children, which is essential to motivate them to return over multiple days of evaluation. During some recess periods, counselors and subjects play group games, such as Charades, I Spy, Twenty Questions, Super Silent Speed Ball, Radioactive Eraser, Taboo, Win-Lose-Draw, or Pictionary. Some individual games are provided, too, such as Trouble, Jenga, Don't Break the Ice, Connect Four, Legos, or card games. Equipment is provided for computer games, such as Gameboy,® Nintendo,® and Playstation® systems. On each test day, the recess staff conducts arts and crafts activities, in which the subjects make objects such as Popsicle stick creations, lanyards, sand art, tie-dye shirts, wooden block cars, mosaics, origami paper creations, decorative picture frames or boxes, or planters. When the weather is appropriate, outdoor recess on the playground is allowed, and subjects choose from a number of supervised group activities (e.g., basketball or soccer) or individual use of playground equipment (swings, slides, etc.). At times during the day, children have the opportunity to participate in outdoor activities on the playground or indoor games in the game room. Counselors are preassigned to each station to ensure proper supervision of specific activities and to make sure the games are controlled and do not involve excessive contact.

The recess staff also serves meals and snacks. In some clinical trials, meals are served in closable "takeout" containers. The food technician prepares a meal for each child by placing a specific amount of food in the container, labeling the container with each child's name and subject number, and weighing the container with the food. These containers are delivered to the children at mealtime, and counselors monitor the meal to enforce some basic rules: no sharing of food, no food is to be thrown away, and additional food may be requested but must be noted and weighed for each child. At the end of the meal, counselors make sure that all remaining food is placed in the appropriate containers. After the meal, the food technician collects the containers and weighs each one. The difference in weight before and after the meal is taken as the estimate of amount of food consumed by each subject.

Medical staff

A medical staff, made up of physicians, nurses, phlebotomists, and trained technicians, is necessary for obtaining safety measures, blood samples and monitoring adverse events. The counselors may assist the medical staff in taking vital signs or temperature at times specified by the protocol. The results are checked to ensure that they fall within specified safety ranges and are monitored by a study physician throughout the day. For blood pressure measurements, either manual systems or automatic systems (e.g., DynaMap) can be used to obtain blood pressure and pulse rate. For some trials, serial electrocardiograms (EKGs) are specified in the protocol, so additional equipment is required. For clinical trials that include PK components, nurses have the responsibility to draw blood samples at each of the scheduled times, and technicians have the responsibility to process the samples. Because multiple blood samples are required for a PK study, an indwelling catheter system is used. After each blood sample is drawn, a centrifuge is used to separate the sample. The serum is transferred to a tube that must be frozen, so a freezer is needed for storage.

To facilitate keeping to a tight schedule, counselors bring the children to the medical room in the same order each cycle. Counselors accompany the children to the nurses' station and engage in a distraction activity (e.g., looking at an I Spy book) during catheter insertion and blood draws. A token system is established for the blood samples, even though token systems are not used in other components of the protocol, because they might interfere with the measurement of behavior that is affected by medication. Each child has an opportunity to earn "stamps" for attempting each blood draw throughout the day. Colorful stamps are placed on the individual child's "stamp card," which is turned in at the end of the day for a prize.

Table 4. Academic Games for the LSP Classroom

At the beginning of the study day, the students are split into two "teams." The teams earn points during the academic and transition games. The team with the most points at the end of each game wins and is excused from class first.

Sound Baskets

During this game, students will observe phonics flash cards. The teacher will call on students (alternating between both teams) and prompt them to suggest a word using the sound-symbol displayed on the card. As students from a team correctly suggest words, they move a chosen student (the "shooter") from that team closer to a basket. Each word moves the student approximately one step closer. After (up to) five steps, the "shooter" will try for a basket. Points are scored for each basket made.

Materials needed

20 index cards with initial consonants written on them (for the younger group); the older group should use index cards with consonant blends

3 Baskets with a Nerf ball or bean bag

Chalk or tape to mark shooting positions

Math Bingo

Students choose 9 numbers between 1 and 20 and write them on a 9-cell grid. The teacher hands out 9 "counters" to each child. Each student is instructed to place a counter on the number on a grid if it matches the answer to a math problem. The teacher calls out addition problems and the students solve them, covering the spaces on their bingo sheets if they are the correct answer to the problems. Points are scored when a member gets the type of bingo specified by the teacher.

Materials needed

20 index cards with simple addition problems on the front with answers (between 1 and 20) on the back

Math bingo sheets for each child (9-cell grid)

Counters to cover bingo numbers

A pocket chart to display cards

Hangman

Each table of students will try to guess letters forming a word. If letters called out are not parts of the word, portions of a hangman picture will be added to the board. Each team will try to determine its word before the entire picture is finished. Subsequent words are made until the period ends. Points are scored when a team discovers its word.

Materials needed

Marking pens or chalk

A chalkboard, dry-erase board, or easel

Concentration

Two sets of matching cards are used. One set will be arranged on the board in a 5 × 5 matrix with column headings A–E and row headings 1–5 (face down). The other set is placed in a bag. Students attempt to match a card drawn by the teacher with the corresponding card on the board matrix. All matches are removed from the board and a point is given for each correct match.

Materials needed

A chalkboard, dry-erase board, or easel, or pocket chart

A card set with matching pairs of pictures or symbols

Row and column heading cards A–E and 1–5

(*continued*)

Scramble Words
As with the Hangman activity, each team will try to determine a "mystery word." The letters for each team's word are visible and out of sequence. Students attempt to unscramble the word by taking turns calling the letters in sequence. Points are awarded as each team unscrambles its word. Subsequent words are made until the period ends.

Materials needed
A chalkboard, dry-erase board, or easel

Marking pens or chalk

Phonics Jeopardy
Students choose from a collection of topics written on the chalkboard (i.e., animals, cartoons, fruits, and vegetables). Using the same phonics cards prepared for the sound baskets game, the teacher will call on students and prompt them to choose topics and think of up to 5 answers within each chosen topic that begins with a sound shown on a phonics card. Points are awarded for each correct answer. The game continues until the period ends.

Materials needed
20 index cards with initial consonants written on them (for the younger group); the older group should use index cards with consonant blends.

Index cards displaying topics

Zoom In
Students will attempt to guess an unknown "mystery" number between 1–20 chosen by the teacher. As the teacher shuffles a deck of 20 index cards, a student will prompt the teacher to stop shuffling and show a number. The teacher will tell students if the number chosen is greater or less than the "mystery number." As the students continue to choose numbers and the teacher reveals those numbers to the group, the range of possible answers will decrease. If a student prompts the teacher to show a card and it is the mystery number then that team scores points.

Materials needed:
20 index cards with the numbers 1–20 written on them.

A pocket chart to display cards

Phonics Bingo
Each student chooses 9 initial consonants (consonant blends are used for students in the older group) and writes them on a 9-cell grid. The teacher hands out 9 "counters" to each student. Students are instructed to place counters on the letters on their grids if they match the beginning sound of word announces to the group. A team scores points when a member gets the type of bingo specified by the teacher.

Materials needed
20 index cards with initial consonants written on them (for the younger group); the older group should use index cards with consonant blends.

Phonics bingo sheets for each child (9-cell grid)

Counters to cover bingo letters

Family Feud
Students will attempt to estimate the top answers to surveys conducted among the adult staff at the study site. Surveys may include such topics as favorite desserts, colors, lunch foods, or sports. Teams are assigned points for correct answers. The team with the most points wins.

Materials needed
Survey questions and answers for 3–4 rounds of play for each of the 6 study days.

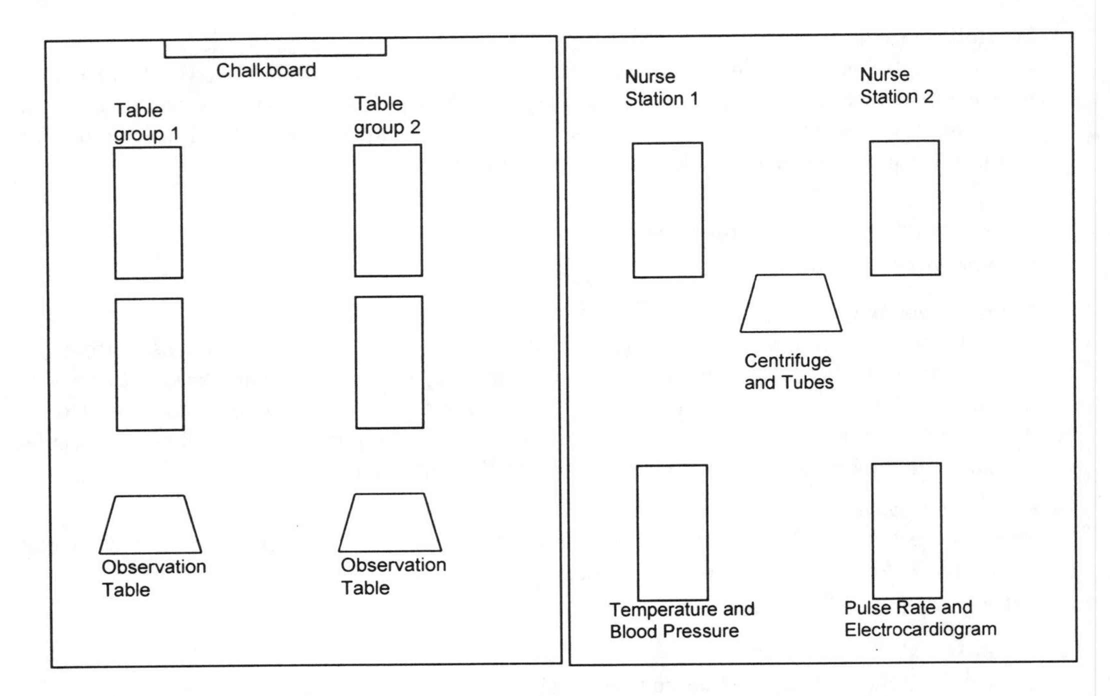

FIG. 1. The recommended analog classroom setting and medical staff room.

Space requirements

The space required for the LSP should accommodate the four types of activities (administrative, educational, medical, and recreational). At UCI, a reception area and a large room is used for the administrative activities of checking in up to 32 families in the morning and checking them out at the end of the day. For the educational component, a classroom of about 600 square feet is recommended. As shown in Figure 1, the classroom should include a chalkboard or easel, tables and chairs for seating two groups of students, and two observation desks or tables for observation stations. A room for medical staff is necessary, to take vital signs (temperature, blood pressure, heart rate, etc.) and, for PK studies, to take blood samples (see Figure 1). The room should provide stations for nurses to insert catheters and draw blood, and each station should provide a place for a child to sit and for a nurse to have access to the child's arm. A station is needed for processing the blood. This station could be a large table with multiple racks for tubes and room for a centrifuge. Also, depending on the particular trial, a separate room or station may be needed for serial physical exams, and this may require space for equipment to take blood pressure, EKGs, or other measurements of vital signs.

For the recreational component of the LSP, space (e.g., a 600-square-foot room) for inside activities (arts and crafts, games, movies, etc.) is recommended. Also, outside space for a playground or a gym is recommended to allow activities typical for a school playground. A staff room is recommended (another 600-square-foot room), where counselors can complete forms, eat meals, take breaks, rest, and engage in other activities as required for a specific trial.

Cycle of activities and daily schedule

Precise timing of activities is an essential part of the control provided by the LSP, and minute-by-minute responsibilities are specified for staff members to provide the timing and settings required for this control. All counselors wear watches that are synchronized at the start of the day, and each counselor carries a detailed schedule on a clipboard throughout the day. In the LSP, a specific sequence of events defines a cycle, which is repeated across the day to provide opportunities to measure the time course of effects of medication. A typical cycle includes time for preparation for each event (a buffer to allow the group to stay on schedule), time to conduct a classroom session that includes a seatwork assignment (to engage in written work such as the 10-minute Math test), group activities (to play a 10-minute academic game such as Phonics Bingo), time to perform a phlebotomy (to take blood samples from the indwelling catheter), and time for recess (to provide a break between the classroom probes and to entertain the children).

The detailed schedule for a specific clinical trial is determined by the set of observations (i.e., the number of activities in a cycle) and the number of cycles across the day. The length of time covered by a cycle is set by the purpose of the study. For example, a 1-hour cycle may be used for frequent observations in a clinical trial that is designed to capture the peak effects of a single dose of a short-acting medication, while a 1.5-hour cycle may be used to capture less time-sensitive information in studies with multiple doses (e.g., bid or tid). Examples of these two cycle times are shown in Table 5. Each classroom session starts and ends with a transition game, to allow for some students to enter late or leave early to participate in other scheduled activities.

Some variations in the cycles repeated across the day are allowed for meals and other periodic activities. In Table 6, two examples are shown to demonstrate repetition of the short and long cycles across the day to measure effects of a tid dosing regime. These schedules provide multiple probe times to obtain PK and PD measurements at precise times after each dose.

In some instances, two groups of children are assessed over the same day. To accomplish this, a schedule of activities is prepared to allow the groups to alternate in using the classroom, recess, and medical facilities. An example schedule is presented in Table 7 for a two-group PK/PD assessment using a 1-hour cycle time to evaluate a typical bid–dosing regime. Some variations across cycles are shown, which allow for dense PK sampling at the times when peak serum concentrations are expected (see 9:00 to 9:30 A.M. and 1:00 to 1:30 P.M.) and sparse PD sampling during the postpeak periods to reduce the demand on subjects and staff (see 10:30 to 11:00 A.M. and 2:30 to 3:00 P.M.).

Measurement instruments

The primary outcome measures used in the LSP are obtained from the classroom session of each cycle. Two instruments have been developed for the multiple repeated measurements: the Math test, which provides an objective measure of performance (the number of

TABLE 5. CYCLE TIME AND ACTIVITIES WITHIN A CYCLE

Short, 1-hour cycle	*Long, 1.5-hour cycle*
Preparation (10 minutes)	Preparation (15 minutes)
Classroom period (20 minutes)	Classroom period (30 minutes)
Phlebotomy (10 minutes)	Phlebotomy (15 minutes)
Recess (20 minutes)	Recess (30 minutes)

TABLE 6. REPETITION AND VARIATION IN CYCLES ACROSS THE DAY

Time of day	*Activity*	*Time after dose*	*1-hour cycle*	*1.5-hour cycle*
7:00 A.M.	Arrival			
7:30	Catheter inserted			
8:00			Cycle 1	Cycle 1
8:30	Dose 1	0		
9:00		.5	Cycle 2	
9:30		1.0		Cycle 2
10:00	Snack	1.5	Cycle 3	
10:30		2.0		
11:00		2.5	Cycle 4	Cycle 3
11:30	Dose 2	3.0		
12:00 P.M.		3.5/.5	Cycle 5	
12:30	Lunch	4.0/1.0		Cycle 4
1:00		4.5/1.5	Cycle 6	
1:30		5.0/2.0		
2:00		5.5/2.5	Cycle 7	Cycle 5
2:30	Dose 3	6.0/3.0		
3:00		6.5/.5	Cycle 8	
3:30		7.0/.1.0		Cycle 6
4:00	Snack	7.5/1.5	Cycle 9	
4:30		8.0/2.0		
5:00		8.5/2.5	Cycle 10	Cycle 7
5:30		9.0/3.0		
6:00	Dismissal	9.5/3.5		

problems worked correctly), and the SKAMP rating scale, which provides subjective ratings of behavior (subscale scores for attention and deportment). They are intended as surrogate measures of response to medication to measure efficacy in a controlled setting rather than effectiveness in the natural environment (see Hoagwood et al., 1995).

The Math test is a 10-minute written test given as seatwork in the classroom. Performance is measured by a permanent product score (the number of problems worked correctly). In studies of medication effects (see Pelham et al., 1995; Swanson et al., 1998), the improvement from placebo on an effective dose of medication has been shown to be about 50% (e.g., from 50 problems to 75 problems worked correctly).

The initial version of the Math test (see Pelham et al., 1995) consisted of one page of each of the mathematical operations (+ , – , × , ÷) arranged in an ascending order of difficulty (i.e., page 1 with 100 addition problems, page 2 with 100 subtraction problems, page 3 with 100 multiplication problems, and page 4 with 100 division problems). Students are instructed to work all problems on each page before moving on to the next page, so the difficulty level of work increases with time on the test. Performance on this version of the Math test will vary across age and ability (e.g., older children will work more problems than younger children). This may not matter for crossover designs in which each subject is his or her own control, but it will matter in between subject designs. We developed another version of the Math test to adjust for age and ability. For our first strategy, we developed a test using "blackline masters" of grade-appropriate math problems, but this was unsuccessful. We found that the speed of working some advanced problems is often greater than for basic problems (e.g., for some children, doing multiplication is faster than addition or subtraction), so older children still worked more problems than younger children.

TABLE 7. SCHEDULE OF ACTIVITIES ACROSS THE DAY FOR TWO COHORTS

Time	*Hr*	*PK*	*Cycle*	*Group 1 activities*	*Hr*	*PK*	*Cycle*	*Group 2 activities*
6:45 A.M.				Arrival—physical				
7:00				Catheter insertion				Arrival—physical
7:30	0	S1	C1	Dose 1, Class 1				Catheter insertion
8:00	0.5			Recess	0	S1	C1	Dose 1, Class 1
8:30	1.0	S2	C2	Class 2	0.5			Recess
9:00	1.5	S3		Recess	1.0	S2	C2	Class 2
9:30	2.0	S4	C3	Class 3	1.5	S3		Recess
10:00	2.5			Snack	2.0	S4	C3	Class 3
10:30	3.0	S5	C4 (skip)	Recess	2.5			Snack
11:00	3.5			Recess	3.0	S5	C4 (skip)	Recess
11:30	4.0	S6	C5	Dose 2, Class 4	3.5			Recess
12:00 P.M.	4.5			Lunch—weigh food	4.0	S6	C5	Dose 2, Class 4
12:30	5.0	S7	C6	Class 5	4.5			Lunch—weigh food
1:00	5.5	S8		Recess	5.0	S7	C6	Class 5
1:30	6.0	S9	C7	Class 6	5.5	S8		Recess
2:00	6.5			Recess	6.0*	S9*	C7	Class 6
2:30	7.0	S10	C8 (skip)	Recess	6.5			Recess
3:00	7.5			Recess/snack	7.0	S10	C8 (skip)	Recess
3:30	8.0	S11	C9	Class 7	7.5			Recess/snack
4:00	8.5			Recess	8.0*	S11	C9	Class 7
4:30	9.0	S12	C10	Class 8	8.5			Recess
5:00	9.5			Snack—measure food	9.0	S12	C10	Class 8
5:30	10.0		C11 (skip)	Recess	9.5			Snack—weigh food
6:00	10.5			Recess	10.0		C11 (skip)	Recess
6:30	11.0	S13	C12 (skip)	Dismissal	10.5			Recess
7:00					11.0	S13	C12 (skip)	Dismissal

Our second strategy used addition and subtraction problems mixed on a page, and difficulty level was varied by requiring (or not) "renaming" (carrying and borrowing) and by the number of digits (2 or 3) per problem. These combinations generate four levels of difficulty for the New Math test. Examples of this test are provided in Table 8.

During screening, an 8-minute pretest (1 minute per page, for 2 test pages at each level of difficulty) is used to select for each individual the difficulty level that produces about 10 problems per minute. For subsequent 10-minute tests in the classroom sessions of each cycle of the LSP, children are given 4 pages of 100 problems at the selected difficulty level. Because the Math test will be administered multiple times each day across multiple days, different versions of equivalent tests are prepared. In some clinical trials with repeated measures on subjects, a large number of tests must be generated (e.g., eight per day for 4 days, or a total of 32 tests).

Other primary outcome measures are derived from the SKAMP rating scale. The original SKAMP rating scale (Swanson, 1992) was based on ten items describing behaviors that are expected of students during each classroom session. A factor analysis confirmed two factors (McBurnett et al., 1997), which we called Attention (getting started, staying on task, completion of work, accuracy and neatness, attending to discussion, transition to next period) and Deportment (interactions with peers, interactions with staff, remaining quiet, remaining seated). The SKAMP was revised for the Multimodality Treatment study of chil-

TABLE 8. EXAMPLES FROM THE NEW MATH TEST

Basic test (1 digit without renaming):				
5	9	8	7	8
+ 2	− 4	− 5	+ 2	− 6
9	3	5	4	4
− 3	+ 2	− 1	+ 5	+ 1
Easy test (2 digits without renaming):				
66	35	85	86	52
+ 23	− 24	+ 12	− 45	+ 33
39	85	69	93	32
− 25	− 62	+ 20	− 42	+ 54
Moderate test (2 digits with renaming):				
56	78	29	30	41
+ 27	− 59	+ 34	− 22	− 18
91	45	27	83	66
− 58	+19	+ 37	− 69	+ 24
Difficult test (3 digits with renaming):				
459	492	482	847	742
− 384	+263	+ 139	+ 163	+ 268
528	498	572	554	622
− 459	+263	− 399	+ 455	− 338

dren with ADHD (MTA) (Greenhill et al., 1996) by adding two items ("following directions of the teacher" and "following rules of the school") and expanding the rating categories from four levels of symptom presence (Not at All = 0, Just a Little = 1, Quite a Bit = 2, and Very Much = 3) to 7 levels of impairment (None = 0, Slight = 1, Mild = 2, Moderate = 3, Severe = 4, Very Severe = 5, and Maximal = 6). The items for the two subscales (Attention and Deportment are averaged to obtain a score reflecting the average rating per item.) A copy of the version of the SKAMP recommended for use in the LSP is presented in Table 9.

We have presented multiple versions of the SKAMP over the last several years (Swanson, 1992; Swanson et al., 1998b; Wigal et al., 1998c). However, the version presented in this chapter provides direct correspondence between coded items for frequency counts to be converted to SKAMP ratings. One way to use the SKAMP is to use only the first 8 items which relate to the factors of Attention and Deportment and not to additional inspection of written work, as we have done in some applications of the LSP (e.g., Swanson et al., 1998b). To be consistent with other versions (e.g., Wigal et al., 1998c), the version presented here includes written work and general items (e.g., following the rules, child-specific items) although they are separated out from the other two factors. We now consider this to be the standard version of the SKAMP.

In the LSP, the time (a 30-minute period), place (the classroom), and setting (schoolwork) are specified for each SKAMP rating. Thus, the SKAMP rating scale differs from

TABLE 9. THE SKAMP RATING SCALE

Child's Name: ______________________ Rater's Initials: ____________
Date: ___/___/____ Time: ______________ Session: ____________

READ EACH ITEM BELOW CAREFULLY, AND CHECK THE BOX THAT BEST DESCRIBES THIS CHILD DURING THE CLASS PERIOD.

	Level of impairment:						
	No impairment	*Slight*	*Mild*	*Moderate*	*Severe*	*Very severe*	*Maximal impairment*
Classroom Behavior:							
1. Getting started on assignments for classroom	⓪	①	②	③	④	⑤	⑥
2. Sticking with tasks or activities for the alloted time	⓪	①	②	③	④	⑤	⑥
3. Attending to an activity or discussion of the class	⓪	①	②	③	④	⑤	⑥
4. Stopping and making transition to next period	⓪	①	②	③	④	⑤	⑥
5. Interacting with other children (e.g., other students)	⓪	①	②	③	④	⑤	⑥
6. Interacting with adults (e.g., teacher or aide)	⓪	①	②	③	④	⑤	⑥
7. Remaining quiet according to classroom rules	⓪	①	②	③	④	⑤	⑥
8. Staying seated according to classroom rules	⓪	①	②	③	④	⑤	⑥
Written Work:							
9. Completing assigned work	⓪	①	②	③	④	⑤	⑥
10. Performing work accurately	⓪	①	②	③	④	⑤	⑥
11. Being careful and neat while writing or drawing	⓪	①	②	③	④	⑤	⑥
General:							
12. Complying with teacher's usual requests or directions	⓪	①	②	③	④	⑤	⑥
13. Following the rules established for the school	⓪	①	②	③	④	⑤	⑥
14. Individual item A	⓪	①	②	③	④	⑤	⑥
15. Individual item B	⓪	①	②	③	④	⑤	⑥

Comments:

TABLE 10. UCI-CDC OBSERVATIONAL CODES

Behavior	*Observation Guidelines*	*Code*
Getting Started		
Not initiating	Refuses to comply with initial request to begin an activity or clean up materials within 5 seconds	Ni (record 1 for each 5 second interval)
Not following directions	Refuses to comply with verbal or nonverbal requests of staff within 5 seconds, while getting started on activities (other than the initial request to get started)	Xg (record 1 per incident)
Directions		
Not following directions	Refuses to comply with verbal or nonverbal requests of staff within 5 seconds	X (record 1 per incident)
School Rules		
Interruption (verbal)	Speaks and interferes with someone addressing the group	i (record 1 per incident)
Not sitting properly	Fails to sit with all legs of chair on the ground, "bottom on chair," facing forward unless given permission otherwise	s (record 1 per incident or record 1 for each 30 second interval)
Out of seat	Leaves chair without permission	o (record 1 per incident)
Disruptive body language	Manipulates body causing interference with the participation of others	d (record 1 per incident)
Noise making	Makes noises other than speech without permission	n (record 1 per incident)
Inappropriate language	Curses, words, statements, or phrases tending to provoke authority	L (record 1 per incident)
Calling out	Blurts, yells answers solicited by teacher without being called to do so	c (record 1 per incident)
Destructive behavior	Attempts to break and/or destroy materials	Da = anger Dc = careless (record 1 per incident)
Relationships		
Teasing (verbal or nonverbal)	Provokes peers through statements or actions	T (record 1 per incident)
"Mean," aggressive voice/body	Addresses others in a nonassertive style characterized by raised volume of voice, threatening tone, tensed muscles in the face or body, clenched fists, or glaring eye contact	M, Ms = toward staff (record 1 per incident)
Passive, whiney voice/body	Addresses others in a nonassertive style characterized by low volume of voice, distressful tone, overrelaxed slumping posture	W, Ws = toward staff (record 1 per incident)
Touching without permission	Touches others or materials without permission (to be recorded as teasing if provocation is apparent)	(T) (record 1 per incident)

(*continued*)

TABLE 10. (*continued*) UCI-CDC OBSERVATIONAL CODES

Behavior	*Observation Guidelines*	*Code*
Aggression	Attempts or succeeds in assaulting peers or staff (may include hitting, kicking, biting, spitting, pushing, restraining)	A (record 1 per incident)
Not accepting (frustration tolerance)	Demonstrates frustration in statements or actions in response to denial or perceived inequities (to be scored as passive or aggressive if directed toward others)	Ac (record 1 per incident)
Rudeness to staff	Provokes adults through statements or actions	R (record 1 per incident)
Lying	Attempts to deceive peers or adults through statements or actions	Ly (record 1 per incident)
On task		
Poor eye contact	Directs eyes toward objects or people other than the intended speaker or action	E (record 1 for each 30 second interval)
Playing	Avoids attending to activity or task by playing with materials or peers not directed by the teacher	P (record 1 for each 30 second interval)
Talking	Avoids attending to activity or task by talking when not directed by the teacher	t (record 1 for each 30 second interval)
Staring	Looks at directly and fixedly objects or people other than the intended speaker or activity for a duration of 5 seconds or longer	S (record 1 for each 30 second interval)
Cleaning Up		
Not initiating	Refuses to comply with initial request to begin an activity or clean up materials within 5 seconds	Ni (record 1 for each 5 second interval)
Not following directions	Refuses to comply with verbal or nonverbal requests of staff within 5 seconds, during clean up activities (other than the initial request to clean up)	Xc (record 1 per incident)
Other	This code corresponds to anecdotal notes on behaviors not covered by coding system	Ot

other rating scales, which are designed to capture typical school behaviors across a longer interval of time (e.g., an entire day, week, or month). In the LSP, each observer/rater has the difficult task of rating up to 8 students each cycle on the SKAMP rating scale. For a protocol with 6 classroom probes across the day, the rater would complete up to 48 SKAMP ratings, which would overwhelm memory for specific classroom sessions. Therefore, the

TABLE 11. ALGORITHM FOR CONVERTING FREQUENCY COUNTS TO SKAMP RATINGS

SKAMP Item	*Ratio (Frequency Counts to Rating Scale)*	*Relevant Codes*
Attention		
1. Getting started	Ni = 2:1 any other = 1:1	Ni, Xg under getting started
2. Sticking with tasks	2:1	E, P, T, S, Ot under task
3. Attending to topic	2:1	E, S under task
4. Making transitions	2:1	Xc, Ni under clean up
Deportment		
5. Interacting with students	1:1	M, W, (T), As, Ac, Rs, Ly, Ot
6. Interacting with staff	1:1	T, M, W, (T), A, Ac, Ly, Ot
7. Remaining quiet	1:1	n, i, c under rules
8. Staying seated	1:1	s, o under rules
Written work		Computer generated by a scoring program
9. Completing assigned work		Number of problems
10. Performing work accurately		Number of errors
11. Being careful and neat		By visual inspection
Other		
12. Complying with directions	1:1	X under directions
13. Following rules	1:1	l, s, o, d, n, L, c, Da, Dc, Ot under rules

rating is done immediately after each classroom session. To keep track of up to 8 students, an observer/rater uses an observation code (see Table 10) to note behaviors observed during a classroom session. The observation code was developed as part of the UCI-CDC school-based day-treatment program (Swanson et al., 1991), and the observation categories used are linked to the items of the SKAMP rating scale (Swanson, 1992).

Observational codes are written next to the appropriate category title (i.e. for an interruption, "i" would be written next to School Rules), with marks made from left to right across the tally sheet with dividing lines marking the beginning of each classroom activity (e.g., Math test or classroom game). In addition to the specific codes, a space is provided on the right side of the frequency count tally sheet for notes. This space is used to note additional information on the intensity of behavior, time out of classroom, and/or observed symptoms. At the end of each classroom period, the observer/rater uses the observations recorded on the tally sheet as a record of behavior of all students being observed during a specific classroom period. The observer/rater consults these notes and completes a SKAMP rating scale for each student being observed and rated. An algorithm has been formulated for the conversion of frequency counts to SKAMP ratings (see Table 11). Some items are converted with a 1:1 ratio (i.e., 1 frequency count = 1 point on the SKAMP severity scale) while other items are converted with a 2:1 ratio (i.e., 2 frequency counts = 1 point on the SKAMP severity scale).

Although the use of frequency counts and a conversion algorithm will tend to quantify the SKAMP ratings, it is not intended to be a measure without qualitative elements. The SKAMP ratings are based on both the frequency of behaviors (objective quantitative counts of specific behavior described in the observation code) and the quality of behaviors (subjective impressions of overall behavior throughout the rating interval based on intensity, context, emotional content, or other factors not specified in the code). For each item, the rater is guided by the frequency counts, but based on recalled observations and anecdotal notes on behavior, the rater may elect to modify the rating on any item. Based on these methods, the test–retest reliability (about 0.75) and concurrent validity (about 0.8) has been established for the SKAMP (see Swanson et al., 1998).

EXAMPLES OF USE OF THE LSP AT UCI

Effects of drug delivery patterns on efficacy: Evidence of acute tolerance

The first study based on the LSP was supported by ALZA Corporation and addressed the impact of drug delivery patterns on behavior and cognition (Swanson et al., 1995; Gupta, 1997; Swanson et al., 1998b; Swanson et al., 1999; Swanson et al., 1999). Thirty-one children (each with a clinical history of a favorable response to methylphenidate and a confirmed *Diagnostic and Statistical Manual of Mental Disorders, 4th Edition* diagnosis of ADHD) completed a double-blind study of four conditions with weekly assessments in the LSP on four Saturdays. On each test day, a 1-hour cycle was used to evaluate two cohorts of children at the expected peaks and troughs of bid dosing of MPH (i.e., at about 1.5 and 3.5 hours after each dose). On each test day, capsules were administered at 30-minute intervals, with contents varied to establish experimental drug delivery patterns based on known PK properties of MPH (Chan et al., 1980 and 1983; Shaywitz et al., 1982; Gualtieri et al., 1982; Patrick et al., 1989). Two control conditions were established: an inactive (Placebo) control condition with lactose in each capsule and an active (bid) control condition in which each child's usual clinical doses of MPH were pulverized and mixed with lactose to fill the capsules administered at 7:30 A.M. and 12:00 noon. Two experimental drug-delivery patterns were established to produce either a rapid rise followed by a flat serum concentration across the day (Flat) or a rising serum concentration across the day achieved without a bolus administration (Ascending). These 4 conditions, labeled Placebo, Bid, Flat, and Ascending, were designed to evaluate the clinical impression that sustained-release (SR) form of MPH was not as effective as the immediate-release (IR) form of this drug (Greenhill and Osman, 1991; Birmaher et al., 1989).

In the classroom probes, students performed individual seatwork and group activities to simulate typical schoolwork, and the SKAMP and Conners, Loney and Milich (CLAM) rating scales (see Swanson, 1992; Swanson et al., 1999) were completed after each session for each child. The Math test was not used. Instead, after each classroom session, a laboratory task of attention and memory was administered (the Memory-Display Scanning Task that required button press responses to visually presented target and nontarget stimuli). Also, physiologic measures were obtained [blood pressure (BP) and heart rate (HR)]. So, for each cycle of the LSP these procedures generated ten measures: Attention and Deportment ratings from the SKAMP; IO, AD, and Mixed ratings from the CLAM; False Alarms and Misses from the memory scanning test; S-BP, D-BP, and HR from the vital signs). The traditional analysis of variance of these measures has been reported (Swanson et al., 1999). These group analyses revealed significant effects for Drug Delivery Condition (Placebo, BID, Flat, and Ascending), Time of Cycle (9:00, 11:30, 1:00, and 3:30), and the interaction of these two factors (Condition × Time).

The initial analyses were used to estimate the magnitude of effect for the groups of subjects. To do this, we quantified the difference between drug and placebo conditions expressed in standard deviation units (i.e., an "effect size"). Because so many studies have contrasted IR MPH and placebo, the effect size for the Placebo and Bid control conditions in the LSP was used to validate this first application of the LSP (see Swanson, et al., 1999; Wigal et al., 1998). The effect size for the teacher ratings were in the expected range of about 1 SD unit in the Bid condition (i.e., for the IOWA)-Conners Inattention/Overactivity subscale the effect sizes were 0.84, 0.62, 1.22, and 0.90 at the four cycle times). This effect can be used as a "Ritalin® ruler" for evaluating the magnitude of the effects of the experimental conditions. For example, this study was specifically designed to evaluate the efficacy of MPH in the afternoon after different histories of medication during the day, so the effect sizes across the four cycle times for the Flat (0.60, 0.60, 0.67, 0.68) and Ascending (0.24, 0.64, 0.96, and 0.90) can be expressed as a percentage of the standard effect size for the Bid treatment with time held constant. The Flat condition achieved about the full standard effect size in the morning (98% at 8:00 A.M.) but does not maintain the full effect size in the afternoon (55% at 1:00 P.M. and 76% at 3:30 P.M.). On the other hand, the full effect size was approximated late in the afternoon in the Ascending condition (79% at 1:30 P.M. and 100% at 3:30 P.M.). This study led to two conclusions: that a constant drug delivery did not maintain the full clinical response over time and that a bolus administration was not necessary to elicit a clinical response to MPH. A second study provided a wider variation in serum concentrations, and suggested that these effects were caused by acute tolerance (tachyphylaxis) to MPH (see Swanson et al., 1999).

Effects of time and dose in the LSP: documentation of efficacy of Adderall®

The second study based on the LSP (supported by Richwood Pharmaceutical Company) addressed the PD effects of Adderall® in 29 children with ADHD and histories of clinical responses to MPH (see Swanson et al., 1998a,b; Wigal et al., 1999). Time (defined by six classroom sessions spaced at precise intervals related to dosing: 0, 1.5, 3.0, 4.5, 6.0, and 7.5 hrs) and Dose (defined by placebo and 4 doses of Adderall®: 0, 5, 10, 15, and 20 mg) factors were included in the design, and a positive control condition was also specified by each subject's clinically titrated dose of methylphenidate. A 6 × 6 Latin Square was used to randomize the order, and each of the six conditions was administered for 1 week as single daily doses. At the end of each week the subjects spent 10 hours (from 7:00 A.M. to 5:00 P.M.) in the LSP. A 1.5-cycle time was used, which generated six probe classroom sessions in which the Math test and the SKAMP ratings were obtained.

Analysis of variance revealed significant main effects of Time and Dose, and significant Time × Dose interactions for these surrogate outcome measures of efficacy (see Swanson et al., 1998a,b). This study demonstrated several important reasons why the tight control provided by the LSP is especially important for short-acting stimulants. First, a pronounced effect over time was documented in the placebo control condition. Ratings of Deportment on the SKAMP and performance on the Math test deteriorated across the day, so placebo adjustments are essential for the interpretation of time-course effects. Even though last measures of the day in the treatment conditions were higher than the first measures of the day, this does not support the notion of a "rebound" effect of medication, because it appears to be caused by the expected time course effects in the nonmedication condition. Also, the LSP allows for some precision in the documentation of peak PD effects of Adderall®. The peak effect in the intermediate-dose condition (15 mg) was slightly greater than in the high-dose condition (20 mg), so even though the average PD effect across the day was greater in the high-dose condition, the best drug level to be maintained throughout the day may be achieved by a lower dose. In fact, a variant of the Sprague and Sleator (1977) hypothesis is supported by these data, which suggest that the use of higher doses to maintain effects for longer periods between dosing may be inappropriate. As pointed out by Levy (1964) long ago, the dose–response relationship should be defined at

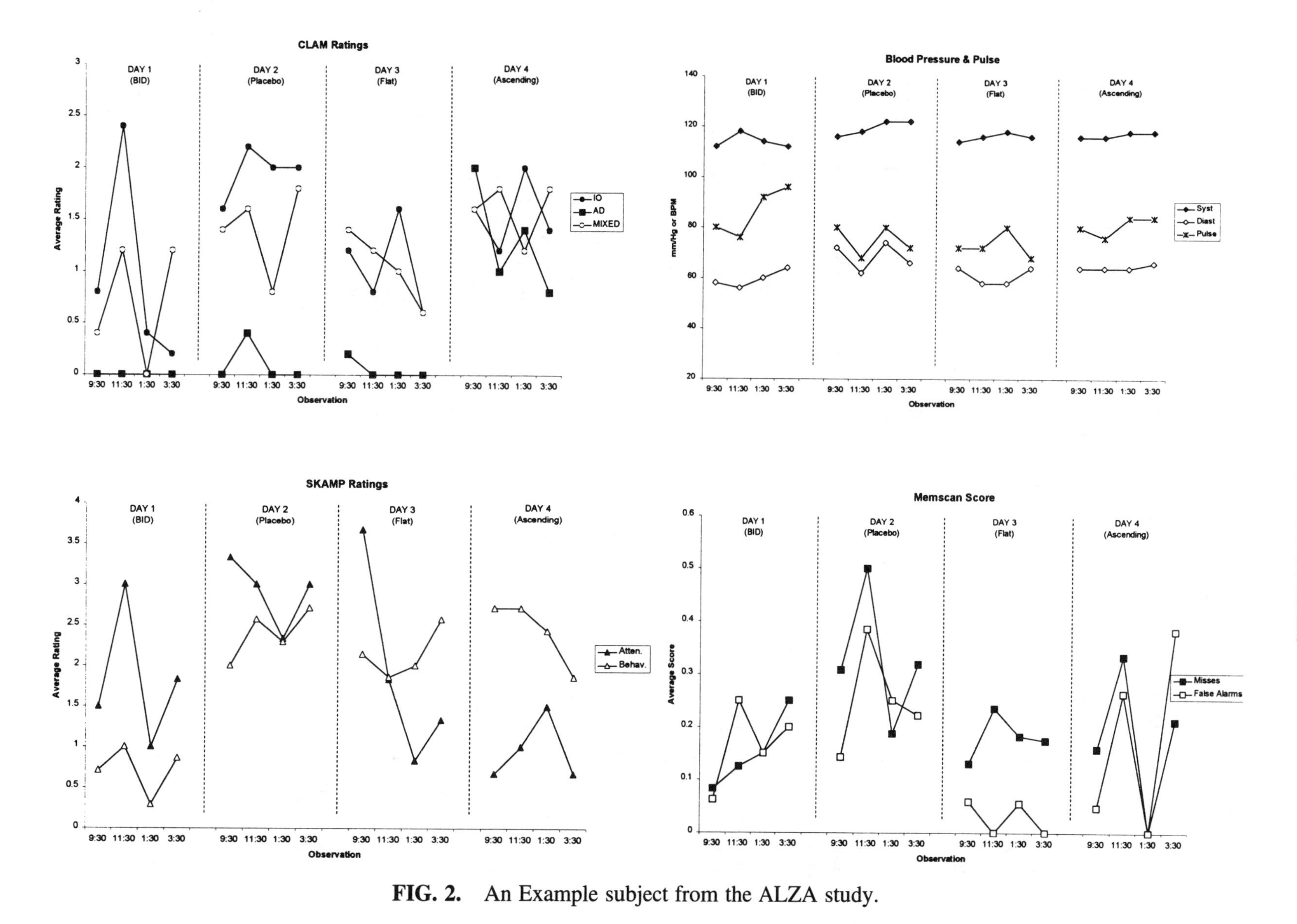

FIG. 2. An Example subject from the ALZA study.

the time of peak efficacy to understand the PD effect of a drug. The LSP provides a way to accomplish this.

Analysis of response of individual subjects

The traditional analysis of average group effects was the primary purpose of the first two studies based on the LSP, which we described above. However, in our application of the LSP we have used these data to develop new analyses for evaluating individual subjects in this controlled setting (Swanson et al., 1999), which we review here.

Our procedures were based on clinical evaluation of the multiple measures of efficacy obtained from a within-subject design. Some procedures use multiple observations of each individual in each condition and calculate an effect size for each individual (see Pelham et al., 1995; Greenhill et al, 1996). However, in most clinical trials, each subject experiences each condition only once. Some researchers (e.g., Rapport et al, 1994) have recommended the use of group statistics to evaluate "reliable change" (see Jacobson and Truax, 1991), but even when adjusted for regression to the mean (Speer and Greenbaum, 1995), this procedure may be flawed (Kraemer et al., personal communication). We have made use of the multiple measures obtained in each condition in the LSP (i.e., the PD effects) to capture an individual pattern of response. The richness of the multidimensional data make integration by formula impractical (see Kleinmuntz, 1990), so we constructed figures to present the data. In out studies, these data are presented to "expert judges," who are asked to inspect each figure, integrate the information over the cycles and test days, filter this by clinical experience, and rank the test days (from best to worst) for each individual subject.

To evaluate overall response for each individual in the first study on drug delivery patterns, we prepared a figure for each individual that contained a set of multidimensional graphs (see Figure 2). This example figure displays sixteen observations of each of the ten measures of response. The sixteen repeated observations are from four cycles of the LSP (i.e., the four time points within each test day) for each of the four drug conditions (i.e., the four test days). The figure has four sections: (1) in the top left panel, the teacher ratings on the CLAM scale (IO, AD, and Mixed); (2) in the bottom left panel, the teacher ratings on the SKAMP (Attention and Deportment); (3) in top right panel, the vital signs (systolic and diastolic BP and HR); (4) in the bottom right panel, performance on the memory scanning task (false-positive and false-negative errors).

The drug condition associated with each test day was not specified on the graphs, so the double-blind code was not revealed to the judges (as it is in Figure 2). The judges understood that clinical doses of stimulants typically produce time-limited decreases in teacher ratings on the CLAM and the SKAMP as well as decreases in errors on the memory scanning task that were associated with symptoms of Inattention (i.e., false-negative responses or Misses) and symptoms of Impulsivity (i.e., false-positive responses or False Alarms).

TABLE 12. RANKINGS OF CONDITIONS FOR AN EXAMPLE SUBJECT BY ALL 4 JUDGES, WITH A CALCULATION OF KENDALL'S W (COEFFICIENT OF CONCORDANCE), AND r_{SW} (AVERAGE OF SPEARMAN RANK CORRELATION COEFFICIENTS)

Judge	*BID*	*Placebo*	*Flat*	*Ascend*	S_W	*W*	r_{SW}	p-*value*
1	1	4	2	3	68	0.85	0.80	0.01
2	2	4	1	3				
3		3	2	4				
4	1	4	2	3				

The judges also understood that clinical doses of MPH usually produced small, insignificant increases in blood pressure and pulse rate but could, in unusual cases, produce large unacceptable increases.

The reader is invited to inspect Figure 2, to ignore the label specifying the condition for

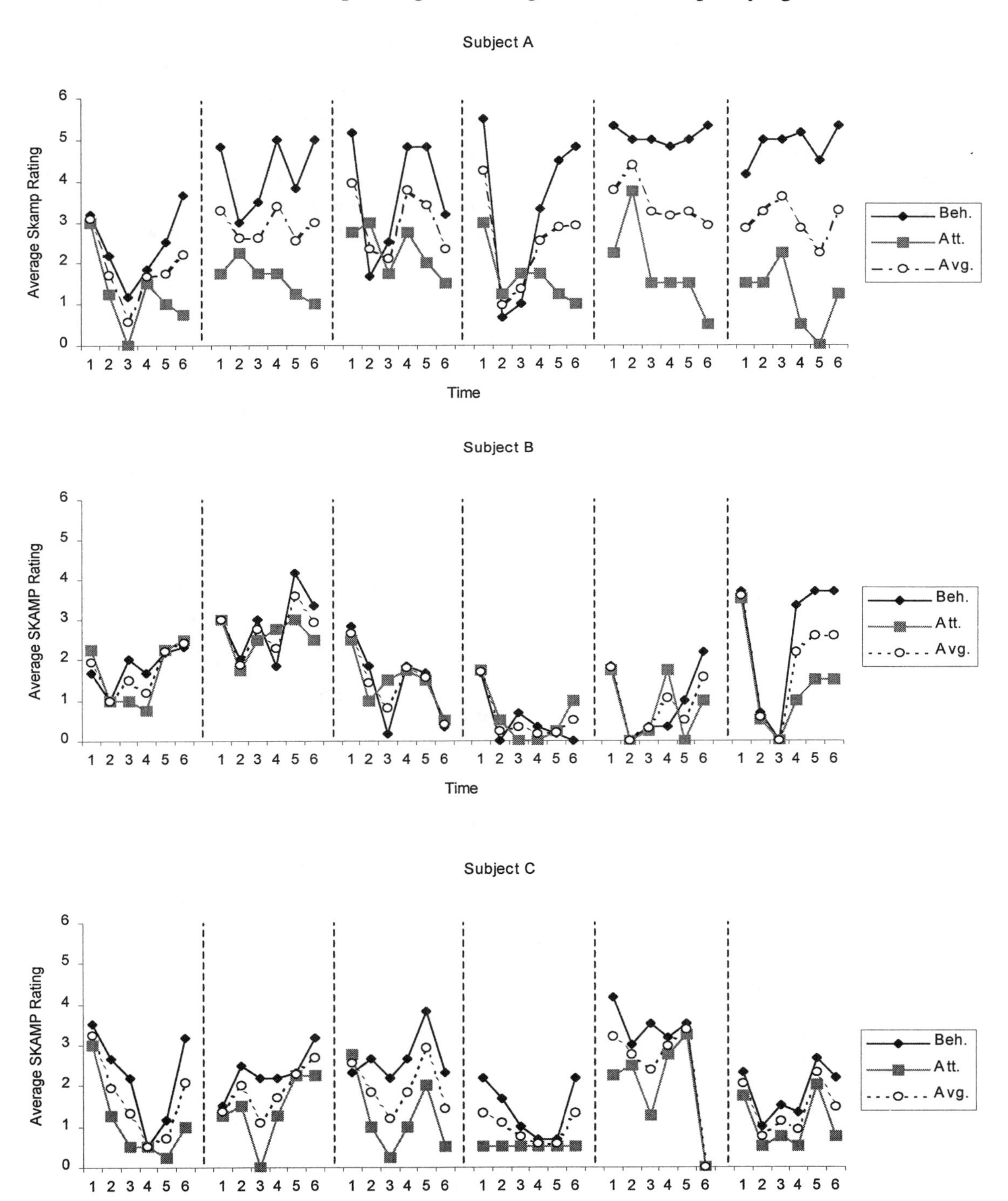

FIG. 3. Ratings from the SKAMP scale for 3 example subjects.

each test day, and to act as an "expert judge" by ranking the test days from best to worst. We chose an example in which agreement across the judges was not perfect. As shown in Table 12, all four judges ranked Days 1 and 3 better than Days 2 and 4, but did not agree whether Day 1 or 3 was the best or whether Day 2 or 4 was the worst.

An inspection of Figure 2 suggests that disagreements reflected in Table 12 may be the result of differences across judges in emphasis on the multiple outcome measures (for which interpretation is invited by the definition of the dependent variables shown on the ordinates of the graphs) or a different interpretation of time-course effects (for which interpretation is invited by the definition of the independent variables shown on the abscissa of the graphs). As shown in Table 12 (see rows 2 and 3), different rankings were offered by judge 2 (who ranked Day 3 as better than Day 1), probably because of an emphasis on the low scores on the cognitive task and high late-morning scores on the I/O and Attention subscales on Day 1) and judge 3 (who ranked Day 4 as worse than Day 2, probably because of an emphasis on the high A/D ratings).

Our statistical procedures for individual subject analysis are based on W, Kendall's Co-

TABLE 13. KENDALL'S W AND r_{sw} FOR 3 EXAMPLE SUBJECTS FROM THE ADDERALL STUDY

		Order of Presentation					
Subject	Judge	1ST	2ND	3RD	4TH	5TH	6TH
A	BW	1	4	3	2	5	6
	DC	1	4	3	2	5	6
	JS	1	4	3	2	5	6
	LG	1	4	3	2	5	6
	SW	1	4	3	2	5	6
	Sum of Ranks	5	20	15	10	25	30
		(A15)	(R)	(A10)	(A20)	(A5)	(P)
	SS = 437.5						
	W = 1						
		Order of Presentation					
Subject	Judge	1ST	2ND	3RD	4TH	5TH	6TH
B	BW	4	6	5	1	2	3
	DC	4	6	5	1	2	3
	JS	3	6	5	1	2	4
	LG	4	6	5	1	2	3
	SW	4	6	3	1	5	2
	Sum of Ranks	19	30	23	5	13	15
		(R)	(P)	(A15)	(A20)	(A10)	(A5)
	SS = 371.5						
	W = .849143						
		Order of Presentation					
Subject	Judge	1ST	2ND	3RD	4TH	5TH	6TH
C	BW	2	5	4	1	6	3
	DC	3	5	4	1	6	2
	JS	3	5	4	1	6	2
	LG	1	5	4	2	6	3
	SW	1	3	4	5	6	2
	Sum of Ranks	10	23	20	10	30	12
		(A20)	(A10)	(R)	(A15)	(P)	(A5)
	SS = 335.5						
	W = .766857						

efficient of Concordance (see Swanson et al, 1999), as well as a transformation, r_{SW}, that represents the average correlation between all pairs of judges. In this study, for each subject the r_{SW} was significant, verifying that the judges were concordant. The average rank was used to specify the consensus ranking of conditions across judges. When the double-blind code was broken, it revealed that 2 of the 31 subjects were “placebo responders,” that most subjects responded best to their clinical (bid) dosing, and that the two experimental conditions were considered best for approximately an equal number of subjects.

For the second application of the LSP to evaluate the PD effects of Adderall,® we prepared a set of graphs for each subject based on subjective behavior ratings that were completed for each subject after each of six classroom sessions and on the permanent product scores from the 10-minute Math tests. A figure for each subject was given to 5 judges who were instructed to rank the conditions from 1 (best) to 6 (worst). In Figure 3, example graphs from 3 subjects are shown. The graphs on the top are based on subjective behavior ratings ($SKAMP_{attention}$ and $SKAMP_{deportment}$), and the graphs on the bottom are based on the permanent product scores from the 10-minute Math tests ($PERMP_{attempted}$ and $PERMP_{correct}$).

We choose these 3 subjects to demonstrate some variation in the concordance across judges, and the rankings of conditions for these three example subjects are shown in Table 13. In the first example subject, the judges agree, and $W = 1$. In the second example subject, the judges agree on the best and worst conditions, but there is some disagreement in the rankings of the other conditions, and $W = 0.849$. In the third example, there is agreement of the worst conditions, but some disagreement about the best condition and the other conditions, too, and $W = 0.76$. However, in this study the concordance of the judges is statistically significant for each subject.

Based on the consensus ranks, 3 of the 29 subjects were “placebo responders.” We were tempted to use the consensus ranks to specify the “optimal dose” for each individual, but these graphic presentations reminded us that the comparison across conditions is complicated by time-course effects. The optimal condition may reflect the average effects across the day rather than optimum peak effect that, if maintained over time, might be the best target for delivery of medication across the day. In subsequent studies, we have attempted to establish optimal drug delivery across the day and then compare conditions based on the pattern rather then the peak effects or the average effects.

SUMMARY

The primary purpose of the laboratory school protocol is to measure time-course effects of medications. As described in this chapter the outcome measures are surrogates that are related to behavior at school and performance in the regular classroom. We have established tight control over the time and the content of regular probes, and we have used these measures as primary outcome variables in the LSP.

The surrogate measures from the SKAMP ratings and the permanent product scores have high face validity. We are currently evaluating the relationship between surrogate measures in the laboratory and traditional outcome measures in the real-world settings.

REFERENCES

Birmaher, B., Greenhill L.L., Cooper, T.B., Fried, J., Maminski, B. (1989), Sustained release methylphenidate: Pharmacokinetic studies in ADDH males. *J. Am. Acad. Child Adoles. Psychiatry*, 28(5):768–772.

Chan, Y.P., Soldin, S.J., Swanson, J.M., Deber, C.M., Thiessen, J.J., Macleod, S. (1980), Gas chromatographic/mass spectrometric analysis of methylphenidate (ritalin) in serum. *Clin. Biochem.*, 13(6):266–272.

Chan, Y.P., Swanson, J.M., Soldin, S.S., Thiessen, J.J., Macleod, S.M., Logan, W. (1983), Methylphenidate hydrochloride given with or before breakfast: II. Effects on plasma concentration of methylphenidate and ritalinic acid. *Pediatrics,* 72(1):56–59.

Collier, C.P., Soldin, S.J., Swanson, J.M., MacLeod, S.M., Weinberg, F., Rochefort, J.G. (1985), Pemoline pharmacokinetics and long term therapy in children with attention deficit disorder and hyperactivity. *Clin. Pharmacokinet.*, 10(3):269–278.

Greenhill, L.L., Abikoff, H.B., Arnold, L.E., Cantwell, D.P., Conners, C.K., Elliott, G., Hechtman, L., Hinshaw, S.P., Hoza, B., Jensen, P.S., March, J.S., Newcorn, J. Pelham, W.E., Severe, J.B., Swanson, J.M., Vitiello, B., Wells, K. (1996), Medication treatment strategies in the MTA study: Relevance to clinicians and researchers. *J. Am. Acad. Child Adolesc. Psychiatry*, 35(10):1304–1313.

Greenhill, L.L., Osman, B.B., eds. (1991), *Ritalin: Theory and Patient Management*. Larchmont, NY: Mary Ann Liebert Publishers, Inc.

Gualtieri, C.T., Wargin, W., Kanoy, R., Patrick, K., Shen, C.D., Youngblood, W., Mueller, R.A., Breese, G.R. (1982), Clinical studies of methylphenidate serum levels in children and adults. *J. Am. Acad. Child Psychiatry*, 21(1):19–26.

Gupta, S. Acute tolerance to methylphenidate. Presentation at the Annual Meeting of the American Academy of Child and Adolescent Psychiatry, Toronto, October 1997.

Hoagwood, K., Hibbs, E., Brent, D., Jensen, P. (1995), Introduction to the special section: Efficacy and effectiveness in studies of child and adolescent psychotherapy. *J. Consult. Clin. Psycho.*, 63(5):683–687.

Jacobson, N.S., Truax, P. (1991), Clinical significance: A statistical approach to defining meaningful change in psychotherapy research. *J. Consult. Clin. Psychol.* 59(1):12–29.

Jensen, P.S., Vitiello, B., Leonard, H., Laughren, T.P. (1994), Design and methodology issues for clinical treatment trials in children and adolescents: Child and adolescent psychopharmacology. Expanding the research base. *Psychopharmacol. Bull.*, 30(1):3–8.

Kleinmuntz, B. (1990), Why we still use our heads instead of formulas: Toward an integrative approach. *Psychol. Bull.* 107(3):296–310.

Kraemer, H.C., Stice, E., Kazdin, AE., Offord, D. (1999), Kupfer, D. How do risk factors work? Mediators, moderators, independent, overlapping, and proxy-risk factors. Department of Psychiatry, Stanford University. (Unpublished manuscript).

Levy, G. (1964), Relationship between elimination rate of drugs and rate of decline of their pharmacologic effects. *J. Pharmaceutical Sci.*, 53:342–343.

McBurnett, K., Swanson, J.M., Pfiffner. L.J., Tamm, L. (1997), A measure of ADHD-related classroom impairment based on targets for behavioral intervention. *J. Attention Dis.*, 2:63–76.

Patrick, K.S., Straughn, A.B., Jarvi, E.J., Breese, G.R., Meyer, M.C. (1989), The absorption of sustained-release methylphenidate formulations compared to an immediate-release formulation. *Biopharmaceutics Drug Disposition*, 10(2):165–71.

Pelham, W.E., Jr., Carlson, C., Sams, S.E., Vallano, G., Dixon, M.J., Hoza, B. (1993), Separate and combined effects of methylphenidate and behavior modification on boys with attention deficit-hyperactivity disorder in the classroom. *J. Consul. Clin. Psychol.*, 61:506–515.

Pelham, W.E., Jr., Swanson, J.M., Furman, M.B., Schwindt, H. (1995), Pemoline effects on children with ADHD: A time-response by dose–response analysis on classroom measures. *J. Am. Acad. Child Adolesc Psychiatry*, 34(11):1504–1513.

Rapport, M.D., Denney, C., DuPaul, G.J., Gardner, M.J. (1994), Attention deficit disorder and methylphenidate: Normalization rates, clinical effectiveness and response prediction in 76 children. *J. Am. Acad. Child Adolesc. Psychiatry*, 33:882–93, 1994.

Safer, D,. Zito, J., Fine, E. (1996), Increased methylphenidate usage for ADD in the 1990s. *Pediatrics*, 98:1084–1088.

Shaffer, D., Campbell, M., Cantwell, D., Bradley, S., Carlson, G., Cohen, D., Denckla, M., Frances, A., Garfinkel, B., Klein, R. (1989), Child and adolescent psychiatric disorders in *DSM-IV*: issues facing the work group. *J. Am. Acad. of Child Adoles. Psychiatry*, 28(6):830–835.

Shaywitz, S.E., Hunt, R.D., Jatlow, P., Cohen, D.J, Young, J.G., Pierce, R.N., Anderson, G.M., Shaywitz, B.A. (1982), Psychopharmacology of attention deficit disorder: Pharmacokinetic, neuroendocrine, and behavioral measures following acute and chronic treatment with methylphenidate. *Pediatrics*, 69(6):688–694.

Soldin, S.J., Chan, Y.P., Hill, B.M., Swanson, J.M. (1979), Liquid-chromatographic analysis for methylphenidate (Ritalin) in serum. *Clin. Chem.* 25(3):401–404.

Soldin, S.J., Hill, B.M., Cahn, Y.P., Swanson, J.M., Hill, J.G. (1979), A liquid-chromatographic analysis for ritalinic acid [alpha-phenyl-alpha-(2-piperidyl) acetic acid] in serum. *Clin. Chem.*, 25(1):51–54.

Speer, D.C., Greenbaum, P.E. (1995), Five methods for computing significant individual client change and improvement rates: support for an individual growth curve approach. *J. Consul. Clin. Psychol.*, 63(6):1044–1048.

Sprague, R.L., Sleator, E.K. (1977), Methylphenidate in hyperkinetic children: Differences in dose effects on learning and social behavior. *Science*, 198:1274–1276.

Swanson, J.M. (1985), Attention deficit disorder: Current perspectives. In: Kavanaugh, J & Truss, TJ (eds.), *Learning Disabilities: Proceedings of the National Conference*, eds., J. Kavanaugh & T.J. Truss. Maryland: York Press.

Swanson, J.M. (1997), Hyperkinetic disorders and attention deficit hyperactivity disorders. *Curr. Opinion. Psychiatry*, 10:300–305.

Swanson, J.M. (1985), Measures of cognitive functioning appropriate for use in pediatric psychopharmacological research studies. Psychopharmacol. Bull. 21:887–890.

Swanson, J.M. (1992), *School-Based Assessments and Interventions for ADD Students*. Irvine, CA: K.C. Publishing.

Swanson, J.M., Cantwell, D., Lerner, M., McBurnett, K., Hanna, G. (1991), Effects of stimulant medication on learning in children with ADHD. *J. Learn. Disabil.*, 24(4): 219–30, 255.

Swanson, J.M., Gupta, S., Guinta, D., Flynn, D., Agler, D., Lerner, M., Williams, L. Shoulson, I., Wigal, S. (1999) Acute tolerance to methylphenidate in the treatment of attention deficit hyperactivity disorder in children. *Clin Pharmacol. Ther.* 66(3).

Swanson, J.M., Lerner, M., Williams, L. (1995), Letter to the editor: More frequent diagnosis of attention deficit-hyperactivity disorder. *N. Eng. J. Med.*, 333(14):944.

Swanson, J.M., McBurnett, K., Christian, D.L., Wigal, T. (1995), Stimulant medications and the treatment of children with ADHD. In: *Advances in Clinical Child Psychology*, eds., T.H. Ollendick & R.J. Prinz. New York: Plenum Press.

Swanson, J.M., Wigal, S., Greenhill, L.L., Browne, R., Waslik, B., Lerner, M., Williams, L., Flynn, D., Agler, D., Crowley, K., Fineberg, E., Baren, M., Cantwell, D.P. (1998a), Analog classroom assessment of Adderall in children with ADHD. *J. Am. Acad. Child Adolesc. Psychiatry*, 37(5):519–526.

Swanson, J.M., Wigal, S.B., Greenhill, L., Browne, R., Waslik, B., Lerner, M., Williams, L., Flynn, D., Agler, D., Crowley, K., Fineberg, E., Regino, R., Baren, M., Cantwell, D.

(1998b), objective and subjective measures of the pharmacodynamic effects of Adderall In the Treatment of Children with ADHD in a controlled laboratory classroom setting. *Psychopharamcol. Bull.*, 34:55–60.

Swanson, J.M., Sunohara, G.A., Kennedy, J.L., Regino, R., Fineberg, E., Wigal, T., Lerner, M., Williams, L., LaHoste, G.J., Wigal, S. (1998c), Association of the dopamine receptor D4 (DRD4) gene with a refined phenotype of attention deficit hyperactivity disorder (ADHD): A family-based approach. *Molec. Psychiatry*, 3:38–41.

Swanson, J.M., Wigal, S.B., Udrea, D., Lerner, M., Gupta, S. (1999), Evaluation of relative response of individuals in the analog classroom setting: I. Effects of different drug delivery patterns of methylphenidate. *Psychopharmacol. Bull.* (in press)

Tomkins, C.P., Soldin, S.J., MacLeod, S.M., Rochefort, J.G., Swanson, J.M. (1980), Analysis of pemoline in serum by high performance liquid chromatography: Clinical application to optimize treatment of hyperactive children. *Ther. Drug Monitor.* 2:255–260.

Wigal, S.B., Gupta, S., Guinta, D., Swanson, J. (1998), Reliability and validity of the SKAMP rating scale in a laboratory school setting. *Psychopharmacol. Bull.* 34:47–53.

Wigal, S.B., Swanson, J.M., Greenhill, L., Waslick, B., Cantwell, D., Clevenger, W., Davies, M., Lerner, M., Regino, R., Fineberg, E., Baren, M., Browne, R. (1999) Evaluation of relative response of individuals in the analog classroom setting: II. Effects of dose of amphetamine (Adderall®). *Psychopharmacol. Bull.*, (in Press).

Subject Index

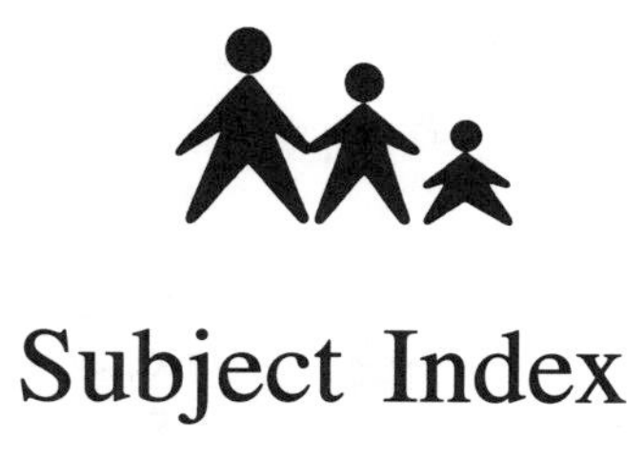

Subject Index

A

Academic games, types, 410
Academic performance
  direct measures, 199
  outcome measures, 47
  Ritalin effect, 219, 229
  test scores, 229
Achenbach-Conners-Quay Project, 116
Acquired immunodeficiency syndrome (AIDS)
  children, 165
  dementia complex, 166
  Ritalin treatment, 13
  stimulant drugs, 166
  see also Human immunodeficiency virus
Activity level
  ADHD children, 347–353
  measuring, 346
Acute tolerance, classroom evidence, 420
Adderall
  ADHD children, 385–396
  efficacy, 421
  psychodynamics, 421
  rating scales, 417
  time and dose, 421
Additive factor method (AFM), 324
Adolescents
  ADHD treatment, 119, 175, 193
  assessment problem, 114
  conduct disorders, 341
  Conners Rating Scales, 120
  coordinating care, 175–186
  medication responses, 244
  rating scales, 114, 119
  Ritalin, 175–186
  self-reporting, 119
  see also Children
Adrenergic overdrive, 401
Adults
  ADHD treatment, 13, 121, 141
  diagnosis, 141
  rating scales, 121
  Ritalin effects, 145
  symptoms, 121
  validity and prevalence, 144
Age-specific therapy, 13
Aggression
  ADHD children, 237, 245, 329
  amphetamines, 135
  conduct disorders, 352
  eruptive vs. hostile, 238
  laboratory studies, 241
  measuring, 239
  multidimensional, 238
  naturalistic, 242–244
  neurobiology, 350–352
  parent ratings, 247
  peers vs. adults, 238
  physical, 238
  public schools, 242
  rating scales, 247
  Ritalin effects, 237–247
  specificity and dosage, 239
  stimulant drugs, 240
  verbal, 238
Alcohol abuse, ADHD adults, 143
Alternative Uses and Instances Test, 228
Alternative medicine
  ADHD children, 185
  international perspective, 19
Alza Corporation, 405, 419
American Academy of Child and Adolescent
    Psychiatry, 175
American Academy of Pediatrics, 175
American Medical Association, 2
American Psychological Association, 116
Amphetamines
  ADHD treatment, 130–136
  animal models, 28, 128
  case report, 202
  central processing, 326
  controlled substance, 27
  encoding studies, 325
  HIV children, 167
  language problems, 267
  motor organization, 327
  neurochemistry, 127
  noradrenergic function, 351
  pharmaceutical promotion, 17
  relative strengths, 135
  responder summary, 135
  vs. Ritalin, 127–137
  side effects, 136
  sleep problems, 287
  tic response, 311
  Tourette's syndrome, 127, 137
  see also Dextroemphetamine

Anger
  rating scales, 119
  see also Aggression
Anorexia, 136
Antidepressant drugs
  ADHD children, 79
  anxiety disorders, 79
  prescribing rate, 1
  see also Tricyclic antidepressants
Antiretroviral therapy, HIV children, 170
Antisocial behavior
  measuring, 134
  neurobiology, 352
  overt and covert, 238, 241
  parent ratings, 247
  Ritalin effects, 237–247
  substance abuse, 143
Anxiety
  Ritalin effects, 258
  stimulant-induced, 146, 151
  type-specific, 255n
Anxiety disorders
  ADHD children, 74–78
  antidepressants, 79
  clinical diagnosis, 72, 348
  comorbid ADHD, 77–80
  desipramine, 79
  family studies, 75
  fluoxetine, 80
  imipramine, 79
  incidence, 71
  overview, 71
  physiology, 77
  Ritalin treatment, 71–80
  substance abuse, 143
Archives of General Psychiatry, 375
Attention
  ADHD children, 348–350
  clinical assessment, 348–350
  cognitive-energetic model, 323–325
  measuring, 341, 346
  outcome measures, 47
  paper-and-pencil tests, 344
  rating scales, 420
  see also Inattention
Attention deficit disorder (ADD)
  diagnostic changes, 12
  history and derivation, 253
  media interest, 1
  rating scales, 116
  Ritalin response, 258–260
Attention deficit hyperactivity disorder (ADHD)
  activity level, 348–350
  adolescents, 120
  adults, 14, 120
  age variation, 257
  aggression, 350–352
  antisocial behavior, 242
  anxiety disorders, 74–77
  attention, 348–350
  auditory processing, 272
  behavioral intervention, 210
  central processing, 326
  child vs. adult, 147
  classification, 19
  clonidine and methylphenidate, 401–404
  cognitive impairment, 226, 341, 350
  combined treatment, 95–98
  comorbidity, 77, 254, 341
  conduct disorders, 341–353
  Conners Rating Scales, 120
  core symptoms, 345–349
  demographics, 257
  diagnosis, 1, 353
  differential diagnosis, 178–180
  empiric findings, 258–260
  encoding studies, 325–327
  familial, 76, 142
  gender-specific, 142, 151, 257
  genetic aspects, 142
  heterogeneity, 353
  history and derivation, 253
  impairment, 254–256
  impulsivity, 222, 348
  inattention, 260, 350
  incidence, 87, 175
  increased recognition, 404
  issues and challenges, 1–3
  judicial decisions, 18
  laboratory school protocol, 405
  language problems, 266–270
  learning and memory, 224
  legislation, 17
  motor organization, 327
  neurobiology, 349–351
  neurochemistry, 341
  neuropsychology, 145, 345
  pathophysiology, 77, 345
  persistent features, 16
  physician specialty, 17
  plasma studies, 370
  prevalence, 1, 145, 257
  psychopharmacology, 1–3
  public health concern, 87
  rating scales, 118, 148, 196
  reading disorders, 270–273
  Ritalin effects, 321–332
  school setting, 179
  sleep problems, 287–297
  subject recruitment, 406

substance abuse, 143
teacher ratings, 19
tic disorders, 301
Tourette's syndrome, 301–303
types, 253–260
United States, 1
validity, 132
ADHD treatment
academic thought, 17
Adderall, 385–396
adults, 141
age-specific, 14
amphetamines, 130–136
antidepressants, 79
clinical response, 45–50
consumer advocacy, 17
coordinating care, 175–186
desipramine, 79, 152
drug trials, 122
economic status, 14
educational setting, 12, 185
efficacy and effects, 117
fluoxetine, 80
future research, 157
gender-specific, 13
HIV children, 165, 167
imipramine, 79
interdisciplinary, 176
long-duration stimulants, 385–396
Medicaid data, 13
medication prevalence, 10–18
multimodal, 175
nonmedical, 185
nonstimulant drugs, 152–155
outpatient assessment, 210–212
parent training, 87, 178
parochial schools, 12
patient demographics, 13–15
pemoline, 151, 156
pharmaceutical promotion, 18
pharmacoepidemiology, 7
pharmacology, 88
planning and monitoring, 180–184
private schools, 12
psychosocial interventions, 91
public schools, 12
race and ethnicity, 14
referrals and assessment, 176
responder summary, 134
Ritalin, 77, 130, 147, 253
special education classes, 12
stimulant drugs, 165, 167
tamoxetine, 152–156
United States, 19
Auditory Continuous Performance Test, 145
Auditory processing
ADHD children, 273
clinical implications, 277
Ritalin effects, 273
Australia
ADHD children, 19
drug prevalence, 17
Azidothymidine (AZT), 169

B

Barkley's Home Situations Questionnaire, 46
Beck Depression Inventory, 148
Behavior
ADHD children, 185
drug delivery patterns, 419
intervention, 210–212
modification, 200
specificity and prediction, 61
see also Attention deficit disorder
Body mass, Ritalin response, 50–57
Brain
activity, 378
function, 376
imaging, 375–382
pharmacodynamics, 376
Ritalin and cocaine, 375–382

C

Caffeine
alternative therapy, 185
sleep problems, 287
California Verbal Learning Test, 145
Canada
ADHD treatment, 19
rating scales, 118
Case report forms, 407
Catecholamines, 127
Central processing, cognitive-energetic model, 326
Central auditory processing disorder (CAPD), 272
Cerebral blood flow (CBF), 379
Child Behavior Checklist, 79, 180
Child psychiatry, 123
Children
ADHD treatment, 175–186
clinical trials, 56–66
conduct disorders, 341
Conners Rating Scales, 119
coordinating care, 175–186
rating scales, 113–123
Ritalin, 175–186
schizophrenia, 323
see also Adolescents

Chlorpromazine, 130
Cholinergic agents, 157
Chronic fatigue syndrome, 14
Classrooms
  academic games, 409
  analog setting, 413
Clinical Global Impression Scale, 149
Clonidine
  bounce back effect, 401
  and methylpenidate, 401–404
  pediatric practice, 402
  safety and efficacy, 401
  Scott-Levin report, 403
  sudden death, 401
  tic disorders, 306
  usage patterns, 401–404
Cocaine
  action mechanism, 376
  administration routes, 375
  animal models, 28
  brain imaging, 375–382
  CBF studies, 379
  controlled substance, 27
  dopaminergic effect, 374–376
  pharmacokinetics, 376
  pharmacology, 375–377
  vs. Ritalin, 375–382
Cognition
  ADHD children, 227, 341, 349
  constriction, 227–230
  drug delivery patterns, 419–422
  impairment, 349–351
  focusing, 269
  performance, 76
  Ritalin effects, 219, 269
Cognitive-behavioral therapy, 185
Cognitive-energetic model
  central processing, 326
  encoding studies, 325
  motor organization, 330
  Ritalin effects, 325
Color naming, 272
Columbia Impairment Scale, 395
Combined treatment, 95–99
  design and methodology, 95, 99
  effects, 97, 100
  identifying studies, 96
  implications, 98–100
  pharmacoepidemiology, 8
  single-factor design, 95, 99
Communication disorders, 266
Comorbidity
  ADHD children, 254, 341
  diagnostic, 341–343
  Ritalin effects, 71–80
Complex Figure Test, 144
Concentration, academic game, 410
Conduct disorders
  ADHD children, 242–244
  aggression, 242, 352
  case report, 206
  clinical assessment, 343, 348
  disruptive behavior, 238
  vs. hyperactivity, 118n
  Ritalin vs. amphetamines, 135
  Ritalin effects, 246, 322
  substance abuse, 144
Conners Rating Scales
  Child and Adolescent, 121
  Parent, 78
  restandardized, 118–120
  Teacher, 46, 199
Constriction, cognitive, 227–231
Consumer advocacy, 16
Contingency Naming Task, 227
Continuous Performance Task (CPT), 76, 199
  impulsivity, 224
  Ritalin effects, 321–323
Controlled Substances Act, 27
Convergent thinking, 227
Coordinating care, adolescents, 175–186
Core symptoms, ADHD children, 346–350
Crossover trials, Ritalin vs. amphetamines, 132
Curvilinear dose-response, 220

D

Daily report cards, outpatient assessment, 210–213
Daydreaming, gender-specific, 184
Dementia, antiretroviral therapy, 170
Deportment, rating scales, 420
Depression
  Ritalin vs. amphetamines, 34
  stimulant-induced, 147, 153
Desipramine
  academic thought, 18
  ADHD adults, 152, 156
  safety issue, 20
  sudden death, 79
  tic disorders, 306, 310
Dextroamphetamine
  ADHD children, 385–396
  adverse events, 388
  clinical trials, 385–396
  crossover trials, 391
  language problems, 268
  limitations, 389
  long-duration, 385–396
  parallel trials, 391
  parent training, 88

vs. Ritalin, 127
sales data, 8
sleep problems, 287
tic response, 310
Diagnosis criteria, 115
Diagnostic and Statistical Manual of Mental Disorders, 253
Diagnostic Interview for Children (DISC), 72
Didanosine, 169
Discrimination, Ritalin abuse, 30
Disruptive behavior disorders (DBD)
ADHD children, 342
clinical assessment, 242, 348
Disruptive Behavior Disorders Scale, 198
Divergent thinking, 227
Dopamine
changes, 381
genetic aspects, 144
Ritalin, 127, 372
synaptic cleft, 381
Dopamine transporter
binding kinetics, 379
cocaine effect, 377
regional distribution, 379
Ritalin target, 376, 379
Dopaminergic transmission, 379–381
Dose-response curves
cognitive measures, 219
curvilinear, 220
implications, 231
rating scales, 196
Ritalin, 219
types, 220
Drowsiness, parent perceptions, 289
Drug abuse, 36, 143
Drug Abuse Warning Network, 36
Drug delivery patterns
button-press responses, 419
efficacy effects, 420
Drug Enforcement Administration (DEA)
database, 10
Ritalin, 7, 17, 38
sales data, 15
Drug prevalence
academic thought, 18
ADHD estimates, 10–16
clinical factors, 15–18
consumer advocacy, 18
diagnostic changes, 15–19
educational setting, 11
future research, 20
geographic variation, 17
lifetime, 9
medical setting, 17
mentally retarded, 18
patient demographics, 13–15
payment sources, 17
pharmaceutical promotion, 18
special groups, 17
United States, 19
Drug trials
behavioral response, 122
children, 121
progress chart, 123
rating scales, 135
symptom changes, 122
Dyslexia, 271

E
Education for All Handicapped Children Act (1975), 18
Educational therapy, 185
Effort, cognitive model, 329
Electrocortical potential, 322
Emotionality, rating scales, 120
Encoding, cognitive model, 325
Endocarditis, 35
Energetic factor. *See* Cognitive-energetic model
Executive function
ADHD children, 331, 348
working memory, 275
Expressive language disorders, 266
Externalizing behavior, 238

F
Family feud, academic game, 411
Family studies
ADHD children, 76
rating scales, 119
Ritalin use, 76
Fatigue, 14
Fluoxeine, anxiety disorders, 80
Frequency counts, converting algorithm, 421

G
Gender-specific therapy, 13
Generalized anxiety disorder (GAD), 72
Glucose metabolism, Ritalin and cocaine, 378
Go-No-Go Task, 321–323
Government regulation, 18

H
Hallucinations, 171
Halo errors, rating scales, 114
Haloperidol, 128
Hamilton Anxiety Scale, 149
Hamilton Depression Scale, 149
Hangman, academic game, 410

Harvard University, 385
Health maintenance organization (HMO)
drug prevalence, 17
usage patterns, 11
Hemiplegia, 35
Homeopathy, 19
Human immunodeficiency virus (HIV)
ADHD children, 165–172
amphetamines, 167
antiretroviral therapy, 169
clinical data, 166–171
Ritalin use, 167
stimulant drugs, 165–172
5–Hydroxytryptamine (5–HT), 350
Hyperactivity
clinical assessment, 348–350
vs. gender specific, 184
index, 118, 122
see also Attention deficit hyperactivity disorder
Hyperkinetic disorder, 15, 19
Hypomania, 171

I
Imaging. *See* Brain imaging
Imipramine, anxiety disorders, 79
Impairment
ADHD children, 254–256
types and dimensions, 254
Impulsivity
ADHD children, 348–352
clinical assessment, 348–350
cognitive, 224
vs. inattention, 178
measuring, 325
neurobiology, 340–342
rating scales, 347
Ritalin vs. amphetamines, 135
type-specific, 220
Inattention
ADHD children, 184
case report, 292
gender-specific, 184
vs. impulsivity, 178
measuring, 314
neurobiology, 350–35
rating scales, 347
Ritalin vs. amphetamines, 135
type-specific, 254n
Individual Disability Education Act (1990), 19
Information processing
paradigm, 329
stages, 328
Insomnia, 288
Institutional review boards, 408
Intelligence quotient (IQ), 271, 344

L
Laboratory school protocol (LSP)
academic games, 410
activity cycle, 412
Adderall efficacy, 421
button-press responses, 420, 422
daily schedule, 412
drug delivery patterns, 420
generic manual, 406
implementing, 406–420
math test, 413–416
measuring instruments, 413–420
medical staff, 409
methylphenidate, 405
multiple sites, 405
observational codes, 418
pemoline, 405
pharmacodynamics, 405
questionnaire, 414
rating scale, 417
recess staff, 408
school staff, 408
space required, 412
staff and facility, 407–412
subject recruitment, 406
time and dose, 421
typical schedule, 406
usage examples, 420–427
Language disorders, 252
Language problems
ADHD children, 266–270
clinical implications, 277
comprehension, 274
Ritalin effects, 266–277
stimulant effects, 266–270
Learning problems
amphetamines, 136
Ritalin effects, 219, 225, 258
tests, 224–226
type-specific, 257
Leniency error, rating scales, 114
Linear dose-response, 220
Logical errors, rating scales, 114
Long-duration stimulants
clinical trials, 385–396
comorbid patients, 394
control studies, 391
fidelity and compliance, 395
impairmemnt measures, 394
intent-to-treat analysis, 396
length of trials, 393
limitations, 378–382
multiple informants, 395
optimizing dosage, 352
outcome measures, 415

parallel trials, 391
patient samples, 393
trial methodology, 388–396

M
Magnetic resonance imaging (MRI)
ADHD adults, 143
brain, 375–382
diagnosis, 178
executive function, 345
neurobiology, 143
Massachusetts General Hospital, 147
Math bingo, academic game, 410
Matching Familiar Figures Test, 195, 224, 345
Media impact, 18
Medications
additive effect, 94, 98
ADHD treatment, 9–17
adherence and satisfaction, 18
case reports, 15
combination therapy, 8
discontinuing, 89
educational setting, 11
encapsulated, 212
ethical issues, 89
limitations, 88
nonadditive effect, 93, 98
outpatient assessment, 211–213
parent training, 87, 93
prevalence estimates, 9–17
regimen and dosage, 17
scheduling, 212
synergistic effect, 94, 99
types, 8
usage patterns, 10
see also Specific medications
Megavitamin therapy, 185
Memory
ADHD children, 75
Ritalin effects, 219, 225
scanning, 326
tests, 224–226
see also Working memory
Mental retardation, drug prevalence, 18
Methadone patients, 35
Methodology of Epidemiology in Children and Adolescents Study, 2
Methoxyhydroxyphenylglycol (MPG), 351
Methylphenidate. *See* Ritalin
Monitoring the Future (Institute of Social Research), 36
Mood disorders, substance abuse, 143
Motor behavior, 74
Motor organization, 327
Multivariate studies, stimulant responses, 183–193

N
Naming
color, 272
rapid automatized, 271
Ritalin effects, 274
Narcolepsy, 14
Narcotic abusers, 34
National Institute of Mental Health (NIMH), 120
National Physician's Drug and Diagnosis Audit, 10
Naturalistic aggression, 242
Nebraska, Ritalin theft, 36
Negative predictive power (NPP), 60, 62
Neurobiology, adults and children, 143, 349
Neurochemistry, ADHD children, 341
Neuropsychology tests, 345
Neurotransmitters, pharmacodynamics, 376
Nightmares, parent perceptions, 289
Noncompliant behavior, 238
Nonstimulant drugs, 152–156
Noradrenergic function, 349
Northwestern University, 406
Novartis (Ciba-Geigy), 18
Nuclear medicine, 378

O
Observational codes, 418
Obsessive-compulsive disorder (OCD), 314
Ohio, Ritalin theft, 36
Oppositional defiant disorder (ODD)
ADHD children, 341
aggression, 242
case reports, 204, 292
clinical assessment, 343, 348
disruptive behavior, 238
rating scales, 118
Ritalin vs. amphetamines, 135, 137
Oral language, stimulant effects, 266–271
Outpatient assessment, 211–213
Overanxiety disorder, 71

P
Paired-Associate Learning Task, 77, 199, 225
Parent training, 91–96
additive effect, 94, 99
ADHD children, 87
aggression, 247
combined treatment, 91–95
competence-based, 99
courses, 91
didactic, 91, 98
effectiveness, 91, 99
experimental, 91, 97
implications, 99
interviews, 179

Parent training (*continued*)
  medications, 95–97
  nonadditive effect, 93
  psychotherapy, 91
  rating scales, 121
  Ritalin use, 93–95
  synergistic effect, 94, 99
  tailoring and timing, 100
  transactional effect, 94, 99
Parochial schools, 11
Peabody Picture Vocabulary Test, 46, 227
Pemoline
  ADHD treatment, 151, 156, 385
  adverse events, 387
  case report, 202
  clinical trials, 385–396
  limitations, 389
  long-duration, 385–396
  sales data, 8
  tic response, 310
Pentazocine, 35
Personality Inventory for Children, 77
Pharmacoepidemiology, 7–10
  data sources, 10
  population-based, 8
  research methods, 8
  stimulant drugs, 7
Phonics jeopardy, academic game, 411
Phonological processing, 270, 275
Phytopharmaceuticals, 19
Polysomnography, 291
Positive predictive power (PPP), 60
Positron emission tomography (PET)
  ADHD adults, 143
  basic principles, 378
  executive function, 345
  neurobiology,143
  Ritalin mechanism, 371
Pragmatic language disorders, 266
Preclinical discrimination, 28
Prefrontal cortex, executive function, 345
Prevalence. *See* Drug prevalence
Private schools, 11
Proactive behavior, 238
Progress charts, drug trials, 123
Promotion, pharmaceutical, 18
Psychiatry, child and adolescent, 1–3
Psychoactive substance use disorders (PSUD), 143
Psychopharmacology, pediatric, 1–3
Psychosocial interventions, 91
Psychostimulants. *See* Stimulant drugs
Psychotherapy, parent training, 91
Psychotic episodes, 35
Psychotropic drugs, prescribing rates, 1
Public schools, 11, 243
Pulmonary hypertension, 35

Q

Quadratic dose-response, 220

R

Race and ethnicity, ADHD treatment, 14
Rapid eye movement (REM), 291
Rating scales
  adolescents, 120
  adults, 122, 149
  Canada, 119
  cautionary remarks, 114
  children, 122
  clinical trials, 113–123
  data collection, 119
  diagnostic use, 122, 179
  domains, 115
  dose-response curves, 197
  drug trials, 121
  history and development, 117–122
  long and short, 119, 123
  parents, 116
  replicability, 119
  restandardized, 118–120
  symptoms, 122
  teachers, 118, 121
  United States, 119
  see also Specific scales
Reactive behavior, 238
Reading disorders
  ADHD children, 271–275
  comorbidity, 272
  developmental, 271
  implications, 277
  neurochemistry, 272
  neuropsychology, 272, 345
  research, 277
  Ritalin effects, 271–275
  see also Dyslexia
Recency errors, rating scales, 114
Receptive language disorders, 266
Referrals, ADHD treatment, 176
Reserpine, 128
Ritalin (methylphenidate)
  academic performance, 219, 229
  action mechanism, 147
  adherence and satisfaction, 17
  administration, 182, 375
  adverse events, 387
  vs. amphetamines, 127–137
  animal models, 128
  behavioral specificity, 60
  between-dose differences, 58

bioequivalent products, 363–367
body mass, 50
brain imaging, 375–382
case reports, 202, 206
central processing, 326
chemistry, 369
clinical use, 111
and clonidine, 401–404
vs. cocaine, 375–382
cognitive constriction, 226–229
cognitive-energetic model, 324
cost and efficacy, 367
criteria, 85
d-isomer role, 369–372
delivery patterns, 418
dependence, 34
diagnostic issues, 43
discriminative effects, 31
effort measurements, 312
encoding studies, 325
energetic factor, 321–332
family studies, 76
future research, 361
generic vs. brand, 363–367
government regulation, 18
immediate-release, 364
length of trials, 391
limitations, 389
long-duration, 385–396
media impact, 1, 18
metabolism, 370
motor organization, 327
narcotic abusers, 33
neurochemistry, 127
parent training, 93–95
pharmacodynamics, 376
pharmacokinetics, 365, 376
pharmacology, 375–382
plasma studies, 370
predicting behavior, 60
prescription and use, 175–186
prevalence data, 36
production and consumption, 37
psychomotor stimulant, 34
psychopharmacology, 1
rating scales, 148
relative strengths, 135
sales data, 8
safety and efficacy, 401
sensitization, 34
side effects, 136
status determination, 49
sudden death, 401
sustained-release, 183, 366, 385
theft, 36
threat of lawsuits, 18
tolerance, 34
trend analysis, 53, 58
withdrawal, 34
see also Stimulant drugs

Ritalin abuse
animal models, 28
case reports, 35
children, 36
complications, 35
discrimination, 27–30
diversion, 36–38
high school survey, 37
liable and actual, 27–36
preclinical, 28–30
Sweden, 35

Ritalin effects
adolescents, 175–186
ADHD types, 191, 258
aggression, 237–247
antisocial behavior, 237–247
auditory processing, 272
biochemistry, 198
case reports, 202–212
CBF studies, 379
children, 321–332
comorbidity, 258
conduct disorder, 246
crossover study, 197
direct measurement, 199–201
dopaminergic function, 379–381
electrophysiology, 198
empiric findings, 258–260
executive function, 331
impulsivity, 223
language problems, 266–271
learning and memory, 219, 225, 258
measuring, 193, 321
multivariate studies, 201–211
noradrenergic function, 351
predicting, 193
rating scales, 321–323
reading disorders, 271–274
reinforcement, 31, 33
sleep problems, 287–290
stimuli, 29
subjective, 32, 380
working memory, 331

Ritalin treatment
ADHD types, 253–260
adults, 146–152
aggression, 237–247
anxiety disorders, 71–80
children, 56, 130, 175, 385
clinical trials, 45, 71, 147, 385

Ritalin treatment (*continued*)
  comorbidity, 77–79
  conduct disorder, 246
  control studies, 49, 391
  coordinating care, 175–186
  crossover trials, 391
  dosage and results, 48–56, 193–199
  dose-response curves, 52, 182, 219
  HIV children, 167
  implications, 135–137
  outpatient assessment, 211–213
  parallel trials, 391
  parent-teacher communication, 185
  planning and monitoring, 180–183
  protocols, 195
  vs. psychosocial therapy, 242
  rating scales, 195
  responders, 58
  scheduling, 182
  school nurses, 182
  self-administration, 31–34
  terminating, 186
  tic disorders, 301
  Tourette's syndrome, 127, 137, 301
  unlabeled, 14

S

Scramble words, academic game, 411
Schizophrenia, childhood, 45, 323
School nurses, 183
Schools
  ADHD treatment, 12
  Baltimore County, 8
  parochial and private, 12
  stimulant drugs, 8
  survey, 8
  see also Public schools
Scientology, media campaign, 18
Seizure disorders, 171
Selective Reminding Test, 226
Self-administration, 31–34
Self-Control Rating Scale, 118
Self-talk, Ritalin effects, 270
Separation anxiety, 75
Serotonergic function, 350
Severity errors, rating scales, 114
Single-Dose Questionnaire (SDQ), 30
Single-photon emission computed tomography (SPECT), 143
Sleep
  delayed or disturbed, 287–297
  objective measures, 290
  Ritalin effects, 287–297
Sleep problems
  case reports, 292–298
  parent perceptions, 288
  tic disorders, 294
  see also Insomnia
Social behavior
  direct measurement, 200
  stimulant effects, 268
  type-specific, 256
Sound baskets, academic game, 410
Special diets, alternative therapy, 185
Special education classes, 11
Specific developmental disorders (SDD), 341
Speech disorders, 266
Spontaneous flexibility, 228
Stereoisomers, Ritalin vs. amphetamines, 137
Stimulant drugs
  ADHD children, 266–271, 385–396
  adverse effects, 171, 386
  aggression, 240
  case reports, 202–212
  clinical trials, 166, 385
  cognitive effects, 201
  comorbidity, 387
  dose selection, 193–199
  duration and effects, 89
  efficacy, 171, 405
  government caution, 7
  HIV children, 165–172
  immediate-release, 385
  increased use, 7
  international perspective, 19
  language problems, 266–271
  learning and memory, 224
  length of treatment, 171
  limitations, 389–396
  long-duration, 385–396
  media criticism, 7
  multivariate studies, 201–211
  outpatient assessment, 211–213
  rating scale, 8
  school survey, 8
  short-acting, 405
  therapeutic effects, 386
  trial methodology, 388–397
  see also Amphetamines; Ritalin
Stop Signal Task, 224, 329
Story comprehension, 411
Substance abuse, ADHD adults, 143
Sudden death
  clonidine, 401
  desipramine, 79
Summer treatment programs (STP), 202–212
Supplemental Security Income, 19
Sweden, Ritalin abuse, 35
Synaptic cleft, dopamine changes, 381
Synergistic effect, parent training, 94, 99

T
Tachyphylaxis. *See* Acute tolerance
Talc granulomatosis, Ritalin abuse, 35
Target Detection Test, 345
Teacher Rating Scale, 117, 121
Teachers
  ADHD diagnosis, 179
  outcome measures, 47
  see also Schools
Thinking, convergent and divergent, 228
Tic disorders
  ADHD children, 301
  alternative drugs, 306
  case reports, 292, 312
  clinical survey, 307–312
  comorbid symptoms, 310
  familial, 313
  medication, 310
  parent history, 311
  patient behavior, 309
  Ritalin controversy, 303, 307
  sleep problems, 294
  treatment, 311
  see also Tourette's syndrome
Tolerance, preclinical studies, 34
Tomoxetine, ADHD adults, 152
Tourette's syndrome
  ADHD children, 301–303
  case studies, 305, 312
  clinical survey, 307–312
  familial, 302
  neuropsychiatry, 302
  patient behavior, 309
  psychiatric symptoms, 308
  Ritalin vs. amphetamines, 127, 137, 301
Trail-Making Test, 228
Transactional effect, parent training, 94, 99
Tricyclic antidepressants, 79, 152

U
United Nations, 36
United States
  psychopharmacology, 1
  rating scales, 118
University of California (Irvine), 401
University of Michigan, 37
University of Pittsburgh, 244
Unlabeled treatments, 14

V
Validity, ADHD adults, 145
Visual analog scales, 30
Visuomotor disorders, 135
Visuospatial sketchpad. *See* Working memory

W
Werry-Weiss-Peters Activity Scale, 46
Wechsler Intelligence Scale for Children, 130, 145
Wide Range Achievement Test, 145
Wisconsin Card Sorting Test, 145, 228
Withdrawal symptoms, 34
Word identification, 272
Working memory
  ADHD children, 331
  explanatory model, 275–277
  neuroimaging studies, 276
  stimulant drugs, 270, 276
  visuospatial sketchpad, 276

Y
Yale Neuropsychoeducational Assessment Scale, 167

Z
Zidovudine. *See* Azidothumidine
Zoom, academic game, 411